Manual of Equine Anesthesia and Analgesia

# Manual of Equine Anesthesia and Analgesia

*Second Edition*

*Edited by*

*Tom Doherty, MVB, MSc, DACVAA*
*Retired from the College of Veterinary Medicine, University of Tennessee*
*Knoxville, TN, USA*

*Alex Valverde, DVM, DVSc, DACVAA*
*Ontario Veterinary College, University of Guelph*
*Guelph, Ontario, Canada*

*Rachel A. Reed, DVM, DACVAA*
*College of Veterinary Medicine, University of Georgia*
*Athens, GA, USA*

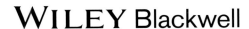

*Registered Office*
John Wiley & Sons, Inc., 111 River Street, Hoboken, NJ 07030, USA

*Editorial Office*
111 River Street, Hoboken, NJ 07030, USA

For details of our global editorial offices, customer services, and more information about Wiley products visit us at
www.wiley.com.

Wiley also publishes its books in a variety of electronic formats and by print-on-demand. Some content that appears in
standard print versions of this book may not be available in other formats.

*Library of Congress Cataloging-in-Publication Data*
Names: Doherty, T. J. (Tom J.), editor. | Valverde, Alex, editor. | Reed,
   Rachel A., editor.
Title: Manual of equine anesthesia and analgesia / edited by Tom Doherty,
   Alex Valverde, Rachel A. Reed.
Description: Second edition. | Hoboken, NJ : Wiley-Blackwell, 2022. |
   Includes bibliographical references.
Identifiers: LCCN 2021034858 (print) | LCCN 2021034859 (ebook) |
   ISBN 9781119631286 (paperback) | ISBN 9781119631293 (Adobe PDF) |
   ISBN 9781119631323 (epub)
Subjects: MESH: Equidae–surgery | Horses–surgery | Anesthesia–veterinary
   | Analgesia–veterinary | Handbook
Classification: LCC SF951 (print) | LCC SF951 (ebook) | NLM SF 951 |
   DDC 636.10897–dc23
LC record available at https://lccn.loc.gov/2021034858
LC ebook record available at https://lccn.loc.gov/2021034859

Cover Design: Wiley
Cover Images: © Photo Credit/Tom Doherty, Alex Valverde, Greg Hirshoren, Usama Hagag

Set in 9.5/12.5pt STIXTwoText by Straive, Pondicherry, India

Printed in Singapore
M102081_271021

# Contents

# List of Contributors

**Dr. Pia Haubro Andersen, DVM, PhD**
Department of Veterinary Clinical Sciences
Section of Medicine & Surgery
University of Copenhagen
Denmark

**Dr. Regula Bettschart-Wolfensberger, Dr. med. vet. PhD, DECVAA**
Vetsuisse Faculty
Department of Diagnostics and
Clinical Services
Section of Anaesthesiology
University of Zurich
Zurich 8057
Switzerland

**Dr. Suzanne L. Burnham, DVM**
Department of Veterinary Pathobiology
College of Veterinary Medicine
Texas A&M University
College Station
TX 77843-4474, USA

**Dr. Genevieve Bussieres, DVM, MSc**
Department of Small Animal
Clinical Sciences
The University of Tennessee
College of Veterinary Medicine
Knoxville
TN 37996-4545, USA

**Dr. Luis Campoy, LV, Cert VA, DECVAA, MRCVS**
Department of Clinical Sciences
Cornell University College of Veterinary
Medicine
Ithaca
NY 14853, USA

**Dr. Nigel Caulkett, DVM, MVSc, DACVAA**
Veterinary Clinical & Diagnostic Sciences
University of Calgary,
Calgary
Alberta, Canada

**Dr. Natalie S. Chow, DVM**
Department of Small Animal Clinical Sciences
The University of Tennessee
College of Veterinary Medicine
Knoxville
TN 37996-4545, USA

**Dr. Catherine M. Creighton, DVM, MS, DACVAA**
Department of Companion Animals
University of Prince Edward Island
Charlottetown
Prince Edward Island
C1A 4P3, Canada

**Dr. Carrie A. Davis, DVM, DACVAA**
Irving
TX, USA

**Dr. Machteld van Dierendonck, PhD**
Equine Behaviour Clinic
Department of Equine Sciences
Faculty of Veterinary Medicine
Utrecht University, the Netherlands

**Dr. Tom Doherty, MVB, MSc, DACVAA**
Knoxville
TN, USA

**Dr. Lydia Donaldson, DVM, PhD, DACVAA**
Middleburg
VA 20118, USA

**Dr. Bernd Driessen, DVM, DrMedVet., DACVAA, DECVPT**
University of Pennsylvania
New Bolton Center
Kennett Square
PA 19348, USA

**Dr. Tanya Duke-Novakovski, B VetMed, DACVAA**
Department of Veterinary Anesthesia
Radiology and Surgery
Western College of Veterinary Medicine
University of Saskatchewan
Saskatoon
Saskatchewan
S7N 5B4, Canada

**Dr. Christine Egger, DVM, MVSc, DACVAA**
Department of Veterinary Anesthesia,
Radiology and Surgery
Western College of Veterinary Medicine
University of Saskatchewan
Saskatoon
Saskatchewan
S7N 5B4, Canada

**Dr. Kira L. Epstein, DVM, DACVS-LA, DACVECC**
University of Georgia
College of Veterinary Medicine
Athens
GA 30602, USA

**Dr. Flavio SA. Freitag, DVM, MSc**
Department of Clinical Studies
Ontario Veterinary College
The University of Guelph
Ontario, Canada

**Dr. Kirsty Gallacher**
School of Animal and Veterinary Sciences
Roseworthy Campus
The University of Adelaide
Adelaide 5371
Australia

**Dr. Benjamin Gingold, DVM, DACVAA**
Turner
ACT
Australia, 2612

**Dr. Karina B. Gleerup, DVM, PhD**
Elleorevej 9
4000 Roskilde
Denmark

**Dr. Diego E. Gomez, MV, MSc, MVSc, PhD, DACVIM**
Department of Clinical Studies
Ontario Veterinary College
The University of Guelph
Ontario, Canada

**Dr. Meggan Graves, DVM**
Department of Large Animal Clinical Sciences
The University of Tennessee
College of Veterinary Medicine
Knoxville
TN 37996-4545, USA

**Dr. Tamara Grubb, DVM, PhD, DACVAA**
Uniontown
WA 99179, USA

**Dr. Usama Hagag, Dr. med. vet, PhD**
Faculty of Veterinary Medicine
Department of Surgery, Anesthesiology and Radiology
Beni-Suef University
Beni-Suef 62511, Egypt

**Dr. Chiara E. Hampton, DVM, MS, DACVAA**
School of Veterinary Medicine
Baton Rouge
LA 70803, USA

**Dr. Allana N. Johnson, DVM, DACVAA**
Department of Comparative, Diagnostic &
Population Medicine
University of Florida
Gainesville
FL 32608, USA

**Dr. Philip D. Jones, DVM, MS, DACVS-LA**
Department of Large Animal Clinical Sciences
The University of Tennessee
College of Veterinary Medicine
Knoxville
TN 37996-4545, USA

***Dr. Ron Jones, MVSc, FRCVS, DVA, DrMedVet,***
***DECVAA, DACVAA (Hon)***
Oxton, Prenton
Merseyside CH43 5UF
England

***Dr. Daniel G. Kenney, VMD, DACVIM***
Health Sciences Centre
Ontario Veterinary College
The University of Guelph
Ontario, Canada

***Dr. Carolyn Kerr, DVM, DVSc, PhD, DACVAA***
Department of Clinical Studies
Ontario Veterinary College
The University of Guelph
Ontario, Canada

***Dr. Stephanie Kleine, DVM, PhD, DACVAA***
Department of Small Animal Clinical Sciences
The University of Tennessee
College of Veterinary Medicine
Knoxville
TN 37996-4545, USA

***Dr. Leigh Lamont, DVM, MS, DACVAA***
Department of Companion Animals
University of Prince Edward Island
Charlottetown
Prince Edward Island
Canada

***Dr. Hui Chu Lin, DVM, MS, DACVAA***
Department of Clinical Sciences
College of Veterinary Medicine
Auburn University
AL 36849, USA

***Dr. Casper Lindegaard, DVM, PhD, DECVS***
Department of Veterinary Clinical Sciences
Section of Medicine & Surgery
University of Copenhagen
Denmark

***Dr. Thijs van Loon, DVM, PhD, DACVAA***
Division of Anaesthesia and Intensive Care
Department of Equine Sciences
Faculty of Veterinary Medicine
Utrecht University, The Netherlands

***Dr. Manuel Martin-Flores, MV, DACVAA***
Department of Clinical Sciences
Cornell University College of Veterinary
Medicine
Ithaca
NY 14853, USA

***Dr. Krista B. Mitchell, DVM, DACVAA***
Department of Clinical Studies
Ontario Veterinary College
The University of Guelph
Ontario, Canada

***Dr. Joanna C. Murrell, BVSc, PhD, DECVAA***
Highcroft Veterinary Referrals
Whitchurch
Bristol, UK

***Dr. Patricia Queiroz-Williams, DVM, MS***
School of Veterinary Medicine
Baton Rouge
LA 70803, USA

***Dr. Rachel A. Reed, DVM, DACVAA***
University of Georgia
College of Veterinary Medicine
Athens
GA 30602, USA

***Dr. Robert Reed, DVM, PhD***
Department of Biomedical and Diagnostic
Sciences
The University of Tennessee
College of Veterinary Medicine
Knoxville
TN 37996-4545, USA

***Dr. Simone K. Ringer, PD, Dr. med. vet.***
***PhD, DECVAA***
Department of Clinical Diagnostics and
Services
Section of Anaesthesiology
Vetsuisse Faculty
University of Zurich
Zurich
Switzerland

**Dr. Daniel M. Sakai, MV, DACVAA**
University of Georgia
College of Veterinary Medicine
Athens
GA 30602, USA

**Dr. Luiz Santos, DVM, MS, MANZCVS, DACVAA**
School of Animal and Veterinary Sciences
Roseworthy Campus
The University of Adelaide
Adelaide 5371
Australia

**Dr. Jim Schumacher, DVM, MS, DACVS**
Department of Large Animal Clinical
Sciences
The University of Tennessee
College of Veterinary Medicine
Knoxville
TN 37996-4545, USA

**Dr. John Schumacher, DVM, MS, DACVIM**
Department of Clinical Sciences
College of Veterinary Medicine
Auburn University
AL 36849, USA

**Dr. Reza M. Seddighi, DVM, PhD, DACVAA**
Department of Large Animal Clinical Sciences
The University of Tennessee
College of Veterinary Medicine
Knoxville
TN 37996-4545, USA

**Dr. Alicia Skelding, DVM, MSc, DVSc, DACVAA**
Toronto Animal Health Partners Emergency
and Specialty Hospital
North York, Ontario
Canada

**Dr. Christopher K. Smith, DVM, DACVAA**
Department of Small Animal Clinical
Sciences
The University of Tennessee
College of Veterinary Medicine
Knoxville
TN 37996-4545, USA

**Dr. Tanner Snowden, DVM**
Oklahoma Equine Hospital
Washington
OK 73093, USA

**Dr. Carla Sommardahl, DVM, PhD, DACVIM**
Department of Large Animal Clinical Sciences
The University of Tennessee
College of Veterinary Medicine
Knoxville
TN 37996-4545, USA

**Dr. Tena L. Ursini, DVM, DDACVSMR**
Department of Large Animal Clinical Sciences
The University of Tennessee
College of Veterinary Medicine
Knoxville
TN 37996-4545, USA

**Dr. Neal Valk, DVM, DACVS**
Department of Large Animal Clinical
Sciences
The University of Tennessee
College of Veterinary Medicine
Knoxville
TN 37996-4545, USA

**Dr. Alex Valverde, DVM, DVSc, DACVAA**
Department of Clinical Studies
Ontario Veterinary College
The University of Guelph
Guelph
Ontario NIG 2W1, Canada

**Dr. Daniel S. Ward, DVM, PhD, DACVO**
Department of Small Animal Clinical Sciences
The University of Tennessee
College of Veterinary Medicine
Knoxville
TN 37996-4545, USA

**Dr. Ray Wilhite, MS, PhD**
Department of Anatomy, Physiology and
Pharmacology
College of Veterinary Medicine
Auburn University
AL 36849, USA

## Preface

The second edition of the *Manual of Equine Anesthesia & Analgesia* has been updated and rearranged. Most topics have been expanded and new chapters added. Chapters devoted to the sedation and anesthesia of horses undergoing imaging procedures, anesthesia of donkeys and mules, and recognition of pain in horses and donkeys are now included. Case examples of the pharmacologic control of pain are provided, and information on non-pharmacologic treatment of acute and chronic pain using acupuncture and physical rehabilitation techniques have also been added. In addition, a suggested reading list is included for the reader who wishes to seek further information on the topic.

This edition of the *Manual of Equine Anesthesia & Analgesia* strives to deliver relevant information on the physiologic and pharmacologic principles underpinning the anesthesia of equids, in addition to providing useful information on the clinical practice of anesthesia. The *Manual* has retained the same easily accessible format of the first edition, and we believe that it will be a useful guide to all those involved in the anesthesia of equids.

Tom Doherty
Alex Valverde
Rachel A. Reed

## Acknowledgments

We wish to acknowledge our contributors for providing their expertise, and we greatly appreciate the time and effort they expended on this project. A special word of thanks to the staff at John Wiley & Sons, especially Ms. Erica Judisch, Ms. Susan Engelken, and Ms. Merryl Le Roux, for making this project possible.

# 1

# Preoperative Evaluation and Patient Preparation

## The Risk of Equine Anesthesia

*Tanya Duke-Novakovski*

- Risks of equine anesthesia have been linked with various conditions and situations and are reviewed in detail elsewhere and summarized in this chapter.

## I   Risk of equine anesthesia

- Anesthesia of the horse always involves an assessment of risk.
- Potential complications range from the less serious (e.g. skin wounds) to the more serious (e.g. long bone fractures, myopathies, and peripheral neuropathies), and to death in some cases.
- There is also risk of injury to personnel and safe handling should be practiced.
- The *goal of the anesthetist* is to minimize the adverse effects (ideally at minimum cost) by:
  ○ Identifying and defining the risk(s).
  ○ Selecting the best strategy for controlling or minimizing the risk(s).
- Data from single clinics have cited mortality rates of 0.24–1.8% in healthy horses.
- Data from multicenter studies cite the death rate for healthy horses undergoing anesthesia at around 0.9% (approximately 1 : 100).
- The overall death rate, when sick horses undergoing emergency colic surgery are included, has been reported to be 0.12% when fatalities were directly related to anesthesia in one study, and 1.9% in another study.

## II   Classification of physical status (see Box 1.1)

- Classification of health status is generally based on the American Society of Anesthesiologists (ASA) system.
- This system uses information from the history, physical examination, and laboratory findings to place horses into one of five categories.
- The classification allows for standardization of physical status only.
- The ASA system does *not* classify risk, although increased risk of complication is associated with a high ASA status.
- These classifications are not always useful for horses: nevertheless, the system serves as a guide to case management.

*Manual of Equine Anesthesia and Analgesia*, Second Edition. Edited by Tom Doherty, Alex Valverde, and Rachel A. Reed.
© 2022 John Wiley & Sons, Inc. Published 2022 by John Wiley & Sons, Inc.

| Box 1.1 | ASA Classification System |
|---|---|
| *ASA 1* | Healthy horse does not require intervention (e.g. castration). |
| *ASA 2* | Horse with mild systemic disease (e.g. mild anemia, mild recurrent airway obstruction) or localized injury (e.g. wound repair). |
| *ASA 3* | Horse with moderate systemic disease (e.g. stable colic, infected joint). |
| *ASA 4* | Horse with severe systemic disease (e.g. recent ruptured bladder, endotoxemia). |
| *ASA 5* | A moribund horse not expected to survive longer than 24 hours (e.g. unstable colic, ruptured bladder of several days duration). |
| *E* | The letter E is added to status 2–5 under emergency conditions. |

## III   Risk factors

### A   Age and physical status

- The risk increases with age, and horses aged 12 years or older are at an increased risk of mortality.
- Older horses may be more prone to fracture of a long bone in the recovery period, which could result in euthanasia.
- Foals have an increased risk of fatality and this is probably associated with unfamiliarity with neonatal anesthesia, an immature cardiovascular system, and presence of systemic illness.
- Pregnant mares have increased risk of mortality in the last trimester of pregnancy and this is probably associated with a need for emergency surgery. Otherwise, there is no difference between sexes.
- Horses with a high ASA physical status have increased risk of mortality.

### B   Type of surgery and recovery

- In otherwise healthy horses, the risk of mortality (euthanasia) following fracture repair is highest from repair failure or from fracture of another bone.
- However, long periods of anesthesia typical of fracture repair have also been associated with increased mortality, and horses presented for fracture repair may be dehydrated and stressed.

  *Emergency surgery* (non-colic) carries a 4.25 times higher risk of mortality compared with elective surgery, and for emergency abdominal surgery the risk of fatality is 11.7%.

  *Colic surgery* is associated with increased mortality because of a higher ASA physical status, emergency procedure with less time for stabilization, and use of dorsal recumbency possibly with episodes of hypotension.

  *Eye surgery*, in one institution, resulted in longer recovery times and risk of complications and were associated with long anesthesia time compared to non-ophthalmic procedures. *Fluconazole* (microsomal P450 enzyme inhibitor) use was associated with increased risk of postoperative colic and longer recovery time. The use of the lowest effective volume of local anesthetic for a retrobulbar block was also recommended (10 ml/500 kg horse). Ophthalmic procedures have been associated with unsatisfactory recovery quality.

- Assisted recovery with ropes can decrease the risk of fracture and dislocation, although the benefit of assisted-recovery is still debatable.

## C Time of day

- Performing anesthesia outside of normal working hours carries an increased risk for horses. This increase in risk is separate from the fact that most of these cases are emergency in nature.
- Surgeries performed between midnight and 6 a.m. carry the highest risk of mortality. This may be due to the nature of the emergency, as well as to staff shortages and personnel fatigue.

## D Body position

- Dorsal recumbency was found to increase risk compared to either lateral recumbency, but most "*colic*" surgeries are performed with the horse in dorsal recumbency.
- An increased risk of postanesthetic myelopathy has mostly been associated with draft breeds between 6 and 24 months of age and dorsal recumbency.

## E Drug choice

- Using total inhalational anesthesia regimen in foals (<12 months of age) *without premedication* carries the highest risk.
- Halothane sensitizes the myocardium to circulating catecholamines. Fewer cardiac arrests occurred when isoflurane was substituted for halothane, although overall mortality did not differ between groups because limb fracture in recovery was prevalent for the isoflurane group.
- Isoflurane and sevoflurane may be associated with unsatisfactory recovery, and sedation is often used following anesthesia to reduce the risk of excitable recovery.
- Use of isoflurane and sevoflurane was linked with increased mortality, but this was because these drugs are more likely to be selected for sick horses.
- Not using any premedication is associated with the highest risk, probably owing to increased circulating catecholamines from stress. It may be prudent to premedicate foals before induction of anesthesia, especially when using halothane.
- *Acepromazine* lowers the risk of mortality when used alone as a premedicant, because it reduces the incidence of ventricular arrhythmias in the presence of halothane.
- No particular injectable induction regimen is associated with greater risk when used with inhalational anesthesia.
- Total intravenous anesthesia (TIVA) is associated with the lowest risk of all, but TIVA is often used for short procedures. TIVA has been associated with reduced stress response.

## F Duration and management of anesthesia

- Long periods of anesthesia (>2 hours) with volatile anesthetics are often associated with cardiovascular depression and poor tissue perfusion, leading to problems such as cardiac arrest or postanesthetic myopathy.
- Intraoperative *hypotension* during anesthesia has clearly been associated with postanesthetic myopathy, and can still occur with short anesthetic periods. Direct arterial pressure monitoring should be used during lengthy anesthetic periods.
- *Postanesthetic myopathy* may lead to bone fracture or dislocation.
- Postanesthetic airway obstruction and pulmonary edema may be prevented by keeping the head in a normal position thereby reducing the risk of laryngeal nerve paralysis, and with good airway management in the recovery period.

## Suggested Reading

Arndt, S., Hopster, K., Sill, V. et al. (2020). Comparison between head-tail-rope assisted and unassisted recoveries in healthy horses undergoing general anesthesia for surgeries. *Vet. Surg.* 49: 329–338.

Bidwell, L.A., Bramlage, L.R., and Rood, W.A. (2007). Equine perioperative fatalities associated with general anaesthesia. *Vet. Anaesth. Analg.* 34: 23–30.

Niimura del Barrio, M.C., David, F., Hughes, J.M.L. et al. (2018). A retrospective report (2003–2013) of the complications associated with the use of a one-man (head and tail) rope recovery system in horses following general anaesthesia. *Ir. Vet. J.* 71: 1–9.

Curto, E.M., Griffith, E.H., Posner, L.P. et al. (2018). Factors associated with postoperative complications in healthy horses after general anesthesia for ophthalmic versus non-ophthalmic procedures: 556 cases (2012–2014). *J. Am. Vet. Med. Assoc.* 252: 1113–1119.

Donaldson, L.J., Dunlop, C.S., Holland, M.S., and Burton, B.A. (2000). The recovery of horses from inhalant anesthesia: a comparison of halothane and isoflurane. *Vet. Surg.* 29: 92–101.

Dugdale, A.H.A. and Taylor, P.M. (2016). Equine anaesthesia-associated mortality: where are we now? *Vet. Anaesth. Analg.* 43: 242–255.

Dugdale, A.H.A., Obhrai, J., and Cripps, P.J. (2016). Twenty years later: a single-centre, repeat retrospective analysis of equine perioperative mortality and investigation of recovery quality. *Vet. Anaesth. Analg.* 43: 171–178.

Duke, T., Filsek, U., and Read, M.R. (2006). Clinical observations surrounding an increased incidence of post-anesthetic myopathy in halothane-anesthetized horses. *Vet. Anaesth. Analg.* 33: 122–127.

Grandy, J.L., Steffey, E.P., Hodgson, D.S., and Woliner, M.J. (1987). Arterial hypotension and the development of postanesthetic myopathy in halothane-anesthetized horses. *Am. J. Vet. Res.* 48: 192–197.

Johnston, G.M., Taylor, P.M., Holmes, M.A., and Wood, J.L.N. (1995). Confidential enquiry of perioperative equine fatalities (CEPEF-1): preliminary results. *Equine. Vet. J.* 27: 193–200.

Johnston, G.M., Eastment, J.K., Wood, J.L.N., and Taylor, P.M. (2002). The confidential enquiry into perioperative equine fatalities (CEPEF): mortality results of phases 1 and 2. *Vet. Anaesth. Analg.* 29: 159–170.

Johnston, G.M., Eastment, J.K., Taylor, P.M. et al. (2004). Is isoflurane safer than halothane in equine anaesthesia? Results from a prospective multicenter randomized controlled trial. *Equine. Vet. J.* 36: 64–71.

Leece, L., Corletto, F., and Brearley, J.C. (2008). A comparison of recovery times and characteristics with sevoflurane and isoflurane anaesthesia in horse undergoing magnetic resonance imaging. *Vet. Anaesth. Analg.* 35: 383–391.

Parviainen, A.K.J. and Trim, C.M. (2000). Complications associated with anaesthesia for ocular surgery: a retrospective study 1989-1996. *Equine. Vet. J.* 32: 555–559.

Ragle, C., Baetge, C., Yiannikouris, S. et al. (2011). Development of equine post anesthetic myelopathy: thirty cases (1979-2010). *Equine. Vet. Educ.* 23: 630–635.

Santos, M., Fuente, M., Garcia-Iturralde, P. et al. (2003). Effects of alpha$_2$ adrenoceptor agonists during recovery from isoflurane anaesthesia in horses. *Equine. Vet. J.* 35: 170–175.

Senior, M. (2005). Post-anesthetic pulmonary oedema in horses: a review. *Vet. Anaesth. Analg.* 32: 193–200.

Young, S.S. and Taylor, P.M. (1990). Factors leading to serious anaesthetic related problems in equine anaesthesia. *J. Ass. Vet. Anaesth.* 17: 59. (abstr).

Young, S.S. and Taylor, P.M. (1993). Factors influencing the outcome of equine anaesthesia: a review of 1,314 cases. *Equine. Vet. J.* 25: 147–151.

# Patient Preparation
*Tanya Duke-Novakovski*

## I Preparation of the horse

### A Evaluation

- *History* and *physical examination findings* help with evaluation of health.
- Many emergency cases, especially intestinal emergencies, are in cardiovascular shock and must be stabilized as much as possible prior to induction of anesthesia.

### B Laboratory tests

- In normal horses undergoing elective surgery, there is generally no value in performing extensive laboratory tests.
- In emergency cases, performing laboratory tests such as electrolyte and metabolic acid-base status may be vital to the management of the case (e.g. a foal with uroabdomen).

### C Physical examination

- During the examination, attention should be directed to the neurological, cardiovascular, and respiratory systems.
- Musculoskeletal problems, which may affect recovery, should be considered, and a plan should be made to assist recovery if deemed necessary.

### D History

- May reveal information that affects case management.
- A recent history of coughing may indicate a viral infection of the airway, in which case elective surgeries should be postponed until one month following resolution of clinical signs.
- Owners might report that the horse previously had a "bad" or "over" reaction to an anesthetic or sedative drug. These concerns should be investigated.

### E Fasting

- Fasting (~12 hours) was previously advised because of the potential benefits for lung function and the reduced risk of stomach rupture from trauma at induction or recovery.
- Many equine hospitals *do not fast* horses prior to elective surgery. In one study, the $PaO_2$ values during anesthesia were not significantly better in fasted versus non-fasted horses, and not fasting might reduce the incidence of postanesthetic colic due to changes in gastrointestinal motility.
- However, it is generally the case that grain is removed.
- Water should be made available up to the time of surgery.

## F   Medications

- It is best to administer all ancillary drugs (e.g. antimicrobials, anti-inflammatories) prior to sedation. Sodium penicillin can reduce systolic arterial pressure by 8–15 mmHg in anesthetized horses. If antimicrobials are administered during the anesthetic event, this effect can be minimized by administering the drug slowly.

## G   Jugular catheter

- An intravenous (IV) catheter should *always* be placed prior to anesthesia.
- This reduces the likelihood of perivascular injection and provides ready access for further IV anesthetic or emergency drugs.

## H   Flushing the oral cavity

- It is important to flush food debris from the oral cavity, especially if the airway is to be intubated (see Figure 1.1).

## I   Removal of shoes

- Removal of shoes prevents damage to the horse and hospital flooring.
  - However, removal of shoes is not popular with owners. An alternative is to apply bandage material or tape to improve grip and to cover metal points.
- Certainly, loose shoes and nails should be removed.
- Removal of shoes and metallic debris is necessary when an MRI is to be performed.

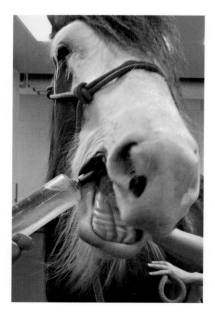

Figure 1.1   Rinsing of the mouth with water prior to induction of anesthesia using a large dosing syringe.

## Suggested Reading

Bailey, P.A., Hague, B.A., Davis, M. et al. (2016). Incidence of post-anesthetic colic in non-fasted adult equine patients. *Can. Vet. J.* 57: 1263–1266.

Dobromylskyj, P., Taylor, P.M., Brearley, J.C. et al. (1996). Effect of pre-operative starvation on intra-operative arterial oxygen status in horses. *J. Vet. Anaesth.* 23: 75–77.

Hubbell, J.A.E., Muir, W.W., Robertson, J.T., and Sams, R.A. (1987). Cardiovascular effects of intravenous sodium penicillin, sodium cefazolin, and sodium citrate in awake and anesthetized horses. *Vet. Surg.* 16: 245–250.

Toews, A.R. and Campbell, J.R. (1997). Influence of preoperative complete blood cell counts on surgical outcomes in healthy horses: 102 cases (1986-1996). *J. Am. Vet. Med. Assoc.* 211: 887–888.

# 2

## Serum Chemistry and Hematology
*Carla Sommardahl*

- As previously mentioned, there is little value in performing laboratory tests for healthy horses undergoing elective procedures.
- However, when indicated, the appropriate tests should, ideally, be performed before general anesthesia is induced. Nevertheless, this may not always be feasible in emergency situations.

## I   Complete blood count (CBC)

### A   Erythrocytes

- Evaluation of erythrocyte numbers can begin with a determination of the packed cell volume (PCV) or hematocrit (HCT), which measure the percentage of the volume of whole blood that the red blood cells (RBCs) occupy.
- Erythrocyte numbers are $6.9-10.7 \times 10^{12}$/l, which represent a normal PCV of 35–45% and a normal hemoglobin of 12–15 g/dl.
- A stained blood smear can be used to evaluate RBC morphology and the presence of infectious organisms on the RBCs.
- Increased RBC numbers (*erythrocytosis*) is most commonly associated with hemoconcentration – this is called a *relative erythrocytosis* as there is no increase in RBC mass.
  - *Splenic contraction* can cause a transient increase in circulating RBC mass.
- In rare cases, there is an increase in numbers due to an increase in RBC production, *absolute erythrocytosis*.
  - *Absolute erythrocytosis* is further categorized as *primary*, as in *polycythemia vera*, and *secondary*, as results from *chronic hypoxemia*.
- Decreased RBC numbers (*anemia*) can be caused by increased removal from the circulation by blood loss or destruction (*hemolysis*); or by decreased production by the bone marrow.
  - Intravascular hemolysis is accompanied by a decrease in hemoglobin concentration; however, extravascular hemolysis is harder to confirm.
  - Decreased production with iron deficiency secondary to chronic inflammation is a common cause of nonregenerative anemia in the horse, and is characterized by microcytic hypochromic RBCs and decreased RBC indices.

*Manual of Equine Anesthesia and Analgesia*, Second Edition. Edited by Tom Doherty, Alex Valverde, and Rachel A. Reed.
© 2022 John Wiley & Sons, Inc. Published 2022 by John Wiley & Sons, Inc.

- Red cell distribution width (RDW) – a measure of RBC variation in size and volume - is used to detect RBC regeneration and is interpreted in conjunction with other values on the complete blood count (CBC).

## B Leukocytes

- Granulocytes (neutrophils, eosinophils, basophils, and mast cells), monocytes, macrophages, and lymphocytes are important for immune function, and changes in their numbers reflect a response to a disease process.
- Total leukocyte count is $5.1–11.0 \times 10^9/l$.
- Neoplasia, bone marrow disease, or functional defects can cause a decrease or increase in leukocyte numbers.

*Neutrophils*

- Changes in numbers and morphology are important in evaluating the response to systemic inflammation, infection, and stress.
- However, the neutrophil count can be normal in the presence of inflammation or infection.
- Reference values include $2.8–7.7 \times 10^9/l$ segmented neutrophils and $0.0–0.2 \times 10^9/l$ bands.
- *Neutrophilia* is often associated with chronic bacterial infections.
- *Neutropenia* in adult horses is most often associated with endotoxemia (and other bacterial by-products).
- *Neutropenia* in foals is most commonly associated with sepsis and systemic inflammation.

*Eosinophils*

- Reference values are $0.0–0.7 \times 10^9/l$.
- Eosinophilia is rare in horses. Conditions to rule out include:
  - Parasitism with cyathastomes.
  - Eosinophilic colitis, enteritis, or multisystemic disease.

*Lymphocytes*

- Reference values are $1.3–4.7 \times 10^9/l$.
- Lymphopenia: Glucocorticoid release or administration, viral infection, old age, and immunodeficiency in foals (e.g. combined immunodeficiency disease in Arabian or Arabian crossbred foals).
- Lymphocytosis: epinephrine release or administration, exercise, equine herpesvirus 2 (foals), leukemia.

*Monocytes and Basophils*

- Reference values for monocytes are $0.1–0.8 \times 10^9/l$.
- Monocytosis: Chronic inflammation, use of corticosteroids.
- Reference values for basophils are $0.0–0.1 \times 10^9/l$.

## C Platelets

- The normal platelet count for horses is $75\,000–300\,000/\mu l$.
- Platelets function in hemostasis, inflammatory responses, immunity, tissue regeneration, and disease pathology.

*Thrombocytosis* (platelet count >400 000/μl)
  Reactive or Secondary:
      – Age < 3 years, intact males, pyrexia, infectious, or inflammatory conditions.
      – Platelet count: 400 000–850 000/μl.
  Primary or Clonal:
      – A rare chronic myeloproliferative disorder.
      – Platelet count >1 000 000/μl.

*Thrombocytopenia* (platelet count <75 000/μl)
  Increased platelet destruction:
      – Immune mediated.
      – Causes include:
          ▪ Equine infectious anemia, anaplasma phagocytophilum.
          ▪ Drugs, toxins, snake bites.
  Increased use:
      – Hemorrhage.
      – Disseminated intravascular coagulation.
  Decreased production:
      – Myelosuppressive drugs (e.g. phenylbutazone).
      – Bone marrow disease.
      – Idiopathic.

## II  Blood chemistry interpretation

- Point of care (POC) analyzers have made the evaluation of chemistry, electrolyte, and blood gas values available rapidly as stall-side or immediate vicinity testing (see Figures 2.1 and 2.2).

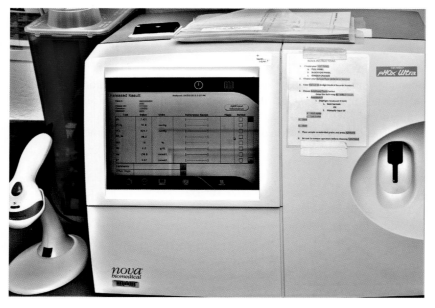

Figure 2.1    Bench top point-of-care blood analyzer, *Source:* NOVA Biomedical.

Figure 2.2   Stall-side point-of-care blood analyzer, *Source:* Abbott point-of-care iSTAT system.

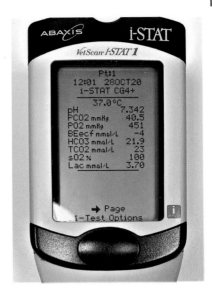

- Specific reference ranges from the laboratory or analyzer conducting the analysis should be utilized.
  - Reference ranges for foals should be used based on age.
  - Reference ranges for donkeys (asses, burros), mules, and hinnies should be used accordingly.

## A   Creatine kinase (CK)

- Also called creatine phosphokinase (CPK).
- The reference range for the horse is 108–430 U/l.
- CK is a specific indicator of muscle damage.
  - It is a "*leakage*" enzyme released secondary to *myocyte* damage or death.
- Serum concentrations *increase quickly* following myocyte damage.
  - In contrast to aspartate aminotransferase (AST) concentrations which increase more slowly and persist for longer (see below).
- CK has a short half-life (hours); thus, serum concentrations *decrease quickly* after an episode.
- Urine will be positive for blood on test strips if *myoglobin* is present.
  - *Myoglobin* and *free hemoglobin* have peroxidase-like activity, which results in oxygen liberation from organic peroxide in the reagent strip, causing a color change in the strip.
  - The urine may be "*coffee*" colored.

*Mild increases* in CK (1000–5000 U/l) may result from:
  - Recumbency, trailer ride, recent exercise, or intramuscular injections.
  - Consider a diagnosis of mild exertional rhabdomyolysis (ER) and/or polysaccharide storage myopathy (PSSM) if the above conditions are not applicable.

*Moderate* (~5000 U/l) to severe increases in CK (>10 000 U/l):
  - *Severe cases* of ER may have associated CK values >100 000 U/l.

- These high values may be associated with a traumatic event, but may occur following general anesthesia.

*Note:* Because myoglobin may cause renal tubular damage, treatment may be indicated.

## B   Aspartate aminotransferase (AST)

- AST is a "*leakage*" enzyme released secondary to *myocyte* or *hepatocyte* damage or death.
  - Small amounts are also present in *myocardial* cells.
- Increased AST values in horses are most commonly associated with skeletal muscle damage.
  - The reference range for the horse is 160–400 U/l.
- Serum AST may also increase significantly in horses in early training.
- AST values in foals may be greater than adult values for many months.
  - This increase may be related to muscle growth.
- Small amounts are present in RBCs.
  - Thus, hemolysis can cause small increases in serum AST.
- AST in serum increases more slowly (peak 6–12 hours) than does CK after muscle injury.
- It has a long half-life (~seven days) in horses compared to other domestic species, and serum concentrations fall slowly (three to four days to return to normal) after an episode.

*Note*: AST activity will remain increased after CK activity has returned to normal.

- AST values should be interpreted in association with CK and other liver enzymes (Sorbitol (Iditol) dehydrogenase [SDH], Gamma glutamyl transferase [GGT]).
- Serum AST activity can also increase with *in vivo* or *in vitro* hemolysis.

## C   Gamma glutamyl transferase (GGT)

- GGT resides in the cell membranes of all somatic cells, but its greatest activity is in biliary epithelial cells, pancreatic acinar cells, and renal tubular epithelial cells.
- GGT is a cell surface glycoprotein and is a liver canalicular enzyme, and it is induced by dilation of the biliary tree.
- It has multiple functions including the regulation of the anti-oxidant glutathione.
- Increased GGT activity in serum is usually an indication of hepatobiliary toxicity, especially cholestasis.
- Bile accumulation (cholestasis), biliary hyperplasia, and some drugs (e.g. phenobarbital, furosemide, phenytoin, and cimetidine) increase serum GGT activity.
- GGT has a long half-life (approximately three days), thus serum concentrations fall slowly after an episode.
- Chronic liver disease associated with hepatocyte destruction, fibrosis, and biliary hyperplasia are associated with severe increases in GGT.
- Right dorsal displacement of the colon causes an increase in serum GGT activity by impeding the outflow of bile.
- Proximal enteritis causes increases in AST and GGT activity secondary to ascending infection of the biliary tract and/or liver damage from systemic effects such as endotoxemia and hypovolemia.
- Reference range: Adult horses 6–30 U/l.
- The normal range for burros, donkeys and asses may be 2–3 times higher, and mules and hinnies may be two times higher than values for horses.

○ Foals have a higher reference range than adults for the first one to two months of life.
  – Unlike in ruminant neonates, this is not due to ingestion of *colostrum* as GGT activity is low in mare's colostrum.
  – The increased serum GGT activity in foals in the first month of life seems to be due to *endogenous* sources.

Note: *Idiopathic* increases in GGT occasionally occur in young, apparently healthy Thoroughbred horses. The cause is unknown. These horses may exhibit poor performance.

*Urinary GGT*

○ GGT is not excreted by glomerular filtration; thus, its presence in urine indicates acute damage to *tubular epithelial cells.*
○ GGT appears early in the urine when there is acute tubular damage, and this occurs prior to the development of azotemia.
○ However, urinary GGT activity decreases quickly after an acute episode of tubular injury, even in the presence of ongoing tubular impairment.
○ To allow for the effect of urine flow, GGT concentrations in the urine are generally expressed as a *ratio* to urinary creatinine concentrations.

D **Alkaline phosphatase (ALP)**

○ ALP is present in *biliary epithelial cells*, *hepatocytes*, *bone*, *placenta*, and *intestine.*
○ The reference range for the horse is 119–329 U/l.
○ Activity originates from induction similar to GGT, but it is *not liver specific.*
  – However, most serum ALP is derived from the liver, and the remainder is from bone, and a small amount from intestine.
○ Increase in ALP activity indicates *cholestasis* from intra or extrahepatic causes.
  – But increases are more likely if the obstruction is extrahepatic.
○ Intestinal lesions can also increase ALP activity.
○ Bone growth causes an increase in serum ALP activity.
○ ALP in serum is highest at birth and decreases over the first month to adult range by two to four years.
  – The increased ALP activity in neonatal foals may be of *placental* origin.

E **Sorbitol (Iditol) dehydrogenase (SDH)**

○ SDH is a cytoplasmic enzyme, and it acts as a catalyst in the conversion of sorbitol to fructose.
○ SDH activity is low, and the majority comes from the *hepatocyte.*
○ SDH is a *"leakage"* enzyme released when hepatocytes are damaged.
○ Thus, SDH is considered a specific indicator of *liver damage,* especially acute damage.
○ SDH has a short half-life (hours), so serum concentrations fall quickly.
  – It is generally not increased in chronic liver disease.
○ It is a *labile* enzyme, and its activity decreases with time.
  – However, it is stable in serum for up to five hours when refrigerated.
○ Reference range: 1–8 U/l.

F **Total bilirubin (TBIL)**

○ Increased TBIL in serum is an indicator of *hepatic dysfunction, hemolysis,* or *reduced feed intake.*

- TBIL may be subdivided into *unconjugated* (indirect) bilirubin, and *conjugated* (direct) bilirubin.
- The reference range for the horse is 21–57 µmol/l for TBIL; 2–10 µmol/l for conjugated bilirubin, and 18–52 µmol/l for unconjugated bilirubin.
- *Hepatic dysfunction* causes both indirect and direct concentrations to rise.
    - If *direct* is greater than 8% of total, liver disease should be suspected as a contributor to the increase.
- *Biliary obstruction* (e.g. cholelithiasis) increases the direct to indirect ratio.
- *Hemolysis* raises the serum indirect concentration.
- *Reduced feed intake* raises the serum indirect concentration as a result of slowed clearance of bilirubin from the blood rather than from its overproduction. However, the cause is uncertain.
    - *Ligandin*, a protein responsible for bilirubin uptake into the liver may be decreased in the fasting horse, as has been demonstrated in rats.
    - *Free fatty acids* may play a role in fasting hyperbilirubinemia, and horses develop significant hyperlipidemia during fasting. This may result in competition for carrier proteins.
    - Increases in unconjugated bilirubin occur after 12 hours of fasting.
- *Neonates* have higher bilirubin values due to immaturity of liver processing.
    - This can lead to *kernicterus,* resulting from unconjugated bilirubin causing neurologic damage. However, this condition is extremely rare in foals, and may be more likely to occur in a foal with *neonatal isoerythrolysis.*

## G Serum bile acids (SBA)

- Bile acids are synthesized and secreted by the liver.
- Bile acids are removed from the portal blood by hepatocytes, and SBA concentrations increase as hepatic function decreases.
- Increase in SBA concentration is an indicator of *hepatic* dysfunction.
- Reference range: 0–20 µmol/l.
- Bile acids are not affected by fasting.
- Only a single blood sample is required instead of pre- and post-feeding samples, as bile is released continuously because the horse lacks a gallbladder.

## H Blood urea nitrogen (BUN) and creatinine (Cr)

- Increased BUN and or Cr indicates that the horse suffers from either pre-renal, renal, or post-renal azotemia.
- Reference range for BUN is 4.2–8.9 mmol/l and for Cr is 80–130 µmol/l.
- In contrast to urea nitrogen, Cr is *not reabsorbed* within the tubules, so serum Cr concentrations provide a more accurate measurement of glomerular filtration rate (GFR) than does BUN.
- *Neonates* have higher Cr values, and the value declines over the first week of life.

### Pre-renal azotemia

- Occurs when the increases in BUN and Cr results from a decrease in renal blood flow and the associated decrease in GFR.

○ Significant (>75%) decreases in GFR are required before the BUN is increased, especially early in disease.
  – Most commonly results from dehydration and circulatory shock.
○ When renal function is adequate (pre-renal), azotemia is accompanied by a urine specific gravity (USG) > 1.025.
  – This indicates that the kidney has the ability to concentrate the urine.
○ Uroperitoneum secondary to *bladder rupture in foals* also causes pre-renal azotemia.

*Renal azotemia*
  ○ Occurs when the GFR is low due to acute or chronic kidney injury.
  ○ BUN may be low because less of the filtered urea is re-absorbed in the proximal tubule.
  ○ Serum Cr increases as filtration decreases.
  ○ Diagnosed by concurrently measuring the USG.
    – The presence of azotemia in a patient that cannot concentrate their urine (USG < 1.020) indicates kidney injury.

*Post-renal azotemia*
  ○ Is associated with mechanical (e.g. *uroliths*) or functional (e.g. *neurogenic bladder dysfunction*) obstruction of the urinary tract.
  ○ It is uncommon in horses.

## III Plasma proteins

- Blood consists of plasma and solid components.
- Plasma comprises about 55% of the blood volume.
- Plasma contains about 90% water, and the remaining 10% consists of ions, proteins, dissolved gases (primarily *nitrogen*, *oxygen*, and *carbon dioxide*), nutrients, and wastes.
- Total protein reference range for adult horse: 6.5–7.5 g/dl.
  ○ Plasma protein value is approximately 0.3–0.5 g/dl greater than serum protein.
- The proteins in plasma include the *globulins*, *albumin*, *fibrinogen*, and *coagulation factors*.
- A hand-held *refractometer* can be used to measure total solids, which are an estimate of total protein; however, the readings can be affected by other substances in the plasma.
  ○ This is because refractometer scales are calibrated against normal serum, and values of many non-protein solutes (e.g. electrolytes) vary in the population.
  ○ Thus, it may be prudent to evaluate *albumin* and *globulin* concentrations separately in some disease states.

### A Albumin

  ○ Albumin is the main protein present in plasma.
  ○ The reference range is 2.7–3.7 g/dl.
  ○ Its main function is the regulation of the colloidal osmotic pressure (COP) of blood.
  ○ It accounts for 75–80% of the COP of normal plasma, although it only comprises 50–60% of the total protein content of plasma.
  ○ The oncotic effect of albumin is enhanced by its ability, due to its negative charge, to attract cations, particularly $Na^+$.
    – This is termed the *Gibbs-Donnan* effect.

- Albumin is the smallest plasma protein in molecular weight (~66 kDa).
- Albumin binds water, ions, fatty acids, hormones, bilirubin, and therapeutic compounds.
- It is synthetized by the liver and has a plasma half-life of approximately 19 days in the horse.
- Albumin is classified as a *negative acute phase reactant* because its production is down-regulated during inflammation.

*Hypoalbuminemia can result from:*
- Increased loss (most common cause).
  - Gastrointestinal (GI) (e.g., bacterial-induced colitis).
  - Vasculitis, peritonitis, and pleuritis.
  - Renal – due to glomerular disease.
- Reduced synthesis.
  - End-stage or diffuse liver disease.
  - Chronic inflammation.
- Excessive catabolism
  - Most likely due to starvation.
  - Plasma proteins are a rapid source of replacement for tissue proteins.
- Low dietary protein intake.
- Hypoalbuminemia may result in *edema* depending on the severity of albumin loss and rapidity of onset.

## B Globulins

- The reference range is 2.1–3.2 g/dl.
- The globulin fraction of plasma proteins comprises dozens of proteins including:
  - Carrier proteins.
  - Complement.
  - Immunoglobulins (IgGs).
  - Enzymes.
- Includes $\alpha$, $\beta$, and $\gamma$ globulins, from smallest to largest.
- Globulins are large molecules (~90–150 kDa) in comparison to albumin.
- Reference range for $\alpha 1$ is 0.1–0.2 g/dl and for $\alpha 2$ is 0.6–0.8 g/dl.
- Reference range for $\beta 1$ is 0.3–0.8 g/dl and for $\beta 2$ is 0.2–0.9 g/dl.
- Reference range for $\gamma$ is 0.5–1.3 g/dl.
- $\alpha$ and $\beta$ globulins are synthetized in the liver.
- $\gamma$ globulins are synthetized in lymphoid tissue by plasma cells.
- $\gamma$ globulins are a major class of IgG.

*Hyperglobulinemia*
- Is associated with chronic disease, such as the presence of as an abscess, intestinal parasites, or a tumor.

*Hypoglobulinemia*
- Malnutrition can result in a decrease in total globulins due to decreased synthesis.
- In rare cases, a congenital immune deficiency might be the cause of hypoglobulinemia.

## C Fibrinogen

- ○ Fibrinogen is an important soluble glycoprotein that is synthetized by the liver.
- ○ It is a plasma clotting factor precursor which is converted to fibrin on contact with a sticky surface.
  - – The fibrin threads formed in this way trap platelets to form the primary platelet clot on which a stable blood clot is formed by the process of coagulation.
- ○ Fibrinogen is a *positive acute phase reactant*, and it can be used to diagnose and monitor inflammatory conditions.
- ○ Reference range is 2–4 g/l.
- ○ Plasma fibrinogen concentrations can increase up to 10-fold in an inflammatory process.
  - – The half-life of fibrinogen is ~three days.
- ○ Foals may have increased concentrations up to six months of age.
- ○ Pregnant mares may have increases of up to 40%, and fibrinogen may further increase in the immediate postpartum period, before returning to normal in about two weeks post-foaling.

## IV Lactate

- ● **Hyperlactatemia (>2 mmol/l)**
  *Type A*
  - – Is due to inadequate tissue perfusion and oxygen depletion.
    - ■ e.g. hypovolemia, septic shock, anemia.
  *Type B*
  - – Is associated with increased lactate production in patients with underlying diseases, but with normal tissue perfusion.
  *Type B1*
  - – Is associated with sepsis, neoplasia, endocrine disease, hepatic disease, and renal failure.
  *Type B2*
  - – Is associated with a number of toxins and pharmaceuticals.
    - ■ e.g. salicylates, epinephrine, norepinephrine, bicarbonate.
  *Type B3*
  - – Results from genetic metabolic abnormalities.
    - ■ e.g. glycogen storage disease.
- ● **L-lactate**
- ○ It is produced by mammalian cells, and can be used as a marker of hypoxia or decreased tissue perfusion.
- ○ It is the form of lactate measured by POC analyzers.
- ○ In colic cases, a high lactate concentration in blood and peritoneal fluid is indicative of a surgical lesion.
- ○ In horses with colic, increases in L-lactate concentrations in the peritoneal fluid and plasma are associated with intestinal ischemia and increased mortality.
- ○ L-lactate measurement has potential application for diagnosis, monitoring, and prognostication.

- **D-lactate** (*not routinely measured*)
  ○ It is a stereoisomer of mammalian L-lactate.
  ○ It is not produced by mammalian cells.
  ○ Rather, it is product of bacterial fermentation.
  ○ D-lactate is not metabolized in mammals.
    – D-lactate produced in the gut can be measured unchanged in peripheral blood.
  ○ D-lactate concentrations in the blood may increase in patients with intestinal ischemia.
  ○ In colic cases, plasma D-lactate is poorly correlated with plasma L-lactate.
  ○ On the other hand, peritoneal D-lactate concentration has a strong correlation with peritoneal L-lactate.
  ○ Furthermore, peritoneal fluid D-lactate is highly sensitive in detecting horses with strangulating obstructions of the intestine.

## Suggested Reading

DeNotta, S. and Divers, T. (2020). Clinical pathology in the adult sick horse: the gastrointestinal system and liver. *Vet. Clin. North Am. Equine. Pract.* 36: 105–120.

Lester, S., Mollat, W., and Bryant, J. (2015). Overview of clinical pathology and the horse. *Vet. Clin. North Am. Equine. Pract.* 31: 247–268.

Newman, A. (2020). Practical tips on sample handling for hematology, chemistry, and cytology testing for equine patients: getting more bang for your buck. *Vet. Clin. North Am. Equine. Pract.* 36: 1–14.

Tennet-Brown, B. (2012). Interpreting lactate measurement in critically ill horses: diagnosis, treatment, and prognosis. *Compend. Contin. Educ. Vet.* 34: E2.

# 3

# The Cardiovascular System

## Physiology of the Cardiovascular System

*Tamara Grubb*

- The cardiovascular system consists of three components (heart, vessels, blood/plasma) whose ultimate goal is to work in concert with the respiratory system to deliver oxygen to the working cells.
- Tissue oxygen delivery ($DO_2$) is determined by both the volume of blood pumped to the cells (cardiac output or "Q") and the oxygen content of the blood ($CaO_2$).
- Anesthetic drugs can drastically alter cardiovascular function and have a global impact on organ function via decreased $DO_2$.

## I  Anatomy

### A  Chambers

- The equine heart is a typical mammalian heart with four chambers: two atria and two ventricles.

*Atria*

- Primary function is to receive and store blood that will empty into the ventricles during early diastole.
- Oxygen depleted blood from the body is delivered to the right atrium via the cranial and caudal vena cavae and from the myocardium via the coronary sinus and cardiac veins.
- Oxygen rich blood from the lungs is delivered to the left atrium via pulmonary veins.

*Ventricles*

- The primary function is to pump blood into the high-pressure systemic (left ventricle) and low-pressure pulmonary (right ventricle) circulations.
- As described by the *Law of LaPlace* (see Table 3.1), the thick-walled, conical left ventricle is better suited for high-pressure pumping than the thin-walled, flattened right ventricle.

*Manual of Equine Anesthesia and Analgesia*, Second Edition. Edited by Tom Doherty, Alex Valverde, and Rachel A. Reed.

**Table 3.1** Summary of physiologic laws pertaining to the cardiovascular system.

| Name of Law | Formula | Formula components | Application |
|---|---|---|---|
| LaPlace | $T = P \times R$ | <ul><li>$T$ = Tension</li><li>$P$ = pressure</li><li>$R$ = radius</li></ul> | For any given pressure, the tension developed by the wall of the ventricle increases as the radius of the cylinder increases. |
| | | <ul><li>The left ventricle has a much greater radius than the right ventricle and thus is able to develop greater tension (or force).</li><li>($LV$ = left ventricle; $RV$ = right ventricle)</li></ul> | |
| Ohm's | $Q = \Delta P / R$ | <ul><li>$Q$ = blood flow</li><li>$\Delta P$ = the pressure difference (P1-P2) between the two ends of the vessel.</li><li>$R$ = resistance</li></ul> | Blood flow is directly proportional to pressure difference and inversely proportional to resistance. |
| | | $P = 100$ mmHg ➡ $Q = 0\%$ ⬅ $R = 100$mmHg<br><br>$P = 100$ mmHg ➡ $Q = 50\%$ ⬅ $R = 50$mmHg | <ul><li>Thus, the *difference in pressure* between the two ends of the vessel determines the rate of flow and not the absolute pressure in the vessel.</li></ul> |
| Poiseuille's | $Q = \pi \Delta P r^4 / 8\eta l$ | <ul><li>$Q$ = blood flow</li><li>$\Delta P$ = the pressure gradient</li><li>$r$ = the radius of the vessel</li><li>$\eta$ = the viscosity of the blood</li><li>$l$ = the length of the vessel</li><li>$\pi$ relates to the vessel radius</li></ul> | <ul><li>Blood flow is directly proportional to the $4^{th}$ power of the radius of the vessel as long as the flow is laminar.</li><li>Slight changes in the diameter of a vessel cause tremendous changes in flow because blood flowing in the middle of the vessel flows freely, whereas blood at the periphery flows slowly because of friction caused by the endothelium of the vessel wall. In a small vessel, a large percentage of the blood is in contact with the vessel wall so the rapidly flowing central stream of blood is absent.</li></ul> |
| | | Perfusion pressure (P) is constant ⟹ <br>$r = 1$  ⟹ $r^4$ (Q) = 1<br>$r = 2$  ⟹ $r^4$ (Q) = 16<br>$r = 4$  ⟹ $r^4$ (Q) = 256 | <ul><li>Changes in vessel diameter greatly influence blood flow (Q).</li></ul> |
| Starling's | None | None | <ul><li>Within physiological limits, stretched cardiac muscle (and other forms of striated muscle like skeletal muscle) will contract with greater force.</li></ul> |
| | | | <ul><li>The force of contraction of the cardiac muscle is proportional to its initial length.</li><li>When the diastolic filling of the heart is increased or decreased with a given volume, the displacement of the heart increases or decreases with this volume.</li><li>Excessive stretch can result in decreased contractility.</li></ul> |

*Atrio-ventricular valves*
- They connect atria and ventricles.
- Tricuspid valve is between the right atrium and right ventricle.
- Mitral valve is between the left atrium and left ventricle.

*Semilunar valves*
- They connect ventricles to the outflow tracts.
- Aortic valve is between the left ventricle and aorta.
- Pulmonary valve is between the right ventricle and pulmonary artery.

**B    Structural or "skeletal" components of the heart**

- *Myocardium* – muscle layer (striated muscle) of atria and ventricles.
- *Endocardium* – internal lining of the heart chambers, valves and blood vessels.
- *Epicardium* – external lining of the myocardium, continuous with pericardium; secretes pericardial fluid.

**C    Neural input to the heart**

- Atria are highly innervated by sympathetic and parasympathetic fibers.
  - Controls heart rate (HR) and contractility.
  - Parasympathetic fibers – decrease rate and contractility.
  - Sympathetic fibers – increase HR and contractility.
- Ventricles are primarily innervated by *sympathetic* fibers.
  - They continually discharge to maintain a strength of ventricular contraction 20–25% greater than what would occur with no sympathetic input.

## II    Cardiac contractions

**A    Initiation**

- Unlike most physiologic systems, neither the autonomic nor motor neurons are necessary for *initiating* cardiac contractions.
- The heart can continue beating in the absence of outside neural control because the cells of the *specialized electrical conducting system* of the heart are capable of automatic rhythmical depolarization or "self-excitation." This is due to:
  - Cell membranes that are "leaky" or permeable to sodium ions.
  - Increased permeability to potassium and calcium ions also plays a role in the spontaneous depolarization of the pacemaker cells.
  - A *resting* cell membrane potential that is not adequately negative to keep sodium channels closed.
  - The resting membrane potential of cardiac conducting cells is −60 to −70 millivolts (mV) and that of the SA node is −55 to −60 mV (compared to −90 mV for other cell membranes).

B    Components of the specialized electrical conducting system

- Sinoatrial (SA node)
  - Has the fastest rate of spontaneous depolarization and is the *pacemaker*.
  - Located at the junction of the cranial vena cava and the right auricle.
- Atrioventricular (AV) node
  - Slows the rate of impulse transmission as it conducts impulses from the atria to the ventricles.
- Internodal pathways – conduct impulses through the atria to the AV node.
- Right and left bundle branches and His-Purkinje system.
  - Conduct impulses throughout ventricles and ventricular septum.

## III   Unique features of the equine heart

- Large SA node.
  - A "wandering pacemaker" is common.
    - Seen as *variably shaped P waves* on electrocardiogram (ECG).
- Large atria that may depolarize slightly asynchronously.
  - Result in *biphasic P or bifid waves* on the ECG.
- Deeply penetrating His-Purkinje system.
  - Facilitates movement of electrical impulses throughout the large ventricular muscle. Often called Type II Purkinje system.
- Ossa cordi.
  - In all species there is a connective tissue "skeleton" that separates the atria from the ventricles.
  - In cattle and in older horses, these structures may ossify and create two bones, the "ossa cordi."

## IV   Circulatory systems

- The *systemic* (high pressure) and *pulmonary* (low pressure) circulatory systems are separate but coupled (in series) and interdependent so that dysfunction of one will lead to dysfunction of the other.
- The circulatory systems are not just mere conduits, but are active and, through dilation and constriction, control distribution of blood throughout the body and in localized tissue beds.
- The *lymphatic system* is often included as a component of the circulatory system.

A    Components of the systemic circulation

Aorta → Arteries → Arterioles → Capillaries → Venules → Great veins → Right atrium

- The elastic wall of the aorta *recoils* following ventricular contraction, creating a force that maintains blood flow throughout systole and diastole.

- *Arterioles* provide the greatest *resistance* to circulation and, via dilation or constriction, control blood flow to each tissue capillary bed.
- *Capillaries* are the site of exchange of nutrients and waste products.
- The majority of the circulating blood volume (approximately 80%) is generally "stored" in the *venules* and *great veins*.

### B Components of the pulmonary circulation

Pulmonary artery → Arterioles → Capillaries → Pulmonary vein → Left atrium

- The pulmonary artery is the only artery in the body that carries deoxygenated blood, and the pulmonary vein is the only vein that carries oxygenated blood.
- Although the pulmonary circulation receives the same cardiac output as the systemic circulation, the pulmonary system remains a low-pressure system due to the:
  - Tremendous dispensability of the thin-walled vessels.
  - The large number of vessels that are not normally perfused but that can be recruited in times of increased output.
- Distribution of pulmonary blood vessels is an important component of ventilation/perfusion (V/Q) distribution and gas exchange.
- Unlike most tissues in the body, pulmonary tissues constrict when hypoxic (*hypoxic pulmonary vasoconstriction*) in an attempt to divert blood away from poorly ventilated alveoli. This phenomenon can contribute to V/Q mismatch, especially during anesthesia since atelectasis is common in anesthetized horses.
- The lung also receives blood flow through the *bronchial circulation*, a branch of the systemic circulation that perfuses the tissues of the respiratory system.

### C Blood

- Consists of plasma and cellular components.
- Normal equine hematocrit or packed cell volume (PCV) is approximately 35–45% and normal hemoglobin is approximately 15 g/dl.
  - Most oxygen is transported bound to hemoglobin (see section on $DO_2$)
  - When saturated, equine hemoglobin binds 1.36–1.39 ml of oxygen per gram of hemoglobin (Hüfner's constant).

## V Cardiovascular physiology

- The *cardiac cycle* can be described as a period of ventricular contraction (*systole*) followed by ventricular relaxation (*diastole*).
- The electrical, mechanical and audible events that occur during the cardiac cycle are depicted in the *Wigger's* diagram (see Figure 3.1) and described below.

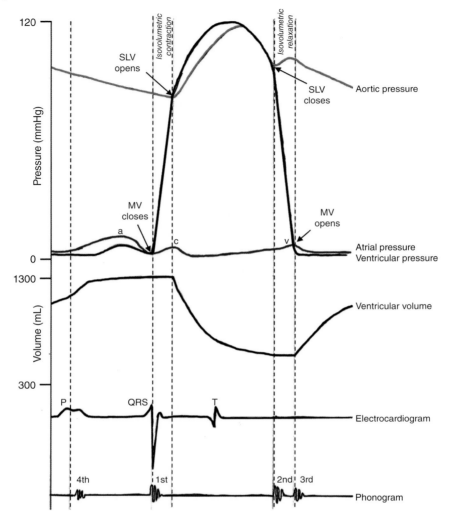

**Figure 3.1** The Wigger's diagram depicts the electrical, mechanical and audible events of the cardiac cycle. SLV, semilunar valve; MV, mitral valve; a, atrial contraction; c, tricuspid bulge; v, atrial filling.

## A Events occurring during late diastole

- The cardiac cycle begins with the spontaneous discharge of the pacemaker, the SA node.
- Discharge is followed quickly by electrical activation of the right atrial muscle and then the left atrial muscle.
  - This results in the *P wave* on the ECG.

- Passive filling of the ventricles occurs during this period.
- Because electrical activation always precedes mechanical activity (termed the *electrome-chanical delay*), the actual atrial contraction occurs shortly after the P wave is generated.
  ○ The rapid flow of blood from atrium to ventricle following atrial contraction generates the *atrial* or *fourth heart sound (S4)* and adds blood to the ventricles so that *end-diastolic blood volume* (or *preload*) is reached.
    - The atrial contribution to the ventricular blood volume is generally minimal and not affected by atrial arrhythmias such as atrial fibrillation.
    - However, during high HRs when the diastolic filling time is shortened and in patients with impaired contractility and decreased stroke volume (SV) the atrial contribution becomes a significant percentage of the total ventricular volume and subsequent ejection fraction.
  ○ Atrial contraction causes a rise in atrial pressure (*"a" wave*) which is transmitted up the systemic venous system and often produces a normal *jugular pulse*.
  ○ The atrial excitation wave reaches the medial wall of the right atrium and is conducted slowly through the *AV node*.
    - This results in the *PR interval* on the ECG.
    - *AV block* occurs when the impulse from the atria is not conducted through the AV node to the ventricles.
      ■ This is reflected on the ECG as a P wave that is not followed by a QRS.
      ■ In the horse, AV block is generally normal due to inherently high *vagal tone*, and is considered benign if the block is abolished by exercise or excitement.

## B    Events occurring during systole

  ○ The impulse exits the AV node and electrical activation of the ventricles occurs.
    - This results in the *QRS complex* on the ECG.
  ○ Ventricular contraction begins shortly after electrical activation.
    - Ventricular pressure quickly exceeds atrial pressure.
  ○ The AV valves are forced closed, producing the high-frequency *first heart sound* (S1).
    - Following closure of the AV valves and prior to the onset of ventricular ejection, the ventricle contracts on a constant volume of blood (*isovolumetric contraction*).
  ○ When left ventricular pressure exceeds aortic and pulmonary artery pressure the *semilunar valves open* and ventricular ejection (the *ejection period*) begins.
    - The time between the onset of the QRS and the opening of the semilunar valves (the *pre-ejection period)* can be measured by echocardiography and is an index of ventricular myocardial contractility.
    - Normal functional systolic "flow" or *ejection murmurs* may occur during the early part of the ejection period.
    - The *arterial pulse* can be palpated during the ejection period, but the actual timing of the pulse depends on the proximity of the palpation site relative to the heart.

○ The audible "cardiac impulse" or "apex beat" occurs during early systole when the contracting heart twists slightly, causing the left ventricle to strike the chest wall just caudal to the left olecranon.

– A "c" wave will be observed during early systole due to bulging of the tricuspid valve into the right atrium or possibly due to pulsations from the carotid artery.

– Ventricular contraction causes the atria to collapse toward the ventricles (*ventricular "suction"*), which causes a brief collapse of the jugular vein and a decrease in atrial pressure (the "x" *descent*).

○ Following this event, atrial filling begins.

– This generates the positive "v" *wave*.

## C   Events occurring at the end of the ejection period (late systole/early diastole)

○ Ventricular pressure rapidly drops below the pressure in the aorta and pulmonary artery, causing a reversal of the direction of blood flow and closure of the *semilunar valves*.

– This produces the high-frequency *second heart sound (S2)*.

– In horses, the pulmonary valve may close either slightly after or slightly before the aortic valve, resulting in an audible "splitting" *of S2*. This splitting is normal but can be dramatic in horses with pulmonary disease.

– Along with aortic recoil, valve closure produces the *incisura* of the arterial pressure curve.

*Comment:* The volume of blood ejected during systole is called *SV*, and the ratio of the SV to the end-diastolic volume is the *ejection fraction*, which is a commonly used measure of systolic function.

## D   Events occurring during early diastole

○ Ventricular pressure continues to fall with no change in ventricular volume (*isovolumetric relaxation*).

○ This proceeds until the ventricular pressure drops below atrial pressure, when the AV valves open and the phase of *rapid ventricular filling* begins.

– Ventricular pressure rises slowly but ventricular volume increases rapidly as blood that accumulated in the atria during ventricular systole flows rapidly into the ventricle.

– Rapid filling may be associated with a *functional protodiastolic murmur* and the termination of rapid filling results in the low-frequency *third heart sound* (S3).

– The rapid decline in both atrial volume and pressure results in the "y" *descent* on the atrial pressure curve and may be visualized as a collapse of the jugular vein.

○ The period of rapid ventricular filling is followed by a period of low velocity filling (*diastasis*) which extends until the next atrial systole.

– In the resting horse with a normal HR, diastasis is the longest period of diastole.

– During diastasis, jugular vein filling may occur, especially during periods of bradycardia.

○ *SA node firing* followed by *atrial contraction* occur during the last phase of ventricular diastole and start the cardiac cycle again.

## VI   Cardiovascular function and clinical applications

- Clinically, cardiovascular function is determined by measurable components such as HR, blood pressure (BP) and cardiac output (see Table 3.2).
- Anesthetic drugs, surgical positioning, surgical events (e.g. hemorrhage) and pathology prior to surgery (e.g. sepsis) can have a profound effect on cardiovascular function.

### A   Cardiac output

$$\text{Cardiac output}\left(Q\right) = HR \times SV$$

- Defined as the volume of blood ejected by the ventricles per minute (l/min).
- Equals the product of HR (beats/min) and SV (l/beat).
- In a normally functioning heart, cardiac output equals venous return.
- Cardiac output in the conscious resting horse (400–500 kg) is 32–40 l/min.
- To standardize cardiac output among individuals, it is often normalized for body surface area or body weight and reported as *cardiac index.*
  - Cardiac index in the conscious, resting horse is 70–90 ml/kg/min.

*Factors affecting cardiac output:*
- HR.
- Preload.
- Afterload.
- Contractility.

### B   Heart rate

- Horses have a wide HR range.
  - A resting rate of 24–50 beats/min to a high of 220–240 beats/min at exercise.
- Increased HR will generally result in increased cardiac output if SV is constant.
  - In horses, the greatest changes in cardiac output generally occur due to a change in HR (rather than in SV).

Table 3.2   Summary of formulas for cardiovascular variables.

| Name | Formula |
| --- | --- |
| Cardiac output (Q) | Heart rate $\times$ Stroke volume |
| Mean arterial blood pressure | Cardiac output $\times$ Systemic vascular resistance |
| Systemic vascular resistance (SVR) | $\dfrac{\text{Mean arterial pressure - Mean right atrial pressure}}{\text{Cardiac Output}}$ |
| Pulmonary vascular resistance (PVR) | $\dfrac{\text{Mean pulmonary arterial pressure} - \text{Mean pulmonary wedge pressure}}{\text{Cardiac output}}$ |
| Arterial oxygen content ($CaO_2$) | $CaO_2 = ([Hb] \times SaO_2\% \times 1.36) + (PaO_2 \times 0.003)$ |
| Oxygen delivery ($DO_2$) | Cardiac output $\times$ arterial oxygen content |

- Extreme *tachycardia* may actually decrease cardiac output because diastolic filling time is decreased, resulting in decreased SV.
- Extreme tachycardia can cause arrhythmias and worsen cardiac disease since the rapidly beating heart spends less time in diastole, the period of the cardiac cycle in which the myocardium is perfused.
- During tachycardia, *myocardial oxygen delivery* is decreased at a time when *myocardial oxygen consumption* is increased, resulting in inadequate oxygen delivery to the myocardium (i.e. *oxygen debt*).

*Factors influencing HR:*
- HR is primarily regulated by autonomic input.
  - Parasympathetic (decreases) and sympathetic (increases) HR.
  - Horses have inherently *high vagal tone* which contributes to the slow HR and normally occurring intermittent second-degree AV block.
- HR is also affected by factors such as ambient temperature, body temperature, exercise, pain, fever and anemia, and reflexively controlled by BP through *baroreceptor* responses.
- Various other activities affect HR.
  - For instance, the *Bainbridge reflex* is an increase in HR secondary to increased right atrial volume and stretching of the SA node.
- Anesthetic drugs can affect HR either directly or indirectly.
  - Anticholinergics (e.g. *atropine*) decrease parasympathetic tone and increase HR.
  - Alpha$_2$ agonists (e.g. *xylazine*) decrease HR via direct effects on the SA node and indirect effects via the baroreceptor response.
    - Alpha$_2$ agonists cause vasoconstriction and hypertension.
  - *Acepromazine* and *inhalant anesthetic gases* may cause hypotension, which can, in turn, cause a baroreceptor-mediated increase in HR.

## C  Stroke volume (SV)

- Defined as the volume of blood ejected by the ventricles per beat.
- SV is the product of *preload, afterload* and *contractility* (inotropy).
  - These components are interlinked and interdependent.

*Preload*
- Is the force acting to stretch the ventricular fibers at the end of diastole.
- It may be described as either *end-systolic volume* or *end-systolic pressure*.
- The volume or pressure in the *left* ventricle is generally used to determine preload.
- It is dictated in large part by *venous return*.
  - The venules serve as *capacitance vessels* or reservoirs, storing the majority of the circulating blood volume. They constrict during times of increased demand, thereby increasing venous return and preload. The great veins and the spleen also act as reservoirs for blood.
  - Anesthetic drugs that can change venous return include *acepromazine* (via vasodilation) and *alpha$_2$ agonists* (via vasoconstriction).
  - Venous return is affected by a number of factors including circulating blood volume, body position, phase of respiration and respiratory disease (due to changes in intrathoracic pressure) and valvular regurgitation.
- Ideally, an appropriate preload will cause stretch of the myocardium, which will improve contractility and increase SV due to *Frank-Starling's Law* of the heart (see Table 3.1).

*Afterload*

- o Is the pressure or resistance against which the ventricle must pump in order to eject blood.
- o Although *aortic impedance* is the most accurate measurement, *arterial BP* is the most commonly used index of afterload. (see section on BP for more information.)
  - – Aortic impedance = Aortic pressure/Aortic flow.
- o End-systolic *ventricular wall stress* is also used to describe afterload.
  - – At the end of systole, with the aortic valve open, increased resistance in the vascular system will be imposed on the ventricles and will increase ventricular wall stress.
- o Anesthetic drugs that can affect afterload include *acepromazine* (vasodilation decreases afterload) and *alpha$_2$ agonists* (vasoconstriction increases afterload).

*Contractility (inotropy)*

- o Defined as the ability of cardiac muscle fibers to shorten or develop tension.
  - – Cardiac muscle contraction is initiated by an action potential which triggers the release of intracellular calcium and the flux of extracellular calcium into the cell, ultimately resulting in cross bridging of *actin* and *myosin* and a shortening of the sarcomere.
- o *Ejection fraction* is a simple measurement of contractility.
  - – Ejection fraction is the ratio of the SV to the end-diastolic volume.
  - – Normal ejection fraction is 60–70%.
- o Other indices used to evaluate contractility include the rate of change of ventricular pressure with respect to time (dP/dt), ventricular function curves, and pressure-volume loops.
- o Increased contractility causes an increase in *myocardial oxygen consumption*.
- o Factors that affect contractility include:
  - – Autonomic tone.
  - – Acidosis, hypoxia.
  - – Thyroid disorders.
  - – Electrolyte imbalance.
  - – Anesthetic drugs.
- o Anesthetic agents that affect contractility include:
  - – Barbiturates, *propofol* and inhalant anesthetic gases cause a decrease in myocardial contractility.
  - – *Ketamine* causes an indirect increase in myocardial contractility via stimulation of the sympathetic nervous system (the direct effect of ketamine is decreased contractility).

*Relaxation (lusitropy)*

- o Corresponds to the extrusion/reuptake of calcium and relaxation of the sarcomere.
- o Imperative for normal diastolic function.
- o Impaired by conditions like hyperthyroidism and heart failure, and by anesthetic drugs such as most inhalational anesthetics.

**D   Blood Pressure** (see Table 3.2)

- o Although *cardiac output* is a more precise measure of cardiovascular function, BP is easier to measure and is often used for evaluation of the cardiovascular system. (See Chapter 19.)
- o BP = Cardiac output (Q) × Systemic vascular resistance (SVR)

$$SVR = \frac{\text{Mean arterial pressure} - \text{Mean right atrial pressure}}{\text{Cardiac output}}$$

*Note*: SVR is often referred to as *total peripheral resistance* (TPR).
- Pulmonary vascular resistance (PVR)

$$PVR = \frac{\text{Mean pulmonary arterial pressure} - \text{Mean pulmonary wedge pressure}}{\text{Cardiac output}}$$

- Arterial BPs are recorded as *systolic, diastolic and mean values.*
  - Systolic pressure = Peak pressure.
  - Diastolic pressure = Nadir pressure.
  - Mean pressure = 1/3 (Systolic pressure − Diastolic pressure) + Diastolic pressure.
- Reference values in conscious adult horses are:
  - Systolic pressure of 147–169 mmHg.
  - Diastolic pressure of 92–110 mmHg,
  - Mean pressure of 115–131 mmHg.
- These values should be maintained at not lower than a 40–50% decrease in the anesthetized horse.

## E Physics of flow

- Blood in the middle of the vessel flows freely, whereas it flows slowly at the periphery because of the friction with the endothelium.
  - In a small vessel, a large percentage of the blood is in contact with the vessel wall so the rapidly flowing central stream is absent.
- Although capillaries have the smallest vessel diameter, *arterioles* pose the highest resistance to blood flow (i.e., there is greater perfusion pressure drop across the arterioles than across any other segment of the systemic circulation).
  - Due to the fact that each arteriole distributes blood to numerous capillaries, thus making the *net resistance* of the capillaries less than the resistance of the single arteriole delivering blood to them.
  - Thus, dilation and constriction of the arterioles dictates organ and tissue blood flow.
- BP is dictated by the laws of Ohm and Poiseuille (see Table 3.1 and described below).

### Ohm's law

- Demonstrates the relationship between current (I), resistance (R), and voltage (V) in an electrical circuit and can be expressed in three ways:
- It can also be used to describe blood flow (cardiac output, Q), resistance (R), and pressure difference across vessels (Δ) in the cardiovascular system.
  - So blood flow is *directly* proportional to the pressure gradient across the vessel and *inversely* proportional to the resistance.
  - The absolute pressure in the vessel is therefore less important than the ΔP across the vessel determining the flow.

### Poiseuille's law (Hagan-Poiseuille)

- Gives the relationship between resistance to flow and vessel dimensions and is analogous to Ohm's Law.
- It applies to laminar flow of incompressible uniformly viscous fluids (described as "Newtonian Fluids") in uniform vessels.

The law does *not* apply to pulsatile flow.
- ○ Its main application is in peripheral vessels where flow is almost steady.
- ○ The Poiseuille equation can be derived by inserting the factors which affect resistance (R) into Ohm's Law.

$$Q = \frac{\Delta P}{R} \quad \text{and} \quad R = \frac{8\eta l}{\pi r^4}$$

(for laminar flow in a vessel of length *l*, radius *r* and blood viscosity η)

So, with substitution, $Q = \dfrac{\Delta P \pi r^4}{8\eta l}$

- ○ Significance of Poiseuille's Law:
  - – Because *r* in this equation is raised to the fourth power, slight changes in vessel diameter (radius) cause tremendous changes in flow.
  - – An increase in viscosity (e.g., with dehydration) will contribute to a decrease in blood flow.

*Laplace's law*
- ○ States that for any given pressure (P), the tension (T) developed by the ventricular wall increases as the radius (R) of the cylinder increases.
  - – For a cylindrical vessel $T = P \times R$.
  - – For a spherical vessel $T = (P \times R)/2$.
  - – So for any given radius and internal pressure, a spherical vessel will have half the wall tension of a cylindrical vessel.
- ○ In the case of the heart, the left ventricle has a much greater radius than the right ventricle and thus is able to develop greater tension (or force).

*Starling's law (Frank-Starling mechanism,* see Table 3.1)
- ○ Describes the intrinsic capability of the heart to increase its force of contraction in response to an increase in venous return.
  - – This response occurs in isolated hearts indicating that it is independent of humeral and neural factors.
- ○ Preload *directly* determines cardiac output when the HR is constant.
- ○ An increase in preload, up to a certain point, increases cardiac output.
- ○ At the end-diastolic volume, cardiac output *will not increase further* and may actually decrease.

## F   Tissue oxygen delivery

- ○ As stated, the ultimate responsibility of the cardiovascular system is to provide adequate oxygen to the working cells.

$$\text{Tissue } O_2 \text{ delivery}\left(DO_2\right) = \text{Cardiac output}\left(Q\right) \times \text{Arterial } O_2 \text{ content}\left(CaO_2\right)$$

- ○ $CaO_2 = ([Hb] \times SaO_2\% \times 1.36) + (PaO_2 \times 0.003)$
  - – [Hb] = concentration of hemoglobin in the blood in gr/dl
  - – $SaO_2$ = percent saturation of hemoglobin with oxygen
  - – 1.36 = a constant (Hüfner's) describing the amount of oxygen bound by 1 g of Hb
  - – $PaO_2$ = the partial pressure of oxygen in arterial blood
  - – 0.003 = the solubility coefficient of oxygen in blood (ml/mmHg of oxygen/dL of blood)

*Note*: The effect of decreases in [Hb] and $SaO_2$ on $CaO_2$ are shown in Box 3.1.

---

**Box 3.1    Effects of Decreases in [Hb] and SaO$_2$ on CaO$_2$**

- Normal [Hb](15 g/dl) and normal SaO$_2$ (SaO$_2$ 98%, PaO$_2$ 95 mmHg):

$$(15 \times 0.98 \times 1.36) + (95 \times 0.003) = 20.29 \text{ml} / \text{dl}$$

- Normal [Hb](15 g/dl) and *decreased* SaO$_2$ (SaO$_2$ 85%, PaO$_2$ 60 mmHg):

$$(15 \times 0.85 \times 1.36) + (60 \times 0.003) = 17.52 \text{ml} / \text{dl}$$

- *Decreased* [Hb] (6 g/dl) and normal SaO$_2$ (SaO$_2$ 98, PaO$_2$ 95 mmHg):

$$(6 \times 0.98 \times 1.36) + (95 \times 0.003) = 8.29 \text{ml} / \text{dl}$$

*Comment*: Although adequate Hb saturation with O$_2$ is important, a critical mass of circulating red cells is *imperative* for tissue oxygenation.

---

## VII    Anesthesia

### A    Effects of anesthetic drugs (see Table 3.3)

- Most drugs used for sedation/tranquilization and anesthesia cause some degree of dose-dependent cardiovascular changes which may manifest as changes in HR, preload, afterload, contractility or a combination of these factors.
- Regardless of which drugs are used, drug dosages in *compromised patients* should almost always be reduced.
  - Most adverse effects, like the cardiovascular depression caused by inhalational anesthetic gases, are dose-dependent.
  - A greater percentage of administered drug may reach the brain (see below).

### B    Effects of cardiovascular disease

- Depending on the severity of the cardiovascular disease, changes *in HR, preload, afterload* and *contractility* can range from barely noticeable to life threatening.
- *SV* decreases due to decreased contractility and increased afterload.
- *Decreased contractility* due to:
  - Direct effects of the disease (e.g. myofibril damage from ischemia).
  - Indirect effects of electrolyte imbalance (e.g. decreased ionized calcium), acid–base imbalance, or sepsis.
- *Increased afterload* due to:
  - A hypotension-mediated increase in sympathetic activity, which results in excessive vasoconstriction in an attempt to maintain BP in the face of decreased cardiac output.
  - A hypotension-mediated decrease in arterial baroreceptor inhibition of autonomic centers in the brain stem, which stimulates the release of *renin*, which increases vascular resistance and promotes salt and water retention through release of *aldosterone*.
- *Decreased SV* due to decreased contractility and increased afterload.
  - This causes *cardiac output to become more HR dependent.*
  - HR generally increases, thereby increasing myocardial O$_2$ consumption.
- *Increased preload* due to reduced SV, accumulated venous return and an increase in fluid retention secondary to activation of the renin/angiotensin system.

Table 3.3 Cardiovascular effects of some commonly used anesthetic drugs.

| Drug | Heart rate | Heart rhythm | Pre-load | After-load | Contractility | Cardiac output |
|---|---|---|---|---|---|---|
| Acepromazine | ↑ | — | ↓ | ↓ | − or ↓ | ↑or ↓ |
| Alpha$_2$ agonists | ↓↓ | + | ↑ | ↑ | − or ↓ | ↓ |
| Benzodiazepines | — | — | — | — | — | — |
| Opioids | − or↓ | — | ↓ | — | − or ↓ | − or ↓ |
| Thiopental | ↑ | + | ↓ | ↓ | ↓ | ↓ |
| Ketamine and Tiletamine | ↑ | + | ↑ | ↑ | ↑ or ↓ | ↑ or ↓ or − |
| Propofol | − or↓ | ± | ↓ | ↓ | ↓ | ↓ |
| Halothane | ↓ | + | ↓ | ↑ | ↓↓ | ↓ |
| Isoflurane | ↓ | — | ↓ | ↓ | ↓ | ↓ |
| Sevoflurane | ↓ | — | ↓ | ↓ | ↓ | ↓ |

↑ = increased; ↓ = decreased; — = no change; + = potentially arrhythmogenic.
*Source:* Adapted from Muir (1998).

- – If the myofibrils can respond, this initially leads to improved contractility via the Frank-Starling law.
  - – It eventually leads to over-distension of the ventricle, which impairs contractility and increases myocardial O$_2$ demand.
- o Circulation becomes "centralized" in patients with moderate to severe cardiac disease, resulting in greater delivery of blood (and drugs carried by the blood) to highly perfused tissues, including the brain.
  - – However, cardiac output is often decreased in these patients, resulting in *slower* drug delivery to the brain.
  - – Thus, the dosage of anesthetic drugs administered to patients with cardiac disease should be *decreased* and drugs should be administered *slowly* and with ample time between doses for delivery to the brain.
- o Congestion of blood and lack of forward flow leads to the *development of edema.*
  - – Pulmonary edema can seriously impair gas exchange.
- o *Myocardial O$_2$ demand increases* (due to tachycardia, increased afterload and overdistended or hypertrophic myocardium) yet O$_2$ supply decreases (due to decreased myocardial perfusion), possibly resulting in O$_2$ debt and further myocardial injury.

## VIII Cardiovascular disease in horses presented for anesthesia

### A Diseases of the conducting system

- o Include irregularities of the SA node (e.g. sinus tachycardia and vagally-mediated bradycardia), the atrial conduction system (e.g. atrial fibrillation), the AV node (e.g. first-, second-, or third-degree AV block) and the bundle branch or His-Purkinje system (e.g. bundle branch block).

○ Because the equine atrial muscle mass is large, the equine heart is predisposed to the development of re-entrant rhythms like *atrial fibrillation*.

*Atrial fibrillation*
- ○ *The most common pathologic arrhythmia encountered in horses.*
- ○ Atrial contribution to ventricular filling may be significant during anesthesia.
- ○ Some anesthetic drugs are arrhythmogenic and should be avoided.
- ○ Patients may need to be converted to normal sinus rhythm prior to anesthesia, although conversion is not always achieved with current options.

**B  Congenital disease**

- ○ Includes patent ductus arteriosus, ventricular septal defects and tetralogy of Fallot.
- ○ *Patent ductus arteriosus*
  - – The most commonly encountered congenital disease in horses.
  - – The ductus arteriosus may be patent for up to 72 hours in normal foals.
  - – Anesthetic-induced hypotension may reverse blood flow through the PDA and create pulmonary hypertension.

**C  Primary myocardial disease**

- ○ Rare in horses.
- ○ *Congestive heart failure* (CHF) is associated with limited cardiac output, increased neurohumoral activity, sodium retention, edema in tissues and transudation of fluid into body cavities.
  - – *Valvular disease* is the most common cause of (CHF) in the horse.
  - – Horses with CHF are at an extremely high anesthetic risk.

**D  Secondary cardiovascular compromise**

- ○ Common in horses presented for anesthesia.
- ○ Causes include circulatory shock (e.g. severe hemorrhage), sepsis (e.g. colic) and profound electrolyte imbalance (e.g. uroabdomen in foals).
- ○ Cardiovascular changes that occur in sepsis include:
  - – Decreased cardiac output resulting from a direct decrease in cardiac contractility and a decrease in preload due to splanchnic pooling and vascular leakage.
  - – Pulmonary hypertension (with subsequent hypoxemia).
  - – Complex alterations in systemic BP (initial hypertension followed by hypotension with loss of vascular tone).
  - – Drastic alterations in hematologic function, including hypercoagulability followed by hypocoagulability.

## IX  Anesthetic plan for horses with cardiovascular disease

**A  Patient preparation**

- ○ All patients scheduled for anesthesia should have a thorough physical examination.
- ○ Because anesthetic drugs can drastically alter cardiovascular function, techniques to evaluate the cardiovascular system should be emphasized, especially in patients with

primary cardiovascular disease or cardiovascular compromise secondary to other systemic disease (e.g. sepsis).
  – Laboratory tests should include serum chemistry and a complete blood count.
- Regardless of the cause of cardiovascular compromise, the patient must be stabilized prior to anesthesia. This includes:
  – Restoration of circulating blood volume (use of whole blood if necessary).
  – Intravenous fluids must be used judiciously in horses with heart failure.
  – Restoration of electrolyte balance.
    ▪ Serum $[Ca^{++}]$ and $[K^+]$ are often decreased.
  – Promotion of cardiovascular function (e.g. IV fluids, positive inotropes, and analgesics).

## B  Sedation and induction

- Following stabilization, the patient should be sedated with low dosages of sedatives (e.g. *alpha₂ agonists, acepromazine*).
- Pre-emptive analgesic drugs should be utilized (e.g. *opioids, alpha₂ agonists,* NSAIDs) to decrease the horse's stress and to decrease the dosages of induction and maintenance drugs.
- A balanced induction technique should be used (e.g. *guaifenesin + ketamine*) and low dosages of the drugs should be administered to effect.
- Intubation and oxygen administration should occur as soon as possible.

## C  Maintenance

- Inhalational anesthetics are generally used for maintenance but dosages should be kept as low as possible to minimize the hypotensive effects of the drugs.
  – Balanced anesthesia (e.g. inhalational agent plus a *ketamine* and/or *lidocaine* infusion) should be considered.
- Analgesia is imperative and can be supplied via systemic administration of drugs or by the use of local anesthetic blockade, or ideally, by using both techniques.
- *Monitoring is extremely important* and should include arterial BP, ECG, and arterial blood gases.
  – A cardioselective inotrope (e.g. *dobutamine*) is recommended for correction of hypotension.
- Fluid therapy should include evaluation and support of PCV, total protein (TP), acid–base balance and electrolyte concentrations.

## D  Recovery

- Is as critical as the other steps of anesthesia.
- Patient support (including monitoring, fluid administration, oxygen administration and provision of analgesia, should be maintained, when possible, throughout the recovery period.

### Evaluation of the Cardiovascular System

*Daniel G. Kenney*

- Evaluation of the horse should include detailed evaluation of the medical and performance history. Of particular note for the cardiovascular system is whether there is an unexplained decrease in body condition, the presence of respiratory abnormalities, edema formation, and decreased exercise tolerance.
- A thorough physical examination should be performed in a systematic fashion, including detailed assessment of the cardiovascular system.

## I   Cardiovascular evaluation

### A   Body condition

  - Poor body condition and decreased exercise tolerance may indicate cardiovascular disease.

### B   Edema

  - Presence of edema in ventral areas (abdomen, thorax, prepuce, udder, limbs) may be indicative of cardiovascular disease.

### C   Mucous membranes

  - Assess for hydration, color, and capillary refill time.
  - The oral mucous membranes are readily assessed in most horses.
  - Vulva membranes and sclera (observation only) may also be assessed.

*Color:*

  - The mucous membranes are visually assessed; normal membranes are pink.
  - Pale membranes (pale pink to whitish) may be due to poor cardiac output/poor perfusion and/or anemia.
  - Dark membranes (deep pink, red, brown, purple) may be due to poor perfusion, vascular congestion, septicemia, and/or toxemia.
  - Bluish membranes may indicate poor perfusion.
  - Yellow membranes occur with elevated bilirubin concentrations (icterus/jaundice). Horses with reduced feed intake often have a mild yellow component to the membrane color. Icterus also occurs to a more severe extent with hemolysis (intravascular or extravascular) or with liver disease.
  - Hemorrhagic membranes may present as "pinpoint" to "expansive" lesions (petechiae to ecchymosis). These may occur with thrombocytopenia, coagulopathies or microangiopathies.

*Moistness:*

  - Hydration is assessed by:
    - Observation and by touching the membranes.
    - Normal membranes are moist.
    - Tacky to dry membranes can occur due to dehydration resulting from many disease processes. The effects of dehydration can be categorized into three groups:

*Mild dehydration* (~5% of body weight) – slight tacky membranes. Skin turgor is normal and eyes are not sunken.

*Moderate* dehydration (6–8% of body weight) – moderately tacky membranes and increased duration of skin tenting (decreased turgor). Eyes are not sunken.

*Severe* dehydration (10–12% of body weight) – markedly tacky membranes, decreased skin turgor (prolonged tenting), eyes are sunken.

*Note*: Caution should be used when assessing sunken eyes as this may also occur with a decrease in the retrobulbar fat pad due to weight loss. The sunken appearance may also occur with ocular disease. Decreases in skin turgor may occur in the neonate, the very old horse, and animals with marked weight loss.

*Exposure:*
- Mucous membranes may be tacky to dry with exposure secondary to swelling, trauma, neurologic dysfunction or other cause.

*Capillary refill time (CRT):*
- Is assessed by rapid light touch of the observer's finger or thumb to the membranes resulting in blanching of the tissue, and the time to reestablish color is noted (see Figure 3.2).
- Normal CRT is <2 seconds. A prolonged CRT may occur due to dehydration, toxemia/septicemia and/or decreased cardiac output. Prolongation usually reflects systemic problems but may also occur due to local disease processes.

**D    Peripheral arteries (pulses)**
- Peripheral pulses can be assessed at the head or on the limbs of a horse.
- Caution must be used when palpating the hind limb arteries to avoid injury to the examiner.

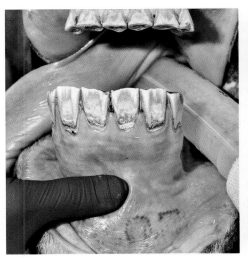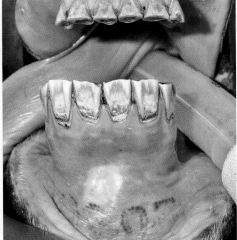

Figure 3.2    Normal mucous membrane color, blanching of mucous membranes with pressure for assessment of capillary refill time.

*Sites for palpation:*
- ○ **Transverse facial artery**
  - – Runs horizontally on the lateral aspect of the head, behind the zygomatic arch, cranio-ventral to the ear.
- ○ **Facial (submandibular artery)**
  - – Can be palpated at the ventral aspect of the mandible, just cranial to the ramus, easy to palpate by "trapping" the somewhat movable artery between the skin and medial aspect of the mandible.
- ○ **Maxillary artery**
  - – Rostral to the infraorbital canal.
  - – This is a useful site in foals to palpate the pulse.
- ○ **Posterior digital and abaxial sesamoid arteries**
  - – Located at the caudolateral and caudomedial aspects of the pastern and fetlock, respectively.
  - – Palpable in all limbs.
- ○ **Radial artery**
  - – Located at the medial aspect of the carpus.
- ○ **Median artery**
  - – Located at the medial aspect of the forearm.
- ○ **Great metatarsal artery**
  - – Caudolateral aspect of the hind limbs, runs vertically in the groove formed by the apposition of the canon and lateral splint (MT 3 and 4) bones.
- ○ **Femoral artery**
  - – Deep palpation at the medial aspect of the thigh. Not a practical site for palpation in the adult horse.
- ○ **Coccygeal artery**
  - – More readily palpable in foals than adult horses.

*Assessment of the pulse:*
- ○ **Pulse rate**
  - – Normal rate is similar to the HR (24–50 pulses per minute).
  - – Assess the pulse while auscultating the heart to determine whether there are any heart beats without pulse generation ("dropped beats" or "pulse deficit").
- ○ **Pulse rhythm**
  - – The normal rhythm is regular. Slight irregularities may occur in the normal horse due to irregularities in the sinus firing (inherent or respiration associated).
  - – Rhythm assessment can be difficult when palpating the head arteries if there is head or chewing motions.
- ○ **Pulse strength**
  - – The normal pulse pressure is usually moderate in the healthy horse at rest; however, a very mild pulse may be present, especially in the distal limbs, when the horse is at rest.
  - – Decreased pulse strength may occur with peripheral vasoconstriction due to inactivity or cool ambient temperatures. May also be due to disease processes resulting in decreased perfusion or decreased cardiac output (e.g. hypovolemia, cardiac disease).
  - – Increased pulse strength occurs with increased peripheral vascular demand such as excitement, exercise or transportation. Examples of disease-associated increases in pulse pressure include *laminitis* (may have increased pulse pressure in the distal limbs) and *aortic valve regurgitation* (common in older horses).

- ○ **Pulse profile**
  - – The normal pulse profile consists of an initial rapid increase in the pulse pressure during systole, followed by a decreased pressure in very early diastole, then another increase in pressure due to the elastic-recoil properties of the aorta and a subsequent decrease in pressure to baseline. The transition from the initial decrease to the second increase is termed the *dicrotic notch*. This second increase is typically palpable in the normal horse. An increase in pulse pressure above normal and a loss of the dicrotic notch occurs in horses with *aortic valve* regurgitation (see below).

## E Peripheral veins

- ○ The jugular veins are the main veins assessed in the horse; however, all regions of the body should be observed and potentially palpated for vascular abnormalities.
- ○ The following are recommendations for jugular vein assessment:
  - – Examine the jugular veins for signs of inflammation (heat, pain, swelling) and obstruction (thrombosis/thrombophlebitis).
  - – Cranial neck and head swelling may occur, especially with acute venous obstruction.
  *Note*: IV injections of various drugs and compounds are commonly given to performance horses of most all disciplines, so careful evaluation of the jugular veins is important as partial to complete obstructions are commonplace.

*Jugular vein waveforms*
- ○ It is common to see fluid waves in the distal jugular vein (at the thoracic inlet) in the normal horse.
- ○ These waveforms are due to the presence of blood within the distal jugular vein, as the vein serves as a reservoir when the heart chambers are full and during systole.
- ○ The waveforms are generated in the blood column by the continuous flow of blood from the periphery to the jugular veins, carotid artery pulsation, and atrial & ventricular contractions.
- ○ These typically extend one-third of the way up the neck when the horse is at rest and has its head and neck elevated.
- ○ The waveforms may extend one-half of the way up the neck if the head and neck are held in a lower position or may go the length of the entire jugular vein if the head and neck are lowered such as when eating off the ground.

*Occluding the jugular vein*
- ○ Occlude each jugular vein in turn just caudal to the angle of the jaw (cranial jugular furrow) and *milk* the luminal blood distally toward the thoracic inlet; the vein should empty readily. Examine the vein for any spontaneous filling from the heart while the vein is still occluded (see jugular waveforms, above). Retrograde filling (jugular pulse) occurs with marked *right AV valve regurgitation*. A "true" jugular pulse is rare in the horse.
- ○ Next occlude the jugular vein distally at the thoracic inlet and observe the time for the vein to refill. The jugular vein will normally fill with blood over several seconds in the normal resting horse. Then release the vein and watch for rapid emptying.

## F Heart

*Cardiac silhouette*
- ○ Refers to the region of the chest where the heart can be auscultated or palpated. An increased area of auscultation occurs due to cardiac enlargement or (caudal) displacement, thoracic masses or pulmonary/pleural disease.

*Heart rate*
- The normal HR in the resting adult horse is 24–50 beats/min.
- Some older, unfit horses may have a slightly higher resting HR.
- The neonatal foal will have a resting HR of 80–100 beats/min and this rate will decrease as the animal ages.
- The horse is very reactive to autonomic input to the heart, and some normal horses will have resting HRs less than 24 beats per/min due in part to parasympathetic nerve input (vagal stimulation).

*Heart rhythm*
- The heart rhythm is typically regular with even timing between beats. Slight irregularity may normally occur spontaneously or in response to the respiratory cycle.

*Auscultation*
- Heart sounds are generated by the turbulence in blood flow resulting from closure of the heart valves. The valves do not have sufficient mass to generate sounds.
- Auscultation on the left side is performed between the third and fifth intercostal spaces (ICS) on the lower third of the chest. Sounds associated with the aortic, pulmonic, and mitral valve closure are heard at the base of the heart, the mitral sound is located in a more caudal position.
- Auscultation on the right side is performed between the fourth and fifth ICS on the lower third of the chest. Sound associated with closure of the tricuspid valve is heard at the base of the heart.

*Left side heart sounds*:
- Mitral valve at fifth ICS, caudal to the elbow.
- Aortic valve at fourth ICS, just dorsal to the elbow.
- Pulmonic valve at third ICS, under the triceps muscle, just below the level of the elbow.

*Right side heart sounds*:
- Tricuspid valve at fourth ICS, just under the triceps muscle.

*Normal heart sounds* (see Figure 3.1)
- Two to four heart sounds may be heard in the horse.
- S1 and S2 are usually louder than S3 and S4.
- S1 may be "split" (two sounds) due to slight variation in contraction in the right and left sides of the heart (uncommon).
  - S1 is associated with closure of the left and right AV valves.
  - S2 is associated with closure of the aortic and pulmonic valves.
  - S3 is associated with rapid ventricular filling.
  - S4 is associated with atrial contraction.

*ECG* (see Section III below)
- Information acquired from an equine ECG is limited to the HR, rhythm and presence or abnormalities of electrical complexes. This is due to the rapid depolarization of the horse heart (ventricles) because of the almost complete penetration of nerve Purkinje fibers across the ventricular myocardium (Type II Purkinje system).
- Lead placement – A base-apex lead is commonly used in the horse. One method of applying the ECG leads for this is as follows:

- Negative lead (RA) White on Manubrium.
- Positive lead (LA) Black on Xyphoid.
- Ground lead (LL) Red on loose skin of neck cranial to the scapula.

*Note*: Europe, RA red, LA yellow, LL green.

## II Heart murmurs

- Murmurs are a result of turbulent blood flow within the heart.
- Murmurs may result from normal or abnormal blood flow.

### A Location

- The point-of-maximal intensity (PMI) and distribution over which the murmur is heard should be defined.
- First defined as left- and/or right-sided.
- Left-sided murmurs are further defined as to the location on the chest wall.
- The murmur is further defined on how widely the sound is heard over the cardiac silhouette.
  - Examples of this are *very focal*, *focal*, *radiating*, *widely radiating*.
  - Very focal, valve-associated murmurs may be detected at expected anatomic locations.

### B Timing in cardiac cycle

- The occurrence of the murmur in the cardiac cycle is identified as systolic, diastolic or continuous.
- Many clinicians assess systole as the short portion of the cardiac cycle when the horse is at rest and diastole as the longer duration.
  - Caution should be used because the systolic and diastolic periods may be equal in length or the diastole period shorter with excitement, exercise or disease.
- Systole is readily identified if a cardiac impulse is palpated while auscultating the heart (common in foals or horses in thin body condition). If the cardiac impulse cannot be felt, simultaneous palpation of a peripheral pulse while auscultating the heart should be performed.
  - An example of this is palpation of the transverse facial artery while listening to the heart. This may be difficult in larger framed horses whereby palpation of the radial artery at the medial aspect of the carpus while listening to the heart may be done.
- Systolic murmurs should be further defined as to when the murmur occurs, i.e. throughout, early, middle or late.
  - Holosystolic murmurs occur throughout systole and S1 and S2 are distinct from the murmur.
  - Pansystolic murmurs overlie one or both S1 and S2.

### C Intensity

- Murmur intensity is categorized on a scale of 1 (very quiet) to 6 (very loud).
- In general, soft murmurs (grade 1 and 2) are non-pathologic while the louder murmurs are associated with pathology in the heart. However, there are exceptions to this rule-of-thumb.

*Grade 1*
- Very soft, small area; the heart must be auscultated for several minutes to detect.

*Grade 2*
  ○ A faint murmur. The heart must be auscultated for a short period to detect.
*Grade 3*
  ○ The murmur is readily heard when auscultation begins. It is localized.
*Grade 4*
  ○ A loud murmur which is widespread (radiates), but there is no palpable *thrill* (vibration felt on the chest wall).
*Grade 5*
  ○ A loud, widespread murmur with a palpable thrill.
*Grade 6*
  ○ A very loud widespread murmur with a palpable thrill. The murmur can still be heard when the stethoscope is lifted slightly off of the chest wall.

*Sounds*
  ○ The murmur sound quality may be categorized as soft, moderate or coarse; other terms may include blowing, rumbling, musical or other such descriptor.
  ○ Sound contour may be described as *band-shaped* (equal sound intensity over time), *crescendo* (gets louder), *decrescendo* (gets softer) or a *combination* of these.

**D   Physiologic (non-pathologic) murmurs**

  ○ Occur due to normal blood flow from the ventricles to the aorta and pulmonary artery.
  ○ This type of murmur is usually holo- or early-systolic, soft blowing, band-shaped murmur.
  ○ The PMI is at the left heart base (forth ICS).
  ○ Diagnosis is based on ruling out abnormal flow through the heart valves and heart defects with the use of ultrasonography.

**E   Pathologic murmurs**

  ○ Initially assessed by auscultation.
  ○ Further definition with echocardiography is indicated.
  ○ Murmurs are generated by turbulent blood flow often due to back flow through a heart valve or flow through an abnormal or persistent anatomic opening (e.g. a ventricular septal defect (VSD), patent foramen ovale).

**Left-sided systolic murmurs**
  ○ **Left AV (mitral) valve regurgitation**
    – Usually occurs as a holosystolic, soft blowing murmur.
    – May be focal or radiate mildly to widely. PMI at the left heart base.
  ○ **Ventricular septal defect (VSD)**
    – Murmurs are pansystolic, sound quality may be anywhere from soft-blowing to a coarse, rumbling murmur.
    – May be focal or they may radiate widely.
    – Usually loudest on right side but may be heard on the left; may be louder on the left if there is right to left shunting.
    – Less commonly, a VSD may be located such that there is shunting from the left ventricle to the right ventricular outflow tract. The PMI with this type of defect is at the left-third ICS, under the triceps muscle.

○ **Valvular endocarditis**
  – Can occur at any or a combination of heart valves.
  – Left-sided lesions are more common in the horse than right-sided lesions.
  – Murmurs are due to both altered blood flow passing by the lesion (anterograde) as well as regurgitant flow through the valve.
  – The quality generally depends on the size and location of the valvular lesion(s).

**Left-sided diastolic murmurs**
○ **Aortic valve regurgitation** (AVR)
  – A very common condition in older horses, usually over 15-years-of-age.
  – This is classically a *decrescendo* murmur which may be soft to coarse in quality.
  – The sound may be quite profound and has been termed a "*dive bomber*" murmur.
○ **Aortic valve endocarditis** – similar to AVR.

**Right-sided systolic murmurs**
○ **Right AV (tricuspid) valve regurgitation**
  – The PMI is usually at the fourth ICS due to flow from the right ventricle to the right atrium.
  – Typically, a holosystolic, soft, blowing murmur.
○ **Aortic valve regurgitation**
  – The PMI is usually left-sided, but the murmur is often heard to a lesser degree on the right side (see above).
○ **Ventricular septal defect**
  – The murmur is usually loudest on the right side of the chest as there is shunting from the left-to-right side of the heart.
  – The common defects are located high in the interventricular septum.
  – Occurs most commonly in Arabian or Arabian cross-breed horses, indicating that this breed is genetically predisposed to the condition.

**Continuous (systolic and diastolic) murmurs**
○ **Patent (persistent) ductus arteriosus** (PDA)
  – This type of murmur may be heard in the newborn foal but usually resolves in the first days-to-weeks of life.
  – It may persist beyond this period; however, this condition is very uncommon to rare in horses.

## III  Electrocardiogram

### A  The elements of the ECG (see Figure 3.3)

○ P wave – depicts atrial depolarization.
  – Due to the horse's large atria, the P wave may be biphasic, or bifid (notched).
○ The QRS complex follows the P wave, and it depicts ventricular depolarization.

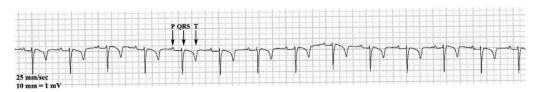

25 mm/sec
10 mm = 1 mV

**Figure 3.3**  Normal sinus rhythm.

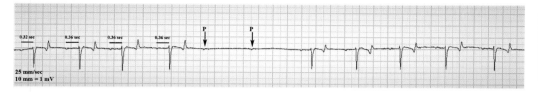

Figure 3.4   Second-degree atrioventricular blockade.

 – The Q, R, and S wave are not always present.
 – The T wave follows the QRS, and it depicts ventricular repolarization.
 – The T wave may be positive or negative at rest.
 – During exercise or stress, the T-wave polarity is opposite to that of the QRS complex.
 – Tall T waves may be mistaken for QRS complexes.

## B   Evaluation of the ECG

 ○ Evaluation of the ECG should be performed in a systematic manner.

*Is each QRS complex preceded by a P wave?*
 ○ Absence of a P wave indicates sinoatrial block.
 ○ P waves may be absent or "hidden" in the following conditions.
   – *Hyperkalemia*: No P wave, tall T waves and wide QRS complexes.
   – *Atrial fibrillation*: No P wave and the rate is irregular, and f waves are present.
   – *Ventricular tachycardia*: P waves hidden in QRS complexes, and presence of wide and bizarre QRS complexes.
     ▪ P wave may be "hidden" in the previous QRS complex during atrial or sinus tachycardia. The morphology of the QRS complex is normal.

*Is each P wave followed by a QRS complex?*
 ○ Second-degree heart block (see Figure 3.4).
   – Occasional absence of AV conduction.
   – P wave is not followed by a QRS complex (see below Section IV, C).
 ○ Third-degree heart block.
   – The condition is rare in horses.
   – P waves not followed by a QRS complex.
   – This is a "complete heart block" and atrial impulses are not conducted through the AV node.
   – The condition is most likely related to pathology of the AV node.
   – The HR is slow because the ventricles are contracting at their intrinsic rate (*escape rhythm*).
   – P waves have normal morphology but have no relationship with QRS complex.
   – The QRS complex can be normal or have a bizarre shape depending on its location of origin.

## IV   Arrhythmias

 • Horses have a high incidence of arrhythmias compared to other domestic animals and this is due to their high degree of vagal tone.

- *Physiologic* arrhythmias usually resolve during exercise or excitement when there is an increase in sympathetic tone and/or a decrease in vagal stimulation.
- Conversely, some arrhythmias may be exacerbated by exercise.

## A Bradycardia

- Sinus bradycardia is considered to be present when the HR is <24 beats/min, but the RR interval is regular.
  - The normal HR is between 24 and 50 beats/min.
- Usually, bradycardia is due to increased vagal stimulation.
  - Generally, disappears with exercise.
- HRs lower than 24 beats/minute may occur in a fit horse, but may also reflect cardiac disease, such as sinus abnormalities and/or infiltrative processes.

## B Tachycardia

- Characterized by a resting HR > 50 beats/min.
  - The RR intervals are normal (variations >20% are considered to be abnormal).
  - The relationship between the P waves and QRS complexes is normal.
- May be due to excitement or exercise in the normal horse.
- The maximal HR is between 220 and 240 beats/min.
- Abnormal increases at rest occur with many extra-cardiac as well as cardiac disease processes.
  - Extra-cardiac causes include external stimuli to the heart, and are often due to one or a combination of the following: pain, hypovolemia, toxemia, septicemia. The "drive" may be a need for increase blood flow.
  - Tachyarrhythmias have many causes and may be multifactorial. The origin may be atrial (SA node-related or extra-nodal, such as atrial fibrillation), supraventricular tachycardia (SVT) or ventricular tachycardia (VT).

## C Second-degree AV blockade (see Figure 3.4)

**Type 1** (Mobitz type1, Wenckebach phenomenon)
- This is the most common type of second-degree block in the horse.
- Progressive prolongation of the PR interval until a dropped beat occurs. The ECG shows a P wave not followed by a QRS complex.
- Often associated with increased vagal tone and is common with administration of $\alpha_2$ agonists.
- Normal sinus rhythm can be restored with this type of arrhythmia by exciting or exercising the horse to increase sympathetic tone and decreasing parasympathetic tone. Elevation of the HR above 60–80 beats/min may be required to resolve the block.

**Type 2** (Mobitz type 2)
- Regular PR interval and then sudden absence of a QRS after a P wave.
- Persistence of the heart block, despite exercising the horse to increase the sympathetic tone, may indicate a pathologic condition such as disease of the AV node, which is often the case for this type of block.

**D    Atrial fibrillation** (see Figure 3.5)

- Atria are not contracting in a coordinated manner.
- It is relatively common in horses due to their large atria and high degree of vagal tone.
  - There is a higher incidence in Standardbreds, Draft horses and Warmbloods.
- *Paroxysmal* atrial fibrillation has been reported in Thoroughbreds during racing, and sinus rhythm returns spontaneous within 72 hours. In most cases however, atrial fibrillation does not spontaneously convert to sinus rhythm.
- No "P" waves are present. Fibrillation (f) waves are evident and they may have a frequency up to 500 beats/min, but few are conducted through the AV node to the ventricle.
  - The f wave morphology can be *course* or *fine*.
- The RR interval is irregularly irregular and QRS complexes are normal if there is no underlying disease.
- Cardiac function can be relatively normal at rest or during mild to moderate exercise if the finding is incidental.
- Decreased cardiac function occurs if there is associated heart disease or at high levels of performance.

*Treatment of atrial fibrillation*

- If cardiac function is otherwise normal, atrial fibrillation can generally be converted to sinus rhythm with *quinidine*. Prognosis for conversion is poor if atrial fibrillation has been present for over four months.
- Transvascular electrical conversion under general anesthesia is reported to have good success in converting atrial fibrillation of longer duration.

**E    Atrial flutter**

- Similar to atrial fibrillation but less common in horses.
- Baseline sinusoidal wave with more frequent "f" waves, referred to as saw-tooth pattern, between two consecutive QRS complexes.
- Uncommon in horses.
- Treatment is the same as for atrial fibrillation.

**F    Premature atrial contractions (PACs)**

- A normal QRS complex appears before expected; therefore, the R–R interval is shorter between the previous normal beat and the premature beat.
- The "P" wave can be absent (hiding) if the PAC occurred to soon after the normal beat.
- Can be incidental or associated with heart disease that has caused enlarged atria, or myocarditis or hypokalemia.
- A solitary PAC is not likely to be significant if not associated with clinical signs and does not occur during exercise.

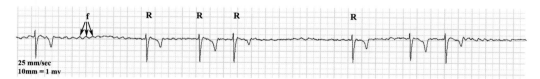

25 mm/sec
10mm = 1 mv

**Figure 3.5**    Atrial fibrillation.

*Treatment*

- o Not necessary to treat unless the PACs become frequent and the horse develops clinical signs or atrial fibrillation is triggered.
- o *Quinidine* can be used to terminate the arrhythmia.
- o *Digoxin* can be used to control the arrhythmia if there is underlying cardiac disease.

### G Premature ventricular complexes (PVCs) (see Figures 3.6 and 3.7)

- o Large, abnormal morphology QRS complexes that appear before a normal beat was expected. Therefore, the R–R interval is shorter.
- o The depolarization from the PVC travels retrograde and blocks the next impulse from the SA node, which can result in a compensatory pause after the abnormal beat.
  *Note*: Singular to several PVCs are often identified in normal horses.
- o The PVC is not conducted via the normal conduction pathway; hence, its morphology is different and it is of longer duration than a normal QRS complex.
- o The PVC is not associated with the preceding P wave.
- o Runs of PVCs are of concern and may result in weakness, syncope, ventricular tachycardia and death.
- o PVCs do not allow for complete and normal filling of the ventricle, which affects the SV and results in a lower cardiac output and/or hypotension.

*Treatment of single PVCs*

- o Treatment should be administered if PVCs:
  - – Are multifocal.
  - – Are frequent and the pulse quality is poor.

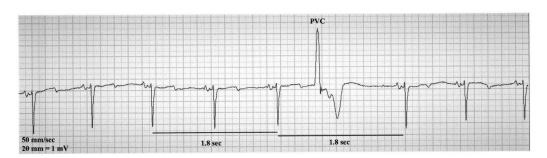

Figure 3.6   Premature ventricular complex.

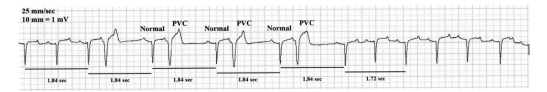

Figure 3.7   Ventricular bigeminy; every other complex is ventricular in origin.

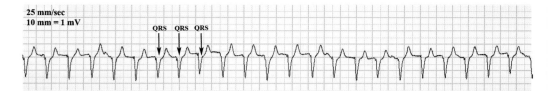

**Figure 3.8** Ventricular tachycardia.

  – Are on top of the preceding T wave, as this scenario may result in ventricular fibrillation.
  ○ Administer *lidocaine* (0.5–2 mg/kg, IV).

*Treatment of multiple PVCs*
  ○ *Lidocaine* (0.5–2 mg/kg, IV) for immediate control of PVCs.
  ○ Treat underlying cause (e.g. hypoxia, electrolyte abnormalities [$K^+$, $Ca^{++}$, $Mg^{++}$]).
  ○ *Quinidine gluconate* (1.1–2.2 mg/kg, IV) for short-term control of PVCs.
  ○ Lidocaine (25–50 µg/kg/min) for longer term control.

H  **Ventricular tachycardia (VT)** (see Figure 3.8)

  ○ A group of *four* or more consecutive PVCs.
  ○ Characterized by abnormal QRS complexes that are not associated with P waves.
    – P waves, if present, may be hidden in the QRS complexes.
  ○ VT may be paroxysmal or sustained for minutes or hours and may lead to ventricular fibrillation.
  ○ The ventricular rate may be slow (slightly above normal rate) or fast (up to 200 beats/min).
  ○ The QRS complexes may be monomorphic or polymorphic.
  ○ SV is decreased especially if the ventricular rate is high, and this results in a lower cardiac output and/or hypotension.

*Treatment*
  ○ A slow ventricular rate usually does not need to be treated.
  ○ Multifocal ventricular tachycardia should be treated.
  ○ Treatment should be initiated if the HR is >100 beats/min.
  Treatment is similar to that for PVCs.
  ○ Diagnose and treat underlying cause.

## Suggested Reading

Durando, M. (2019). Cardiovascular causes of poor performance and exercise intolerance and assessment of safety in the equine athlete. *Vet. Clin. North Am. Equine Pract.* 35: 175–190.

Hubbell, J. and Muir, W. (2015). Oxygenation, oxygen delivery and anaesthesia in the horse. *Equine Vet. J.* 47: 15–25.

van Loon, G. (2019). Cardiac arrhythmias in horses. *Vet. Clin. North Am. Equine Pract.* 35: 85–102.

McGuirk, S.M. and Muir, W.W. (1985). Diagnosis and treatment of cardiac arrhythmias. *Vet. Clin. North Am. Equine Pract.* 1: 353–370.

McGurrin, M. (2015). The diagnosis and management of atrial fibrillation in the horse. *Vet. Med. (Aukl)* 26: 83–90.

Muir, W.W. (1998). Anesthesia for dogs and cats with cardiovascular disease - Part II. *Compend. Contin. Educ. Vet.* 20: 473–484.

Reef, V.B. (1985). Evaluation of the equine cardiovascular system. *Vet. Clin. North Am. Equine Pract.* 1: 275–288.

Sage, A., Keating, S., Lascola, K. et al. (2018). Cardiopulmonary effects and recovery characteristics of horses anesthetized with xylazine-ketamine with midazolam or propofol. *Vet. Anaesth. Analg.* 45: 772–781.

Shih, A. (2019). Cardiac monitoring in horses. *Vet. Clin. North Am. Equine Pract.* 35: 205–215.

# 4

# The Respiratory System

## Anatomy of the Equine Respiratory System

*Robert Reed*

## I    Organization of respiratory system

- The respiratory system is primarily a collection of tubular organs designed for the conduction of air and gas exchange.
- The respiratory system can be divided into:
  - *Conducting* components.
  - *Gas exchange* components.

### A   Conducting components

- Consist of the nasal cavity, paranasal sinuses, pharynx, larynx, trachea, bronchi, and bronchioles.

### B   Gas exchange components

- The gas exchange components include the respiratory bronchioles, alveolar ducts, alveolar sacs, and alveoli.

## II   Tubular organs

- The tubular organs that comprise the respiratory system are made up of four layers.

### A   Tunica mucosa

- Contains the epithelial layer that lines the internal surface of the organ.
- The function of the organ determines the type of epithelial cells present in this layer.

*Manual of Equine Anesthesia and Analgesia*, Second Edition. Edited by Tom Doherty, Alex Valverde, and Rachel A. Reed.

B   **Tunica submucosa**

    ○ The tunica submucosa is a layer of collagenous connective tissue that supports glands, blood vessels, and nervous structures.

    ○ The glands are responsible for secretions, which moisten the epithelial surface or assist with movement of materials.

    ○ The submucosa acts as a flexible surface on which the tunica mucosa can attach.

C   **Tunica muscularis**

    ○ Is the thickest layer of the tubular organ.

    ○ It acts to regulate lumen size and tone.

D   **Tunica adventitia**

    ○ A loose collagenous connective tissue layer that anchors organs to surrounding tissues.

## III   Nasal cavity

- Each half of the nasal cavity is divided into four regions or *meatuses* by the mucous membrane covered dorsal and ventral *conchae*.
  - Conchae serve to warm and humidify inspired air.
  - Conchae also clean the inspired air by trapping particulate matter in mucus secretions.

## IV   Paranasal sinuses

- Paranasal sinuses of the equine are found within the *frontal, maxillary, palatine* and *sphenoid* bones as well as the dorsal and ventral *conchae*.
- Paranasal sinuses are mucous-membrane lined, air-filled cavities within bones, which serve to decrease the weight of the skull. Connections exist between the middle nasal meatuses and the paranasal sinuses that allow for increased exposure of air to mucous membrane.

## V   Pharynx

- The wall of the pharynx contains cartilage and skeletal muscle and is lined with a mucous membrane.
- The pharynx is sub-divided into three regions (nasopharynx, oropharynx, and laryngopharynx).
- The opening of the auditory tubes is located in the lateral walls of the nasopharynx.

*Guttural pouch*

    ○ In the equine, each auditory tube has an expanded caudoventral diverticulum called the guttural pouch.

    ○ The internal carotid arteries are closely associated with the medial compartments of the guttural pouches.

○ It is believed that the air inside the pouches cools the blood within the internal carotid arteries before the blood reaches the brain.

## VI   Larynx (see Figure 4.1)

- The larynx is, in part, composed of skeletal muscle and five individual, mucous membrane-lined cartilages.
- The opening into the larynx is called the *rima glottis*.
- The muscles which attach to the larynx are used for swallowing and phonation.

### A   Cartilages

- ○ *Epiglottic* cartilage functions to occlude the rima glottis during swallowing.
- ○ *Thyroid* cartilage is a trough-shaped cartilage, which forms the majority of the lateral and ventral extremities of the larynx.
- ○ *Arytenoid* cartilages (paired) are associated with the actions of the vocal ligaments and *phonation.*
- ○ *Cricoid* cartilage is the caudal-most cartilage of the larynx and forms a complete ring. It is responsible for maintaining patency of the larynx.

### B   Innervation of the larynx

- ○ Nervous supply to the muscles of the larynx is provided by the *cranial laryngeal* and *recurrent laryngeal* nerves.
- ○ The recurrent laryngeal nerves innervate the *cricoarytenoideus dorsalis.*
  - – The cricoarytenoideus dorsalis abducts the arytenoid cartilages out of the lumen of the larynx to allow the passage of air.

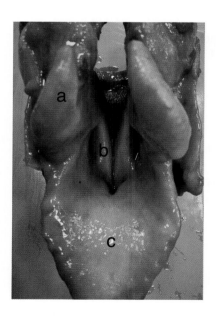

Figure 4.1   Normal equine larynx: arytenoid cartilage (a), vocal fold (b), epiglottis (c). *Source:* Dr. Corrie Brown, DVM, PhD, DACVP University of Georgia, College of Veterinary Medicine.

## VII  Trachea

- Is formed from "C-shaped" cartilaginous rings whose incomplete dorsal aspects are bridged by the *trachealis* muscle.
  - The trachealis muscle is composed of smooth muscle fibers.
- The tracheal cartilages prevent collapse of the trachea.
- The trachea terminates near the hilus of the lungs as it bifurcates into the left and right principal bronchi.
- The esophagus is located dorsal to the trachea in the cranial and caudal portions of the cervical region and to the left of the trachea in the middle portion of the cervical region.

## VIII  Lungs and pulmonary circulation

- The lungs are a paired organ found within the thoracic cavity.
- The left and right lungs are each divided into *cranial* and *caudal lobes* by a large fissure called the *cardiac notch*.
- The right lung also possesses an *accessory lobe*.

### A  Blood supply

- The lungs receive two forms of blood supply (*pulmonary*, *bronchial*).
- The *pulmonary* circulation involves blood that is delivered to the lungs for the purpose of oxygenation.
- The *bronchial* circulation involves blood that supplies $O_2$ and nutrients to the lung parenchyma.

### B  Nerve supply

- The lungs receive *sympathetic* nerve fibers from the *sympathetic trunks*.
- The lungs receive *parasympathetic* nerve fibers from the *vagus nerves*.
- These autonomic nerve fibers control smooth muscle and glands within the lung.

## IX  Bronchi and bronchioles

- Primary bronchi branch within the lung into lobar (secondary) bronchi, which correspond to the lobation of the lungs.
- Secondary bronchi branch into tertiary bronchi.
- The branching of tertiary bronchi gives rise to the *bronchiolar system*.
- The bronchiolar system branches into primary, secondary and tertiary components in the same fashion as did the bronchi.
- Tertiary bronchioles give rise to *terminal bronchioles*, which are the final segment of the conducting components of the respiratory system.
- Lumen diameter of the airway decreases with each incidence of branching.

## X   Respiratory epithelium

- Is the primary epithelial-type lining the conducting components of the respiratory system.
- Classified as *ciliated, pseudostratified columnar epithelium with goblet cells.*
- The *goblet cells* secrete mucus, which serves to trap inhaled particles.
- *Cilia* on columnar cells move this mucus layer out of the respiratory tract.
- This epithelium changes to simple columnar and eventually to simple cuboidal epithelium as the conduction system branches toward the gas exchange components.

## XI   Alveolar region

- Terminal bronchioles divide into several *alveolar ducts.*
- Alveolar ducts end in *alveolar sacs.*
- Alveolar sacs are dilatations of the airway lined with hemispherical chambers called *alveoli.*
- Gas exchange occurs between the blood and inspired air across the wall of the alveolus.

### A   Alveoli

- Alveoli are lined with two cell types classified as *type I* and *type II pneumocytes.*

### B   Type I pneumocytes

- Type I pneumocytes are simple squamous cells with extremely thin processes.
- They are more abundant than type II pneumocytes.
- They are a component of the blood–air barrier.

### C   Type II pneumocytes

- Type II pneumocytes are cuboidal cells.
- They function to secrete *pulmonary surfactant.*
- Pulmonary surfactant stabilizes alveoli during inflation by keeping them uniform in size thus preventing collapse.

## XII   Blood–air barrier

- The partition between inspired air and the pulmonary capillary system.
- Formed by the processes of type I pneumocytes, a small amount of connective tissue and capillary endothelial cells.
- Gas molecules must cross this barrier to enter or exit the blood vascular system.

## XIII   Muscles of respiration

- The *diaphragm* is the primary muscle of respiration.
  - It is innervated by the *phrenic nerves*, which originate from the 4th, 5th, and 6th cervical spinal nerves pairs.

- ○ Contraction produces the negative pressure within the thoracic cavity involved with inspiration.
- *Scalenus, serratus dorsalis cranialis*, and *intercostal muscles* are also involved with inspiration.
- *Serratus dorsalis caudalis* muscles are involved with expiration.

## Suggested Reading

Froydenlund, T.J., Dixon, P.M., Smith, S.H. et al. (2015). Anatomical and histological study of the dorsal and ventral nasal conchal bullae in normal horses. *Vet. Rec.* 177: 542.

Johnson, L., Montgomery, J.B., Schneider, J.P. et al. (2014). Morphometric examination of the equine adult and foal lung. *Anat. Rec.* 297: 1950–1962.

Pekarkova, M., Kircher, P.R., and Konar, M. (2009). Magnetic resonance imaging anatomy of the normal equine larynx and pharynx. *Vet. Radiol. Ultrasound.* 50: 392–397.

## Physiology of the Respiratory System

*Carolyn Kerr*

- The primary function of the respiratory system is the transport of $O_2$ from the environment to the pulmonary capillaries and the transport of $CO_2$ from the pulmonary capillaries to the environment.
- Many processes are involved in achieving gas exchange. These include:
  - ○ Ventilation.
  - ○ Perfusion.
  - ○ Matching of ventilation and perfusion within the lung.
  - ○ Diffusion of gases across the alveolar capillary membrane.
  - ○ Carriage of gases to and from the alveoli to the tissues.

## I  Alveolar ventilation (VA)

- *Ventilation* refers to the movement of gas into and out of the lung. In the normal spontaneously breathing horse, inspiration and expiration are *active* processes utilizing metabolic energy.
- Alveolar ventilation is regulated by the CNS through chemoreceptors that sense $CO_2$ and $O_2$ partial pressures in the blood, and through pulmonary reflexes and non-pulmonary neural input.

### A   Mechanics of ventilation

- *Intrapleural pressure* is approximately $-5\,cm\ H_2O$ at rest, resulting in a transpulmonary pressure of $5\,cm\ H_2O$.
- *Inspiration* is characterized by expansion of the chest, (due to contraction of the diaphragm and the external intercostal muscles) which results in a *decrease* in intrapleural pressure and an *increase* in the transpulmonary pressure gradient. As a result, gas moves from the atmosphere into the respiratory passages.

- *Gas flow* ceases at the end of inspiration, as there is no longer a gradient between the atmospheric and alveolar pressure.
- *Expiration* is characterized by relaxation of the inspiratory muscles, elastic recoil of the lung, and contraction of the internal intercostal and abdominal muscles. These processes result in an increase in the transpulmonary pressure, and movement of gas from the lung to the ambient atmosphere.
- In horses, both inspiration and expiration have a biphasic pattern. The first phase of inspiration is passive, from a forced and active contraction of abdominal muscles at the end of expiration that forces the respiratory system below its equilibrium. The second part of inspiration is active through contraction of the diaphragm and other inspiratory muscles. The first part of expiration is passive through recoil of the respiratory system down to its equilibrium position, but then is active so that the next inspiration begins with relaxation of the abdomen.
- *Contraction of muscles* in the nares, pharynx and larynx is necessary to prevent collapse of structures into the air passages in the presence of the negative pressures generated in the respiratory tract during inspiration,
  - *For example, muscle relaxation secondary to the effects of sedatives/anesthetics or as a consequence of nerve dysfunction can impair airflow.*

## B   Work of breathing

- The work or energy expended in ventilation is due to the forces required to overcome the *elasticity* of the lung and *frictional resistance* to air flow.
- The relative amount of energy spent on these two forces in addition to the total amount of energy spent to achieve ventilation can be altered by the *pattern of breathing*.
- In the normal horse at rest, gas flow rate within the airways is slow, and the majority of the work of breathing is due to the *elastic resistance* of the lung.
- As flow rates increase during more rapid respirations, a greater amount of energy is spent overcoming the frictional resistance within the airways.

## C   Lung and airway resistance

- *Elastic resistance* is a result of surface tension forces at the alveolar air-liquid interface in addition to the elastic properties of the lung tissue matrix.
- *Frictional resistance* is primarily influenced by airway radius and length.
  - The *upper airways* (nasal cavity, pharynx, and larynx) provide approximately 60% of the total resistance to breathing.
  - The *lower airway* resistance primarily resides in the trachea and bronchi.
  - The *bronchioles* provide only a small fraction of the total resistance due, in large part, to the low airflow in a high cross-sectional area.
- *Airway radius* or diameter can be altered due to changes in the smooth muscle tone within the walls of airways.
  - In the horse, smooth muscle extends from the trachea to the alveolar ducts.
  - In general, parasympathetic mediated smooth muscle contraction results in airway narrowing and an increase in airway resistance.
  - β-adrenergic and nonadrenergic noncholinergic activation results in bronchodilation and a decrease in airway resistance.

## II   Lung volumes (see Figure 4.2)

### A   Minute ventilation ($V_E$)

$$V_E = f \cdot V_T$$

○ Is the total volume of air breathed each minute. It is the product of the respiratory rate ($f$) and the tidal volume ($V_T$).
○ On average, a normal adult horse breathes at a rate of 14 breaths per minute with a tidal volume of 12 ml/kg. This results in a minute ventilation of approximately 170 ml/kg/min.

### B   Tidal volume ($V_T$)

$$V_T = V_A + V_D$$

○ Each breath or tidal volume, is composed of:
  – *Alveolar ventilation* ($V_A$). The portion of gas that enters the respiratory zone of the lung.
  – *Physiologic dead space* ($V_D$). The portion of gas that remains in the part of the respiratory system that does not participate in gas exchange.

### C   Dead space

○ *Anatomic* dead space is the volume of gas that ventilates conducting airways.
○ *Alveolar* dead space is the volume of gas not taking part in effective gas exchange at the alveolar level.
○ *Physiologic* dead space is the sum of anatomical and alveolar dead space.
○ The fraction of a tidal volume breath that occupies the physiologic dead space is commonly expressed as the $V_D/V_T$ ratio.
○ In normal adult horses, the $V_D/V_T$ ratio is 50–75%, a value significantly greater than the $V_D/V_T$ ratio in humans (15–20%).

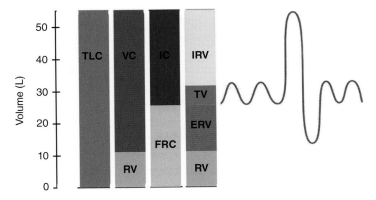

Figure 4.2   Lung volumes in an adult horse (500 kg). TLC, Total lung capacity (55 l); VC, Vital capacity (44 l); RV, Residual volume (11 l); IC, Inspiratory capacity (29.5 l); FRC, Functional residual capacity (25.5 l); IRV, Inspiratory reserve volume (23.5 l); TV, Tidal volume (6 l); ERV, Expiratory reserve volume (14.5 l).

**D Measurement of dead space – Bohr equation**

- ○ The ratio of physiologic dead space to the tidal volume ($V_D/V_T$) can be calculated using *Enghoff's* modification of the *Bohr* equation, which substitutes alveolar $CO_2$ ($PACO_2$) with arterial $CO_2$ ($PaCO_2$):

$$\frac{V_D}{V_T} = \frac{PaCO_2 - PECO_2}{PaCO_2}$$

- ○ This measurement is based on the fact that all expired $CO_2$ comes from perfused alveoli and none from dead space.
    - – $PECO_2$ in this equation is the $CO_2$ content in the mixed expired gas, which is obtained under experimental conditions by sampling a mixture of the expired gas collected from a large bag or through a device that measures of expired $CO_2$ content and expired volume over time.
    - – In clinical practice, end-tidal $CO_2$ can be used to follow trends in the $V_D/V_T$ ratio.
- ○ An increase in dead-space ventilation necessitates an increase in minute ventilation in order to maintain alveolar ventilation. This results in an increase in the work of breathing required to maintain normal gas exchange in a spontaneously breathing patient. In a mechanically ventilated patient, an increase in dead space requires an adjustment in minute ventilation by increasing the respiratory rate or tidal volume settings. In a hemo-dynamically compromised patient, the latter changes may have negative cardiovascular consequences.

*Factors that increase dead space include*
- ○ Decreased pulmonary artery pressure (e.g. decreased cardiac output).
- ○ Loss of perfusion to ventilated alveoli despite normal pulmonary artery pressure (e.g. pulmonary embolus).
- ○ Increased airway pressure.
- ○ Equipment (e.g. endotracheal tubes (ET) protruding excessively beyond the lips).
- ○ Rapid, short inspirations.

**E Functional residual capacity (FRC)**

- ○ At the completion of a tidal volume breath, the lung does *not empty*. The volume of gas remaining in the lung is referred to as the FRC (see Figure 4.2).
- ○ The volume of the FRC is important as it acts as a *reservoir* for gas exchange and is esti-mated at 51 ml/kg in the horse.
- ○ A reduction in FRC alters lung mechanical properties (see pulmonary compliance below) as well as increasing pulmonary vascular resistance.
- ○ In the horse, the FRC is reduced with recumbency and general anesthesia.
- ○ If the FRC is very low, one can see from the shape of the pressure-volume curve (see Figure 4.3), that the change in lung volume for a given change in pressure is very small.

## III Pulmonary compliance

- • Compliance ($\Delta V/\Delta P$) is the change in lung volume ($\Delta V$) per unit change in transpulmonary pressure ($\Delta P$) and it has been estimated as 22.7 l/kPa (3.0 l/mmHg).

- Lung compliance can be measured in an awake spontaneously breathing horse in a laboratory setting by measuring the mouth to intrathoracic pressure and lung volume change using a pneumotachograph (device that measures airflow over time) attached to a facemask. In anesthetized horses, pulmonary compliance and pressure volume curves are determined using positive pressure to achieve a change in lung volumes from FRC to total lung capacity. (see Figure 4.3)
- *Compliance* is the slope of the pressure-volume curve and, due to the non-linear shape of the curve, it fluctuates with lung volume.
- In the spontaneously breathing animal with normal lungs, tidal volume breathing occurs on the steep portion of the curve. As a result, for a given change in intrapleural pressure, there is a greater change in lung volume than would occur if tidal volume breathing occurred at the extremes of the curve.

## A  Distribution of alveolar ventilation

- ○ The distribution of alveolar ventilation, or the change in alveolar size with each breath, is not uniform throughout the lung due to differences in the mechanical properties of the lung and chest wall.
- ○ In the *standing horse*, the intrapleural pressure is more sub-atmospheric in the dorsal part of the lung relative to the ventral part, due to the effect of gravity on lung tissue. The alveoli in the dorsal part of the lung are therefore more distended, and less compliant than in the ventral part of the lung. As a result, alveolar ventilation per unit change in pressure is greater in the ventral compared to the dorsal part of the lung.
  - – The alveoli in the dorsal aspect of the lung would be at a location further to the right on the curve. (see Figure 4.3)

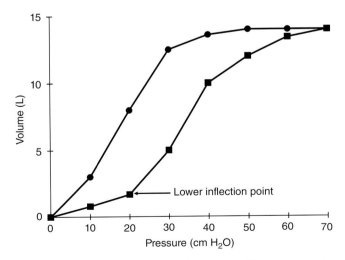

**Figure 4.3**  Pulmonary pressure-volume curve; illustrating greater pressure difference required for inspiration than for expiration (squares = inspiration; circles = expiration).

B   **Factors decreasing pulmonary compliance**

- Atelectasis resulting in a loss of lung volume.
- Pulmonary edema and/or pulmonary surfactant dysfunction.
- Pleural, interstitial or alveolar disease.
- Airway occlusion.
- Pleural and/or pericardial effusion.
- Rigidity of the chest wall or diaphragm (e.g. secondary to abdominal distension).

## IV   Alveolar perfusion

A   **Lung blood flow**

- The lung receives blood from two circulations, the *pulmonary artery* and the *bronchial artery*.
- The pulmonary artery receives the total output of the right ventricle, and perfuses the alveolar capillaries.
- The bronchial artery is a branch of the aorta and perfuses the parenchymal structures of the lung (e.g. airways).
- The pulmonary arterial systolic, diastolic, and mean pressures in the horse average 42, 18, and 22 mmHg, respectively. This indicates a *low vascular resistance* compared to the systemic circulation.
- For gas exchange to occur across an alveolar membrane, the alveoli must be perfused. Optimal gas exchange occurs when the alveolar ventilation and blood flow are equally distributed in the lung.

B   **Distribution of blood flow in lung**

- The distribution of pulmonary blood flow within the lung of the horse was previously thought to be primarily influenced by gravity; however, there is *not* a consistent vertical gradient to blood flow in the lungs of horses.
- This implies that gravity does not play a major role in blood flow distribution.
- *Endogenous vasoactive mediators* (e.g. *nitric oxide* and *endothelin-1*) are now thought to play a major role in the distribution of perfusion within the lung.

C   **Hypoxic pulmonary vasoconstriction**

- Vasoconstriction and shunting of blood away from alveoli with low oxygen content, is a result of *vasoactive mediators* acting on pulmonary vasculature.

D   **Ventilation/perfusion (V/Q) ratio** (see Figure 4.4)

- In the normal horse, the V/Q ratio is close to 1.0.
- This normal V/Q relationship may be altered by the distribution of ventilation, perfusion and/or a change in their relative distribution.
  - When a lung unit has low or no ventilation relative to perfusion, blood leaving the unit will have lower $O_2$ content than units with optimal V/Q relationships.

**Figure 4.4** Blood entering the pulmonary capillaries associated with non-ventilated alveoli is termed "shunt," and represents a V/Q ratio of 0. Alveoli that are ventilated but not perfused are termed "deadspace" and represents a V/Q ratio of infinity. Alveoli that are equally perfused and ventilated represent a V/Q ratio of 1.

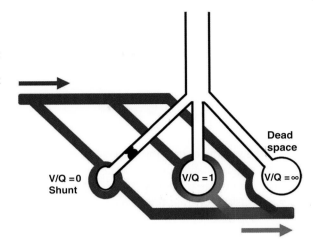

- If the V/Q relationship is 0, the blood leaving this unit will have $O_2$ content similar to pulmonary artery blood.
  - In this situation, the blood leaving this unit is referred to as an *intrapulmonary shunt* and is most commonly a result of atelectasis, partial or complete airway obstruction.
- The other extreme, a V/Q ratio of infinity, is *dead space* ventilation.

## V Alveolar gas exchange

### A Composition of gases

- The composition of gases in a mixture can be described by their *fractional composition* or their *partial pressures*.
- The composition of gas within the alveoli is determined by the movement of gas into and out of the alveoli via the airways or across the alveolar capillary membrane and into or out of the pulmonary capillaries.

### B Movement of gases

- *Bulk transfer* describes the movement of gases during inspiration and expiration within the *proximal large airways*.
- *Diffusion* is the passive movement of gases down the concentration gradient in the *distal small airways* to the alveolus. It is the process by which gases move (i) in and out of the alveoli into the terminal airways, (ii) across the alveolar capillary membrane, and (iii) between the blood and tissues.

### C Factors influencing diffusion

- The surface area available for diffusion.
- The physical properties of the gas.
- The thickness of the air-blood barrier.

○ The driving pressure of the gas between the alveolus and capillary blood as described by *Fick's law of diffusion.*

---

**Fick's Law**

$$V_{gas} = \frac{A}{T} \cdot D \cdot (P_1 - P_2)$$

$V_{gas}$ = the volume of gas transferred across a membrane or barrier.
A = the area available for diffusion.
T = the membrane thickness.
D = a diffusion constant that is dependent on the physical properties of the gas.
$P_1$-$P_2$ = the partial pressure difference of the gas across the membrane.

---

*Note: $CO_2$ is approximately 20 times more soluble than $O_2$, and therefore its diffusion across a membrane is less likely to be impaired, relative to $O_2$, by a change in membrane thickness.*

○ In the normal lung, equilibration of $O_2$ and $CO_2$ across the alveolar capillary membrane occurs within 0.25 seconds; approximately one third of the time the blood is in the capillary.

## D   Carbon dioxide

○ Carbon dioxide is the end product of aerobic metabolism. There is a continuous gradient of $CO_2$ from the mitochondria in peripheral cells to venous blood and then to the alveolar gas.
○ Carbon dioxide is transported in the blood in several forms including:
  – Dissolved in physical solution (~5%).
  – As carbonic acid (~90%).
  – Combined with proteins (~5%) such as carbaminohemoglobin.
○ Carbon dioxide moves from the blood to the alveoli in its dissolved form only.
○ Alveolar $CO_2$ partial pressures are directly proportional to $CO_2$ production and indirectly proportional to alveolar ventilation.

---

$$PACO_2 \propto \frac{VaCO_2}{V_A}$$

$VaCO_2$ = Rate of $CO_2$ production.
$V_A$ = Alveolar ventilation.

---

○ Clinically, the adequacy of alveolar ventilation is evaluated by measuring arterial $CO_2$ partial pressures ($PaCO_2$).
○ The normal values for $PaCO_2$ and $PACO_2$ are between 35 and 45 mmHg.

## E   Oxygen

- ○ The partial pressure of oxygen in the alveoli can be determined using a simplified version of the *alveolar gas* equation:

$$PAO_2 = FiO_2\left(PB - PH_2O\right) - \frac{PaCO_2}{R}$$

- – $FiO_2$ = Fraction of inspired oxygen $\approx 0.21$.
- – PB = Atmospheric pressure (760 mmHg at sea level).
- – $PH_2O$ = Water vapor pressure (mmHg) in airway (~50 mmHg at body temp of horse).
- – R = Respiratory gas exchange ratio (~0.8).
- ○ This calculation emphasizes the significance of $FiO_2$ and $PaCO_2$ on the alveolar gas partial pressure.
- ○ Clinically, this equation highlights the significance of *$O_2$ supplementation* for patients with impaired ventilation.

*Example 1.* Horse breathing room air (21% $O_2$) with a $PaCO_2$ = 35 mmHg.

$$PAO_2 = 0.21\left(760 - 50\right) - 35/0.8\left[50 = \text{water vapor pressure}\left(\text{mmHg}\right)\text{in airway}\right]$$

$$= 149 - 44$$

$$PAO_2 = 105\,\text{mmHg}$$

*Example 2.* Horse breathing 100% $O_2$ with a $PaCO_2$ = 35 mmHg.

$$PAO_2 = 1.0\left(760 - 50\right) - 35/0.8$$

$$= 710 - 44$$

$$PAO_2 = 666\,\text{mmHg}$$

*Example 3.* Anesthetized horse hypoventilating on room air ($PaCO_2$ = 70 mmHg)

$$PAO_2 = 0.21\left(760 - 50\right) - 70/0.8$$

$$= 0.21\left(760 - 50\right) - 88$$

$$PAO_2 = 149 - 88 = 61\,\text{mmHg}$$

- – Although this horse is hypoxemic, a $PaO_2$ of <60 mmHg is fairly typical for anesthetized horses breathing room air.
- – This example emphasizes how an increase in $PaCO_2$ affects $PAO_2$ and hence $PaO_2$.

*Example 4.* Anesthetized horse hypoventilating on 100% oxygen ($PaCO_2$ = 70 mmHg)

$$PAO_2 = 1.0\left(760 - 50\right) - 70/0.8$$

$$= \left(760 - 50\right) - 88$$

$$PAO_2 = 710 - 88 = 622\,\text{mmHg}$$

- This example emphasizes the importance of providing $O_2$ during anesthesia to prevent hypoxemia.

## F Alveolar-arterial oxygen gradient [P(A-a)$O_2$]

- A small gradient in oxygen partial pressure normally exists between the alveoli (A) and the arterial blood (a).
- This gradient is due to:
  - Normal physiologic shunting of blood through bronchial and coronary veins that drain deoxygenated blood directly into the left side of the heart.
  - Normal ventilation-perfusion gradients within the lung.
- The magnitude of the gradient (A-a) can be calculated using the alveolar gas equation and by measuring the $PaO_2$.
- Knowledge of the magnitude of the difference in the P(A-a)$O_2$ can indicate whether a functional deficit in $O_2$ exchange exists.
- The significance of a calculated gradient is, however, dependent on the $FiO_2$.
- *Examples*:
  - A normal horse breathing room air, the P(A-a)$O_2$ gradient is <10 mmHg.
  - A normal horse breathing 100% $O_2$ may have a gradient up to 70 mmHg.
- Increases in P(A-a)$O_2$ may be due to:
  - Anatomical shunting.
  - V/Q mismatching.
  - Diffusion impairment due to a thickened alveolar-capillary membrane.

## G Arterial/alveolar ratio

- To eliminate the impact of variable $FiO_2$ on the assessment of ventilation-perfusion relationship in the lung, the arterial/alveolar ratio of oxygen can be calculated.
  - Normal $PaO_2/PAO_2$ ratio should be >0.75 regardless of $FiO_2$.

## H Oxygen carriage

- In blood, $O_2$ exists in two forms:
  - Dissolved in plasma.
  - Combined with hemoglobin.
- $O_2$ is poorly soluble, so the majority of $O_2$ in the blood is carried in combination with hemoglobin (Hb).
- *Oxygen content* of the blood (Ca$O_2$) is calculated as the sum of the $O_2$ bound by Hb and that dissolved in the plasma.

$$CaO_2 \left( mL/dL \right) = \left[ 1.36 \times Hb \left( g/dL \right) \times \frac{Hb\%Sat}{100} \right] + \left( 0.003 \times PaO_2 \right)$$

*Note*: $PaO_2$ is expressed in mmHg.

- *Oxygen delivery* to tissues (D$O_2$) is a function of the arterial $O_2$ content (Ca$O_2$) and cardiac output.

D$O_2$ (ml/min) = Cardiac Output (l/min) x Ca$O_2$ (ml/l)

*Note*: it is important to convert Ca$O_2$ to (ml/l)

I   **Oxygen binding to Hb**

- ○ Several factors can influence the binding of $O_2$ to hemoglobin.
- ○ The $O_2$-Hb dissociation curve demonstrates the relationship between $PO_2$ and saturation of Hb with oxygen ($SO_2$) (see Figure 4.5).
  - – A *left-shift* to the curve indicates a higher affinity of Hb for $O_2$ and thus a higher saturation at a given $PaO_2$.
  - – A *right shift* in the curve results from a lower affinity of Hb for oxygen.
- ○ The position of the curve is usually described by the position at which Hb is 50% saturated ($P_{50}$).
  - – $P_{50}$ is approximately 24 mmHg in the adult horse.

J   **Shunting and oxygenation**

- ○ *Intrapulmonary shunts* can result in the delivery of poorly oxygenated blood into the pulmonary venous blood.
- ○ The fraction of cardiac output that passes through a shunt is expressed as the shunt fraction (Qs/Qt), and can be calculated using the *Berggren* equation:

$$\frac{Qs}{Qt} = \frac{CcO_2 - CaO_2}{CcO_2 - CvO_2}$$

- ○ $CcO_2$ = the $O_2$ content in pulmonary capillary blood (Calculated based on $PaO_2$, assuming 100% saturation of Hb).
  - – $CaO_2$ and $CvO_2$ = the $O_2$ content in arterial and mixed venous blood (obtained from a pulmonary artery catheter), respectively.
  - – In order for this calculation to be accurate, measurements must be performed when the horse is breathing 100% $O_2$.

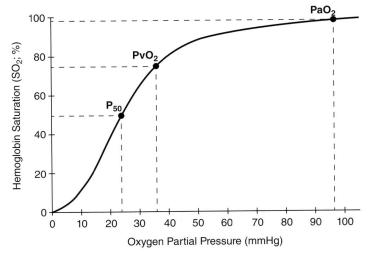

**Figure 4.5**   The oxy-hemoglobin dissociation curve illustrates the relationship between the partial pressure of oxygen in arterial blood and the percent of hemoglobin that is bound by oxygen. The sigmoid shape of the curve illustrates the cooperative binding of oxygen to hemoglobin. The $P_{50}$ indicates the partial pressure of oxygen at which hemoglobin is 50% saturated.

- Estimates of (Qs/Qt) can be determined using the F-shunt equation where a fixed arterial to mixed venous oxygen content difference [C(a-v) $O_2$] of 3.5 ml/dl is assumed.
  ○ *Normal* shunt fraction is <5%.
    - Clinically insignificant shunts are 10–19%.
    - Clinically significant shunts are 20–30%.
    - Potentially *fatal* shunts are >30%.
  ○ *Physiologic* shunts are the *most common* type of shunt and they arise secondary to atelectasis or consolidation of alveoli.
  ○ *Anatomic* shunts include bronchial, mediastinal, pleural, and coronary veins.
  ○ *Pathologic anatomic* shunts include shunts secondary to congenital or traumatic anomalies and intrapulmonary tumors.
  ○ Shunts and V/Q inequalities have a greater impact on $O_2$ uptake than $CO_2$ removal from the lungs due to the shapes of their respective dissociation curves.
    - Specifically, blood passing under-ventilated alveoli tends to retain its $CO_2$, and blood passing over-ventilated alveoli gives off an excessive amount of $CO_2$.
    - The amount of the retained $CO_2$ and the excessively lost $CO_2$ are proportional due to the relatively linear relationship of $CO_2$ to $V_A$.
    - On the other hand, blood passing under-ventilated alveoli does not take up enough $O_2$, and blood passing over-ventilated alveoli cannot take up a proportionately increased amount of $O_2$ owing to the flatness of the $O_2$-Hb dissociation curve in this region.

## VI  Effects of sedation and anesthesia on respiratory function

### A  Sedation

  ○ In the horse, the effects of sedatives on lung function are relatively minor although differences do exist among agents.
  ○ In general, with *acepromazine* and $\alpha_2$ adrenergic agonists, ventilation changes include a *decrease in rate* and an *increase in tidal volume*.
  ○ $\alpha_2$ agonists increase the work of breathing.
    - Due to a decrease in tone of the abductor muscles of the upper respiratory tract, thus leading to collapse of the external nares and/or laryngeal structures during inspiration.
    - The effects of increased work of breathing are insignificant in the normal horse, but may be significant in the horse with airway obstruction.
    - Heavy sedation with $\alpha_2$ agonists (e.g. *detomidine* 0.01 mg/kg, IV) decreases the gas exchange function of the lungs.
    - The decrease in oxygenation with *detomidine* sedation is due, in part, to an increase in the V/Q maldistribution within the lung.

### B  General anesthesia

  ○ General anesthesia dramatically alters the function of the respiratory system.
  ○ Changes result from the *direct* effects of the anesthetic drugs on the respiratory system and the *indirect* effects of recumbency.
  ○ In the anesthetized recumbent horse, $PaO_2$ can markedly decrease, and arterial $CaO_2$ and $DO_2$ may become critically impaired.

– These changes are greatest for horses in *dorsal recumbency*.
– Recumbency without anesthesia does not impair gas exchange to the same degree, indicating the role of the anesthetic drugs in this process.
○ The magnitude of the decrease in gas exchange function of the lung does not vary greatly among anesthetic protocols.

## C Mechanisms for decreased oxygenation

○ *V/Q mismatching* and *intrapulmonary shunting* are the major mechanisms responsible for the decrease in oxygenation during anesthesia.
– The distribution of ventilation changes in dorsal or lateral recumbency due to a decrease in FRC and regional differences in pleural pressures.
– Perfusion of the lungs changes due to a decrease in cardiac output, regional changes in vascular resistance, and inhibition of hypoxic pulmonary vasoconstriction.
○ As the degree of right-to-left intrapulmonary shunting increases within the lung, the effect of increasing $FiO_2$ on $PaO_2$ decreases.
○ A decrease in arterial $CO_2$ removal from the lungs (e.g. with hypoventilation) with a resulting increase in $PaCO_2$ is typically observed under general anesthesia.
○ In general, with injectable and inhalational anesthetics, the minute ventilation and $V_T$ are decreased, while the *f* may be increased or decreased.
○ The degree of respiratory depression with anesthetic agents is dose-dependent and results from drug-induced effects on the respiratory control centers.

## Suggested Reading

Clerbaux, T., Serteyn, D., Willems, E., and Brasseur, L. (1986). Determination de la courbe de dissociation standard de l'oxyhemoglobine du cheval et influence, sur cette courbe, de la temperature, du pH et du diphosphoglycerate. *Can. J. Vet. Res.* 50: 188–192.

Drabkova, Z., Schramel, J.P., and Kabes, R. (2018). Determination of physiological dead space in anesthetized horses: a method-comparison study. *Vet. Anaesth. Analg.* 45: 73–77.

Moens, Y. (2013). Mechanical ventilation and respiratory mechanics during equine anesthesia. *Vet. Clin. North Am. Equine. Pract.* 29: 51–67.

Van Loon, J.P., DeGrauw, J.C., and Oostrom, H. (2018). Comparison of different methods to calculate venous admixture in anesthetized horses. *Vet. Anaesth. Analg.* 45: 640–647.

## Evaluation of the Respiratory System

*Tom Doherty*

## A Patient history

○ Should include information on the following:
– Nasal discharge.
– Coughing.

- Abnormal lung sounds.
- Increased respiratory rate and effort.

## B   Physical examination

- The rate, rhythm and character of respiration should be determined.
- Observe the horse from all sides to assess bilateral symmetry and the thoracic and abdominal components of respiration.
- An increase in the abdominal component of respiration may signify recurrent airway obstruction (heaves).
- A reduced thoracic movement is a feature of acute pleuritis.
- Assess airflow through each nostril to check the patency of the nasal passages.
  - Closing each nostril in turn and assessing airflow can verify an obstruction.
  - Airflow can be assessed by placing one's ear close to the nostril.
- Abnormal odors usually signify anaerobic infections (e.g. sinus, dental, lung abscess).
- The pharynx and larynx should be palpated externally for gross abnormalities that may affect airflow or intubation.

*Auscultation*

- In adult horses, it is often difficult to hear lung sounds.
- It may be necessary to "amplify" the sounds by making the horse "re-breathe" prior to auscultation.
- Lungs sounds are generally audible in the foal.

## Airway Management

*Tom Doherty*

- Airway management includes:
  - Maintaining airway patency.
  - Protecting from aspiration.
  - Providing adequate oxygenation and ventilation.
- Intubation of the trachea, either via the oral or nasal passages, requires knowledge of airway anatomy.
- It must be remembered that the horse is an *obligate nasal breather.*
- Although it is generally relatively easy to intubate the trachea of the horse, it is important to recognize situations when it may be difficult.

## I   Larynx

### A   Function

- The primary function of the larynx is to *protect the airway* by preventing the entry of food and foreign materials.
- The *cricoarytenoid dorsalis* is the only muscle of the larynx which abducts the arytenoids and opens the *rima glottidis.*
- *Phonation* is the secondary function of the larynx.

**B    Innervation**

- Motor innervation to the cricoarytenoid dorsalis is provided by the *recurrent laryngeal branch of the vagus nerve.*

**C    Recurrent laryngeal nerve neuropathy**

- Occurs primarily on the left side.
- Is relatively common in larger breed horses.
- Results in an inability to fully abduct the arytenoid cartilages.
- Cases of recurrent laryngeal neuropathy generally do not exhibit signs of airway embarrassment at rest.

**D    Iatrogenic laryngeal neuropathy**

- May result from depositing anesthetic drugs adjacent to the recurrent laryngeal nerve during an attempted jugular vein injection.
- Nerve paralysis can occur with perivascular injection of *α2 agonists* and *local anesthetics.*
- This situation, while temporary, may cause severe airway obstruction necessitating passage of a nasotracheal tube or a tracheostomy.
- *Horner's* syndrome (ptosis, miosis, enophthalmos) may also occur as a result from blocking sympathetic fibers in the vagosympathetic trunk.

**E    Hyperkalemic periodic paralysis (HYPP)**

- Can result in spasm or paralysis of the laryngeal and pharyngeal muscles.
  - May be accompanied by upper airway noise.
- In foals, milk discharging from the nostrils may be due to HYPP.

## II    Assessment of airway

**A    History**

- If intubation was difficult previously, determine if the reason has been resolved or if it was due to anatomical malformations.

**B    Physical examination**

- It is not possible to directly visualize the *larynx* and *pharynx* due to the shape of the horse's head and the minimal opening of the mouth. However, these structures can be visualized using an endoscope.
- Palpation of the *upper trachea* and *intermandibular space* will give an indication of swelling or increased sensitivity.
- *Pharyngeal swelling* (e.g. from abscess formation) may cause obvious signs of airway obstruction.
- *Guttural pouch tympany* in foals may result in distortion of the pharynx.

- ○ Dysphagia resulting from *swelling of the tongue* or *pharynx* may indicate a difficult intubation.
- ○ In cases of *mandibular fracture*, use of a mouth gag may be contraindicated and *nasal* intubation or a temporary tracheostomy may be necessary during surgery.
  - – If nasal intubation is to be performed, determine if the nasal passages are patent by assessing airflow at the nostrils as described above.

## C    Situations in which difficulty is to be expected

*Recurrent laryngeal neuropathy*
- ○ To prevent damage to the adducted arytenoid cartilage it is usually necessary to use a slightly smaller sized endotracheal tube.
  - – A smaller tube will also facilitate the surgical approach and may obviate removal of the tube, intraoperatively, for surgical assessment.

*Pharyngeal abscessation and lymphadenopathy*
- ○ May cause misalignment of oral, laryngeal, and pharyngeal structures.

## III    Airway equipment

- • While it may be considered ideal to intubate the airway at all times in the anesthetized horse, it is *not* routinely practiced under field conditions for procedures of short duration.
- • Airway obstruction is uncommon in the non-intubated horse during short procedures.

### A    Mouth gag

- ○ It is not absolutely necessary to use a gag, but its use facilitates keeping the jaws open to allow passage of an ET tube.
  - – However, there is generally no need to use a gag in neonatal foals as they have minimal jaw tone.
- ○ The gag is fitted between the upper and lower incisors and care must be taken to avoid pressure on the hard palate.
- ○ A variety of gags may be purchased from commercial vendors or a gag may be fashioned from a piece of PVC pipe (see Figures 4.6 and 4.7).
  - – PVC gags are lightweight and unobtrusive.

### B    Laryngoscope

- ○ Laryngoscopes are not used in the horse, as direct visualization of the larynx is not possible with this method. However, endoscopes may be used to assist intubation in some circumstances.

### C    Endotracheal tubes

- ○ Most ET tubes are made from non-toxic plastic or silicone and are numbered according to their internal diameter (mm).

Figure 4.6  PVC mouth gag used to hold mouth open and protect endotracheal tube.

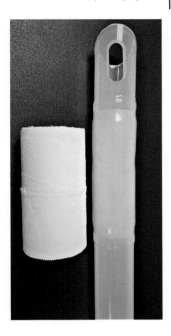

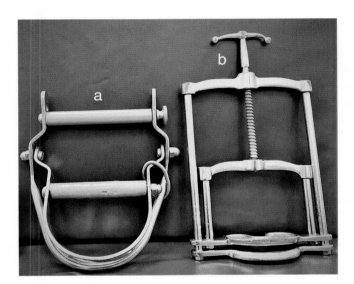

Figure 4.7  Oral speculums used in equine patients: Weingart mouth gag (a), Gunther mouth gag (b).

- ○ Tube selection is generally based on the body mass of the horse.
- ○ It is important that the tube *not* be too tight a fit for the airway.
  - – Most adult, full-size horses (400–500 kg) require a tube size of 24–26 mm.
  - – Larger horses (≥500 kg) require a tube of 26–30 mm or greater.
  - – The airway of the newborn foal (40–50 kg) should accommodate a tube diameter of 10–11 mm.
  - – A newborn miniature horse breed (~10 kg) will need a smaller diameter tube (6–7 mm).
- ○ There is generally little danger of bronchial intubation in horses.

### D   Inflatable cuffs

- Inflation of the cuff creates a seal with the tracheal mucosa.
- This allows the airway to be inflated under positive pressure and protects the lungs from aspiration of foreign material (e.g. gastric contents).
- It is important not to over inflate the cuff.

## IV   Complications of airway intubation

### A   Tissue damage

- To avoid tissue damage, it is important that a gentle technique be employed.
- Even the most seemingly gentle intubation can cause bruising of the tissues of the pharynx, larynx, and trachea.
- A rough technique may result in impaction of the epiglottis into the *rima glottidis*.

### B   Edema

- May result from persistent attempts to pass the tube.
- This causes narrowing of the glottis and hinders air flow.

### C   Over inflation of the cuff

- An increase in cuff pressure will be transferred to the capillaries in the tracheal mucosa and may occlude blood flow.
  - Arteriolar capillary pressure is ~30 mmHg, and during ventilation of adult horses cuff pressures of ~60–70 mmHg are necessary to prevent leaks.
- Ischemia may result in necrosis of the airway mucosa.
- Selection of a suitably sized tube will prevent having to over-inflate the cuff to create a seal.
- *Low-volume* cuffs have an inherently high-cuff pressure once inflated. A problem with low volume, high-pressure cuffs on equine ET tubes is that the pressure measured at the pilot balloon only reflects the elastic force of the cuff, and not the pressure at the mucosa. Thus, checking the cuff pressure with a *manometer* will not prevent over inflation.

### D   Lubrication

- Lubrication of the tube with a water-soluble gel will facilitate its passage.
- It is especially important that a lubricant gel be used liberally for *nasotracheal* intubation.

## V   Intubation of trachea

### A   Difficulty

- Horses are relatively easy to intubate due, in part, to the poor reflex responses of the larynx.
- Flushing the mouth with water prior to induction prevents food materials from being pushed into the airway (see Figure 1.1).
- Foals often have straw or shavings from the bedding in their mouths, and these should be removed.

**B   Position**

- Intubation is usually performed with the horse in *lateral recumbency*.
- However, if there is a likelihood of reflux of gastric contents (e.g. colic case) the horse should be kept *sternal* until the tube is inserted and the cuff inflated (see Figure 4.8).

**C   Technique**

- Intubation is accomplished blindly.
- The head and neck should be extended and the tube advanced into the mouth toward the pharynx.
  - Avoid rubbing the dependent eye on the ground if the horse is in lateral recumbency.
- At this location, the tube may touch the underside of the epiglottic cartilage, which must now be dislodged from its position dorsal to the soft palate.
- Withdrawing the tube slightly and rotating it, will usually reposition the epiglottis and allow the tube to advance. If not, repeat the procedure until successful.
- *Avoid the temptation to force the tube forward.*

**D   Confirmation of tracheal tube placement**

- The tube will advance easily (unless it is too large) if it is in the trachea. If the trachea is held gently in the free hand, the movement of the tube along the tracheal rings can be perceived.
- Gentle compression on the thoracic wall will force air out through a correctly placed tube. However, this is usually unnecessary.

**Figure 4.8**   Intubation of a horse in sternal recumbency if there is a risk of regurgitation and subsequent aspiration of stomach contents.

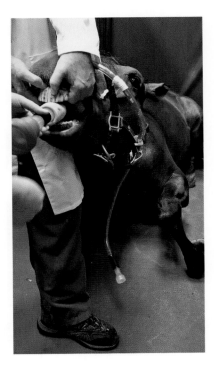

    ○ Esophageal placement of the tube is easily detected, as the tube does not advance easily and will recoil slightly if the driving hand is removed.

        – The esophagus is a "*potential space*" and will not be dilated in the normal state; hence, the slight resistance to advancing the tube.

### E   Intubation of the difficult airway

    ○ On rare situations, when a horse has signs of distress due to of airway obstruction it may be necessary to perform a *tracheostomy* and insert an ET tube prior to sedation.

    ○ In the majority of these cases, the passage of an orotracheal tube can be greatly facilitated by using a narrow-bore tube (e.g. *stomach tube*) as a guide.

    ○ A suitably sized *stomach tube* is inserted into the ET tube and advanced forward into the trachea. The ET tube is then passed into the trachea using the stomach tube as a guide, and the stomach tube is then removed.

        – The stomach tube should be of sufficient diameter and wall thickness that it will not kink as the ET tube is advanced as this will entrap the ET tube and hinder its passage.

## VI   Extubation of the trachea

- *Spontaneous breathing* should have resumed before the tube is removed in recovery.
- Confirm that the horse is taking regular deep breaths.
- Removal of the tube before the horse has regained the swallowing reflex *is* generally acceptable, but many advocate waiting until this reflex has returned.
- It is also acceptable to leave an *orotracheal* or *nasotracheal* tube in place during recovery and this may be indicated under certain circumstances (see Figure 4.9).
  - ○ This is generally indicated if there is a risk of *regurgitation* of gastric contents as in some colic cases.

(a)                (b)

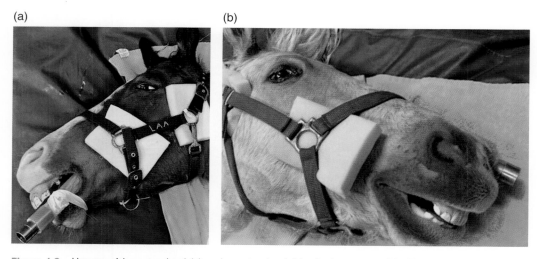

Figure 4.9   Horses with orotracheal (a) and nasotracheal (b) tube in recovery. Ideally, the tube should not protrude beyond the lips as this could lead to kinking of the tube if it were to impact the wall of the recovery box.

- – In these cases, it is also prudent to tilt the head downwards in recovery to facilitate pharyngeal drainage.
  - ○ However, if left in place, the tube should *not* protrude much distance from the mouth to avoid it kinking in the event that it gets impacted against a wall of the recovery stall.
- Horses tolerate orotracheal and nasotracheal tubes well during recovery.
- Since the horse does not produce significant salivary secretions, it is not necessary to drain or suction the oropharynx prior to tube removal. The exception is in cases of reflux of gastric contents into the oropharynx.

## VII   Airway obstruction

- *The importance of preventing airway obstruction cannot be over emphasized.*
- Obstruction in the recovery phase will lead to extreme anxiety in the awakening horse such that it may be impossible to control the horse to establish an airway.
- In extreme cases, airway obstruction may result in *negative pressure pulmonary edema* (NPPE) which can be fatal (see Chapter 38).
- Thus, it is important to have a plan to protect the airway, and to check for airway patency following ET tube removal.
- Because airway obstruction is most likely to result from *nasal edema*, administration of *phenylephrine* intranasally or placement of a *nasal tube* will greatly reduce the incidence of airway obstruction (see Figure 4.10).
  - ○ Airway obstruction, due to *nasal edema* is more likely to occur when the horse has been in dorsal recumbency for long periods.

**Figure 4.10**   Phenylephrine used to resolve nasal edema prior to recovery.

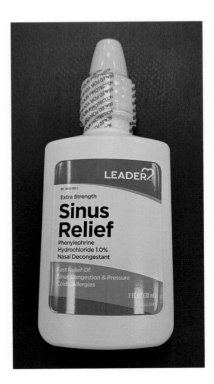

A    **Signs of airway obstruction include:**

- Snoring sounds.
- No evidence of air passage via nostrils or decreased air passage.
- Increased abdominal effort on inspiration and expiration.
- Abnormal abdominal movements (e.g. retraction of abdomen on inspiration).
- Nostril flaring on inspiration.

B    **Laryngospasm**

- Defined as reflex closure of the vocal cords.
- Is uncommon in the horse.
- Indeed, the larynx of the horse is much less sensitive than in other species.

C    **Obstruction of the upper airway**

*At induction*
- Obstruction is a rare occurrence at induction, unless there is a space-occupying mass in the pharynx or nasal passages, or the horse has severe recurrent laryngeal neuropathy.
- However, as previously mentioned, overzealous attempts to intubate may cause a partial obstruction either by causing edema or by displacing the epiglottis.

*Management*
- If obstruction is *anticipated*, a plan should be in place to secure the airway. This may involve performing a tracheostomy or having an endoscope available.
- In some cases of partial obstruction, passing a stomach tube of suitable size into the airway (see Sections V–E) to serve as a guide over which the ET tube can be passed, is usually successful.

*Intraoperative obstruction*
- Obstruction is an uncommon occurrence in the intubated horse.
- However, extreme flexion of the neck may result in kinking and obstruction of the endotracheal tube.
  - The most likely scenario for this occurrence is during radiographic imaging of the cervical vertebrae, during which extreme flexion of the neck is employed.

*At extubation*
- The horse must suddenly change from being a *mouth breather* to having to resume *nasal breathing*, so obstruction of the upper airway is more likely to occur following extubation, especially if the horse is still deeply anesthetized.
- Airway patency should be checked after extubation by placing a hand close to the horse's nostrils and checking for airflow, while at the same time observing thoraco-abdominal excursion. The thoraco-abdominal movements should be smooth, and not accompanied by inspiratory or expiratory effort or upper airway noises indicative of obstruction.
- The epiglottis needs to be re-aligned to its normal position, dorsal to the soft palate, for successful nasal breathing to resume.

*Management*
- *The condition may resolve by flexing and extending the next a few times. Otherwise, gentle passage of a small-bore nasal tube into the larynx may re-align the epiglottis.*

D  **Obstruction of the nasal passages due to edema**

- ○ Is a common occurrence, especially following a prolonged period of anesthesia with the horse in dorsal recumbency.
- ○ Edema develops because of the increased hydrostatic pressure in the nasal mucosa in dorsal recumbency.
- ○ Passage of a nasal or nasotracheal tube is usually effective in the treatment of nasal obstruction.
  - – A 14–16 mm tube will suffice for an adult, and should be left in place for recovery.
  - – Routine use of a nasal tube or orotracheal tube in recovery is recommended following long surgeries, especially if the horse has been in dorsal recumbency.
- ○ *Phenylephrine* instillation, to constrict nasal mucosa, can be used to reduce edema.
  - – *Phenylephrine* can be squirted into the nasal passages via the ventral meatus by elevating the nose and allowing contact with the nasal mucosa.
  - – 5 ml of 0.15% *phenylephrine* (adult, full-sized horse) into each nostril, about 30 minutes before extubation, will reduce nasal edema.
  - – The dose should be reduced proportionally in foals and smaller horses to prevent extreme arterial hypertension.

E  **Obstruction of the nasal passages due to nasal bleeding**

- ○ Bleeding upon removal of a *nasotracheal* or *nasogastric* tube can be quite alarming.
- ○ The author's preference is to remove nasogastric tubes approximately 30 minutes before the end of anesthesia, as this will allow time for bleeding to stop prior to the horse being placed in recovery.
- ○ If bleeding is anticipated, or happening while the horse is still tracheally intubated in recovery, the ET tube should be left in place until the bleeding has ceased or perhaps until the horse is standing.
- ○ If the horse has been extubated, it may be necessary to pass a *nasotracheal* tube down the unaffected nostril to establish an airway.
  - – This can be difficult unless the horse is in a relatively deep plane of anesthesia.
- ○ Some cases necessitate deepening anesthesia to facilitate re-intubation of the trachea and to prevent the horse awakening until the hemorrhage has ceased.
- ○ If the horse is laterally recumbent, the head must be tilted downward to prevent aspiration of blood.

## Suggested Reading

Lukasik, V.M., Gleed, R.D., Scarlett, J.M. et al. (1997). Intranasal phenylephrine reduces post anesthetic upper airway obstruction in horses. *Equine. Vet. J.* 29: 236–238.

Richardson, E. and McMillan, M. (2017). A case of airway obstruction caused by probable nasotracheal tube cuff herniation in a horse. *Vet. Anaesth. Analg.* 44: 191–192.

Touzot-Jourde, G., Stedman, N.L., and Trim, C.M. (2005). The effects of two endotracheal tube cuff inflation pressures on liquid aspiration and tracheal wall damage in horses. *Vet. Anaesth. Analg.* 32: 23–29.

## Tracheostomy

*Tanner Snowden and Jim Schumacher*

## I   Terminology

- A tracheostomy is a surgically-created opening into the trachea. The terms tracheostomy and tracheotomy are used interchangeably.

*Temporary tracheostomy*
- This is performed to temporarily bypass an obstruction of the respiratory tract proximal to the site of tracheostomy.
- The tracheostomy tube is removed when the obstruction has resolved, allowing the tracheostomy to heal.
- A temporary tracheostomy may be an *emergency* procedure when the obstruction is life-threatening.

*Permanent tracheostomy* (see Figure 4.11)
- This is performed to create a permanent tracheal *fistula*, or *stoma*. A tracheal stoma can be created when the obstruction to airflow is severe and permanent.
- Creating a tracheal stoma involves removing a portion of four or five adjacent tracheal rings and suturing the tracheal mucosa and submucosa to the surrounding cutaneous incision.
- The term permanent tracheostomy is sometimes used to describe a stoma that is maintained only during a working season for the horse. This is similar to a temporary tracheostomy but is performed because the obstruction to airflow interferes only with the work of the horse. Though termed a "*permanent*" tracheostomy, this tracheostomy is not actually permanent, because the tracheostomy tube is removed after the working season of the horse, when it is no longer required. The tube is replaced, in preparation for the horse's next working season, after performing another tracheostomy.

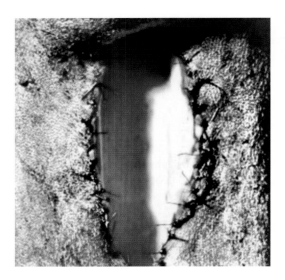

Figure 4.11   Permanent tracheostomy performed to bypass laryngeal obstruction causing severe dyspnea. *Source:* Courtesy of: Dr. Peter Rakestraw, VMD, Dip ACVS.

## II Indications

- To bypass an obstruction of airflow proximal to the site of tracheostomy. The horse is an obligate nasal breather, so severe obstruction of the nasal cavity necessitates creating a tracheostomy.
- To provide access to the trachea for administering an inhalant anesthetic and oxygen, so that surgery of the larynx or pharynx (e.g. resection of the nasal septum, arytenoidectomy, repair of a cleft palate) can proceed unimpeded by the presence of an ET tube.

## III Surgical anatomy

- Structures overlying the site of tracheostomy include the *skin* and *cutaneous coli, sternohyoideus*, and *thyrohyoideus* muscles.
- The site of tracheal incision is the *annular ligament* of the trachea, which attaches one tracheal ring to another.

## IV Tracheostomy tubes (see Figure 4.12)

- J-type tube.
- Dyson tube (self-retaining).
- Bivona silicone tube.
- A temporary tracheostomy tube can be made, in an emergency, from the handle of a one-gallon plastic jug or the cut end of a large stomach tube or garden hose.

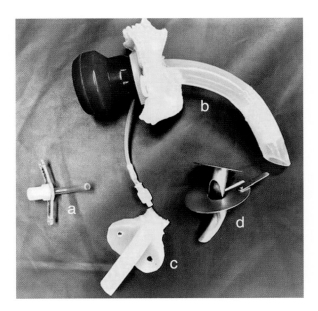

Figure 4.12 Tracheostomy tubes: Bivona silicon tube (a), Dyson tube (b), a tube made from a gallon plastic jug (c), and a J-type tube (d).

## V   Technique

- Tracheostomy is usually performed with the horse standing, but can also be performed under general anesthesia in anticipation of a post-surgical obstruction.
- The procedure is performed most easily with the horse restrained in stocks and sedated with an alpha$_2$ agonist, such as *detomidine* HCl (0.005–0.01 mg/kg, IV) or *xylazine* HCl (0.2–0.5 mg/kg, IV)
  - *Butorphanol tartrate* (0.02–0.03 mg/kg, IV) can be administered after the horse is sedated, if necessary, to provide more profound sedation.
- The usual site is the juncture of the cranial and middle third of the cervical portion of the trachea (3rd to 6th tracheal rings).
  - The trachea can usually be palpated easily at this site.
  - If the surgeon anticipates that the horse may later require a permanent tracheostomy, the site of temporary tracheostomy should be far enough distal on the neck that it does not interfere with creating a permanent tracheostomy.
- Hair at the proposed site of incision is clipped, and the site is scrubbed.
- 8–12 ml of local anesthetic solution is injected subcutaneously at the proposed site of incision (see Figure 4.13).
- A 5–9 cm, longitudinal incision is made through the skin, subcutaneous tissue, and cutaneous coli muscle (see Figure 4.14).
- The juncture between the right and left *sternohyoideus* muscles and the right and left *sternothyroideus* is incised with a scalpel or scissors. Finding the site of the juncture is often difficult and not absolutely necessary.
  - Avoid inadvertently scoring the tracheal rings when the musculature is incised with a scalpel.
- Retracting the skin and musculature with a Weitlaner or Gelpi *retractor* helps to expose the trachea (see Figure 4.15).
  - Inserting a retractor into the wound can be omitted if the tracheostomy is being performed with urgency.

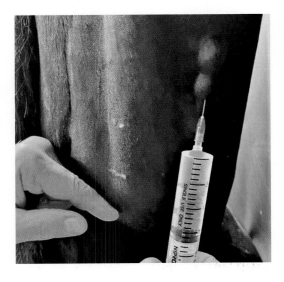

**Figure 4.13**   Local anesthetic is instilled subcutaneously at the proposed site of incision in preparation for performing a temporary tracheostomy.

Figure 4.14 A cutaneous incision is created on the ventral midline of the neck over the palpable trachea. This incision is extended through the cutaneous colli and the right and left sternothyroideus muscles to expose the tracheal rings.

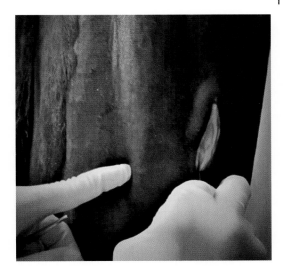

Figure 4.15 The trachea can be better exposed by separating the cutaneous and muscular incision with a self-retaining retractor.

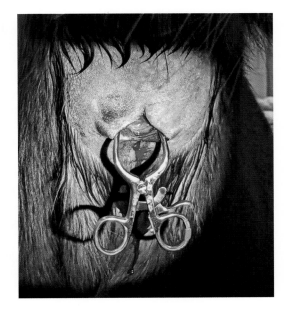

- The annular ligament between two tracheal rings is identified in the center of the incision, and this ligament is incised with a scalpel blade to expose the lumen of the trachea, *being careful to avoid inadvertently incising the mucosa on the dorsal side of the trachea.*
  - The ligament and underlying tracheal mucosa are incised to the right or left, and without removing the blade from the incision, the blade is turned over, and the incision is lengthened in the other direction.
  - Ideally, the tracheal incision should be approximately *one-third* of the circumference of the trachea if a tracheostomy tube is to be inserted. The incision needs to be larger, if it is

created for insertion of an *endotracheal tube* through which an inhalant anesthetic and oxygen are to be administered.

– The tracheal incision should not exceed half of the tracheal circumference.

– Extending the incision beyond one-half of the circumference risks formation of a restrictive cicatrix and transection of an adjacent carotid artery or a nerve, such as the *vagosympathetic* trunk or *recurrent laryngeal nerve*, which lies adjacent to the carotid artery.

*Note:* The scalpel blade should be attached to a scalpel handle, if time allows, so that inadvertent loss of the blade into the lumen of the trachea is avoided.

○ Incision into the tracheal lumen can be recognized by *escape of air* through the wound when the horse exhales. The horse may cough, because of blood entering the tracheal lumen.

- A finger or the jaws of a large forceps are inserted into the lumen of the trachea, through the incised annular ligament and tracheal mucosa, and the *cannula of a tracheostomy tube* is inserted between the two separated tracheal rings, adjacent to the finger or jaws of the opened forceps, into the lumen of the trachea.

○ The *tracheostomy tube* is secured to the site of tracheostomy. Each side of the faceplate (or neck flange) of a J-tube has a slot through which rolled gauze can be threaded and tied around the neck.

○ To ensure that a J-tube does not become dislodged, it can be sutured to the neck through the slot on each side of the faceplate or secured to the neck with elastic adhesive tape.

○ Dyson tubes are self-retaining and need not be secured.

- To ease replacing the tube, a long suture can be placed around each ring adjacent to the tracheal incision. Traction on these sutures widens the tracheal incision for easy insertion of the cannula of the tube and prevents the cannula of the tube from being inserted subcutaneously.

○ The cannula is easily replaced, without the use of sutures, after the wound has developed granulation tissue, usually by day 6.

- Some clinicians, when anticipating a lengthy period of tracheal cannulation, such as for maintaining a tracheal stoma for a working season, remove a crescent-shaped section of cartilage from the distal aspect of the ring proximal to the incision in the annular ligament, and a similar section from the proximal aspect of the ring distal to the incision in the annular ligament (see Figure 4.16).

○ Although removing sections of cartilage may ease daily insertion of the tracheostomy tube, removing cartilage is seldom necessary.

## VI   Post-operative care

- The horse should be administered a *tetanus toxoid* vaccination, if it has not received one within the previous year.

○ It should be administered a *tetanus toxoid* vaccination and *tetanus antitoxin* if it has never been vaccinated against tetanus.

- The horse should be administered a broad-spectrum antibiotic until the tracheal wound begins to develop granulation tissue, usually at five to six days.

- Compressing the tissue at the site of tracheostomy by securing the tracheostomy tube with an elastic adhesive bandage applied around the neck and faceplate, leaving the entrance to

Figure 4.16 To ease daily insertion of a tracheostomy tube, a crescent-shaped section of cartilage can be excised from the distal aspect of the ring proximal to the incision through the annular ligament of the trachea, and a similarly shaped section of cartilage can be removed from the proximal aspect of the adjacent ring. *Source:* Courtesy of Dr. Peter Rakestraw, VMD, Dip ACVS.

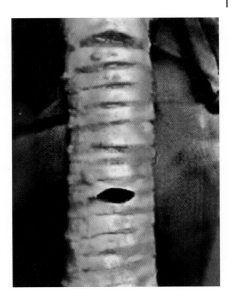

Figure 4.17 Compressing the faceplate of the tracheostomy tube against the tracheal incision diminishes the likelihood of the horse developing excessive subcutaneous emphysema adjacent to the incision.

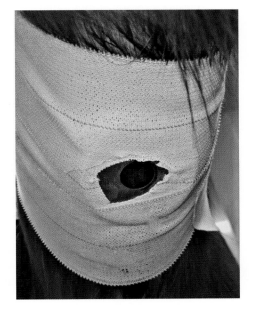

the cannula uncovered, may decrease the severity of subcutaneous emphysema, which frequently develops at the site.

- The tracheostomy tube should be cleaned or replaced with a clean tracheostomy tube, preferably twice daily. More frequent cleaning or replacement may be necessary if the cannula accumulates exudate rapidly.
  - A clean tube should be inserted *as soon as* the soiled tube is removed, if the horse is totally dependent on the tracheostomy to breath.
- The necessity for maintaining a tracheostomy tube can be evaluated by sealing the opening of the tube with tape and evaluating how the horse breaths.

*Note*: Even if the airway proximal to the tube is no longer obstructed, the horse may have difficulty breathing when the opening is sealed, if the tube is so large that an adequate volume of air cannot move around it. This is more likely to happen if the patient is a foal or a miniature horse.

- The wound heals rapidly by second intention after the tube is removed.
  - A tracheostomy that has developed granulation tissue is likely to be healed between two and three weeks after the tube is removed.
  - A thin epithelial scar is often present at the healed site of the temporary tracheostomy.
- The wound should be cleaned of exudate once or twice daily. *Petroleum jelly* should be applied to the skin around the wound, after the wound has been cleaned, to make subsequent cleaning easier.
  - Avoid using soap on the wound.
  - Avoid introducing fluid into the tracheal lumen while cleaning the wound.

## VII  Complications

- When a tracheostomy is performed with the horse anesthetized, the cutaneous and tracheal incisions are sometimes found to be mismatched when the horse stands, because when the horse is recumbent and in dorsal recumbency, with its neck extended, the trachea shifts in relation to the overlying skin.
- Incising the annular ligament more than 180° of the circumference of the trachea may result in an *obstructing cicatrix* when the tracheal incision heals, and the procedure risks transection of a carotid artery or adjacent nerve, such as the vagosympathetic nerve, which lies dorsal to the carotid artery, or the recurrent laryngeal nerve, which lies ventral to the carotid artery.
- The site of tracheostomy may develop a *stricturing cicatrix* if the mucosa on the dorsum of the trachea is incised inadvertently when the tracheostomy is created.
  - This complication is most likely to occur when tracheostomy is performed on a small equid.
  - A tracheostomy tube can be accidentally inserted into the inadvertently-created mucosal incision on the dorsum of the trachea and advanced submucosally, creating a large submucosal pocket.
- When using a Dyson self-retaining, tracheostomy tube, one of the tongues may be inserted inadvertently into the peri-tracheal tissue, rather than into the tracheal lumen. This results in insufficient movement of air through the tube into the tracheal lumen and increases the likelihood of infection at the site of tracheostomy.
- Subcutaneous and peri-tracheal infection.
  - Placing gauze sponges, to which an antimicrobial ointment has been applied, between the faceplate of the tracheostomy tube and the cutaneous incision decreases the likelihood of infection at the wound. Gauze sponges also absorb exudate, preventing excoriation of skin from accumulation of exudate.
- Subcutaneous emphysema often surrounds the site of tracheostomy. This can extend proximally, to involve the head, and caudally, to involve the trunk.
  - Compressing the faceplate of the tracheostomy tube to the wound with elastic adhesive tape decreases the likelihood of subcutaneous emphysema developing at the wound. (see Figure 4.17)

- ○ Severe subcutaneous emphysema is likely to develop if the tracheostomy tube is insufficient in cross-sectional area to relieve high negative intrathoracic pressure. Exaggerated inspiratory effort pulls air through the cutaneous incision.
- *Pneumothorax* can result from migration of subcutaneous air into the mediastinal space and then into the pleural cavities.
  - ○ Inserting a tracheostomy tube insufficient in cross-sectional area to prevent high intrathoracic pressure may contribute to development of pneumothorax.
- *Completely transecting* a tracheal ring leads to enfolding of the ring into the tracheal lumen, because the tracheal rings are incomplete dorsally.
- Leaving the cuff of a cuffed tracheostomy tube *inflated* for more than three hours may lead to mucosal damage, which in turn, may lead to a stricturing cicatrix.

## Suggested Reading

Chesen, A.B. and Rakestraw, P.C. (2008). Indications for and short- and long-term outcome of permanent tracheostomy performed in standing horses: 82 cases (1995-2005). *J. Am Vet. Med. Assoc.* 232: 1352–1356.

Saulez, M.N., Slovis, N.M., and Louden, A.T. (2005). Tracheal perforation managed by temporary tracheostomy in a horse. *J. S. Afr. Vet. Assoc.* 76: 113–115.

# 5

## The Renal System
*Natalie S. Chow*

## I    Role of the kidney

- The functions of the kidney include the following:
  - Elimination of nitrogenous and organic waste.
  - Regulation of body water and electrolytes.
  - Regulation of blood pressure.
  - Maintenance of acid–base status.
  - Production of hormones, including *erythropoietin*, *calcitriol*, and *renin*.

## II    Normal anatomy and physiology

- The equine kidney is unilobar.
- The kidney can be divided into the cortex, medulla, and renal pelvis.
  - The *cortex* is the outer portion between the renal capsule and the medulla.
  - The *medulla* is the inner portion that is responsible for maintaining the salt and water balance of the blood.
  - The *pelvis* is a continuation of the proximal portion of the ureters, carrying urine from the kidney to the urinary bladder.

### A   The nephron

- The nephron is the functional unit of the kidney.
  - It is composed of the *renal corpuscle* and the *renal tubule*.
- The renal corpuscle consists of the glomerulus and Bowman's capsule. These structures are responsible for filtration.
- The *renal tubule* consists of:
- The proximal convoluted tubule (PCT).
  - The loop of Henle (LOH) (composed of descending and ascending limbs).
  - The distal convoluted tubule.
  - The collecting duct.

*Manual of Equine Anesthesia and Analgesia*, Second Edition. Edited by Tom Doherty, Alex Valverde, and Rachel A. Reed.

- These structures are responsible for reabsorbing and secreting electrolytes and water across the tubular lumen.
  o Approximately 95% of urine is water; the remainder is organic and inorganic solutes.

*The glomerulus*
  o It consists of a network of specialized capillaries, which is surrounded by Bowman's capsule.
  o It allows fluid, very small proteins, and electrolytes to be filtered and enter the PCT.
  o The glomerular filtration rate (GFR) can be measured to determine renal function.

*Proximal convoluted tubule*
  o After leaving the glomerulus, the filtrate enters the PCT.
  o The PCT is responsible for the active reabsorption of more than 60% of the filtered substances.
  o Major substances reabsorbed include sodium, potassium, calcium, phosphate, magnesium, chloride, bicarbonate, urea, glucose, and amino acids.
  o The PCT is permeable to water and follows the reabsorption of the electrolytes.
  o The PCT is the major site of ammonia production.

*Loop of Henle*
  o The *descending* limb of the LOH receives filtrate from the PCT.
    - Little to no active transport processes occur here.
    - This part of the LOH is only permeable to water.
    - Water is reabsorbed via osmosis, making the filtrate hypertonic compared to plasma.
  o The *ascending* limb of the LOH receives filtrate from the descending limb.
    - Electrolyte reabsorption via active transport occurs here.
    - It is impermeable to water.
    - This is the major area of solute reabsorption.
    - The filtrate becomes hypotonic relative to plasma.

*Distal convoluted tubule (DCT)*
  o Electrolyte and water reabsorption occurs here.
  o This is the site of the majority of $K^+$ and $H^+$ secretion via active transport.

*Collecting duct*
  o This is the final segment of the nephron, and it has an important role in electrolyte and water absorption.
  o The collecting duct is under the influence of *arginine vasopressin* (anti-diuretic hormone – ADH), which controls the final urine osmolality (concentration).
  o During states of dehydration, ADH is released from the posterior pituitary, resulting in the insertion of *aquaporin* channels into the membrane of the cells of the collecting duct.
    - These channels allow the absorption of water, resulting in a concentrated urine.

*Equine urine*
  o Equine urine can be very *cloudy* and *foamy,* and rather *viscous,* depending on the horse's diet. (see Figure 5.1)
  o The *cloudiness* results from the high concentration of *calcium carbonate* crystals.
    - Diets high in calcium (e.g. alfalfa) are associated with higher concentrations of calcium carbonate crystals in the urine.
    - Excess dietary calcium is eliminated in the urine and feces.
    - The majority of equine uroliths are composed of calcium carbonate.

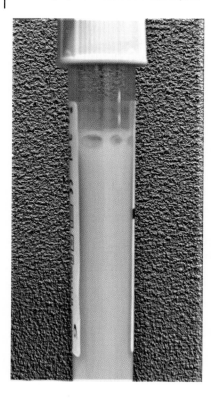

**Figure 5.1** Image of a sample of horse urine. The urine appears cloudy and foamy which is a normal finding.

- ○ The *foamy* and *viscous* nature of equine urine is due to its high concentration of *mucus.*
    - − Gland-like structures in the wall of the equine renal pelvis secrete a mucus-like substance.
    - − Mucus has a lubricant function, and helps in preventing the formation of urinary stones from small calcium carbonate crystals.

## B   Renal blood flow and GFR

*Renal blood flow (RBF)*

- ○ Is approximately 20% of the cardiac output at rest, and is delivered to the kidneys via the renal arteries.
- ○ An uneven distribution exists within the kidney, as the renal cortex receives 90–95% of the blood.
- ○ These activities account for about 10% of the body's oxygen utilization.
    - − Up to 80% of renal oxygen consumption is used for the process of *sodium* reabsorption.
- ○ This high oxygen demand makes the kidney tubules susceptible to hypoxic damage, such as may occur with a decrease in perfusion during anesthesia.

*Renal plasma flow (RPF)*

- ○ Is the volume of plasma that flows through the kidney per unit time.
- ○ Blood cells and most proteins are too large to be filtered through Bowman's capsule.
- ○ The RPF is estimated by multiplying the $RBF \times (1 - \text{hematocrit [HCT]})$

*Filtration fraction (FF)*

- ○ The FF is the fraction of RPF filtered across the glomerulus.
    - − Approximately 20% of the RPF enters the capsule.
    - − The remaining 80% continues through the renal circulation.

*Glomerular filtration rate (GFR)*

- ○ The GFR is the volume of filtrate formed by both kidneys per minute.
- ○ The GFR is equal to the $RPF \times FF$.
- ○ The GFR is determined by:
  - – Renal blood flow.
  - – Neural and hormonal influences.
  - – Intrarenal autoregulation.
  - – Plasma oncotic pressure.

*Autoregulation*

- ○ This is the intrinsic ability of an organ to maintain normal blood flow despite changes in perfusion pressure.
- ○ Autoregulation is intrinsic to the kidneys.
  - – Pressures in the range 80–180 mmHg maintain RBF and GFR at steady states.
- ○ As pressure increases, flow remains constant if resistance increases proportionately, and vice versa.

*Tubuloglomerular feedback (TGF)*

- ○ The TGF is a local intrarenal *negative feedback* mechanism, and is important in regulating the GFR and urine excretion rate.
- ○ Within the distal convoluted tubule, specialized cells called the *macula densa* sense decreased sodium chloride concentrations within the tubular lumen.
- ○ This results in a cascade of events resulting in *renin* release (see Figure 5.2).
- ○ The tone of the glomerular arterioles is adjusted to control GFR.
- ○ *Nitric oxide* and *adenosine* are thought to have an important role in this mechanism.

## C  Urine formation

- ○ The formation of urine involves *three* renal processes:
  - – Glomerular filtration.
  - – Tubular reabsorption of filtrate.
  - – Tubular secretion.
- ○ These processes affect the urine volume and its components.
- ○ Urine formation is controlled by neurohormonal and physiologic factors regulating sodium and water reabsorption.
- ○ These controlling factors include *aldosterone, arginine vasopressin, renin, angiotensin II, atrial natriuretic peptide, prostaglandins, catecholamines, arterial blood pressure, and stress.*

## D  Urine volume in the horse

*Example:* A 450 kg horse (Assume a HCT of 40%)

$$Cardiac\ output = 40\ 1/min \left(approximation\ at\ rest\right)$$
$$Renal\ blood\ flow \left(RBF\right) = 8\ 1/min \left(assume\ 20\%\ of\ cardiac\ output\right)$$
$$Renal\ plasma\ flow \left(RPF\right) = 4.8\ 1/min \left[RBF \times \left(1 - 0.4\right)\right]$$
$$Glomerular\ filtration\ rate = 0.96\ 1/min \left[\left(RPF \times FF \left(\sim 20\%\right)\right)\right]$$
$$= 1382\ 1/day$$
$$Expected\ Urine\ Volume = 13.5\ 1/day \left(assuming\ a\ flow\ rate\ of\ 1.25\ ml/kg/hour\right)$$

*Comments:*

- o The GFR greatly exceeds the urine volume, indicating that about 99% of the filtrate is reabsorbed.
- o Urine production will decrease if there is reduced access to water or food.

## III  Renin-Angiotensin-Aldosterone-System (RAAS) (see Figure 5.2)

- The role of the RAAS is the *long-term* management of blood volume and arteriolar tone.
- This is achieved by increasing reabsorption of sodium and water, and increasing vascular tone.
- In contrast, the *baroreceptor reflex* manages smaller and *short-term* changes.

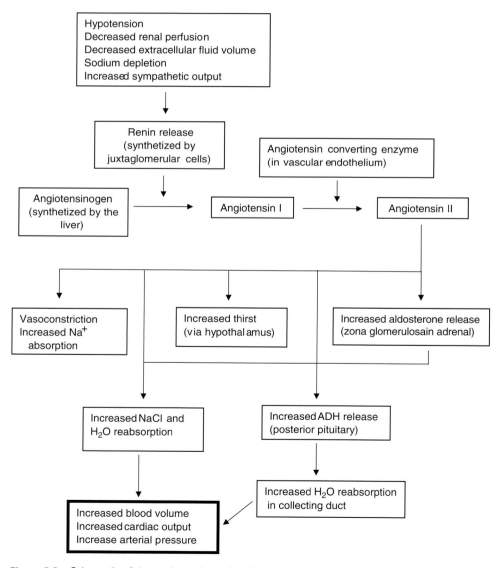

**Figure 5.2**   Schematic of the renin angiotensin-aldosterone-system (RAAS).

- The RAAS has three main components:
  - Renin.
  - Angiotensin II.
  - Aldosterone.
- A decrease in renal blood pressure results in these components acting to increase arterial pressure or decrease salt delivery to the distal convoluted tubule.
- These mechanisms allow for prolonged increases in systemic blood pressure.

*Renin*

- Renin is synthesized by myofibroblast-like cells located in the renal afferent arterioles.
  - These cells are commonly referred to as *juxtaglomerular* cells.
- The primary physiologic *triggers* for renin release are:
  - Decreases in extracellular fluid volume.
  - Sodium depletion.
  - Prostaglandins.
  - Hypotension (MAP < 80 mmHg).
  - Increases in sympathetic output.
- The factors inhibiting renin release are:
  - Angiotensin II.
  - Atrial natriuretic peptide.
  - Vasopressin.
- *Renin* converts *angiotensinogen* (a protein synthesized by the liver) to *angiotensin* I.
  - This is the rate-limiting step of the RAAS.

*Angiotensin I to Angiotensin II*

- *Angiotensin-converting enzyme* (ACE), an enzyme found in vascular endothelium, converts *Angiotensin I* to *Angiotensin II*.

*Effects of Angiotensin II*

- It is a potent *vasoconstrictor*, directly increasing blood pressure by constricting systemic arterioles.
- It increases *sodium* reabsorption, leading to fluid retention and increased extracellular fluid volume.
- *Catecholamines* are released from the adrenal medulla, secondarily affecting systemic blood pressure.
- It diminishes the sensitivity of the *baroreceptor* reflex leading to an increase in blood pressure.
- It increases *thirst* via its effect on the hypothalamus.
- It increases the release of ADH. This leads to the insertion of *aquaporin* channels in the cell membranes of the collecting duct, causing increased water reabsorption.

*Angiotensin III and IV*

- Angiotensin II has a short half-life (one to two minutes) in plasma.
  - It is degraded by peptidases into angiotensin III and IV.
- Angiotensin III has an effect which is equipotent to angiotensin II in causing the release of *aldosterone*, but has less potent pressor effects.
- Angiotensin IV has decreased systemic effects compared to angiotensin II, but has multiple functions in the nervous system.

*Aldosterone*
- o It is released from the zona glomerulosa of the adrenal gland; it promotes sodium retention, leading to fluid retention and increased blood pressure.
- o It increases the excretion of $K^+$ and $H^+$.
- o It increases the release of ADH from the posterior pituitary.

*Angiotensin-converting enzyme (ACE) inhibitors (e.g. enalapril)*
- o Decrease the activity of ACE, resulting in decreased formation of angiotensin II.

## IV Effects of anesthetics on renal function

- Virtually all anesthetic drugs modulate RBF and GFR by direct and indirect effects.
  - o GFR is likely to be reduced due to decreased RBF.
  - o The ability to excrete sodium is reduced. This is thought to be a result of inhibition of Na/K-ATPase.
  - o Urine volume is usually decreased.
- A number of factors are involved in initiating anesthetic-induced changes in renal function, and the contribution of each factor is primarily dependent on the horse's physiologic state and the anesthetic regimen. Factors include:
  - o Decreases in cardiac output and arterial blood pressure.
  - o Increases in sympathetic outflow from renal nerves.
  - o Activation of the RAAS.
  - o Increased release of ADH.
  - o Direct renal effects of anesthetics.
- Many drugs (or metabolites) have some degree of renal metabolism and/or excretion.
  - o Renal dysfunction may, in theory, prolong the effects of anesthetic drugs, but this is rarely of clinical importance.

*Comment:* It is important to consider the co-morbidities associated with renal disease (e.g. azotemia, acid–base imbalance, electrolyte imbalance, anemia, coagulopathy, hypertension) when determining an anesthetic protocol.

### A Changes in RBF with anesthetics

- o May partially result from the systemic changes invoked by anesthetics.
- o A redistribution of cardiac output occurs with an increase in flow to the vessel-rich areas (e.g. brain) and a reduction of flow to the splanchnic system.
- o The effects of anesthetics on autoregulation and intrarenal blood flow are specific to the drug class and depends on renal perfusion pressure.
- o $\alpha_1$-adrenergic receptors are numerous in the renal vasculature and modulate RBF by mediating vasoconstriction.

### B Inhalational anesthetics

- o Most inhalational anesthetics have dose-dependent effects on renal function.
- o In general, RBF is decreased.
- o All inhalants decrease GFR.
- o Urine production decreases with inhalational anesthetics, which increase secretion of ADH and favors fluid retention in the extravascular space.
- o Light planes of inhalational anesthesia can preserve renal autoregulation.

○ Renal vascular resistance increases with most anesthetics.
○ Nephrotoxicity is mainly a problem with "older" inhalants (e.g. *methoxyflurane*).
 – Non-steroidal anti-inflammatory drugs (NSAIDs) and some antibiotics (e.g. *aminogly-cosides*, *tetracyclines*) potentiate the nephrotoxicity of inhalants.

*Methoxyflurane*

○ It undergoes extensive biotransformation (50–75%) in the kidney, producing free fluoride ion and oxalate.
○ Prolonged administration may result in polyuric renal failure.

*Sevoflurane*

○ The fluorinated anesthetics sevoflurane and enflurane have not been associated with a decrease in renal function post-operatively.
○ Sevoflurane undergoes minimal biotransformation (2–5%) in the liver. Nevertheless, hepatic metabolism results in the formation of inorganic fluoride and an organic metabolite.
 – Serum inorganic fluoride concentrations can attain values of 20–40 $\mu$mol/l after 2 MAC hours of exposure in humans, and >50 $\mu$mol/l after prolonged exposure.
 – Values >50 $\mu$mol/l are considered to be nephrotoxic after exposure to *methoxyflurane*, as determined by a decrease in the kidney's concentrating abilities, with clinical signs of toxicity occurring at values >90 $\mu$mol/l.
 – The difference in nephrotoxicity between the two anesthetic agents may be related to *methoxyflurane* undergoing *intrarenal* metabolism, whereas *sevoflurane* is primarily metabolized by the liver.
 – Additionally, *methoxyflurane* is highly soluble in the tissues and takes many hours to be completely cleared from the body. Therefore, the area under the curve of exposure to fluoride is much larger with methoxyflurane than it is with sevoflurane.

*Compound A*

 – Desiccated $CO_2$ absorbents react with sevoflurane to form *compound A*, a vinyl ether.
 – Compound A causes nephrotoxicity in rats following prolonged exposure.
 – The amount of compound A formed is regulated by the concentration of *cysteine conjugate β-lyase*, which transforms cysteine conjugates into toxic products.
 – The pathway of compound A production has not been described in the horse.

C   $\alpha_2$ **adrenergic agonists**

○ Little effect on RBF or GFR.
○ Diuresis results as alpha$_2$-adrenergic agonists:
 – Inhibit ADH release, leading to a redistribution of *aquaporin* channels on the distal tubule and collecting duct.
 – Inhibit *renin* release.
 – Inhibit renal sympathetic activity.
 – Inhibit tubular *sodium* reabsorption.
 – Increase *atrial natriuretic peptide* release.

D   **Other injectable sedatives and anesthetics**

*Phenothiazines*

○ Produce dose-dependent hypotension via antagonism of alpha$_1$-adrenergic receptors.
○ Antagonize *dopamine* receptors, which can prevent dopamine-induced increases in RBF.

*Benzodiazepines*
- ○ Little effect on RBF or GFR.

*Opioids*
- ○ Little effect on RBF or GFR.
- ○ In some species, *morphine* increases the release of ADH resulting in an inhibition of diuresis, and this is accompanied by an increase in *chloride* excretion.

*NMDA antagonists*
- ○ Increase RBF and renal vascular resistance.
- ○ As the dose increases, renal sympathetic nerve activity increases. This decreases RBF while increasing renal vascular resistance.
- ○ *Ketamine* can inhibit *dopamine* transporter proteins in the kidney but the clinical significance is uncertain.
- ○ *Ketamine* and its metabolites are highly dependent on renal excretion.

*Propofol*
- ○ Minimal effects on RBF or GFR.

### E  Intermittent positive pressure ventilation

- ○ Increases in intrathoracic pressure reduce venous return. This decreases right and left ventricular preload.
  - – Cardiac output decreases as a result.
  - – The effect on cardiac output is more pronounced in hypovolemic patients.
- ○ Baroreceptors become activated, initiating a cascade of neurohormonal mechanisms to stimulate the kidney to decrease GFR and increase tubular reabsorption.
- ○ Other mechanisms involved are:
  - – Release of ADH.
  - – Stimulation of the RAAS.
  - – Stimulation of the sympathetic nervous system.
  - – Inhibition of tonic vagal influences.
- ○ This results in decreased urine volume, decreased renal plasma flow, and retention of sodium and water.

### F  Stress

- ○ Stress associated with anesthesia and surgery can result in the release of catecholamines, aldosterone, ADH, and renin.
- ○ This results in decreased RBF and GFR, leading to fluid retention.
- ○ These effects resolve over time after anesthesia.

## V  Diuretics

- There are several different classes of diuretics with different mechanisms of action, ultimately resulting in increased urine production.
- See Table 5.1 for a summary of the diuretic classes.

Table 5.1  Site and mechanism of action of diuretics.

| Diuretic Class | Examples | Site of Action | Mechanism of Action |
|---|---|---|---|
| Osmotic diuretics | Mannitol | PCT | Inhibits $Na^+$ and water reabsorption |
| Carbonic anhydrase inhibitors | Acetazolamide | PCT | Inhibits activity of carbonic anhydrase |
| Loop diuretics | Furosemide | Thick ascending limb of LOH | Inhibits $Na^+$-$K^+$-$Cl^-$ cotransporter |
| Thiazide diuretics | Hydrochlorothiazide | DCT | Inhibits $Na^+$-$Cl^-$ cotransporter |
| Potassium sparing diuretics – Aldosterone inhibitors | Spironolactone | Collecting duct | Inhibits aldosterone receptor |
| Potassium sparing diuretics – Sodium channel blockers | Amiloride | DCT | Inhibits $Na^+$ channel |

PCT – Proximal convoluted tubule.
LOH – Loop of Henle.
DCT – Distal convoluted tubule.

A   **Osmotic diuretics (e.g. *mannitol*)**

- o Inhibit water and sodium reabsorption predominantly at the PCT with some effects on the descending LOH and collecting duct.
- o Expand extracellular fluid and plasma volume, increasing RBF.
  - – This will lead to medullary washout and an inability to concentrate urine.
- o They are filtered through the glomerulus and increase osmotic pressure in the tubule. This reduces transmembrane water flow.

*Note: glucosuria* will also induce an osmotic diuresis.

B   **Carbonic anhydrase inhibitors (e.g. *acetazolamide*)**

- o Acetazolamide is highly protein bound and is not filtered by the glomerulus.
  - – It is secreted by the proximal tubule.
  - – Secretion is GFR dependent.
- o It inhibits the activity of membrane and cytoplasmic carbonic anhydrase in the PCT, preventing reabsorption of bicarbonate. This results in decreased activity of the $Na^+/H^+$ exchanger, causing more sodium to remain in the filtrate.
- o Increases renal excretion of $Na^+$, $K^+$, $HCO_3^-$.
- o Results in a proximal renal tubular acidosis.
- o Can cause *metabolic acidosis.*
  - – Hence, its potential use as a treatment for metabolic alkalosis.
- o Other clinical uses of acetazolamide include glaucoma and neurologic disorders.
- o In equine practice, their main use is in horses likely to be affected by a hyperkalemic periodic paralysis (HYPP) episode.

*Use in potential HYPP episodes:* (see HYPP Chapter 38)
- o Acetazolamide may be administered to horses prone to develop HYPP in order to increase potassium excretion prior to an anesthetic event, for example. It is generally recommended that acetazolamide be administered for a minimum of two days prior to anesthesia.

C   **Loop diuretics** (e.g. furosemide)

- ○ *Furosemide* is the most commonly used diuretic in horses.
- ○ Furosemide inhibits the $Na^+$-$K^+$-$Cl^-$ cotransporter in the luminal membrane of the thick ascending limb of the LOH.
  - – It binds specifically and reversibly to the $Cl^-$ binding site of the transporter's trans-membrane domain.
- ○ Because this transporter reabsorbs about 25% of the sodium load, its inhibition by furo-semide causes an increase in the distal tubular concentration of sodium, leading to a decrease in water reabsorption in the collecting duct.
  - – This inhibits reabsorption of $Na^+$, $Cl^-$, $K^+$, and water.
- ○ It blocks the ability of the kidney to develop a counter-current mechanism, limiting the ability to concentrate or dilute urine.
- ○ Furosemide induces renal synthesis of *prostaglandins*, and this increases RBF and leads to a redistribution of renal cortical blood flow.
- ○ Furosemide reduces plasma and extracellular fluid volume resulting in decreased blood pressure and cardiac output.
- ○ Its use can lead to volume depletion, azotemia, metabolic alkalosis, and electrolyte abnormalities (hyponatremia, hypokalemia).
- ○ The loss of $H^+$ and $K^+$ can be attributed in part to activation of the RAAS secondary to a decrease in blood volume and pressure.
  - – *Aldosterone* causes sodium reabsorption and increases $K^+$ and $H^+$ excretion.
- ○ Can potentiate the toxicity of *aminoglycosides*.

D   **Thiazide diuretics** (e.g. hydrochlorothiazide)

- ○ This group of diuretics is rarely used in horses.
- ○ Thiazides inhibit the $Na^+$/$Cl^-$ cotransporter in the DCT, decreasing sodium reabsorption.
- ○ However, this transporter is only responsible for reabsorbing about 5% of the filtered sodium.
  - – Thus, thiazides are not as effective as loop diuretics in promoting diuresis and natriuresis.
  - – However, like loop diuretics, part of the loss of $H^+$ and $K^+$ is due to activation of the RAAS.
  - – This can result in $K^+$ loss leading to *hypokalemia*.

E   **Potassium sparing diuretics**

- ○ Do not promote secretion of $K^+$ into urine.
- ○ Have a weak diuretic effect because the sites of action are very distal in the nephron.

*Aldosterone inhibitors* (e.g. *spironolactone*)

- – Block effects of aldosterone on aldosterone-receptors leading to reduced $Na^+$ reabsorption.
- – This results in more sodium and water passing into the collecting duct and being excreted.
- – The potassium sparing results from inhibiting sodium reabsorption which causes less $K^+$ and $H^+$ to be exchanged for $Na^+$, and thus not lost in the urine.

*Sodium channel blockers (e.g. amiloride)*

  – Also called "Epithelial Sodium Channel Inhibitors"
  – They directly inhibit sodium channels in distal tubule, reducing $Na^+$ reabsorption.
  – Have similar effects to spironolactone on $H^+$ and $K^+$.

## VI   Nonsteroidal anti-inflammatory drugs

- NSAIDs can affect renal function by a variety of mechanisms.
- The effects of NSAIDs on the kidney are more profound during episodes of hypotension and hypovolemia.
- The renal effects of NSAIDs are discussed in detail in Chapter 16.

## Suggested Reading

Cook, V. and Blikslager, A. (2015). The use of nonsteroidal anti-inflammatory drugs in critically ill horses. *J. Vet. Crit. Care* 25: 76–88.

Geor, R. (2007). Acute renal failure in horses. *Vet. Clin. North Am. Equine Pract.* 23: 577–591.

Toribio, R. (2007). Essentials of equine renal and urinary tract physiology. *Vet. Clin. North Am. Equine Pract.* 23: 533–561.

# 6

# Neurophysiology and Neuroanesthesia
*Tanya Duke-Novakovski*

- Anesthesia for horses with intracranial pathology is not common, but anesthesia for horses with head trauma might be required.
- An understanding of the effects of anesthetic drugs on intracranial pathophysiologic processes is useful in the event that general anesthesia may be required.
- Horses with seizures may have to be anesthetized for diagnostic procedures or for control of seizures.

## I Neurophysiology

### A Membrane potentials

- ○ Nerve cell membrane potentials are maintained through differential distribution of ions across the membrane.
- ○ Depolarization causes movement of sodium and potassium ions, which depolarizes the next segment of the nerve cell. This allows transmission of impulses along nerve axons.

### B Synaptic transmission

- ○ Junctions between nerve cells allow nerve transmission to take multiple pathways.
- ○ Excitatory or inhibitory neurotransmitters are released into the synaptic cleft to activate receptor sites on the post-synaptic cell.
- ○ Excitatory neurotransmitters in the CNS include acetylcholine, norepinephrine, dopamine, 5-hydroxytrytamine, substance P, glutamate, and other amino acids.
- ○ Inhibitory neurotransmitters include glycine, gamma aminobutyric acid (GABA), enkephalins, and endorphins.
- ○ Other transmitters include neurotensin, thyroid-releasing hormone (TRH), gonadotropin-releasing hormone (GnRH), melanocyte stimulating releasing-inhibitory factor, adrenocorticotropic hormone (ACTH), and somatostatin.

*Manual of Equine Anesthesia and Analgesia*, Second Edition. Edited by Tom Doherty, Alex Valverde, and Rachel A. Reed.
© 2022 John Wiley & Sons, Inc. Published 2022 by John Wiley & Sons, Inc.

C  **Brain metabolism**

- The brain almost exclusively uses *glucose* as a source of energy. The brain can also use two ketones, *3-hydroxybutyrate* and *acetoacetate*.
- The selectivity of the blood–brain barrier makes the brain dependent on *glucose* as an energy substrate, and low concentrations decrease the level of consciousness.
- Twenty-five percent of glucose is used for energy, and the remainder is used for protein synthesis (e.g. glutamic and aspartic acid) which are also used for energy in some cell pathways.

D  **Cerebral blood flow**

- Cerebral blood flow increases with cerebral oxygen demand (especially when $PaO_2$ decreases below 50 mmHg) and increases linearly with $PaCO_2$ over the range 20–80 mmHg (see Figure 6.1).
- Hypothermia blunts the response to changing $PaCO_2$.
- The response to $CO_2$ is maintained during volatile and intravenous anesthesia.
- Normal cerebral blood flow in humans is 50 ml/100 g/minute and it has not been quantified in horses.
- Flow is greatest in neonates and declines with age, and within gray matter (80 ml/100 g/minute).
- Autoregulation maintains constant brain–blood flow over a range of mean systemic blood pressures (60–130 mmHg). Autoregulation is dependent on two processes:
  - Vascular smooth muscle responses which occur over 30–40 seconds.
  - Neural mediated vasodilation through cranial nerve VII.
- Arterial hypercapnia or hypoxemia, atropine, and volatile anesthesia administration may attenuate or abolish autoregulation.

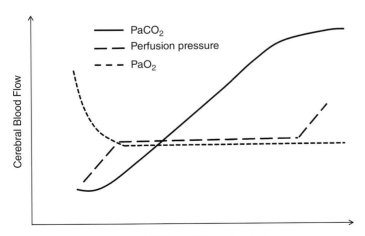

Figure 6.1   The effects of arterial partial pressure of $O_2$ and $CO_2$, and perfusion pressure on cerebral blood flow.

E   Cerebral perfusion pressure (CPP)

- Intracranial pressure (ICP) is maintained at approximately 2 mmHg in conscious healthy horses, even when the head is lowered below heart level.
- Normal neonatal foals in the first 24 hours after birth have ICP between 2 and 15 mmHg and a CPP of in the range 50–109 mmHg.
- Mean (SD) values for ICP in adult standing horses are 2 (4) mmHg and for CPP are 102 (26) mm Hg.
- Cerebral perfusion pressure is the difference between systemic mean arterial blood pressure and ICP, and should be at least 60 mmHg.

$$CPP = MAP - ICP$$

- When CPP is below this value or cardiac output decreases to less than half-normal values, cerebral circulation becomes insufficient.
- In isoflurane-anesthetized horses maintained at 1.2 MAC, ICP increases and is higher in dorsal than in lateral and sternal recumbency (34 *vs* 24 *vs* 19 mmHg, respectively). Head down position for dorsal and sternal recumbency increases ICP further. Because MAP is higher (105 mmHg) in sternal recumbency, CPP is higher (71 mmHg for sternal with head up and 87 mmHg for sternal with head down); intermediate for dorsal recumbency (MAP of 85 mmHg for head level with the thorax and CPP of 51 mmHg; MAP of 76 mmHg for head down and CPP of 55 mmHg); and lower for lateral recumbency (MAP of 72 mmHg and CPP of 48 mmHg).
- Increasing end-tidal concentrations of the inhalational anesthetic causes significant dose-dependent decreases in MAP and CPP, but no change in ICP.
- Mechanical ventilation causes a significant decrease in MAP and ICP but no change in CPP.

F   Cerebrospinal fluid (CSF)

- CSF is continuously formed by the *choroid plexuses* in the lateral and third ventricles and has a specific gravity of 1.002–1.009. The fluid passes into the fourth ventricle, and then into the subarachnoid space around the brain and spinal cord through three foramina.
- Most absorption occurs through the subarachnoid villi which protrude into the venous sinuses of the cranium.
- The subarachnoid space does not communicate with the subdural space, but is continuous with the ventricles of the brain through medial and lateral connections in the roof of the fourth ventricle. Separations of the arachnoid and pia mater form the cerebro-medullary cistern or cisterna magna.
  - Samples of CSF can be obtained from lumbar puncture or through the cisterna magna, although the latter technique carries a higher risk.
- CSF is exchanged every four hours and absorption helps maintain pressure at a constant level.
- CSF acts as a cushion and support for the brain.
- Changes in brain volume can be offset by CSF production and absorption.
- The composition of CSF is tightly regulated. CSF pH remains about 7.33 even with wide changes in plasma pH. Compared to other extra-cellular fluids, CSF contains 7% higher sodium and chloride ion, and 30% and 40% lower glucose and potassium concentrations, respectively.

○ A CSF pH decrease of 0.05 units rapidly results in a fourfold increase in ventilation and reflects the ability of lipid soluble $CO_2$ to cross the blood–brain-barrier, not hydrogen ions. Active transport of bicarbonate ions returns CSF pH to normal with chronic changes in arterial pH.

○ A potential difference between CSF and blood of about +5 mV is the result of an active transport system.

○ $O_2$, $CO_2$, barbiturates, glucose, and lipophilic (anesthetic and sedative) substances effectively cross the blood–brain barrier.

○ Inorganic ions, highly dissociated compounds, amino acids, and sucrose cross very slowly.

○ CSF pressure changes with body position, and expiratory efforts such as coughing or straining can sharply increase the pressure.

## II Central nervous system pathophysiology

### A Seizures

○ Seizures are not common in horses and classification and diagnosis is reviewed elsewhere.

○ Accidental injection of drugs into the carotid artery can cause convulsions.

○ Anticonvulsants raise the seizure threshold, prevent spread of seizure activity, and decrease the level of activity of abnormal neurons while sparing normal cells.

### B Intracranial pressure (ICP) increase

○ As an intracranial mass expands within the bony cranium it can cause an increase in ICP. This increase in ICP can be offset by displacement of CSF, blood flow, and displacement of the brain matter.

 – This effect does not continue, and once a certain point is reached, ICP can rise exponentially (see Figure 6.2).

○ Sudden increases in ICP can increase the risk of brain herniation.

○ During neuroanesthesia, steps are taken to reduce brain volume as much as possible to offset increases in ICP.

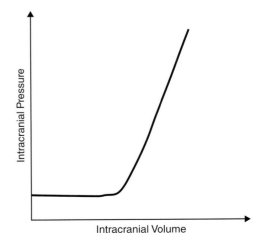

Figure 6.2   The effects of intracranial volume changes on intracranial pressure. At a certain point, the increase in intracranial volume causes a dramatic increase in intracranial pressure as compensatory mechanisms become exhausted.

## III Neuroanesthesia

- Anesthetic drugs and manipulations performed during anesthesia can affect:

### A Cerebral metabolic rate

- In humans, normal $O_2$ consumption is 3–5 ml/100 g/minute, similar to that of working skeletal muscle.
- When the level of consciousness is depressed, the cerebral metabolic rate is decreased.
- Oxygen consumption decreases by approximately 20% during hypoglycemia, 40% during general anesthesia, 3% during sleep, and 15–20% during hypothermia.
- Drugs such as $\alpha_2$ adrenergic agonists and a *propofol* infusion decrease cerebral metabolic oxygen demand and provide some brain protection.
- Isoflurane decreases cerebral metabolic oxygen demand, but causes vasodilation.

### B Cerebral blood flow and perfusion pressure

*Anesthetic drugs*
- Anesthetic drugs can modify cerebral blood flow and cerebral metabolic rate (see Table 6.1).
- These changes can be affected by the presence or absence of intracranial pathology, and may also be influenced by hypoxemic or hypercapnic states.
- *Isoflurane* increases ICP in normal horses, and this is exacerbated by a prolonged duration of anesthesia, by hypoventilation (increased $PaCO_2$), and if the head is positioned below heart level.
- *Isoflurane* preserves autoregulation even at moderate-deep levels of anesthesia in healthy horses and a cerebral blood flow of 33 ml/100 g/minute, regardless of mean arterial pressure in the 60–100 mmHg range.
- *Dobutamine* infusion was not found to increase ICP in normal horses.
- Spinal cord perfusion was found to decrease during *isoflurane* anesthesia, and dobutamine infusion may decrease perfusion further.
- However, *hypotension* and decreased ability to autoregulate cerebral perfusion caused by older volatile anesthetics such as *halothane* may cause rare neurological complications in normal horses.
- Cerebral vasodilation with volatile anesthetics is a problem in disease states when high ICP is already present. The increase in blood volume within the cranium could increase ICP further.
- Drugs which produce a degree of cerebral vasoconstriction may be more useful, especially if they also decrease cerebral metabolic rate (e.g. $\alpha_2$ agonists and *propofol*).

*Increased $PaCO_2$*
- Will increase cerebral blood flow and intracranial volume through vasodilation.
- This could be detrimental in animals with existing increased ICP.
- Mechanical ventilation is required during anesthesia to ensure $PaCO_2$ values are kept between 35 and 40 mmHg (normal $PaCO_2$ in adult horse is approximately 40 mmHg) to reduce the risk of increasing ICP.

Table 6.1 Reported effects of drugs on neurophysiology of the brain.

| Drug | Cerebral blood flow | Cerebral metabolic $O_2$ requirement | Direct cerebral vasodilation | Seizure potential |
|---|---|---|---|---|
| Xylazine | − | ? | Vasoconstriction | High dose: Anticonvulsant Low dose: Proconvulsant |
| Detomidine | ? probably | ? probably | ? probably vasoconstriction | ? |
| Dexmedetomidine | − | − | Vasoconstriction | High dose: Anticonvulsant Low dose: Proconvulsant |
| Acepromazine | − | NC | ? | Possible NC |
| Ketamine | NC with IPPV ++ with hypercapnia | + | With hypercapnia | Proconvulsant or anticonvulsant |
| Thiopental | − | − | No | Anticonvulsant |
| Ketamine/ diazepam | + | + | ? | ? |
| Propofol | − | − | No | Anticonvulsant |
| Alfaxalone (with alphadolone in Cremaphor EL) | − | − | Probably no | Anticonvulsant |
| Midazolam | − | − | No | Anticonvulsant |
| Guaifenesin | ? | ? | ? | Depresses EEG |
| Halothane | +++ | − | Yes | No effect |
| Isoflurane | + or NC with IPPV | − | Yes | No effect |
| Sevoflurane | + or NC with IPPV | − | Yes | No effect |

NC = No change + = Increase − = Decrease.

- Excessive ventilation to below this $PaCO_2$ range will cause excessive vasoconstriction and lead to poor perfusion of some parts of the brain.
- End-tidal capnography often under-estimates $PaCO_2$; therefore, arterial blood gas analysis should be used periodically to check the accuracy of the capnogram.

*Positive pressure ventilation of lungs*
- Although necessary for animals with increased ICP, venous return is impeded during the inspiratory phase, and can cause ICP to rise.
- Avoid high mean airway pressures (long inspiratory time and high-peak inspiratory pressure on the ventilator) as much as possible.

*Venous return*
- In animals with increased ICP, avoid compression of the jugular veins to prevent further increases in ICP.

*Head position*
- The head should be positioned at the level of the heart, and not below, in order to maintain perfusion pressures and avoid increasing ICP.

## C Autoregulation

- ○ It is important to select drugs which will preserve cerebral autoregulation of blood flow as much as possible.
- ○ Direct arterial pressure monitoring should be performed.
- ○ Mean arterial blood pressure should be kept within the range at which autoregulation can function (60–130 mmHg), in order to preserve cerebral perfusion.
  - – A cerebral perfusion pressure of at least 60 mmHg should be maintained.
- ○ During anesthesia, horses should be well oxygenated and hypercapnia prevented with lung ventilation.
- ○ Arterial pressures should be maintained using fluid therapy, inotropes, and volatile anesthetic reduction techniques (see PIVA).

# IV Neuroanesthesia for specific procedures

- • Diagnostic procedures (Imaging is discussed in Chapter 35)

## A CSF withdrawal

- ○ CSF withdrawal using lumbar puncture or from the cisterna magna can be performed in standing horses (see Figure 6.3)
- ○ Horses can be sedated with *xylazine* or *detomidine* with *butorphanol* for this procedure.
- ○ General anesthesia should be avoided in ataxic horses, unless facilities for assisted recovery are available (see Figure 6.4)
  - – *Xylazine* or *detomidine* premedication, followed by induction with *ketamine* combined with *diazepam/midazolam* or *propofol.*

## B Increased intracranial pressure

*Includes head trauma, abscess, and tumor removal.*
- ○ Although, the likelihood that surgery will be required in a horse with increased ICP is rare, it could be performed for tumor resection or for craniotomy to allow drainage of an intracranial abscess.
- ○ Horses may already be mentally depressed due to increased ICP, and drug doses should be reduced accordingly.
- ○ Sedatives might interfere with neurological evaluation, but should be used if the horse is displaying agitation or aggression.

*Preparation*
- ○ *Mannitol* may be required to reduce ICP and can be given before induction (0.15–2.5 g/kg, IV over 20 minutes).
  - – Its routine use has been questioned for emergency treatment of head injury in people.
- ○ Fluid balance should be assessed and corrected if necessary.
  - – Avoid excessive doses of crystalloids in case of worsening cerebral edema.
- ○ Consider using *hypertonic saline* for head trauma patients, especially foals, as it may be more effective than mannitol in reducing ICP.

**Figure 6.3** Lumbosacral spinal tap for collection of cerebrospinal fluid in a standing horse. *Source:* Courtesy of Dr. Erin Beasley.

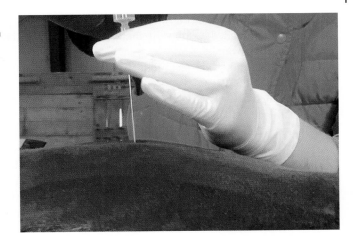

**Figure 6.4** Ataxic horse leaning against stall wall.

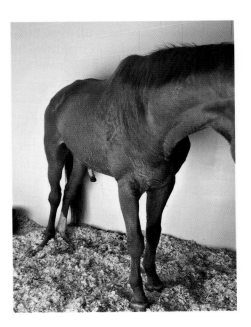

*Sedation, premedication, and induction*
- ○ Neonatal foals sedate well with *diazepam or midazolam* (0.02–0.1 mg/kg, IV).
  - − *Butorphanol* may be added (0.05–0.1 mg/kg, IV).
- ○ Older foals can be sedated with an $\alpha_2$ agonist, but a low dose is recommended if the foal is mentally depressed.
  - − Dexmedetomidine has been shown to reduce ICP.
- ○ *Propofol* sedation can reduce ICP, CBF and oxygen demand. Blood pressure support may be required.

*Induction of anesthesia in foals*
- ○ Excessive stimulation of the larynx during intubation can increase ICP through catecholamine release, although horses appear not to have a strongly reactive airway compared to other species.

- *Lidocaine* (1–2 mg/kg, IV) administration prior to tracheal intubation has been recommended to prevent increases to ICP with brain injury, but its utility remains controversial.
  - A fast induction technique and tracheal intubation allows lung ventilation and rapid control of $PaCO_2$.
  - *Propofol* (2–4 mg/kg, IV) or *alfaxalone* (1–2 mg/kg, IV) can be used for induction of anesthesia in foals, and is fast-acting.
    - A benzodiazepine can be used with these drugs (co-induction technique).
  - *Thiopental* is a good induction agent for adult horses, but should not be used in foals <8 weeks of age. *Thiopental* is not presently available in many countries.
  - *Ketamine*/benzodiazepine combinations have been shown to increase ICP and not obliterate the catecholamine response to intubation, but the neuroprotective benefits of using *ketamine* are now recognized. This technique also allows for rapid tracheal intubation.
  - After prior sedation with a benzodiazepine, gentle nasotracheal intubation or mask-down inhalational techniques using *isoflurane* or *sevoflurane* can be attempted. This technique takes the longest time to perform.
    - Although lung ventilation is possible with nasotracheal intubation, head trauma may preclude the use of nasal tubes.

*Sedation of adult horses*
  - Low doses of *xylazine* or *detomidine* may be used.
  - The head should be kept in a raised position so that a low head carriage does not increase ICP in horses with intracranial pathology.

*Maintenance of anesthesia*
  - *Isoflurane* or *sevoflurane* are better choices than *halothane*. *Halothane* is not available in many countries.
  - $N_2O$ increases cerebral blood flow and cerebral metabolic rate when combined with a volatile agent, and is probably not advisable to use in horses with intracranial pathology. Its use is limited in equine anesthesia, and is usually reserved for use in foals.
  - Since volatile agents increase cerebral blood flow through vasodilation, techniques should be employed to limit this.
    - Use PIVA to reduce *isoflurane* or *sevoflurane* requirements. IV infusions of $\alpha_2$ agonist and/or *lidocaine* can be used.
    - Opioids (*butorphanol, methadone, morphine, remifentanil*) do not reduce *isoflurane* MAC in horses, but can be used for intra-operative analgesia.
    - *Propofol* infusions can be used in horses and can be used alongside *isoflurane* in a similar manner to their use in dogs and humans to provide anesthesia. A disadvantage is the large volume of *propofol* required for TIVA or PIVA in adult horses. In adult horses, *propofol* might reduce $PaO_2$ by an unknown mechanism.
    - *Alfaxalone* infusion can be used for craniectomy, but recovery in foals may result in excitement behaviors.
    - Respiratory and cardiovascular depression during anesthesia requires lung ventilation and blood pressure support.
  - *Hypothermia* should be prevented. Although it can lower cerebral metabolic oxygen demand, it can cause other adverse effects.

**C   Cerebral edema**

- ○ Global edema may result from injury or another cause, such as after a successful resuscitation from cardiac arrest.

*Drug-induced decompression*

- ○ May be achieved through use of:
  - − *Mannitol* (0.15–2.5 g/kg, IV over 20 minutes).
  - − Loop diuretics (e.g. *furosemide* 0.75–1.0 mg/kg, IV).
  - − Hypertonic saline (2–4 ml/kg 7.2%, IV over 10–15 minutes).
  - − *Dimethylsulphoxide* (DMSO) (1.0–2.0 g/kg as a 10% or 20% solution).
  - − Dexamethasone (0.3–0.6 mg/kg, IV) to reduce ICP is controversial and steroid use for treatment of traumatic brain injury is not recommended in people.
    - ■ Steroids stabilize blood–brain barrier permeability, but the gluconeogenic effects may worsen brain injury.
- ○ Further decreases in ICP may be necessary through use of heavy sedation/anesthesia, tracheal intubation and mechanical ventilation with a specialized ventilator. This labor-intensive procedure might not be possible, and is only feasible for foals.
- ○ *Glycemic control.* Hyperglycemia is associated with increased mortality with head trauma. There is debate whether *insulin* should be used to control hyperglycemia, but glucose-containing fluids and gluconeogenic drugs should be avoided.

*Ventilation*

- ○ Anesthetized patients with a high ICP should be ventilated to maintain normocapnia.
- ○ Although hyperventilation has been recommended in the past, it is now recommended that normocapnia should be maintained.
- ○ In small foals, heavy sedation/anesthesia can be obtained using *midazolam* and *propofol* infusions. *Dexmedetomidine* infusion might also help to reduce drug requirements and stabilize ICP.
  - − In any case, normocapnia should be maintained, but this may be difficult to achieve in a sedated foal, and it may be necessary to induce and maintain anesthesia to allow the foal to be intubated and ventilated.
  - − Neonatal foals may have reduced ability to metabolize drugs so signs of deepening sedation indicate a need to reduce the amount of drug administered.
  - − Care should be directed towards life support during long-term sedation, including provision of nutrition.
- ○ The ability to use intermittent positive-pressure ventilation (IPPV) to hyperventilate horses and maintain $PaCO_2$ will be considerably affected by the presence of ventilation/perfusion mismatch and the time required to maintain a horse in recumbency. This technique is probably not feasible in adult horses.

**D   Seizures**

- ○ Sedatives (e.g. *phenobarbital, diazepam*) are used to control seizures.
- ○ IV *phenobarbital* can be used for acute seizures, followed by oral therapy.
- ○ *Diazepam* or *midazolam* (0.1 mg/kg, IV) can be administered for acute seizures because it has a rapid effect. Ataxia may be observed so assistance in standing might be required.
- ○ Oxygen and ventilatory support may be necessary if high doses of diazepam are used in neonates.

- ○ *Propofol* can be used to control seizures and can be given as an infusion. It can be used alongside other anti-seizure medication.

*Anesthesia of horses prone to seizures*
- ○ No study has been published examining these drugs in seizure-prone horses, but the following points are taken from studies performed in other species.
- ○ *Xylazine* (0.5–1.0 mg/kg, IV) or *detomidine* (10–15 μg/kg, IV) can be used as a premedicant.
  - – *Xylazine* has been shown in other species to have proconvulsant activity at low doses and anticonvulsant activity at sedative doses.
- ○ *Acepromazine* was once not recommended because other phenothiazines have been shown to reduce the seizure threshold, but *acepromazine* has been used successfully in seizure-prone dogs.
- ○ *Ketamine* increases the chance of seizures in patients with a known history of seizure activity, although it has been used to treat seizures refractory to conventional treatment. However, ketamine may be the only choice available for induction of anesthesia in adult horses because *thiopental* is now not widely available.
  - – Since *diazepam* is an anticonvulsant, the combined use of *diazepam/ketamine* is safe. Alternatively, *propofol/ketamine* is safe to use.
- ○ *Guaifenesin* may be used in seizure-prone horses. *Triple drip* ($\alpha_2$- agonist/guaifenesin and ketamine combination) may be used for short diagnostic procedures with tracheal intubation and lung ventilation.

## Suggested Reading

Armitage-Chan, E.A., Wetmore, L.A., and Chan, D.L. (2007). Anesthetic management of the head trauma patient. *J. Vet. Emerg. Crit. Care* 17: 5–14.

Brosnan, R.J., LeCouteur, R.A., Steffey, E.P. et al. (2002). Direct measurement of intracranial pressure in adult horses. *Am. J. Vet. Res.* 63: 1252–1256.

Brosnan, R.J., Steffey, E.P., LeCouteur, R.A. et al. (2003). Effects of duration of isoflurane anesthesia and mode of ventilation on intracranial and cerebral perfusion pressures in horses. *Am. J. Vet. Res.* 64: 1444–1448.

Brosnan, R.J., Steffey, E.P., LeCouteur, R.A. et al. (2003). Effects of ventilation and isoflurane end-tidal concentration on intracranial and cerebral perfusion pressures in horses. *Am. J. Vet. Res.* 64: 21–25.

Brosnan, R.J., Steffey, E.P., LeCouteur, R.A. et al. (2002). Effects of body position on intracranial and cerebral perfusion pressures in isoflurane-anesthetized horses. *J. Appl. Physiol.* 92: 2542–2546.

Brosnan, R.J., Esteller-Vico, A., Steffey, E.P. et al. (2008). Effects of head-down positioning on regional central nervous system perfusion in isoflurane-anesthetized horses. *Am. J. Vet. Res.* 69: 737–743.

Brosnan, R.J., Steffey, E.P., LeCouteur, R.A. et al. (2011). Effects of isoflurane anesthesia on cerebrovascular autoregulation in horses. *Am. J. Vet. Res.* 72: 18–24.

Caines, D., Sinclair, M., Valverde, A. et al. (2014). Comparison of isoflurane and propofol for maintenance of anesthesia in dogs with intracranial disease undergoing magnetic resonance imaging. *Vet. Anaesth. Analg.* 41: 468–479.

Chaffin, M.K., Walker, M.A., McArthur, N.H. et al. (1997). Magnetic resonance imaging of the brain of normal neonatal foals. *Vet. Radiol. Ultrasound* 38: 102–111.

Drynan, E.A., Gray, P., and Raisis, A. (2012). Incidence of seizures associated with the use of acepromazine in dogs undergoing myelography. *J. Vet. Crit. Care* 22: 262–266.

Duke-Novakovski, T., Palacios-Jiminez, C., Wetzel, T. et al. (2015). Cardiopulmonary effects of dexmedetomidine and ketamine infusions with either propofol infusion or isoflurane for anesthesia in horses. *Vet. Anaesth. Analg.* 42: 39–49.

Farrell, D. and Bendo, A.A. (2018). Perioperative management of severe traumatic brain injury: What Is New? *Curr. Anesthesiol. Rep.* 8: 279–289.

Flaherty, D., Reid, J., Welsh, E. et al. (1997). A pharmacodynamic study of propofol or propofol and ketamine infusions in ponies undergoing surgery. *Res. Vet. Sci.* 62: 179–184.

Hirota, K., Hashimoto, Y., Sato, T. et al. (2001). Bronchoconstrictive and relaxant effects of lidocaine on the airway in dogs. *Crit. Care Med.* 29: 1040–1044.

Jones, T., Bracamonte, J.L., Ambros, B., and Duke-Novakovski, T. (2019). Total intravenous anesthesia with alfaxalone, dexmedetomidine and remifentanil in healthy foals undergoing abdominal surgery. *Vet. Anaesth. Analg.* 46: 315–324.

Kortz, G.D., Madigan, J.E., Goetzman, B.W., and Durando, M. (1995). Intracranial pressure and cerebral perfusion in clinically normal equine neonates. *Am. J. Vet. Res.* 56: 1351–1355.

Lacombe, V.A. (2015). Seizures in horses: diagnosis and classification. *Vet. Med. Res. Reports* 6: 301–308.

McConnell, J., Kirby, R., and Rudloff, E. (2007). Administration of acepromazine maleate to 31 dogs with a history of seizures. *J. Vet. Emerg. Crit. Care* 17: 262–267.

Miyazaki, Y., Adachi, T., Kurata, J. et al. (1999). Dexmedetomidine reduces seizure threshold during enflurane anaesthesia in cats. *Br. J. Anaesth.* 82: 935–937.

Rasmussen, N.J., Rosendal, T., and Overgaard, J. (1978). Althesin in neurosurgical patients: effects on cerebral hemodynamics and metabolism. *Acta Anaesthesiol. Scand.* 22: 257–269.

Sande, A. and West, C. (2010). Traumatic brain injury: a review of pathophysiology and management. *J. Vet. Emerg. Crit. Care* 20: 177–190.

Serrano, S., Hughes, D., and Chandler, K. (2006). Use of ketamine for the management of refractory status epilepticus in a dog. *J. Vet. Intern. Med.* 20: 194–197.

Spadavecchia, C., Jaggy, A., Fatzer, R., and Schatzmann, U. (2001). Postanaesthetic cerebral necrosis in a horse. *Equine Vet. J.* 33: 621–624.

Steffen, F. and Grasmueck, S. (2000). Propofol for treatment of refractory seizures in dogs and a cat with intracranial disorders. *J. Small Anim. Pract.* 41: 496–499.

Talke, P., Tong, C., Lee, H.W. et al. (1997). Effect of dexmedetomidine on lumbar cerebrospinal fluid pressure in humans. *Anesth. Analg.* 85: 358–364.

Tobias, K.M. and Marioni-Henry, K.A. (2006). Retrospective study on the use of acepromazine maleate in dogs with seizures. *J. Am. Anim. Hosp. Assoc.* 42: 283–289.

Warne, L.N., Beths, T., Fogal, S., and Bauquier, S.H. (2014). The use of alfaxalone and remifentanil total intravenous anesthesia in a dog undergoing a craniectomy for tumor resection. *Can. Vet. J.* 55: 1083–1088.

Zornow, M.H., Fleischer, J.E., Sceller, M.S. et al. (1990). Dexmedetomidine, an alpha 2-adrenergic agonist, decreases cerebral blood flow in the isoflurane-anesthetized dog. *Anesth. Analg.* 70: 624–630.

# 7

# The Autonomic Nervous System
*Christine Egger*

The autonomic nervous system (ANS) is the portion of the central nervous system (CNS) that controls visceral functions such as arterial blood pressure, heart rate, respiratory function, gastrointestinal (GI) motility and secretion, urinary bladder emptying, sweating, body temperature, as well as a number of other important bodily functions.

## I  General organization of the ANS (functional anatomy)

- The ANS is anatomically divided into the *central* and *peripheral* nervous system, and functionally divided into the *sympathetic* (adrenergic) nervous system (SNS) and the *parasympathetic* (cholinergic) nervous system (PNS).

### A  Central autonomic nervous system

- The *hypothalamus* is the principle site of ANS integration (e.g. blood pressure control, thermoregulation, stress response).
- The *medulla oblongata* and *pons* contain the centers for hemodynamic and ventilatory control.

### B  Peripheral autonomic nervous system

- *Pre-ganglionic neurons* are myelinated, rapidly conducting, originate in the CNS, and synapse in an autonomic ganglion.
- *Post-ganglionic neurons* are unmyelinated, slower conducting, arise from the autonomic ganglia, and are distributed to effector organs.
- The *SNS* (paravertebral) *ganglia* are located nearer to the spinal cord than to the innervated organ, and the *PNS ganglia* are located in or near the innervated organ.

*Manual of Equine Anesthesia and Analgesia*, Second Edition. Edited by Tom Doherty, Alex Valverde, and Rachel A. Reed.
© 2022 John Wiley & Sons, Inc. Published 2022 by John Wiley & Sons, Inc.

## C  Afferent input

- The ANS centers in the brain stem act as relay stations for control of activities initiated at higher levels of the brain, such as the hypothalamus and cerebrum.
- Visceral sensory signals entering the autonomic ganglia, spinal cord, brain stem, or hypothalamus elicit reflex responses which control the activity of visceral organs.

## D  Efferent output

- Efferent autonomic signals are transmitted to the body through two major subdivisions of the ANS, the SNS, and PNS. (see later discussion.)

## II  Physiology of the autonomic nervous system

### A  Neurotransmitters

- *Acetylcholine* (ACh) and *norepinephrine* (NE) are the main neurotransmitters.
- All preganglionic neurons are *cholinergic* in both the SNS and PNS nervous systems and secrete ACh.
- Postganglionic neurons of the PNS are *cholinergic*, while most postganglionic SNS neurons are *adrenergic* and secrete NE.
  - The adrenal gland functions like a modified sympathetic ganglion and when stimulated by presynaptic SNS fibers, releases NE and epinephrine (EPI) into the circulation to act on sites distant from the gland; therefore, there is no postganglionic neuron.
  - Sweat glands in horses are mostly apocrine and open into hair follicles. These glands and the piloerector muscles are stimulated by circulating EPI that acts on *adrenergic* ($\beta_2$) receptors.
  - Eccrine sweat glands are common in humans, but are less common in horses. In humans, they constitute 90% of sweat glands and they are stimulated by a postganglionic SNS neuron that secretes ACh.

### B  Synthesis, duration of action, and degradation of ACh

- ACh is synthesized within the axoplasm in the terminal endings of cholinergic nerves.
- The ACh is transported to the interior of the vesicles where it is stored in a highly concentrated form until it is released along with ATP.

$$\text{Acetyl} - \text{CoA} + \text{Choline} \xrightarrow{\text{Choline acetyltransferase}} \text{Acetylcholine}$$

- After release, ACh persists in the tissue for a few seconds, then most of it is split into an *acetate* ion and *choline* by the enzyme *acetylcholinesterase*, which is present in the terminal neuron and the surface of the receptor organ.

### C  Synthesis, duration of action, and removal of NE

- ○ Synthesis of norepinephrine from *phenylalanine* begins in the axoplasm of the terminal nerve endings of adrenergic nerve fibers and is completed inside the vesicles.

$$Phenylalanine \rightarrow L-Tyrosine \rightarrow L-Dopa \rightarrow Dopamine \rightarrow Norepinephrine \rightarrow Epinephrine$$

- ○ In the *adrenal medulla*, this reaction goes one step further and transforms about 85% of the norepinephrine into epinephrine.
- ○ After secretion, NE is rapidly (within a few seconds) removed from the secretory site and taken back to the vesicles, either unchanged or metabolized by monoamine oxidase (MAO). If it reaches the circulation, NE, and also EPI, are metabolized by MAO and catechol-O-methyltransferase (CMT) in the liver and kidney.

### D  Receptors on the effector organs

*Cholinergic* receptors are subdivided into *muscarinic* and *nicotinic*.

- ○ *Muscarinic receptors* are present in all effector cells stimulated by the postganglionic PNS neurons, as well as in those stimulated by the postganglionic SNS cholinergic neurons. Subtypes of muscarinic receptors are described in Table 7.1.
- ○ *Nicotinic receptors* are found in the synapses between the preganglionic and postganglionic neurons of the SNS and PNS, and at the neuromuscular junction.
- ○ ACh is the neurotransmitter at all cholinergic receptors.

*Adrenergic receptors* are subdivided into *alpha* ($\alpha_1$ and $\alpha_2$), *beta* ($\beta_1$ and $\beta_2$), and *dopaminergic* (DA).

- ○ Norepinephrine (NE) excites $\alpha$ receptors more than $\beta$ receptors.
- ○ Epinephrine (EPI) excites $\alpha$ and $\beta$ receptors approximately equally.

*Dopaminergic receptors*

- ○ There are five subtypes of dopaminergic receptors, D1 to D5. Dopaminergic receptors are primarily present in the CNS but are also present in the periphery.
- ○ Dopamine can act by three mechanisms:
  - – It modulates the release of norepinephrine from adrenergic neurons.
  - – It activates $\alpha$ and $\beta$ receptors.
  - – It activates dopaminergic receptors.

Table 7.1  Muscarinic receptor subtypes.

| | M1 | M2 | M3 | M4 | M5 |
|---|---|---|---|---|---|
| Location | CNS Stomach | Heart CNS | CNS Salivary glands; airway smooth muscle | CNS Heart? | CNS |
| Clinical effects | H$^+$ secretion | Bradycardia | Salivation | ? | ? |

## III Function of the adrenal medulla

### A SNS innervation of the adrenals

- Stimulation of the SNS nerves to the adrenal medulla causes large quantities of EPI and NE to be released into the bloodstream.
- Approximately 80% of the secretion is EPI and 20% is NE.

### B Effect of NE release from adrenals

- The circulating NE causes constriction of most blood vessels, increased activity of the heart, inhibition of the GI tract, and dilation of the pupils.

### C Effect of EPI release from adrenals

- EPI, because it has greater affinity for $\beta$ receptors, has a more profound effect on cardiac stimulation than does NE. However, NE is a more potent vasoconstrictor.
- NE and EPI increase systemic vascular resistance, mean arterial pressure and cardiac output through their $\alpha$- and $\beta$-receptor activity. Heart rate is more likely to increase with EPI due to a stronger chronotropic effect, whereas it decreases with NE, as a result of a baroreflex in response to the increase in systemic vascular resistance.

## IV Autonomic effects on the cardiovascular system

### A The heart

- SNS stimulation increases heart rate and contractility.
- PNS stimulation decreases heart rate and can result in asystole.
- Postsynaptic $\alpha_2$ receptors exert a positive inotropic effect and contribute to development of cardiac arrhythmias.
- Postsynaptic $\beta_1$ receptors and presynaptic $\beta_2$ receptors play similar roles in increasing heart rate and myocardial contractility.

### B Systemic blood vessels

- SNS stimulation constricts most systemic blood vessels, especially those of the abdominal viscera and the skin of the limbs.
- PNS stimulation has almost *no effect* on most blood vessels.
- Presynaptic $\alpha_2$ vascular receptors mediate vasodilation, whereas postsynaptic $\alpha_1$ and $\alpha_2$ vascular receptors mediate vasoconstriction.
- Postsynaptic $\alpha_2$-vascular receptors predominate in the venous circulation.
- Postsynaptic $\alpha_2$-receptor activation causes arterial and venous vasoconstriction.
- Postsynaptic $\beta$ receptors are predominantly $\beta_2$ and mediate vasodilation.

### C Effects of SNS and PNS stimulation on arterial pressure

- SNS stimulation increases cardiac contractility and systemic vascular resistance, which usually causes the arterial pressure to increase greatly.

○ PNS stimulation decreases cardiac contractility, but has virtually no effect on systemic vascular resistance.

○ The usual effect of PNS stimulation is a slight fall in pressure.

### D Cardiovascular autonomic reflexes

○ *Arterial baroreceptors* are stretch receptors located in the carotid sinus and aortic arch to detect changes in arterial blood pressure.

○ When arterial blood pressure increases, arterial baroreceptors are stretched and signals are transmitted to the brain stem, which inhibit the SNS impulses to the heart and blood vessels, and increase vagal tone on the SA node of the heart, which results in bradycardia to correct the increase in pressure (*baroreceptor reflex*).

○ When arterial blood pressure decreases, arterial baroreceptors sense the decrease in tension and signal the vasomotor center to facilitate SNS activity in the heart and blood vessels and decrease vagal tone, causing an increase in heart rate to correct the decrease in pressure.

○ *Venous baroreceptors*, located in the right atrium and great veins, increase heart rate when the right atrium is stretched by increased filling pressure *(Bainbridge reflex)*.

## V Autonomic effects on the pulmonary system

• Muscarinic receptors mediate bronchoconstriction and increase mucus secretion.

• $\beta_2$ receptors mediate bronchial smooth muscle *relaxation* and increase mucus secretion (see Table 7.2).

## VI Pharmacology of the ANS

### A Drugs that act on adrenergic effector organs (sympathomimetic drugs)

○ Adrenergic agonists include vasopressors (e.g. *phenylephrine*) and inotropes (e.g. *dobutamine*).

○ Most adrenergic agonists activate both $\alpha$ and $\beta$ receptors, with the predominant pharmacologic effect being the expression of this mixed receptor activation (see Table 7.3).

Table 7.2   Comparative pharmacology of selective $\beta_2$ adrenergic bronchodilators.

| Agent | $\beta_2$ selectivity | Peak effect (minutes) | Duration of action (hours) |
|---|---|---|---|
| *Albuterol* | +++++ | 30–60 | 4 |
| *Metaproterenol* | +++ | 30–60 | 3–4 |
| *Terbutaline* | ++++ | 60 | 4 |
| *Salmeterol* | ++++ | 60 | >12 |
| *Clenbuterol* | ++++ | 30–60 | 8–12 |

Table 7.3   Principal sites of action of adrenergic agonists.

| Agent | $\alpha_1$ | $\alpha_2$ | $\beta_1$ | $\beta_2$ | DA$_1$ | DA$_2$ | Mechanism |
|---|---|---|---|---|---|---|---|
| *Phenylephrine* | +++++ | ? | ± | 0 | 0 | 0 | direct |
| *Norepinephrine* | +++++ | +++++ | +++ | 0 | 0 | 0 | direct |
| *Epinephrine* | +++++ | +++ | +++++ | ++ | 0 | 0 | direct |
| *Ephedrine* | ++ | ? | +++ | ++ | 0 | 0 | indirect + direct |
| *Dopamine* | + to +++++ | ? | +++ | ++ | 0 | 0 | direct |
| *Dobutamine* | ± | ? | ++++ | ++ | 0 | 0 | direct |
| *Isoproterenol* | 0 | 0 | +++++ | +++++ | 0 | 0 | direct |

+ = increase, − = decrease, 0 = no change.

- Hemodynamic effects evoked by adrenergic agonists include changes in heart rate (*chronotropism*), cardiac contractility (*inotropism*), conduction velocity of the cardiac impulse (*dromotropism*), cardiac rhythm, and systemic vascular resistance (see Table 7.4).
- The effects of these drugs on capacitance veins (venous return) may be as important as their inotropic actions and more important than arteriolar effects.

B   **Drugs that cause release of NE from nerve endings**

- Certain drugs have an indirect sympathomimetic action, rather than directly exciting adrenergic effector organs, and cause release of NE from its storage vesicles in the SNS nerve endings (e.g. *ephedrine*).

C   **Drugs that have a PNS potentiating effect (anticholinesterase drugs)**

- These drugs inhibit *acetylcholinesterase*, preventing rapid destruction of ACh so that it accumulates at muscarinic and nicotinic receptors.
- *Neostigmine* and *edrophonium* are mainly used for reversal of non-depolarizing neuromuscular blockade (nicotinic effect). Neostigmine has also been administered parenterally to promote GI motility in horses.
- Simultaneous administration of an anticholinergic prevents unwanted muscarinic signs (bradycardia, salivation, bronchospasm, intestinal hypermotility) without preventing the nicotinic effects of ACh.

D   **Drugs that block cholinergic activity at effector organs (antimuscarinic drugs)**
(see Table 7.5)

- These drugs block the action of ACh on the muscarinic type of cholinergic effector organs, but do not affect the nicotinic action of ACh on the postganglionic neurons or on skeletal muscle (e.g. *atropine, glycopyrrolate*).

Table 7.4  Cardiovascular effects of adrenergic agonists.

| Agent | HR | CO | SVR | VR | MAP | Arrhythmias | RBF | AR | CNS stimulation |
|---|---|---|---|---|---|---|---|---|---|
| Phenylephrine | − | − | +++ | ++ | +++ | 0 | − | 0 | 0 |
| Norepinephrine | − | − | +++ | ++ | +++ | + | − | 0 | 0 |
| Epinephrine | ++ | ++ | + | + | + | +++ | − | − | + |
| Ephedrine | ++ | ++ | ++ | ++ | ++ | ++ | ± | − | + |
| Dopamine | + | ++ | − | +++ | − | + | +++ | 0 | 0 |
| Dobutamine | + | +++ | 0 | ± | + | ± | ++ | 0 | 0 |
| Isoproterenol | +++ | +++ | − | − | ± | +++ | − | − | + |

HR = heart rate, CO = cardiac output, SVR = systemic vascular resistance, VR = venous return, MAP = mean arterial pressure, RBF = renal blood flow, AR = airway resistance. + = increase, − = decrease, 0 = no change.

*Note:* Dopamine decreases SVR and MAP in the horse at clinical doses.

Table 7.5   Comparative effects of anticholinergic drugs.

| Anticholinergic | Salivary and respiratory secretions | HR | Relax smooth muscle | Mydriasis | ↓ Gastric H⁺ secretions | GIT tone | Alter fetal HR |
|---|---|---|---|---|---|---|---|
| *Atropine* | − | +++ | ++ | + | + | − | + |
| *Glycopyrrolate* | − | +++ | +++ | 0 | + | − | 0 |
| *Scopolamine* | − | + | + | +++ | + | − | + |

HR = heart rate, GIT = gastrointestinal tract.
+ = increase, − = decrease, 0 = no change.

## VII   Clinical use of autonomic drugs

- The primary use of autonomic drugs in horses during anesthesia is the support of blood pressure.

### A   Hypotension (see Chapter 38)

- *Dobutamine* and *ephedrine* are "*first-line*" drugs for correcting hypotension in horses.
- *Dopamine*, at clinical doses, increases the cardiac index in horses, but it decreases arterial blood pressure due to a decrease in SVR. Dopamine administration has been associated with the development of ventricular arrhythmias, particularly in *halothane* anesthetized horses.
- *Phenylephrine* administration causes an increase in arterial blood pressure, due to an increase in SVR, but it decreases cardiac index and heart rate.

### B   Cardiac arrest

- *Epinephrine* is primarily used in cardiac arrest and anaphylactic shock.
- It not a "*first-line*" drug for correcting hypotension.

### C   Bradycardia

- *Atropine* and *glycopyrrolate* are indicated for treating patients with intraoperative bradycardia.
  - However, it is rarely necessary to correct bradycardia in horses.
- *Atropine* is considered a "*first-line*" drug in severe bradycardia.

### D   Circulatory shock

- *Norepinephrine* use is reserved for treating patients in circulatory shock.
  - It is not recommended for the treatment of healthy anesthetized horses with hypotension.
- In septic patients, the co-administration of *dobutamine* may improve its effect on splanchnic blood flow.

### E   Bronchodilation

- β$_2$ agonists (e.g. *clenbuterol*) are used to treat recurrent airway obstruction (RAO) in horses, usually in association with a corticosteroid.
- The anticholinergic drugs, particularly *atropine*, cause bronchodilation and can be used during an acute episode of RAO. Administration of *atropine* (0.02 mg/kg, IV) should result in a noticeable decrease in respiratory effort within 30 minutes of administration, and this should aid in confirming the diagnosis of RAO.

### F   Priapism (see Chapter 38)

- *Phenylephrine* can be used to treat priapism.
- *Phenylephrine* HCl: 5–10 mg diluted in 10 ml of physiologic saline solution injected into the corpus cavernosum penis usually results in rapid resolution of the condition.

### G   Reversal of neuromuscular block (see Chapter 15)

- As previously mentioned, *neostigmine* and *edrophonium* are used to reverse non-depolarizing neuromuscular blockade. They should be administered slowly IV, and an anticholinergic drug (e.g. *atropine*) is usually administered concurrently to prevent adverse muscarinic effects, particularly bradycardia.
- When used to treat ileus, *neostigmine* is administered subcutaneously or by a slow IV infusion, thus bradycardia is less likely to occur.

### H   Spasmolytic effect

- *Scopolamine*, also known as *hyoscine-N-butylbromide*, is a competitive antagonist of ACh at muscarinic receptors. It is used clinically in association with the NSAID *dipyrone* to treat horses with spasmodic colic, and to relax the rectum for a *per-rectum* examination of the abdomen, primarily in horses with colic. It has also been used to treat anesthetized horses with bradycardia.

## Suggested Reading

Abraham, G. (2016). The importance of muscarinic receptors in domestic animal diseases and therapy: current and future perspectives. *Vet. J.* 208: 13–21.

Schauvliege, S. and Gasthuys, F. (2013). Drugs for cardiovascular support in anesthetized horses. *Vet. Clin. North Am. Equine Pract.* 29: 19–49.

# 8

# Electrolyte and Fluid Therapy

## Electrolytes

*Rachel A. Reed*

- Electrolytes such as sodium, potassium, chloride, and calcium are present throughout the body and are essential for normal cellular function.
- Abnormalities in electrolyte concentrations will disrupt critical cellular processes including action potential generation, ion channel function, cardiac contractility, and cardiac electrical conduction.

## I  Sodium

- The main extracellular cation.
- Reference values in plasma are 136–144 mEq/l.
- The relatively high extracellular concentration of sodium in comparison to the intracellular concentration is maintained by the Na-K-ATPase pump which moves sodium out of the cell in exchange for potassium.
- Due to the *Gibbs-Donnan* effect the sodium concentration in the intravascular space differs slightly from the concentration in the interstitial space.
    - The physiologic roles of sodium within the body include:
    - Maintenance of extracellular osmolarity and fluid volume.
    - Action potential generation.
- Changes in serum sodium concentration reflect either a change in sodium or a change in total body water.

### A  Hyponatremia (<125 mEq/l)

- *Clinical signs* reflect movement of water from the extracellular space to the intracellular space, resulting in cellular swelling within the central nervous system and development of neurologic signs including lethargy, central blindness, seizures, and tremors.
- *Causes* include disease processes that result in excess free water intake or inability to excrete free water:
    - Loss of high sodium fluids (e.g. diarrhea, sweating, blood loss).
    - Acute renal failure; due to renal loss of sodium.

*Manual of Equine Anesthesia and Analgesia*, Second Edition. Edited by Tom Doherty, Alex Valverde, and Rachel A. Reed.

- Rhabdomyolysis; secondary to renal insult, fluid shifting.
- Adrenal insufficiency; due to decreased mineralocorticoid production.
- Third space loss (e.g. ruptured urinary bladder); low sodium concentration of urine results in movement of sodium into the abdominal fluid.
- Free water intake without access to sufficient sodium.
- Iatrogenic; excessive administration of hypotonic fluids (e.g. 5% dextrose)
○ *Pseudohyponatremia* has been observed due to hyperlipidemia, hyperproteinemia, and hyperglycemia.
○ *Treatment* depends on the duration of hyponatremia.
  - $Na^+$ deficit $=$ (desired $[Na^+]-$ actual $[Na^+])\times0.6\times$ body weight (kg).
  - *Acute hyponatremia* can be rapidly corrected.
    ▪ Hypertonic saline ($3.0–7.2\%$ NaCl, 2–6 ml/kg) can be used to correct the serum $[Na^+]$.
    ▪ The change in $Na^+$ can be determined using *Adrogue's* formula:

$$\text{Change in}\left[Na^+\right]=\frac{\text{Infusate}\left[Na^+\right]-\text{Patient's}\left[Na^+\right]}{\text{Total body water}+1\,\text{L of hypertonic}}$$

Where "Total body water" $=$ Body weight (kg)$\times0.6$ in adults, 0.7 in foals.
*Example:* 70 kg foal with a $Na^+$ of 126 mEq/l, to be corrected with 5% hypertonic saline to 140 mEq/l.
$[Na^+]$ in Hypertonic saline solutions mEq/l:
0.9% NaCl $=$ 154
3.0% NaCl $=$ 513
5.0% NaCl $=$ 855
7.2% NaCl $=$ 1232

$$\text{Change in}\left[Na^+\right]\text{using}\,5\%\text{NaCl}=\frac{855\ \text{mEq/l}-124\ \text{mEq/l}}{\left(0.7\times70\,\text{kg}\right)+11}$$

○ Yields a 14.62 mEq increase in $[Na^+]$ if 1 l of 5% NaCl is administered.
○ To correct the $[Na^+]$ from 126 to 140 mEq/l, would require 14 mEq/l; therefore, 1 l of 5.0% NaCl can correct this deficit, which corresponds to 14 ml/kg.
  - *Chronic hyponatremia* must be corrected slowly. Rapid correction of chronic hyponatremia results in irreparable demyelination of neurons.
    ▪ Serum $[Na^+]$ should be increased slowly at no more than 0.5–1 mEq/l/hr.
    ▪ In hypovolemic patients, isotonic crystalloid replacement solutions with 130–140 mEq/l of sodium can be administered at a rate of 2–4 ml/kg/hr. Recheck serum $[Na^+]$ frequently in order to ensure that it is not being corrected too rapidly.
    ▪ In patients that are hypervolemic, furosemide (0.12 mg/kg/hr, IV) can be administered in combination with isotonic crystalloid replacement fluid. Recheck serum $[Na^+]$ frequently in order to ensure that it is not being corrected too rapidly.

## B  Hypernatremia (>155 mEq/l)

○ *Clinical signs* due to hypernatremia include third eyelid prolapse, myoclonus of the neck, and tail swishing. Chronic hypernatremia results in development of *idiogenic osmoles* that maintain osmolarity within cells in the face of hypernatremia. Too rapid correction of hypernatremia can result in cellular swelling and cerebral edema, as with hyponatremia, due to the presence of idiogenic osmoles.

- o *Causes* can be divided into two categories:
  - – *Pure water loss*:
    - ■ Water deprivation.
    - ■ Respiratory losses (hyperventilation).
    - ■ Lack of thirst mechanism; disease process affecting the thirst center (e.g. neoplasia).
    - ■ Administration of loop diuretics (e.g. furosemide).
  - – *Sodium excess*:
    - ■ Salt intoxication.
    - ■ Feeding electrolytes with not enough free water (e.g., inappropriate preparation of foal milk replacer).
    - ■ Hypertonic fluid administration.
- o *Treatment* depends on the duration of the hypernatremia.
  - – Acute hypernatremia can be corrected rapidly.
  - – Chronic hypernatremia should be corrected slowly. Rapid correction of hypernatremia can result in cerebral edema due to presence of idiogenic osmoles.
    - ■ Serum $[Na^+]$ should be decreased slowly at no more than 0.5 mEq/l/hr.
    - ■ Administration of low $[Na^+]$ solutions (e.g. 0.45% saline) with low $[Na^+]$ concentration will have a dilutional effect on plasma $[Na^+]$.

## II  Potassium

- • Potassium is the major intracellular cation.
- • The relatively high concentration of potassium inside of the cell in comparison to outside of the cell is maintained by the Na-K-ATPase pump which moves sodium out of the cell in exchange for potassium.
- • Reference values in plasma are 3.1–4.3 mEq/l.
- • Potassium is primarily obtained from the diet with high bioavailability (as high 95%).
- • Potassium is primarily eliminated by the kidneys.
  - o Physiologic roles of potassium include:
  - o Maintaining intracellular osmolarity.
  - o Maintaining transmembrane potential.
  - o Developing action potentials in muscles and nerves.

### A  Hypokalemia (<3.1 mEq/l)

- o *Clinical signs* include:
  - – Muscle weakness (most commonly reported clinical sign).
  - – Electrocardiogram changes due to a more negative resting membrane potential (increased P wave amplitude, prolonged PR interval, reduction in T wave amplitude).
  - – Associated with higher incidence of arrhythmias.
  - – Ileus.
- o *Causes* include:
  - – Decreased intake (low potassium diet, anorexia).
  - – Increased loss (diarrhea, sweat, third space loss).

- ○ *Treatment* is aimed at slow replacement of potassium.
  - – Oral or IV administration of potassium.
  - – Do not exceed 0.5 mEq/kg/hr rate of infusion.

**B  Hyperkalemia (>6.0 mEq/l)**

- ○ *Clinical signs* include:
  - ■ Muscle weakness, tremors.
  - ■ Electrocardiogram changes due to less negative resting membrane potential (tall T waves, small/flat P waves, widening of the QRS complex, asystole).
- ○ *Causes* of hyperkalemia can be divided into three categories:
  - – *Increased intake*:
    - ■ Iatrogenic administration of potassium.
    - ■ Oral intake (unlikely cause).
  - – *Transcellular shifts*:
    - ■ *Hyperkalemic periodic paralysis* (HYPP): hyperkalemia due to a defective sodium channel (see Chapter 38).
    - ■ *Rhabdomyolysis*: hyperkalemia due to release of potassium from damaged myocytes, exacerbated by renal injury due to myoglobin.
    - ■ *Hemolysis*: increased plasma potassium due to red blood cell lysis associated with hemolytic anemia, exacerbated by renal injury. Hemolysis is also the source of *pseudohyperkalemia* in blood samples that have been inappropriately handled or stored. The red blood cell $[K^+]$ in healthy horses is approximately 95 mEq/l.
    - ■ *Metabolic acidosis*: theoretically could cause a shift of potassium from within the cell to outside of the cell.
  - – *Vigorous exercise*.
- ○ *Urinary system etiology* (inability to excrete potassium):
  - ■ Renal dysfunction.
  - ■ Uroabdomen/ruptured urinary bladder.
- ○ *Treatment* of hyperkalemia is recommended if plasma [K] exceeds 6 mEq/l.
  - – Identify and correct the underlying cause.
  - – Fluid type and administration rate is dictated by the patient's volume status at the time. All isotonic crystalloid replacement solutions will have a dilutional effect on the plasma potassium concentration. Consider hypertonic saline if $[Na^+]$ is low, for rapid volume expansion.
  - – Shift potassium back into cells.
    - ■ Potassium is transported into the cell with glucose by insulin.
    - ■ *Dextrose* (0.25–0.5 g/kg, IV) to cause release of endogenous insulin, and prevent hypoglycemia associated with insulin administration.
    - ■ Regular *insulin* (0.05–0.1 U/kg, IV).
  - – Protect the heart from arrhythmogenic effect of hyperkalemia.
    - ■ *Calcium gluconate* 23% (0.2–0.4 ml/kg, IV), slowly over 15 minutes.
    - ■ Restores the difference between resting membrane potential and threshold potential.
  - – Recheck potassium and glucose plasma concentrations every 30–60 minutes throughout treatment.

## III  Chloride

- Chloride is the major extracellular anion.
- Reference values in plasma are 95–104 mEq/l.
- Chloride is primarily obtained via the diet and eliminated by the kidneys.
  - Chloride concentrations are generally interpreted relative to sodium concentrations:

$$\text{Corrected}\left[\text{Cl}^-\right] = \text{Measured}\left[\text{Cl}^-\right] \times \frac{\text{Normal}\left[\text{Na}^+\right]}{\text{Measured}\left[\text{Na}^+\right]}$$

### A  Hypochloremia (<90 mEq/l)

- *Clinical signs* often consistent with hyponatremia as the two abnormalities often co-exist.
- *Causes* of hypochloremia can be grouped into three different categories:
  - *Increased loss*:
    - Renal excretion; due to renal failure, *furosemide* administration, or overzealous fluid administration.
    - Metabolic acidosis; causing decreased re-absorption of chloride.
    - Gastrointestinal losses; due to decreased absorption or increased secretion.
    - Chloride sequestration.
    - Sweat; prolonged exercise in hot conditions can result in significant loss of chloride via sweat.
  - *Decreased intake*:
    - Decreased chloride intake in feed can cause mild hypochloremia.
  - *Dilutional effect*, relative water excess:
    - Sequestration of fluid (e.g. uroabdomen).
    - Third space losses (e.g. peritonitis, uroabdomen).
- *Treatment:*
  - Is aimed at correcting the underlying cause of the hypochloremia.

### B  Hyperchloremia (>110 mEq/l)

- *Clinical signs* often attributable to either accompanying acidosis (e.g. depression, anorexia, colic, hyperventilation) or hypernatremia (central nervous system signs).
- *Causes* can are divided into three categories:
  - *Increased intake of chloride*:
    - Feeding diets with low dietary cation-anion balance.
  - *Chloride retention*:
    - Renal tubular acidosis resulting in chloride retention.
    - Acetazolamide therapy for HYPP.
  - *Contraction of total body water*:
    - Water deprivation.
    - Hyperventilation.
- *Treatment:*
  - Is aimed at correcting the underlying abnormality.

## IV  Calcium

- Total body calcium is primarily (>99%) stored in the skeleton. Calcium in tissues and blood is responsible for vital physiologic processes including cardiovascular function (cardiac myocyte action potential and pacemaker activity), muscle contraction, neurotransmission, enzyme function, and blood coagulation.
- Reference values in plasma are 5.4–6.7 mEq/l for total calcium. Ionized calcium represents approximately 50% of these values.
- Calcium is carried in the plasma in three forms:
  - Protein-bound.
  - Ionized.
    - Ionized calcium is considered the "active" form of calcium in the blood.
  - Complexed (in the form of citrate, bicarbonate, lactate, etc.).
- Calcium balance in the body is controlled by parathyroid home, vitamin D, and calcitonin.

### A  Hypocalcemia (<5.4 mEq/l)

- *Clinical signs* include depression, fatigue, synchronous diaphragmatic flutter, tachycardia, tachypnea, muscle fasciculations, recumbency, opisthotonos, and seizures.
- *Causes* of hypocalcemia include:
  - *Gastrointestinal disease*:
    - Colic: decreased gastrointestinal motility results in sequestration of calcium in the intestine.
    - Diarrhea: increased fecal loss of calcium.
  - *Endotoxemia/sepsis*: impaired parathyroid hormone function.
  - *Lactation*: usually within seven days of parturition.
  - *Secondary hyperparathyroidism*: horses fed diets of low Ca : P ratio.
  - *Primary hypoparathyroidism*: decreased parathyroid hormone secretion leading to low circulating calcium.
  - *Cantharidin toxicity*: ingestion of blister beetles from alfalfa hay.
- *Treatment*:
  - Includes administration of calcium gluconate (23%, 0.5–1 ml/kg/hr, IV) or elemental calcium (0.1–0.4 mg/kg/min, IV), and resolution of the inciting cause.

### B  Hypercalcemia (>6.7 mEq/l)

- *Clinical signs* of hypercalcemia include cardiac arrhythmias, muscle weakness, and polyuria. More commonly observed are clinical signs resulting from the primary disease that has caused the hypercalcemia.
- *Causes* include:
  - *Chronic renal failure*: (unique to horses, as most species develop hypocalcemia) high absorption of calcium from the gastrointestinal tract in horses is unable to be excreted by the diseased kidney.
  - *Hypervitaminosis D*: commonly due to toxin ingestion.

– *Malignancy*: tumors that secrete parathyroid hormone related peptide, causing an increase in calcium. Common neoplasms include squamous cell carcinoma and lymphosarcoma.
– *Primary hyperparathyroidism*: increased production of parathyroid hormone secreting cells due to neoplasia or hyperplasia. Rare in horses.
  ○ *Treatment:*
    – Includes administration of calcium free fluids to dilute plasma calcium and *furosemide* to enhance renal excretion of calcium.

## Suggested Reading

Fielding, C.L. and Magdesian, K.G. (2015). *Equine Fluid Therapy*. Oxford, UK: Wiley Blackwell.
Snyder, L.B.C. and Wendt-Hornickle, E. (2013). General anesthesia in horses on fluid and electrolyte therapy. *Vet. Clin. North Am. Equine Pract.* 29: 169–178.
Toribio, R.E. (2011). Disorders of calcium and phosphate metabolism in horses. *Vet. Clin. North Am. Equine Pract.* 27: 129–147.

## Fluid Therapy

### Christopher K. Smith

- A recent systematic review referred to the literature, albeit sparse, regarding fluid therapy in companion animals as "descriptive" and difficult to apply to clinical practice. The following chapter focuses on current, applicable evidence and expert opinion.

## I  Introduction

- The primary goal of administering intravascular (IV) fluids in the peri-anesthetic setting is restoration and maintenance of intra vascular volume to optimize hemodynamics and ultimately tissue perfusion.
  ○ This is particularly important in equine patients who may suffer from *myopathy*, *neuropathy*, and subsequent *poor anesthetic recovery*, if tissue perfusion is compromised.
- In addition to maintenance fluid requirements, some patients will present fluid deplete and will require thorough assessment and fluid replenishment, ideally before anesthesia.
- *Hypotension* and inadequate tissue perfusion can arise from a multitude of causes (e.g. reduced myocardial contractility). However, relative hypovolemia from inhalant anesthetic mediated vasodilation is to be expected when these agents are used for maintenance of general anesthesia.
- Thus, the aim of peri-anesthetic fluid administration should be to restore fluid deficits and combat anesthetic induced alterations in cardiovascular function.
  ○ IV fluid administration should not be the only method employed to combat anesthetic induced cardiovascular depression (see Intraoperative Hypotension Chapter 38)
- Fluid therapy protocols, just as anesthetic protocols, need to be tailored to the individual patient based on findings from the history, physical examination and diagnostic tests. The protocol can then be executed in a goal-directed fashion with measurable endpoints to avoid the detriments of both *hypo* and *hypervolemia*.

## II Total body water

- Approximately 60% of an adult mammal's mass (kg) is comprised of water (total body water [TBW]).
  - Approximately 2/3 (66%) of TBW is intracellular fluid (ICF) and the remaining 1/3 (33%) is extracellular fluid (ECF).
    - Of the ECF, 75% is typically in the interstitial space while the remaining 25% makes up the intravascular plasma volume (see Figure 8.1).
  - Blood volume, which includes red cell mass, is approximately 8% of the animal's mass (kg).
    - However, blood volume varies with the breed, from approximately 6% in Draft horses to 10% in Thoroughbreds.
  - Plasma volume is approximately 5% of body mass (kg).
- TBW in foals is 72–74%, of the body mass (kg) which is lower than the neonates of most other species.
- ECF volume in foals is about 30% greater than per kg than in adult horses.
  - The capillary function and responsiveness of neonatal animals is likely not fully developed:
    - Vasomotor tone is less responsive to stimuli, and capillary oncotic reflection coefficients are typically lower in neonates, allowing more capillary leakage of small and large intravascular solutes as well as fluid.
    - Thus, while neonatal animals may have a higher total body water composition, their ability to handle large intravascular fluid loads, or at least maintain them in the intravascular space, may be reduced.
  - Caution should be taken when administering large volumes of fluids to neonatal foals.

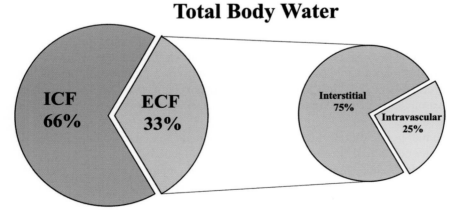

**Figure 8.1** Division of total body water in the healthy adult horse. ECF, extracellular fluid; ICF, intracellular fluid.

## III   Solute distribution

- Solutes are distributed heterogeneously in fluids based on the presence of semi permeable membranes throughout the body (e.g. cell membranes, vascular endothelium) which either exclude or selectively allow solute movement.

*Effective osmoles*
- Are defined as solutes that cannot cross a semi permeable membrane and thus create an osmotic pressure, causing water to move across the membrane in a direction from lower to higher osmotic pressure (i.e. osmosis).

*Effective osmolality*
- Is the difference in pressure generated by osmotic forces between two compartments.

*Osmolality*
- Is defined as the number of osmotically active particles per *kilogram* of solvent.

*Osmolarity*
- Is defined as the number of osmotically active particles per *liter* of solution.
- For clinical purposes, the differences in definition are irrelevant.
- Osmolality is dependent solely on the number of *particles* in solution and *not* their size.
- In plasma, osmolality is largely determined by the ions $Na^+$ and $K^+$, and by glucose and urea.

$$\text{Plasma osmolality}\left(\frac{\text{mOsm}}{\text{kg}}\right) = 2\left(Na^+ + K^+\right) + \frac{\text{Glucose}\left(\frac{\text{mg}}{\text{dL}}\right)}{18} + \frac{\text{BUN}\left(\frac{\text{mg}}{\text{dL}}\right)}{2.8}$$

- Plasma osmolality can be either calculated (see equation) or measured (e.g. freezing point depression), and is normally between 275 and 310 mOsm/kg.

*Colloid oncotic pressure* (COP)
- Proteins, such as albumin, also generate an osmotic pressure and this is termed COP.
- (COP) and can be measured with a colloid osmometer.
- Other than protein concentration, which is typically much higher in plasma than in the interstitial space, these two compartments typically have very similar constituents.
- The subtle, and clinically negligible differences between plasma and interstitial fluid cation and anion concentrations are due to the *Gibbs-Donnan* effect.
- Electroneutrality across a membrane is maintained via slightly different ion concentrations across the membrane because of non-diffusible, negatively charged proteins located in the plasma and much less so in the interstitium.
- The electrochemical gradient produced via this unequal distribution of ions creates a potential difference, and can be calculated using the *Nernst* or, perhaps more completely, by the *Goldman-Hodgkin-Katz* voltage equation.

*ICF versus ECF*
- The largest discrepancy in solute distribution is between the ICF and ECF (see Figure 8.2).
- The major ECF cation and anion is $Na^+$ and $Cl^-$, respectively.

| mEq/L | Plasma | Interstitial | Intracellular |
| --- | --- | --- | --- |
| $Na^+$ | 138 | 145 | 12 |
| $K^+$ | 4 | 4 | 140 |
| $Ca^{2+}$ | 2 | 2 | 4 |
| $Mg^{2+}$ | 2 | 2 | 34 |
| $Cl^-$ | 101 | 112 | 4 |
| $HCO_3^-$ | 24 | 27 | 12 |
| Phosphates | 2 | 2 | 40 |
| Protein | 14 | 1 | 50 |

**Figure 8.2**  Division of charged particles among plasma, interstitium, and intracellular spaces.

- The major ICF cation and anions are $K^+$ and proteins and phosphates, respectively.
- While some membranes are permeable to $Na^+$ and $K^+$, these ions are considered *effective* osmoles due to the activity of cell membrane bound $Na^+/K^+$-ATPase creating significant differences in these solutes' concentrations between intra and extra cellular spaces.
- Most cell membranes are permeable to water, and distribution of these osmotically active solutes is what determines the volume of fluid, and therefore their concentration, in each space.
- At osmotic equilibrium, solute concentrations on either side of a membrane are undisturbed, and thus there is no gradient for osmosis to occur between the two fluid compartments.
- A loss of water results in solute concentration and osmolality changes, and thus osmosis will occur.

## IV  Fluid dynamics

- While separation of the interstitium and intravascular compartments is crucial to maintaining circulating fluid volume, exchange between these compartments, and ultimately the intracellular compartment, must occur in order to maintain delivery and removal of nutrients and waste products, respectively.
- Exchange of fluid and solutes between plasma and the interstitium occurs in *capillary beds*, and is influenced by pressure differentials on both sides of a physiologic membrane (i.e. vascular endothelium).
- *Starling* originally described four forces, whose sum dictated whether fluid was to be filtered or reabsorbed by the capillary:

*Capillary hydrostatic pressure ($P_c$)*
- The blood pressure in the capillary (filtration).

*Capillary oncotic pressure ($\pi_C$)*
- The osmotic pressure generated by the protein molecules within the intravascular compartment (reabsorption).

*Interstitial hydrostatic pressure* ($P_i$)

  ○ The pressure generated by the presence of fluid within the interstitium (reabsorption).

*Interstitial oncotic pressure* ($\pi_i$)

  ○ The pressure generated by the presence of interstitial protein (filtration).

## A  Starling's equation

$$J_V / A = \kappa \left[ \left( P_c - P_i \right) - \sigma \left( \pi_C - \pi_i \right) \right]$$

$J_V/A$ = Volume filtered per unit area
$\kappa$ = Hydraulic conductance
$\sigma$ = Reflection coefficient

  ○ The equation indicates permeability of the capillary wall in regard to protein movement.
  ○ Ultimately, according to *Starling*'s equation, these four forces produced a net filtration at the *arteriolar end* of the capillary bed, and net absorption at the *venular end* (see Figure 8.3).
    – *Filtration* is facilitated by the high $P_c$ at the arteriolar end of the capillary and a relatively low $P_i$.
    – *Reabsorption* of fluid that had previously been filtered back into the intravascular space is facilitated by a high $\pi_C$ at the venular end, and a very low $\pi_i$ due to low protein concentrations in this space.

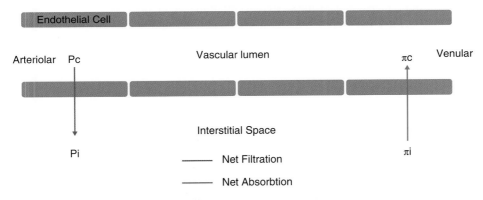

**Figure 8.3** Traditional Starling approach to fluid movement between the vascular and interstitial space.

## B  Revised Starling equation

  ○ Recent literature has shown that Starling's original model described in 1896 is likely to be inaccurate. This is evidenced by:
    – The discovery of significant amounts of protein in the interstitial space; thus, the interstitial space should generate a much more substantial $\pi_i$ than was previously thought.
    – The discovery of the *endothelial surface layer* (ESL).

- The ESL is made up of the following:
  - *Endothelial glycocalyx* – negatively charged, carbohydrate rich layer, which coats the luminal side of vascular endothelium.
  - Glycocalyx bound plasma proteins such as albumin.
  - A volume of fixed plasma.
- Vascular permeability, interactions between circulating blood cells and the vessel wall, rheology, and other factors are all heavily influenced by the ESL.
- Since the non-circulating volume of plasma (*subglycocalyx*) and its constituents in the ESL are in equilibrium with circulating plasma, pressure differentials develop across the *glycocalyx* ultimately producing a small amount of filtrate through small breaks in the ESL.
  - This is why the larger than previously thought protein concentration in the interstitium does not affect the amount of filtrate produced.

*Revised Starling equation:*

$$J_V \,/\, A = \kappa \left[ \left( P_c - P_i \right) - \sigma \left( \pi_p - \pi_{sg} \right) \right]$$

$J_V/A$ = Volume filtered per unit area
$\kappa$ = Hydraulic conductance
$\sigma$ = Reflection coefficient
$\pi_p$ = Oncotic pressure on the plasma side of the ESL
$\pi_{sg}$ = Oncotic pressure in the sub-glycocalyx space
- The net filtration in this "revised" model is much less than originally hypothesized, which is corroborated by studies showing that lymph flow is much lower than the capillary filtration predicted by Starling's original equation (see Figure 8.4).
  - Ultimately, *filtration* occurs from the arteriolar end throughout the length of the capillary bed and is significantly reduced by the end.

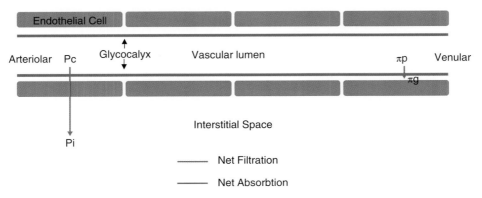

**Figure 8.4** Revised Starling approach to fluid movement between the vascular and interstitial space incorporating the endothelial surface layer.

– *Reabsorption* does *not* occur in most capillary beds, and the volume of fluid filtered is dealt with by the *lymphatic* system ultimately returning fluid to the intravascular space.

## V Administration of exogenous fluids

- When fluid, solutes or both are lost from a compartment, changes occur in the tonicity of that compartment.
- Tonicity is a term which describes the *effective osmolality* of a solution.
  - If water is lost from the ECF in excess of solute, the fluid that is lost is considered *hypotonic*.
  - If solute is lost in excess of water, the fluid lost is *hypertonic*.
  - If both solute and water are equally lost so that osmolality does not change, the loss is considered *isotonic*.

*Dehydration:*
  - The ECF loses water and the osmolality increases (*hypotonic fluid loss*).
  - *Clinically*, this is detectable by an increase in packed cell volume and total solid concentration, and abnormal physical examination findings (e.g. skin tent, tacky mucous membranes).
  - Water from the ICF will diffuse into the ECF until a new equilibrium is established. The net loss of water is from the ICF, and thus needs to be replaced.

*Hypovolemia:*
  - In contrast to dehydration, hypovolemia is loss of fluid from the intravascular compartment.
  - Both situations are encountered commonly in clinical practice and typically require exogenous fluid administration as part of a treatment plan.
  - *Hypovolemia* typically presents with more acute pathology and consequences (e.g. hypotension, inadequate tissue perfusion), and thus fluids are typically administered rapidly.
  - *Dehydration* typically occurs over a longer period and because fluids are ultimately intended to replace losses from the ICF, administration is often over a longer period to allow more gradual re-equilibration.

*Goals:*
  - In the peri-anesthetic setting, the goals of fluid therapy should be to:
    - Restore and maintain circulating volume.
    - Increase the pressure gradient for venous return.
    - Optimize cardiac preload and thus cardiac output.
    - Meet requirements for tissue perfusion.
    - Combat insensible fluid losses (e.g. those lost via the administration of dry respiratory gases).
  - When compared to the compartment of interest (e.g. plasma), a solution can be:
    - *Isotonic*
    - *Hypertonic*
    - *Hypotonic*

A  **Crystalloids**

- o Crystalloids are the most commonly used fluids in companion animals.
- o *Balanced crystalloid* solutions are made up of various electrolyte profiles and water, are relatively isotonic to plasma, contain similar constituents to plasma, and typically are buffered (see Table 8.1).
  - – Examples include: Plasmalyte A, Normosol-R and lactated Ringers.
  - – These solutions are often the fluid of choice for horses needing replacement therapy or undergoing anesthesia, because their electrolyte profile is similar to that of plasma, and they provide a means of maintaining normal body pH through a bicarbonate precursor (e.g. acetate).

*Efficiency ratio*

- o The efficiency ratio is a comparison between the increase in blood volume relative to the volume of IV fluid infused.
- o Isotonic crystalloids rapidly redistribute out of the IV space and into the interstitial fluid.
- o The efficiency ratio of these fluids is typically around 0.4 (in dogs) at 30 minutes after administration.
  - – Only about 25–30% of the volume infused remains in the IV space 30–60 minutes after infusion of isotonic crystalloids.
- o Thus, 3–4x the deficit typically needs to be infused.
- o This may result in a significant volume of fluid entering the interstitium, leading to edema which can have negative sequelae such as:
  - – Ileus.
  - – Impediment for efficient diffusion of oxygen.
  - – Increase morbidity and mortality.
- o Typical rates of administration of isotonic crystalloid solutions in adult, anesthetized equine patients are 5–10 ml/kg/hr.

*Normal saline (NS)*

- o NS is an isotonic crystalloid but is not considered balanced and it can be classified as an acidifying solution.
- o The absence of a buffer and the large concentration of chloride relative to the plasma chloride concentration result in a net pH of around 5.

*Hypertonic saline solutions (HSS)*

- o Consists of water and increased concentrations of electrolytes ($Na^+$ and $Cl^-$) making their osmolality far greater than that of plasma.
- o For example, 7.2% hypertonic saline has an osmolality of 2464 mOsm/l vs. plasma's 300 mOsm/l.
- o Due to an increase in intravascular osmotic pressure gradient, HSS expands the plasma volume by drawing fluid primarily from the intracellular space to the IV space.
- o Because the vast majority of fluid that is expanding the IV space is coming from other locations in the body (e.g. cells), the administration of HSS does very little for TBW deficits.
  - – It is imperative that the administration of HSS is followed by other fluids (e.g. isotonic crystalloids)
- o The *efficiency ratio* for HSS 30 minutes after administration is 2 (in dogs), meaning the effectiveness of plasma expansion is much greater than that of isotonic crystalloids.
  - – E.g. Administration of 2 l of HSS will expand the plasma volume by 4 l.

**Table 8.1** Physicochemical characteristics of commonly used intravenous fluids.

| Fluid | Na$^+$ | Cl$^-$ | K$^+$ | Ca$^{++}$ | Mg$^{++}$ | Lactate | Acetate | Gluconate | Osmolarity | pH |
|---|---|---|---|---|---|---|---|---|---|---|
| Normal saline (0.9%) | 154 | 154 | 0 | 0 | 0 | 0 | 0 | 0 | 308 | 5.0 |
| Lactated Ringer's | 130 | 109 | 4 | 3 | 0 | 28 | 0 | 0 | 272 | 6.5 |
| Normosol-R | 140 | 98 | 5 | 0 | 3 | 0 | 27 | 23 | 294 | 6.5–7.6 |
| Plasmalyte-A | 140 | 98 | 5 | 0 | 3 | 0 | 27 | 23 | 294 | 6.5–7.6 |
| Hypertonic saline (7.2%) | 1232 | 1232 | 0 | 0 | 0 | 0 | 0 | 0 | 2464 | 4.5–7 |

- – This effect of HSS has been corroborated even in animals with clinical dehydration (including horses).
- ○ Therefore, particularly due to the large volume of isotonic crystalloids that would be needed to expand an adult horse's plasma volume effectively, HSS is often considered a mainstay of treatment when addressing hypovolemic horses (e.g. those presenting with colic) even if clinical evidence of dehydration is present.
  - – The recommended dose is 4–6 ml/kg (7.2% NaCl), administered over 10–15 minutes.
  - – It is common practice for the author to administer 2 l of 7.2% HSS (~4 ml/kg) to an adult horse (e.g. 500 kg) suffering from colic and cardiovascular depression prior to induction of anesthesia.
  - – Isotonic crystalloids have resulted in similar outcomes when compared to hypertonic crystalloids, but hypertonic solutions can be administered faster for prompt resuscitation.
- ○ HSS has also been shown to improve myocardial contractility and reduce SVR.
  - – These parameters combined with an increase in *preload* lead to improvements in cardiac output and delivery of oxygen.
- ○ However, the beneficial effects of HSS are typically short lived by virtue of the fact that its composition is just electrolytes and water, both of which will rapidly redistribute out of the IV space.

*Anti-inflammatory effects of HSS:*
- – In addition to its cardiovascular effects, HSS has anti-inflammatory actions.
- – In endotoxemic models, HSS administration was associated with a reduction in LPS-stimulated iNOS expression and nitric oxide release.
- – In an *ischemic* model, HSS *decreased* the activation of NF-κB, TNFα, ICAM-1, and *increased* the expression of the anti-inflammatory cytokine IL-10.

*Hypotonic crystalloids*
- ○ Are rarely used in equine patients but may be considered in patients where both the administration of fluids to replace deficits and a *low sodium* load is desirable.
- ○ Used as a slow infusion or maintenance fluid only (not as a bolus).

## B  Colloids

- ○ Colloids are either natural or synthetic solutions of macromolecules which exert a COP. *Natural colloids include*:
  - – Blood component products (e.g. plasma, albumin, see Chapter 10)
  *Synthetic colloids include*:
  - – Hydroxyethyl starch (HES) and dextrans.
- ○ The key difference between crystalloids and colloids is that the latter contain large molecules, (*synthetic* or *natural*) which cannot easily cross capillary endothelium, and thus typically have longer residence time in the IV compartment while exerting a COP and opposing plasma filtration.
  - – These molecules help to expand and maintain plasma volume.
  - – HES had an efficiency ratio of 1.5 at 30 minutes post administration.
  - – Any disease process that alters the normal activity of the ESL may lead to altered kinetics of synthetic colloids, and thus their IV residence time.

*Synthetic colloids*

- o Are commercially available and utilized when plasma volume expansion with maintenance of COP is desired.
  - – In addition, they can be used in patients with reduced COP (e.g. hypoproteinemia) to improve COP and reduce filtration of fluid into the interstitium (i.e. edema).
- o HES is by far the most common synthetic colloid administered to horses.
- o HES is a solution of synthetic starch polymer (e.g. *amylopectin*) suspended in isotonic crystalloid.
- o HES solutions are typically labeled with several numbers such as 6% HES 130/0.4 in 0.9% NaCl:
  - – 6% = 6 g of HES/100 ml of solution (isotonic).
  - – 130 = mean molecular weight (kDa).
  - – 0.4 = molar substitution of glucose with hydroxyethyl group.
  - – 0.9% NaCl – the above are suspended in normal saline.

*Clinical use of colloids*:

- o A commonly utilized methodology for rapid, effective plasma expansion in horses is to administer a combination of HES and HSS.
  - – E.g. HSS 5 ml/kg and HES 5 ml/kg.
  - – Again, this should be followed by isotonic crystalloids.
  - – This allows for effective plasma expansion, particularly in large, hypovolemic animals where the time required to administer a large volumes would limit the effectiveness of isotonic crystalloids.

*Adverse effects of colloids:*

- o Colloid use in other species (e.g. dogs, humans) has been associated with adverse effects such as:
  - – Bleeding diathesis.
  - – Acute kidney injury.
  - – Increased mortality in septic patients.
- o These adverse effects seem to be dependent on the specific formulation of synthetic colloid used (e.g. tetra vs. hetastarch) and the species they are used in.
- o The veterinary labeled product *Vetstarch* is a commonly used tetrastarch labeled for use in small animals with a recommended dose of 20 ml/kg/day, although some studies report up to 50 ml/kg/day.
- o There is currently no evidence in the equine literature that the use of colloids versus crystalloids has any impact on mortality in critically ill patients.

## Suggested Reading

Dunkel, B. (2020). Science-in-brief: the role of the glycocalyx in critically ill patients with reference to the horse. *Equine Vet. J.* 52: 790–793.

Fielding, L. (2014). Crystalloid and colloid therapy. *Vet. Clin. North Am. Equine Pract.* 30: 415–425.

Pantaleon, L. (2010). Fluid therapy in equine patients: small-volume fluid resuscitation. *Compend. Contin. Educ. Vet.* 32: E1–E6.

Roska, S., Morello, S., Rajamanickam, V., and Smith, L. (2018). Effect of hetastarch 130/0.4 on plasma osmolality, colloid osmotic pressure and total protein in horses anesthetized for elective surgical procedures. *Vet. Rec.* 183: 127.

Snyder, L. and Wendt-Hornickle, E. (2013). General anesthesia in horses on fluid and electrolyte therapy. *Vet. Clin. North Am. Equine Pract.* 29: 169–178.

Van Galen, G. and Hallowell, G. (2019). Hydroxyethyl starches in equine medicine. *J. Vet. Emerg. Crit. Care* 29: 349–359.

Woodcock, T.E. and Woodcock, T.M. (2012). Revised Starling equation and the glycocalyx model of transvascular fluid exchange: an improved paradigm for prescribing intravenous fluid therapy. *Br. J. Anaesth.* 108: 384–394.

# 9

# Acid-Base Physiology

## Traditional Approach

*Alex Valverde and Tom Doherty*

- Acid-base interpretation can be performed using two different methods:
  - The first is the *traditional* approach, which is based on evaluating plasma $[HCO_3^-]$ and/or base excess to measure disturbances in metabolic acid-base balance.
  - The second is the *physicochemical* approach (*Stewart method*) which is based on the quantification of independent variables ($PCO_2$, weak acids, and the strong ion difference) and dependent variables ($HCO_3^-$ and $H^+$ ions).

*Acidemia*
  - Refers to a blood $[H^+]$ above the normal range (36–44 nmol/l or nEq/l) and a corresponding pH below normal (<7.36).

*Acidosis*
  - Is a physiologic condition that would cause acidemia if it were allowed to go uncompensated.

*Alkalemia*
  - Refers to a blood $[H^+]$ below the normal range (36–44 nmol/l) and a corresponding pH above normal (>7.44).

*Alkalosis*
  - Is a physiological condition that would cause alkalemia if it were allowed to go uncompensated.

- Normally, acids and, to a lesser extent bases, are constantly being added to extracellular fluids (ECF), and in order for the body to maintain a physiological pH of 7.4 (a $[H^+]$ of 40 nEq/l) the following three processes are necessary:
  - Buffering by extracellular and intracellular buffers.
  - Alveolar ventilation to regulate $PaCO_2$.
  - Renal $H^+$ excretion to regulate plasma $[HCO_3^-]$.
- *Brönsted-Lowry* Theory
  - An acid is any compound that can donate a proton.
  - A proton is represented by the symbol $H^+$.

*Manual of Equine Anesthesia and Analgesia*, Second Edition. Edited by Tom Doherty, Alex Valverde, and Rachel A. Reed.

## I Traditional approach to acid-base interpretation

### A Henderson-Hasselbalch equation

$$pH = pK_a + \log\frac{[base]}{[acid]}$$

- $pH = -\log_{10}[H^+]$.
- This equation can be applied to any acid-base pair (*Isohydric principle*), although it is most commonly applied to carbonic acid and bicarbonate.
- $pK_a$ is the negative logarithm of the constant of dissociation for plasma carbonic acid.
  - The base is represented by $[HCO_3^-]$ and is regulated by kidney function.
  - The acid is represented by the solubility (expressed as a solubility coefficient $s$) of $CO_2$ and its partial pressure in arterial blood, and is therefore regulated by respiratory function. Thus, pH can be written as:

$$pH = pKa + \log\frac{[HCO_3^-]}{[s \times PaCO_2]}$$

  - The Henderson-Hasselbalch equation is derived from the reversible hydration reaction for $CO_2$ and from the reversible ionization of carbonic acid ($H_2CO_3$).

$$CO_2 + H_2O \overset{CA}{\rightleftarrows} H_2CO_3 \rightleftarrows H^+ + HCO_3^-$$

  - Gaseous $CO_2$ dissolves and combines with water to form $H_2CO_3$.
  - Carbonic anhydrase (CA) in red cells and renal tubular cells allows for this reaction to be up to 1000 times faster than in blood.
  - Carbonic acid is ionized and yields equivalent numbers of $H^+$ and $HCO_3^-$ ions.
  - Bicarbonate acts as an intermediate in removing $CO_2$ via gas exchange in the lungs.
  - Therefore, $HCO_3^-$ concentrations are dependent on the partial pressure of $CO_2$ in plasma.

*Lewis Acid*

*Note*: When $CO_2$ is dissolved in water the solution becomes acidic, this occurs in spite of the fact that $CO_2$ has no $H^+$ to donate, and thus cannot act as a Brönsted-Lowry acid. Carbon dioxide is considered a Lewis acid because of its ability to accept electrons.

*Values for the Henderson-Hasselbalch equation*

- $pKa = 6.1$ (for bicarbonate system).
- $HCO_3^- = 24\,mEq/l$.
- $PaCO_2 = 40\,mmHg$.
- $s = 0.03\,mEq/l/mmHg\ CO_2$ at $37\,°C$.

$$\text{Therefore, } pH = 6.1 + \log\left[24 / (0.03 \times 40)\right]$$
$$pH = 6.1 + \log(24 / 1.2)$$
$$pH = 6.1 + \log 20$$
$$pH = 6.1 + 1.3$$
$$pH = 7.4$$

B    **pH and hydrogen ions** (see Box 9.1)

- Hydrogen ion concentrations in the body are extremely low ($10^{-7}$ to $10^{-9}$ nEq/l).
- [H$^+$] is tightly regulated for enzymatic activities and biochemical reactions.
    - [H$^+$] is regulated by the lungs ($CO_2$) and the kidneys (by altering ion secretion).
- The higher the [H$^+$], the lower the pH.
    - For pH values in the clinical range (7.0–7.5) the relationship between pH and [H$^+$] is fairly linear.
- Hydrogen ions can be formed from water and can be destroyed by the formation of water.
    - It is generally agreed that watery solutions are *neutral* if the concentrations of the hydrogen ions equal the concentrations of the hydroxyl ions.
    - *Neutral* if [H$^+$] = [OH$^-$], *acidic* if [H$^+$] > [OH$^-$], and *alkaline* if [H$^+$] < [OH$^-$].
    - The [H$^+$] is always a dependent variable and is in a non-linear association with PCO$_2$, with the concentration of fully dissociated electrolytes (often termed "strong electrolytes") and weak acids (proteins).

C    **Buffers**

- Buffers serve as the first-line of defense and limit changes in pH resulting from the addition of acids and bases to body fluids.
- Buffers are weak acids or bases that function to minimize changes in pH by accepting or releasing H$^+$.

*The carbonic acid-bicarbonate buffer system*

- This is the main extracellular buffering system.

$$H_2O + CO_2 \leftrightarrow H_2CO_3 \leftrightarrow H^+ + HCO_3^-$$

- The first part of the reaction ($H_2O + CO_2 \leftrightarrow H_2CO_3$) is catalyzed towards the right in the red cell by carbonic anhydrase, but not in plasma, where the reaction is several thousand times slower.
- Carbonic acid is a volatile acid that is controlled by the respiratory system through $CO_2$ elimination.
- The fact that $HCO_3^-$ and PaCO$_2$ can be managed independently (kidneys and lungs, respectively) makes this an effective buffering system.
    - Increased PaCO$_2$ drives the reaction to the right.
    - Decreased PaCO$_2$ drives reaction to the left.

| Box 9.1    Relationship between Hydrogen Ion Concentration and pH | |
|---|---|
| pH | $= -\log_{10}[H^+]$ |
| 6.9 | 125 nEq/l |
| 7.0 | 100 nEq/l |
| 7.1 | 80 nEq/l |
| 7.2 | 64 nEq/l |
| 7.3 | 50 nEq/l |
| 7.4 | 40 nEq/l |
| 7.5 | 32 nEq/l |
| 7.6 | 25 nEq/l |

- *Adding an acid* load results in consumption of $HCO_3^-$ by $H^+$, and formation of $H_2CO_3$.
  - $H_2CO_3$ then forms $H_2O$ and $CO_2$.
- $PaCO_2$ is maintained within a narrow range via the respiratory drive.
- The reaction continues to move to the left as long as $CO_2$ is constantly eliminated or until $HCO_3^-$ is significantly depleted, making less $HCO_3^-$ available to bind $H^+$.
- At equilibrium, the relationship between the three reactants is expressed by the Henderson-Hasselbalch equation, which relates the concentration of dissolved $CO_2$ (i.e. $H_2CO_3$) to $PaCO_2$ ($0.03 \times PaCO_2$) in the following way:

$$pH = 6.10 + \log\left(\left[HCO_3^-\right]/0.03 \times PaCO_2\right)\left(\text{see Henderson} - \text{Hasselbalch equation}\right)$$

### Non-bicarbonate buffer systems

- Includes proteins (especially hemoglobin but also albumin), phosphate, and ammonium.
  - *Hemoglobin* is a more efficient buffer than *albumin* because of its higher concentration in blood and because of its higher buffer value (0.18 vs. 0.12 mEq/g/pH).
- Inorganic and organic phosphate compounds can function as buffers.
- Inorganic phosphates are major urinary buffers.
  - $H_2PO_4^- \rightleftarrows HPO_4^{2-} + H^+$
    - Organic phosphates act as intracellular buffers.
    - Organic phosphates include 2, 3-diphosphoglycerate (2, 3-DPG), glucose-1-phosphate, adenosine monophosphate (AMP), adenosine diphosphate (ADP), and adenosine triphosphate (ATP).

### Role of the renal system in buffering

- To maintain a normal pH, the kidneys must perform two physiologic functions.
  - Reabsorb all the filtered $HCO_3^-$. This mainly occurs in the proximal tubule.
    - Loss of $HCO_3^-$ is equal to the addition of an equimolar amount of $H^+$.
  - Excrete the $H^+$ load. This occurs in the collecting duct.
    - Loss of $H^+$ is equal to the addition of an equimolar amount of $HCO_3^-$.
- Ammonium ($NH_4^+$) is the weak acid of the strong base ammonia ($NH_3$), and it plays an important role in the kidney as a means for removing hydrogen ions from the body.

$$NH_4^+ \rightleftarrows NH_3 + H^+$$

  - Ammonia ($NH_3$), generated by enzymatic actions within the renal tubular epithelial cells, is more diffusible into the tubular lumen than ammonium ($NH_4^+$).
  - The high affinity of $NH_3$ for hydrogen ions produces $NH_4^+$ cations, and because of their nondiffusible properties they are trapped in the lumen and eliminated with the urine.

## D  Base excess

- Defined as the amount (mmol or mEq) of strong acid or strong base required to titrate extracellular fluid (11) to pH 7.40 with $PaCO_2 = 40$ mmHg at normal body temperature (*Accounts for $HCO_3^-$ buffering only*).
- Base excess quantifies the patient's total base excess or deficit from the normal buffer base at any given pH.

○ It is calculated from the measurement of pH, $PaCO_2$, and hematocrit (because red cells contain most of the buffer content, i.e. hemoglobin).
○ The value for base excess is obtained by multiplying the deviation in standard bicarbonate from normal by an empirical factor (1.2) that is related to the buffering capacity of red cells.
○ It is a true non-respiratory reflection of acid-base status.

## E Total $CO_2$ ($TCO_2$)

○ $TCO_2$ is an indirect measure of $HCO_3^-$.
○ It determines the $TCO_2$ in plasma.
○ It includes:
  – Ionized: which consists of $HCO_3^-$ mainly.
  – Un-ionized: $H_2CO_3$ and Dissolved $CO_2$.
○ $TCO_2 = HCO_3^- + \text{Dissolved } CO_2$
  – Dissolved $CO_2$ is approx. $1\,\text{mEq/l}$
  – $(0.03\,\text{mEq/l/mmHg} \times 40\,\text{mmHg} = 1.2\,\text{mEq/l})$
○ $TCO_2 = 24 + 1.2$
$$= 25.2$$

○ $HCO_3^- = \text{is approx.} TCO_2 - 1(25.2 - 1.2)$
$$= 24\,\text{mEq/l}$$

## F Anion gap

○ The anion gap (AG) is the difference between the sums of the positively and negatively charged electrolytes.
○ $\text{AG (mmol/l)} = (Na^+ + K^+) - (Cl^- + HCO_3^-) = (140 + 4) - (105 + 24) = 15$

*Note: $K^+$ is not always included in the calculation.*
○ The reference range is $16 \pm 4$ if $K^+$ is included, and ~12 if $K^+$ is excluded.
○ An AG outside the normal range indicates the presence of excess anions.

*Use of AG:* May signal the presence of an acidotic process, even when there is no base deficit.
○ $(Na^+ + \text{Unmeasured Cations}) - (Cl + HCO_3^-) = \text{Unmeasured Anions}$
  – $Na^+ - (Cl + HCO_3^-) = \text{Unmeasured Anions (UA)} - \text{Unmeasured Cations (UC)}$
  – Anion Gap = UA − UC
○ *Increased AG* – is an indication of the presence of a metabolic acidosis (↓ $[HCO_3^-]$). Thus, the AG is often used to screen for metabolic acidosis – especially in situations where *lactate* determination is not readily available.
○ However, because the AG is due mostly to *albumin*, an unmeasured anion, it is an unreliable indicator of hyperlactatemia in critically ill patients with low albumin concentrations.
  – In these patients, hypoalbuminemia may underestimate the AG.
○ Also, patients with cardiovascular shock can have a normal AG if the $[Cl^-]$ is increased subsequent to a decrease in $[HCO_3^-]$.

**G   Primary disturbances in acid-base** (see Table 9.1)

- ○ Four primary disturbances are recognized:
  - – Respiratory acidosis (increased $PaCO_2$).
  - – Respiratory alkalosis (decreased $PaCO_2$).
  - – Metabolic acidosis (decreased base excess or actual $[HCO3^-]$).
  - – Metabolic alkalosis (increased base excess or actual $[HCO_3^-]$).

  *Note*: *Respiratory acidosis* is the most common acid-base disturbance in healthy horses during anesthesia. *Metabolic acidosis* is most likely, albeit uncommon, to be encountered in horses with cardiovascular compromise presented for emergency intestinal surgery or in foals with bacteremia.
- ○ Combinations of these disturbances can occur as a result of compensatory mechanisms or acid-base derangements.
- ○ The body attempts to maintain the $[HCO_3^-]$ to $PaCO_2$ ratio at 20 : 1 by implementing changes in ventilation or renal function.
  - – In *m*etabolic acidosis, hyperventilation occurs to reduce $PaCO_2$.
  - – In re*spiratory acidosis*, renal conservation of $HCO_3^-$ occurs.

**Acute respiratory acidosis** (pH < 7.35, $PaCO_2$ > 45 mmHg)
- ○ Common in the anesthetized horse due primarily to anesthetic drugs decreasing minute ventilation, but can also result from severe ventilation-perfusion mismatch.
  - – Results in an increase in $PaCO_2$.
- ○ Ventilatory failure can also result from pulmonary disorders, hypoventilation due to CNS depression, and impaired function of respiratory muscles and nerves.
- ○ Increased $PaCO_2$ causes an increase in blood $[H^+]$ and a decrease in pH according to:

Table 9.1   Summary of acid-base disorders.

| Disorders | pH | $PaCO_2$ | $HCO_3^-$ | Base excess | SID |
|---|---|---|---|---|---|
| *Respiratory acidosis* | | | | | |
| Acute (uncompensated) | ↓ | ↑ | N | N | ↑ |
| Partly compensated | ↓ | ↑ | ↑ | ↑ | ↑ |
| Chronic (compensated) | N | ↑ | ↑ | ↑ | ↑ |
| *Respiratory alkalosis* | | | | | |
| Acute (uncompensated) | ↑ | ↓ | N | N | ↓ |
| Partly compensated | ↑ | ↓ | ↓ | ↓ | ↓ |
| Chronic (compensated) | N | ↓ | ↓ | ↓ | ↓ |
| *Metabolic acidosis* | | | | | |
| Acute (uncompensated) | ↓ | N | ↓ | ↓ | ↓ |
| Partly compensated | ↓ | ↓ | ↓ | ↓ | ↓ |
| Chronic (compensated) | N | ↓ | ↓ | ↓ | ↓ |
| *Metabolic alkalosis* | | | | | |
| Acute (uncompensated) | ↑ | N | ↑ | ↑ | ↑ |
| Partly compensated | ↑ | ↑ | ↑ | ↑ | ↑ |
| Chronic (compensated) | N | ↑ | ↑ | ↑ | ↑ |

$$CO_2 + H_2O \rightleftarrows H_2CO_3 \rightleftarrows H^+ + HCO_3$$

- An acute increase in $PaCO_2$ of 20 mmHg decreases the pH by ~0.1.
- An acute increase in $PaCO_2$ of 20 mmHg increases the $[HCO_3^-]$ by ~2 mEq/l.

*Example:* pH = 7.25; $PaCO_2$ = 60 mmHg; $HCO_3^-$ = 26 mEq/l, base excess = 0 mEq/l.

- If normal $PaCO_2$ = 40 mmHg, this case has an excess of 20 mmHg, which increases $HCO_3^-$ by at least 2 mEq/l. Therefore, the $HCO_3^-$ increases to 26 mEq/l, but it does not affect the base excess because the change is respiratory (excess of $CO_2$).

○ *Compensation* occurs by renal retention of $HCO_3^-$, but the process is slow to respond.
- Results in none or just a small change in $[HCO_3^-]$.
- A simple acute respiratory acidosis usually has a $[HCO_3^-]$ between 24–30 mEq/l.
- In an acute respiratory acidosis, the decrease in pH can be drastic as compensatory mechanisms are slow to respond.

*Example*: If $PaCO_2$ acutely increases to 76 mmHg, the $[HCO_3^-]$ will increase by only about 4 mEq/l.

$$Expected\left[HCO_3^-\right] = Normal(24) + Expected\ Increase(4)$$
$$= 28$$

s = 0.03 mEq/l/mmHg $CO_2$ at 37 °C.

$$Expected\ pH = 6.1 + \log(28 / 0.03 \times 76)$$
$$= 6.1 + \log(28 / 2.28)$$
$$= 6.1 + 1.09$$
$$= 7.19$$

- Thus, the pH will decrease dramatically in an acute respiratory acidosis.

○ *Treatment* of acute respiratory acidosis during anesthesia usually includes correcting $PaCO_2$ by instituting mechanical ventilation.
- If it does not correct with mechanical ventilation, other causes of hypoventilation, such as airway obstruction, should be investigated and eliminated.

### Chronic respiratory acidosis

○ A respiratory acidosis with a $[HCO_3^-] > 30$–32 mEq/l signifies a chronic condition (e.g. a horse with recurrent airway obstruction), or a concurrent metabolic alkalosis.

○ If $PaCO_2$ increases by 3, the $[HCO_3^-]$ is expected to increase by 1
- For example, If $PaCO_2$ = 49 (increased by 9 [actual $PaCO_2$ − normal of 40])
- So $[HCO_3^-]$ expected to increase by 3
- Expected $[HCO_3^-]$ = 27 (normal of 24 + 3 increase)

○ In chronic respiratory acidosis, the persistent increase in $PaCO_2$ stimulates increased excretion of titratable acid and $NH_3$, resulting in the addition of new $HCO_3^-$ to the ECF.

*Example*:
- If $PaCO_2$ = 76 mmHg (an increase of 36)
- The expected increase in $[HCO_3^-]$ is $36/3 \times 1.0 = 12$

$$Expected\left[HCO_3^-\right] = 36\ mEq / l$$
$$\left(Normal\ 24 + increase\ of\ 12\ due\ to\ compensation\right)$$

$$\text{Expected pH} = 6.1 + \log(36 / 0.03 \times 76)$$
$$= 6.1 + \log 15.8$$
$$= 6.1 + 1.2$$
$$= 7.3$$

*Note*: Compare the expected pH of 7.3 in *Chronic Respiratory Acidosis* with the expected pH of 7.19 for compensation in *Acute Respiratory Acidosis*. *Renal compensation* offers more significant pH protection in the face of chronic respiratory acidosis in contrast to intracellular buffering in the acute phase.

***Respiratory alkalosis*** (pH > 7.45, $PaCO_2$ < 35 mmHg)
○ Generally, results from a decrease in $PaCO_2$ (<35 mmHg) due to increased alveolar ventilation.
  – Mechanical hyperventilation during anesthesia is a potential cause.
  – Other causes include hypoxia, CNS infection, trauma, pain, and pulmonary edema.
○ The decreased $PaCO_2$ causes a decrease in blood $[H^+]$ and an increase in pH according to:

$$CO_2 + H_2O \overset{CA}{\rightleftharpoons} H^+ + HCO_3^-$$

○ An acute decrease in $PaCO_2$ of 10 mmHg causes the pH to increase by ~0.1. An acute decrease in $PaCO_2$ of 10 mmHg causes $[HCO_3^-]$ to decrease by ~2 mEq/l.
    *Example:* pH = 7.48; $PaCO_2$ = 30 mmHg; $HCO_3^-$ = 22 mEq/l, base excess = +1 mEq/l.
  – If normal $PaCO_2$ = 40 mmHg, this case has a deficit of 10 mmHg, which decreases $HCO_3^-$ by at least 2 mEq/l. Therefore, the $HCO_3^-$ decreases to 22 mEq/l, but it does not affect the base excess because the change is respiratory in origin (deficit of $CO_2$).
○ *Treatment* should address the underlying cause, and during anesthesia this generally involves decreasing alveolar ventilation.

***Metabolic acidosis*** (pH < 7.35, $[HCO_3^-]$ < 20 mEq/l)
Three Main Causes:
1) Increased acid production.
  – Most likely cause is lactic acidosis from hypoperfusion.
2) Loss of $HCO_3^-$.
  – Gastrointestinal (GI) losses from diarrhea (most commonly), or through the kidney. Diarrhea may lead to cardiovascular collapse and tissue hypoxia and lactic acidosis.
  – Bicarbonate loss may occur *indirectly* from an increase in the $H^+$ load from either endogenous or exogenous sources, and from a decrease in the kidney's ability to excrete acid.
    A decrease in $[HCO_3^-]$ of 10 mEq/l decreases the pH by ~0.15
3) Decreased acid excretion.
  – Uncommon finding in horses. Example: chronic renal disease.
  – *Compensation* occurs *initially* by alveolar hyperventilation, but renal compensation ($HCO_3^-$ retention) must also occur to correct metabolic acidosis, and this process may take a few days.
  – If $[HCO_3^-]$ decreases by 1 mEq/l the $PaCO_2$ is expected to decrease by 1 mmHg.

- Metabolic acidosis and AG:
  - Normal AG. $\downarrow[HCO_3^-]$ $\uparrow[Cl^-]$ (Diarrhea, Rapid IV fluid administration).
  - Increased AG. (Added $H^+$, e.g. lactate).
- *Treatment*, by alkali therapy (sodium bicarbonate), is generally recommended to increase the pH to >7.2.
    - A pH of 7.25 is a realistic objective.
    - Complete correction is not recommended as this may lead to a metabolic alkalosis, hypernatremia and an increased risk of cardiac arrhythmias.
- It is important to administer *alkali* therapy if:
  - Plasma pH is <7.20 and a continued decrease in $[HCO_3^-]$ could cause a further decrease in pH.
    - Especially if the $PaCO_2$ is approaching the lower limit of compensation (e.g. ~15 mmHg in healthy human, >15 mmHg in sick or aged individual).
  - Patients in which the metabolic acidosis is compensated but respiratory failure is imminent.
    - In this case, the increased ventilatory drive may result in fatigue of respiratory muscles.
    - An increase in $PaCO_2$ would result in a clinically important decrease in pH.

*Sodium bicarbonate dose* is generally calculated as follows:
  - $NaHCO_3$ (mEq) dose = Body mass (kg) $\times$ $HCO_3^-$ deficit $\times$ 0.3
    - $HCO_3^-$ deficit = normal $[HCO_3^-]$ − actual $[HCO_3^-]$
    - 0.3 represents the volume of distribution of $HCO_3^-$ in extracellular fluid. Higher values (0.4–0.5) are quoted for neonates due to their increased ECF volume.

*Example*: A 500 kg horse with a plasma $[HCO_3^-]$ of 10 mEq/l and pH of 7.15.

$$\begin{aligned} NaHCO_3 \, deficit \left(mEq\right) &= 500 \times \left(24-10\right) \times 0.3 \\ &= 500 \times 14 \times 0.3 \\ &= 2100 \text{ mEq} \end{aligned}$$

  - It is generally recommended to administer one-third to one-half of the calculated deficit over a few hours in association with volume expansion (e.g. balanced electrolyte solutions).
  *Note*: Bicarbonate therapy is only recommended if the cause of the $HCO_3^-$ deficit is related to true $HCO_3^-$ losses (e.g. diarrhea or renal tubular acidosis). Otherwise, fluid support is usually sufficient.

### Determining if compensation is adequate in metabolic acidosis
*Example*: A two-year-old colt with a two-day history of acute severe diarrhea.
- Electrolytes: $Na^+$ = 138 mEq/l, $K^+$ = 3.1 mEq/l, Cl = 110 mEq/l, $HCO_3^-$ = 16 mEq/l, $PaCO_2$ = 30 mmHg, pH = 7.30
- *History*: Based on the clinical signs, the likely acid-base disorders are:
- A normal AG acidosis secondary to diarrhea, or
  - Increased AG acidosis secondary to lactic acidosis as a result of hypovolemia and decreased tissue perfusion.
- The pH is low. Thus, by definition the colt is *acidemic*.
*Note*: it is important to distinguish the initial change from the compensatory response.

○ A low $[HCO_3^-]$ represents acidosis and is consistent with the pH, therefore it must be the initial change.
○ A low $PaCO_2$ represents alkalosis and is not consistent with the pH.
○ The low $PaCO_2$ must be the *compensatory* response.
○ The reduction in plasma $[HCO_3^-]$ results in a decrease in $PaCO_2$, according to:

$$CO_2 + H_2O \overset{CA}{\rightleftarrows} H_2CO_3 \rightleftarrows H^+ + HCO_3^-$$

○ Because the primary change involves $[HCO_3^-]$, this is a metabolic process, i.e. metabolic acidosis.

*Anion gap*
– The AG is $(Na^+ + K^+) - (Cl^- + HCO_3^-) = (138 + 3.1) - (110 + 16) = 15.1$
– The gap is <16, thus, it is considered normal.
  Is compensation adequate?

*Winter's formula for use in metabolic acidosis*
– Calculate the expected $PaCO_2$ for compensation based on the Winter's formula.

$$\begin{aligned} \text{Expected } PaCO_2 &= 1.5 \times \left[ HCO_3^- \right] + 8(\pm 2) \\ &= 1.5 \times 16 + 8(\pm 2) \\ &= 32 \pm 2 \end{aligned}$$

Assessment:
– Since the actual $PaCO_2$ is within the estimated range, the compensation can be considered adequate.
– Thus, there is no separate respiratory disorder present.
– This is a normal AG metabolic acidosis, most likely secondary to severe diarrhea, with adequate respiratory compensation.

**Metabolic alkalosis** (pH > 7.45, $HCO_3^-$ > 30 mEq/l)
○ Is a consequence of the loss or sequestration of gastric contents ($H^+$ loss), the administration of diuretic drugs ($K^+$ loss), and, less frequently, excessive sodium bicarbonate administration.
○ Characterized by:
An increase in $[HCO_3^-]$ of 10 mEq/l increases the pH by ~0.15.
An increase in plasma $[HCO_3^-]$.
– Hypochloremia.
– A reduction in the $PaCO_2/[HCO_3^-]$ ratio.
○ Compensation:
– The body attempts to increase the $PaCO_2$ to match the increase in $[HCO_3^-]$.
– An increase in $PaCO_2$ is accomplished by decreasing alveolar ventilation.
  ■ This happens fairly quickly following the onset of metabolic alkalosis.

*Winter's formula for use in metabolic alkalosis*
○ If $[HCO_3^-]$ increase by 1 mEq/l – the expected $PaCO_2$ increase is 0.7 mmHg
○ Expected $PaCO_2$ = 0.7 $[HCO_3^-]$ + 20 (±5)
– This equation will show if a co-existent respiratory acid-base disorder is present.
– For example, if $PaCO_2$ is less than expected, a respiratory alkalosis is also present.
  *Example:* pH = 7.48; $PaCO_2$ = 62 mmHg; $HCO_3^-$ = 45 mEq/l, base excess = +18 mEq/l.

$$\begin{aligned} \text{Expected PaCO}_2 &= 0.7\left[\text{HCO}_3^{-}\right] + 20\left(\pm 5\right) \\ &= 0.7\left[45\right] + 20\left(\pm 5\right) \\ &= 51.5 \pm 5 \end{aligned}$$

*Assessment*:
- – Since the measured $PaCO_2$ is higher than the expected range, there is a separate respiratory disorder present.
- – This represents a metabolic alkalosis with a concurrent respiratory acidosis.
- ○ Treatment
  Is aimed at removing the underlying cause, such as $H^+$ losses via gastric reflux.

## Physicochemical Approach
### Diego E. Gomez and Alex Valverde

- Also known as the "electrolytes and protein included" approach.
- Details of the mathematical relationship and interdependence of $H^+$ ions activity with electrolytes, $CO_2$ and proteins can be viewed in the textbook "How to Understand Acid-Base" by Peter Stewart, Elsevier, NY, which is available free online at "http://www.acidbase.org/index.php?show=sb."

## I  Brief review of physicochemistry and definitions

- Many substances (e.g. NaCl) when dissolved in water dissociate into charged molecules called *ions*, through a chemical process in which the molecular identity of the original added molecules change.
- These formed ions are called *electrolytes* and it is convenient to subdivide them into *strong* and *weak* electrolytes.

### A  Strong electrolytes

- ○ Strong electrolytes are fully dissociated in a solution; thus the parent substance disappears when dissolved in water. The main electrolytes involved in acid-base balance are $Na^+$, $K^+$, $Cl^-$, $Mg^{2+}$, $SO_4^{2-}$, $Ca^{2+}$, and a few organic acid anions, particularly L-lactate (L-lac$^-$).
- ○ A major feature of these ions is their electrical charge, and the preferred unit is equivalent per liter (Eq/l).
  - – For *univalent* electrolytes, concentration in equivalents per liter is identical to the concentration in moles/l.
  - – For *n valent* electrolytes concentration is *n* times the concentration in moles/l.
- ○ Strong electrolytes (e.g. $Na^+$ component in the bicarbonate solution) present in the solution would determine acid-base changes in the target patient, not the anion $HCO_3^-$ as is often emphasized in textbooks.

### B  Weak electrolytes

- ○ Weak electrolytes (e.g. plasma proteins, phosphates) are substances that only partially dissociate when dissolved in water. Molecules of the parent substance, as well as the products of dissociation, exist together in solution.

○ These molecules are always in the dissociation equilibrium according to their dissociation constant ($K_A$).

○ Weak electrolytes change their degree of dissociation depending on the conditions of the solution.

○ The amount of each component (parent substance and product of dissociation) in any aqueous solution remains constant unless one of the following occurs:

    – A substance is added or removed from the solution.

    – A substance is destroyed or generated by chemical reaction.

○ With regard to $H^+$ ions, the latter is most important. This is the basis of *mass conservation.*

### C   Law of electroneutrality

○ The law of electroneutrality requires that the sum of all cations always equals the sum of all anions ($\Sigma$anions = $\Sigma$cations) and applies to watery biologic solutions (e.g. blood, plasma).

○ An important consequence of this law is that the addition of one single cation or anion to a watery solution is not possible; any aqueous solution is always electrically neutral.

    – It follows that a patient cannot be treated parenterally (IV) with bicarbonate ($HCO_3^-$) *alone*, as is often stated, since there will also always be a neutralizing cation (e.g. $Na^+$) in the solution ($NaHCO_3$).

### D   Strong ion difference (SID) variables

○ The "Strong Ion Difference" approach proposes that three independent variables modify the plasma $H^+$ ion activity:

    – $PaCO_2$.

    – The strong ion difference.

    – Total weak acid concentration.

*PaCO$_2$*

○ The $PaCO_2$ is regulated by the lungs and influences plasma $H^+$ in a linear fashion.

○ See section on "Traditional approach" for additional information on the influence of $PaCO_2$ on pH.

*Strong ion difference*

○ SID accounts for the contribution of the strong cations ($Na^+$, $K^+$, $Ca^{2+}$, $Mg^{2+}$) and strong anions ($Cl^-$, L-lac$^-$), D-lactate$^-$, uremic acids, ketoacids, and unmeasured strong ions (USI) to the changes in plasma pH and $HCO_3^-$

○ Determination of SID requires identification and accurate measurement of all strong ions in plasma. Most commonly, SID can be calculated from the measured plasma concentrations of four strong ions ($Na^+$, $K^+$, $Cl^-$ and L-lac$^-$):

$$SID = (Na^+ + K^+) - (Cl^- + L\text{-lac}^-)$$

○ A normal SID is 38–46 mEq/l.

*Total weak acid concentration ($A_{tot}$)*

○ The total content of albumin, phosphate, and circulating nonvolatile weak acids [HA] and their dissociated anions [A$^-$] is referred to as [$A_{tot}$] in the physicochemical model.

○ Using the full Stewart equation, A⁻ can be precisely calculated as: $[A_{tot}]/[(1 + 10^{(pKa - pH)}]$. However, to estimate the approximate concentration of A⁻ in mEq/l, the concentration of total protein in g/l can be multiplied by a factor of 0.175 (1.75 if the total protein is in g/dl).
  – For example, if the measured protein concentration in a horse is 71.4 g/l (7.14 g/dl), then A⁻ = 71.4×0.175 = 12.5 mEq/l.

## E  Strong ion gap and unmeasured anions

○ A useful clinical application of the physicochemical approach is the calculation of strong ion gap (SIG), which provides an estimate for the difference between the ion charge of plasma non-volatile buffers and unmeasured strong anion (UA) concentration.
○ The SIG can be calculated as:
  – $SIG = SID - [HCO_3^-] - ([A_{tot}]/[(1 + 10^{(pKa - pH)}])$
  *Note: Using assigned values for pK$_a$ of 6.65 in the horse.* Alternatively, the following simplified formula that uses $[A_{tot}]$ instead of $[A^-]$ can be used:
  – $SIG = SID - [HCO_3^-] - (TP\,(g/l) \times 0.175)$
○ The SIG can provide an estimate for the amount of UA that do not include L-lac⁻, if L-lac⁻ has been measured and included in the SID calculation. If L-lac⁻ has not been measured, then SIG is usually mostly represented by L-lac⁻ as an UA.
○ A normal SIG is −2 to 2.
  – However, an SIG <−2 mEq/l would represent an increase in cation concentration, which has not been documented as an acid-base disease. Instead, this would indicate that the electroneutrality law is violated.

## II  Acid-base disorders: definitions

○ With the physicochemical approach, metabolic acid-base disorders are defined as follows:
  – Strong ion acidosis: when SID < 38 mEq/l and SIG > 2 mEq/l.
  – Strong ion alkalosis: when SID > 44 mEq/l.
  – Weak acids acidosis: when $A_{tot}$ > 25 mEq/l.
  – Weak acids alkalosis: when $A_{tot}$ < 13 mEq/l.

## III  Examples of metabolic abnormalities causing acid-base derangements

• Most acute metabolic acid-base disorders result from changes in the concentration of strong ions.
• The major driving forces for interactions between body fluid compartments are strong ion exchanges.

## A  SID acidosis

*Hyperchloremia*
○ Hyperchloremic acidosis is a predictable consequence of a large volume of intravenous normal saline administration, which decreases SID.
  – The excess of Cl⁻ is the cause of the metabolic acidosis.
  – Other causes of hyperchloremic acidosis in horses include renal tubular acidosis because of enhanced renal Cl⁻ conservation in the face of bicarbonate loss. This type

of acidosis has also been demonstrated in adult horses with myopathy, diarrhea, and foals with sepsis.

- ○ The physicochemical approach provides an explanation for the development of hyperchloremic acidosis and therefore a rational treatment for this condition.
    - – Normal plasma SID is 38–46 mEq/l, while the SID of normal saline is 0 mEq/l because $Na^+$ and $Cl^-$ are both strong ions (154 − 154 = 0).
    - – Intravenous administration of normal saline decreases plasma SID, by adding $Cl^-$ to plasma in a greater magnitude than $Na^+$, which will create a strong ion acidosis (assuming that the infusion does not cause a change in $PaCO_2$, plasma albumin, globulin, or phosphate concentrations).
    - – The magnitude of the decrease in plasma SID when normal saline is administered depends on the relative volumes of the extracellular space and the speed of administration.
- ○ The usual treatment is $NaHCO_3^-$ solution to normalize SID.
    - – Eventually, renal handling of $Cl^-$ will correct the hyperchloremia.
    - – Sodium salts of lactate, gluconate, acetate, propionate, or citrate are also used, as $NaHCO_3^-$ precursors.

## B  Lactic acidosis

- ○ L-lactate ($L\text{-}lac^-$) is a strong anion and its increment in plasma lowers the SID leading to strong ion acidosis.
- ○ $L\text{-}lac^-$ accumulation reflects an increased production, reduced catabolism, or a combination of the two.
- ○ Hyperlactatemia ($L\text{-}lac^- > 2\,mEq/l$) has traditionally been attributed to dehydration and tissue hypoxia. Hypoperfusion due to dehydration is responsible for the majority of hyperlactatemia in horses.
- ○ Hyperlactatemia can also occur in presence of proper tissue oxygenation. In critically ill patients, hyperlactatemia is associated with enhanced aerobic glycolytic flux, which is the most important determinant of L-lac production.
- ○ Increased aerobic glycolytic flux in patients with sepsis and septic shock is enhanced by epinephrine secretion and respiratory alkalosis.
- ○ In macrophage-rich organs including the lungs, intestine, and liver (i.e. pneumonia, diarrhea, and hepatitis, respectively), inflammatory cytokines (i.e. TNF and IL-1) promote aerobic glycolytic flux for ATP production required for respiratory burst during sepsis.

## C  SID alkalosis

*Hypochloremic alkalosis*
- ○ $Cl^-$ shifts and hypochloremia occur in patients with GI abnormalities (e.g. gastric reflux).
- ○ Administration of loop diuretics that inhibit the Na-K-Cl cotransporter (NKCC channel) can result in hypochloremia.
- ○ The hypochloremia increases SID and, based on electroneutrality, the change will be balanced by an increase in $HCO_3^-$ concentration.
- ○ Administration of 0.9% NaCl will be an effective treatment.
- ○ If concurrently *hypokalemic*, part of the saline may be replaced with KCl.

### D  $A_{tot}$ acidosis

- Elevated concentrations of total plasma proteins (especially albumin) and phosphates increase plasma $H^+$ activity, and therefore results in non-volatile weak acid ($A_{tot}$) acidosis (> 25 mEq/l).
- $A_{tot}$ acidosis because of hyperproteinemia is associated with reduction in plasma water content due to decreased water intake and loss of protein-poor body fluids (i.e. hypersecretory diarrhea).
- In chronic inflammatory conditions hyperglobulinemia can increase globulin concentration leading to $A_{tot}$ acidosis.
- Treatment of the $A_{tot}$ acidosis should be directed at the underlying cause.

### E  $A_{tot}$ alkalosis

- Decreased concentrations of total plasma proteins (especially albumin) and phosphates increases plasma $H^+$ activity and therefore results in non-volatile weak acid ($A_{tot}$) alkalosis (<13 mEq/l).
- $A_{tot}$ alkalosis because of hypoproteinemia is associated with volume expansion (e.g. fluid overload, pregnancy) and loss of protein-rich body fluids (e.g. protein-losing enteropathy or nephropathy).
- Treatment of the $A_{tot}$ alkalosis should be directed at the underlying cause.

## IV  Examples of the physicochemical approach

*Example 1:*

- A five-day-old Thoroughbred filly presented for acute severe diarrhea and marked depression.
- Diagnosed with sepsis, diarrhea, and pneumonia.
- Laboratory results are provided in Table 9.2.
- The physicochemical approach reveals SID acidosis, SIG acidosis and weak acids alkalosis.
- The $SID_4 = (Na^+ + K^+) - (Cl^- + L\text{-}lac^-)$ is 25 mEq/l, below the normal range of 38–46 mEq/l. Therefore, the diagnosis is *SID acidosis* (see Table 9.3).
- SID acidosis because of hyperchloremia and hyperlactatemia.
  - *Hyperchloremia* has been reported in horses with diarrhea because fecal fluid $[Cl^-]$ losses are lower than those of $[Na^+]$ and urinary excretion of $[Cl^-]$ is also reduced. Plasma $[Cl^-]$ then increases, lowering $SID_4$.
  - Hyperchloremia is commonly detected in septic animals, but the causes are still unknown.
  - Hyperlactatemia can be attributed to dehydration and tissue hypoxia and enhanced aerobic glycolytic flux associated with sepsis.
  - Increased L-lactate lowers the $SID_4$, leading to SID acidosis.
- The $SIG = SID_4 - [HCO_3^-] - ([A_{tot}]/[(1 + 10^{(pKa - pH)})])$ is 10 mEq/l, above the normal range of −2 to 2, which reveals the presence of unidentified strong anions, likely sulfate and other organic anions associated with uremia and sepsis; therefore, an *acidosis* associated to the SID acidosis.

- Alternatively, with SIG = $SID_4$ – [$HCO_3^-$] – (TP in g/l×0.175) is 6 mEq/l, above the normal value.
  o The $A_{tot}$ = TPP×0.175 is 8.8 mEq/l, below the normal range of 13–25 mEq/l, which reveals an $A_{tot}$ *alkalosis* associated with hypoproteinemia, likely as a result of protein-losing enteropathy.
  o The traditional approach indicates that the foal presents with acidemia because of an increase $PvCO_2$ (respiratory acidosis) as a consequence of the respiratory disease (pneumonia and inability to efficiently eliminate $CO_2$). Also, this reveals a decrease in $HCO_3^-$ (metabolic acidosis) as a consequence of its losses through the diarrhea. However, using the traditional approach the mechanism for those acid-base disorders is not apparent.

*Example 2:*
  o A 10-year-old Quarter Horse gelding presented for colic signs.
  o Physical exam revealed a marked dehydration, severe impaction of the large colon and the right dorsal colon displacement was suspected.
  o Initial treatment consisted of a bolus of 20 ml/kg of 0.9% NaCl solution followed by a maintenance rate of 100 ml/kg/day. Twenty-four hours after treatment, the gelding displayed severe signs of colic unresponsive to analgesic therapy.
  o Laboratory results before surgery are provided in Table 9.2.
  o The physicochemical approach reveals SID acidosis (see Table 9.3).
  o The $SID_4$ = ($Na^+$ + $K^+$) – ($Cl^-$ + l-lac$^-$) is 28 mEq/l, below the normal range of 38–46 mEq/l. Therefore, the diagnosis is *SID acidosis.*
  o SID acidosis because of saline-induced hyperchloremic acidosis.
    - 0.9% NaCl has a 1 : 1 ratio of $Na^+$ to $Cl^-$ and contains a proportionately high level of $Cl^-$ (154 mEq/l), higher than the normal plasma concentration.
    - The hyperchloremia lowers $SID_4$, leading to SID acidosis.
    - The acidosis has also resulted in mild hyperkalemia.
  o pH values >7.20 do not seem to have major pathophysiologic implications in the clinical setting described above. However, hyperchloremic acidosis caused by administration of large quantities of 0.9% saline solution should be treated to provide an SID close to that of the horse's plasma (38–46 mEq/l).
    - Sodium salts solutions such as lactate, gluconate, acetate, propionate, or citrate can be used.
  o The SIG = $SID_4$ – [$HCO_3^-$] – ([$A_{tot}$]/[$(1 + 10^{(pKa – pH)})$]) is 1 mEq/l, within the normal range of −2 to 2.
    - Alternatively, with SIG = $SID_4$ – [$HCO_3^-$] – (TP in g/l 0.175) is −2 mEq/l, also within the normal range for unmeasured anions.
  o The $A_{tot}$ = TPP×0.175 is 14 mEq/l, within the normal range of 13–25 mEq/l.
  o The traditional approach indicates that the horse presents with acidemia because of a decrease in $HCO_3^-$ and an increase in base deficit (more negative number); therefore a metabolic acidosis. However, using the traditional approach the mechanism for those acid-base disorders is not apparent.

Table 9.2   Acid-base analysis results for case #1.

| Diagnostic approach | Plasma constituent | Foal | Reference interval (foals three to seven days old) | Interpretation |
|---|---|---|---|---|
| Physicochemical | pH | 6.709 | 7.36 to 7.4 | Acidemia |
| | $Na^+$ (mEq/l) | 138 | 130 to 146 | Normal |
| | $K^+$ (mEq/l) | 5.2 | 3.6 to 5.6 | Normal |
| | $Cl^-$ (mEq/l) | 111 | 96 to 108 | High |
| | L-lactate$^-$ (mEq/l) | 7 | 0 to 2.5 | High |
| | TPP (g/l) | 50 | 44 to 68 | Normal |
| | $SID_4$ (mEq/l) | 25 | 38 to 46 | SID acidosis |
| | $A_{tot}$ (mmol/l) | 8.8 | 13 to 25 | Weak acids alkalosis |
| | SIG (mEq/l) | 10 | −2 to 2 | SIG (unmeasured anions) acidosis |
| Traditional | pH | 6.709 | 7.36 to 7.4 | Acidemia |
| | $PvCO_2$ (mmHg) | 87 | 34 to 42 | Respiratory acidosis |
| | $HCO_3^-$ (mEq/l) | 10 | 25 to 33 | Metabolic acidosis |
| | $BE_{(ECF)}$ (mEq/l) | −31 | −1 to 6 | Metabolic acidosis |

$HCO_3^-$, bicarbonate; BE $_{(ECF)}$ base excess extracellular fluid; TPP, total plasma proteins; $SID_4$, strong ion difference measured using 4 electrolytes as $SID_4 = (Na^+ + K^+) - (Cl^- + l\text{-lactate}^-)$. $A_{tot}$, Total weak acid concentration measured as $A_{tot} = TPP \times 0.175$; SIG, strong ion gap measured as $SIG = SID_4 - HCO_3^- - ([A_{tot}]/[1 + 10^{(6.65 - pH)}])$.

Table 9.3   Acid-base analysis results for case #2.

| Diagnostic approach | Plasma constituent | Horse | Reference interval (adult horses) | Interpretation |
|---|---|---|---|---|
| Physicochemical | pH | 7.22 | 7.32 to 7.44 | Acidemia |
| | $PvCO_2$ (mmHg) | 42 | 38 to 49 | Normal |
| | $Na^+$ (mEq/l) | 149 | 132 to 146 | Normal |
| | $K^+$ (mEq/l) | 5.0 | 2.4 to 4.7 | High |
| | $Cl^-$ (mEq/l) | 124 | 99 to 109 | High |
| | L-lactate$^-$ (mEq/l) | 2 | 0 to 2 | Normal |
| | TPP (g/l) | 79 | 54 to 79 | Normal |
| | $SID_4$ (mEq/l) | 28 | 38 to 46 | SID acidosis |
| | $A_{tot}$ (mmol/l) | 14 | 13 to 25 | Normal |
| | SIG (mEq/l) | 1 | −2 to 2 | Normal |
| Traditional | pH | 7.22 | 7.32 to 7.44 | Acidemia |
| | $PvCO_2$ (mmHg) | 42 | 38 to 49 | Normal |
| | $HCO_3-$ (mEq/l) | 16 | 24 to 28 | Metabolic acidosis |
| | $BE_{(ECF)}$ (mEq/l) | −9.7 | 1.1 to 7.1 | Metabolic acidosis |

$HCO_3^-$, bicarbonate; BE $_{(ECF)}$ base excess extracellular fluid; TPP, total plasma proteins; $SID_4$, strong ion difference measured using 4 electrolytes as $SID_4 = (Na^+ + K^+) - (Cl^- + l\text{-lactate}^-)$. $A_{tot}$, Total weak acid concentration measured as $A_{tot} = TPP \times 0.175$; SIG, strong ion gap measured as $SIG = SID_4 - HCO_3^- - ([A_{tot}]/[1 + 10^{(6.65 - pH)}])$.

## Suggested Reading

Johnson, P. (1995). Electrolyte and acid-base disturbances in the horse. *Vet. Clin. North Am. Equine Pract.* 11: 491–514.

Hughes, J. and Bardell, D. (2019). Determination of reference intervals for equine arterial blood-gas, acid-base and electrolyte analysis. *Vet. Anaesth. Analg.* 46: 765–771.

# 10

## Hemostasis and Hemotherapy

### Hemostasis
*Kira L. Epstein*

## I   Normal physiology

- Hemostasis results in the formation of a blood clot within a vessel. The clot is the combined product of a platelet plug and fibrin meshwork.
  - Formation of a platelet plug is the result of *primary* hemostasis.
  - Formation of a fibrin meshwork is the result of *secondary* hemostasis.
  - The processes of primary and secondary hemostasis are highly interdependent.
  - When vascular trauma occurs, hemostasis is triggered by exposure to subendothelial tissue to maintain circulatory system integrity and prevent excessive blood loss.
  - When infection occurs, hemostasis is triggered by inflamed cells to minimize the systemic spread and limit nutrient/oxygen delivery to pathogens.
- The extent of clot formation within a vessel is limited by inherent properties of normal endothelial cells and anticoagulants. Fibrinolysis removes excessive clots also limiting the extent of clot formation.
- There are multiple mechanisms for feedback between the coagulation (primary and secondary hemostasis), anti-coagulation, and fibrinolysis. Appropriate hemostasis requires maintenance of a delicate balance.

## II   Primary hemostasis

### A   Adhesion

- Adhesion occurs when platelets encounter exposed extracellular matrix or subendothelium.
- Platelets adhere to exposed collagen through von Willebrand factor (vWF) and the GPIbα (GP1b-IX-V complex) platelet receptor in high shear conditions (small and medium arteries) and through *fibronectin* and *laminin* in low shear conditions (veins and large arteries).
- Damaged endothelial cells express P-selectin which is involved in the adhesion process.
- Adhesion results in platelets changing shape and forming interplatelet bridges.

*Manual of Equine Anesthesia and Analgesia*, Second Edition. Edited by Tom Doherty, Alex Valverde, and Rachel A. Reed.

## B   Activation

- ○ Activation is triggered by a number of mechanisms including adhesion/exposure to collagen, exposure to agonists released from other activated platelets like adenosine diphosphate (ADP) and thromboxane $A_2$ (TxA$_2$), and thrombin generated through secondary hemostasis.
- ○ Activated platelets degranulate, releasing agonists for activation and aggregation as well as products involved in localizing and supporting secondary hemostasis on the platelet surface.
- ○ Activated platelets synthesize platelet activating factor (PAF) and TxA$_2$ and express receptors involved in assembling cross-linked fibrinogen during secondary hemostasis.

## C   Aggregation

- ○ Aggregation is stimulated by thrombin, ADP, and TxA$_2$.
- ○ Platelet aggregation is mediated through vWF and the GPIbα (GP1b-IX-V complex) platelet receptor in high shear conditions and through fibrinogen and integrin $\alpha_{II}\beta_3$ (GP IIb-IIIa) platelet receptor in low shear conditions (veins and large arteries).

## D   Thrombin

- ○ Thrombin is an important and potent stimulator of platelets, illustrating the interdependence of primary and secondary hemostasis.

## E   Platelet plug formation

- ○ Plug formation is inhibited by healthy endothelial cells through multiple mechanisms.
- ○ The negative charge of the endothelial cell surface repels negatively charged platelets.
- ○ Nitric oxide and prostacyclin produced by healthy endothelial cells inhibit all stages of primary hemostasis.
- ○ Additionally, thrombin is inactivated by thrombomodulin and heparans and ADP is degraded by ADPases produced by healthy endothelial cells.

# III   Secondary hemostasis

## A   Enzymatic reactions

- ○ Is the end result of multiple coordinated enzymatic reactions *involving serine proteases* cleaving *proenzymes* (factors) to create activated factors that are themselves serine proteases.
- ○ Most of the reactions require *phospholipid* (cell membrane) and *calcium* as cofactors.
- ○ The coordination of the process involves activated factors providing positive and negative feedback by activating other factors and stimulating anticoagulant and fibrinolytic pathways, respectively.

## B   Cascade or waterfall model of coagulation

- ○ Traditionally, this model has been used to explain the process of secondary hemostasis.
- ○ It depicts two separate mechanisms/pathways for initiation (intrinsic and extrinsic) that converge to stimulate the common pathway terminating in the generation of crosslinked fibrin.
- ○ Over time, it has become clear that this is an oversimplification of the process and does not account for interactions between the pathways or the role of cell membranes.

○ Modifications to the cascade model allow for a better representation of the crossover between the two pathways and an increased amount of positive feedback of thrombin on earlier steps but fail to address the key role of cell membranes within the body. Despite these limitations, the cascade model is useful to understanding the enzymatic reactions and *in vitro* plasma coagulation testing.

## C   The cell-based model of coagulation

○ This model was developed to bridge the gap between understanding the plasma-based cascade model and what occurs in the body where endothelial, extravascular, and blood cells are present.

○ Importantly, the cell-based model explains why coagulation *in vivo* is nearly exclusively stimulated by tissue factor (TF) (extrinsic pathway) and the interdependence of primary and secondary hemostasis.

○ The cell-based model is divided into three stages – *initiation*, *amplification*, and *propagation*.

### Initiation stage

○ Initiation occurs on the surface of TF expressing cells, most commonly fibroblast exposed when endothelial cells are injured.

○ Inflamed endothelial cells and monocytes can express TF, but their role in coagulation is less clear.

○ Initiation begins with TF binding circulating FVIIa. Importantly, FVII is the only clotting factor that circulates in any significant quantity (although still only 1% of the total) in the activated/enzymatic form. Initiation generates a small amount of thrombin and FIXa to participate in amplification and propagation, respectively.

### Amplification

○ Amplification occurs on the surface of nearby platelets.

○ The thrombin generated from initiation cleaves vWF from FVIII and activates platelets and factors V, VIII, and XI.

○ The activated platelet localizes factors Va, VIIIa, and XIa.

### Propagation

○ Propagation occurs on the surface of the activated platelets from amplifications and the additional platelets that are recruited, activated, and stimulated to aggregate by the activated platelets.

○ This becomes a large source of localized prothrombinase (FXa-Va) to generate a thrombin burst. Thrombin can then feedback on amplification and participate in generation of fibrin.

## D   Anticoagulants

○ Anticoagulants in circulation and on endothelial cells limit secondary hemostasis.

○ Antithrombin (AT) accounts for ~70% of circulating anticoagulant activity.

○ Heparans produced by healthy endothelium potentiate the anticoagulant activity of AT. AT has the ability to inactivate factors IIa, VIIa, IXa, Xa, XIa, and XIIa.

○ Another important circulating anticoagulant is *tissue factor pathway inhibitor* which inactivates TF-FVIIa complex and FXa.

&#9702; *Thrombomodulin* is an important anticoagulant expressed on the surface of endothelial cells. It has many mechanisms of actions, but most importantly binds thrombin which inhibits thrombin activity and activates protein C leading to inactivation of factors Va and VIIIa.

## IV   Fibrinolysis

- Fibrinolysis is the process of cleaving *fibrin* resulting in degradation of clots.
- Fibrin is cleaved by *plasmin,* which is created when plasminogen, the proenzyme, is cleaved. Healthy endothelial cells produce tissue plasminogen activator (tPA) to convert plasmino-gen to plasmin to help limit clot expansion. Additionally, urokinase and activated factors from the intrinsic pathway (FXIa, XIIa, and kallikrein) activate plasminogen.
- Fibrinolysis inhibition is mediated by several enzymes with differing targets.
  - &#9702; Plasminogen activator inhibitor inhibits tPA and urokinase.
  - &#9702; α2-antiplasmin and α2-macroglobulin directly inhibit conversion of plasminogen to plasmin.
  - &#9702; Thrombin activatable fibrinolysis inhibitor (activated by thrombin, thrombin-thrombomodulin complex, and plasmin) inhibits plasmin cleaving fibrin.

## V   Coagulation testing

- Most tests assessing coagulation evaluate on a portion of the process of hemostasis and can be categorized based on whether they assess primary hemostasis, secondary hemostasis, or fibrinolysis.
- A coagulation profile is a combination of tests and generally contains at least one test in each group.
- Normal values for many coagulation tests vary between laboratories and testing methods. Therefore, laboratory specific reference ranges should be used.

### A   Primary hemostasis

- &#9702; It can be affected by decreases in platelet counts (thrombocytopenia) or deficits in plate-let function (thrombocytopathia).
- &#9702; Buccal mucosal or template bleeding times evaluate primary hemostasis but have *questionable repeatability in horses.*
- &#9702; Thrombocytopenia is diagnosed by a decreased platelet count. More reliable platelet counts are achieved when citrate is used as the anticoagulant compared to ethylenedi-amine tetraacetic acid (EDTA) where pseudothrombocytopenia occurs more frequently.
- &#9702; Laboratory testing for thrombocytopathia is less widely available and, with the exception of measuring vWF activity, must be done within a limited time frame following collec-tion. An automated platelet function analyzer (PFA-100) has been evaluated in horses and aggregometry has been used in horses primarily for experimental studies. PFA-100 closure times will also be prolonged with thrombocytopenia.

### B   Secondary hemostasis

- &#9702; It can be evaluated with clotting times and measurement of activity or number of clotting factors.
- &#9702; Additionally, anticoagulant activity or amount can be measured.

- The most frequently evaluated clotting times are prothrombin time (PT), which detects deficits in the extrinsic and common pathways, and activated partial thromboplastin time (aPTT), which detects deficits in the intrinsic and common pathways.
- Fibrinogen concentration measurement is common and widely available.
- Antithrombin activity is the most common test for anticoagulants.

## C Fibrinolysis

- Is detected by measuring the concentration of the resulting fragments.
- D-dimers are the preferred test for fibrinolysis because they are only produced when cross-linked fibrin (clots) are degraded compared to fibrin(ogen) degradation products (FDPs) which are produced when fibrinogen or cross-linked fibrin are degraded.
- D-dimers appear very sensitive in horses and increase in pathologic and non-pathologic conditions of clot formation.

## D Coagulation profiles

- Profiles vary among laboratories.
- The author prefers a coagulation profile that includes platelet count, PT, aPTT, fibrinogen, AT, and D-dimers.

## E Viscoelastic coagulation tests

- Have been developed with the goal of more global evaluation of coagulation recognizing the complexity of the process compared to previous, individual coagulation test.
- It can evaluate the kinetics (speed) and mechanics (strength) of clot formation and degree of fibrinolysis.
- If performed in whole blood, it provides information on both primary and secondary hemostasis.
- Several testing methods have been evaluated in horses, but they primarily remain tools of research.

# VI Coagulopathy

- Coagulopathies, or abnormalities in coagulation, can result in either excessive bleeding or thrombosis.
- Disseminated intravascular coagulation (DIC) is a coagulopathy that begins with thrombosis and can progress to bleeding.
- Excessive bleeding can be the result of decreased primary or secondary hemostasis (hypocoagulation) or increased fibrinolysis or anticoagulant activity.

## A Defects in primary hemostasis

- Generally, they result in spontaneous bleeding from mucosal surfaces (epistaxis, melena, hematuria, etc.) and/or increased incidence of traumatic (often unrecognized) and iatrogenic (surgical, injection site, etc.) bleeding, ecchymoses, and hematoma formation.
- With thrombocytopenia, petechia are a common clinical sign. Moderate thrombocytopenia (<40000 plt/ul) can result in clinical bleeding with trauma or iatrogenic causes, whereas spontaneous mucosal bleeding occurs only with severe thrombocytopenia (<10000 plt/ul).

B   Defects in secondary hemostasis

- Generally, they result in spontaneous bleeding into body cavities and/or increased incidence of traumatic (often unrecognized) ecchymoses and hematoma formation.
- Clinical signs related to the body cavity affected (e.g. colic from hemoabdomen) and/or blood loss may predominate.

C   Hereditary and acquired causes of hypocoagulation

- Hereditary and acquired causes related to primary and secondary hemostasis have been reported in horses.
- Causes of thrombocytopenia can be separated into three categories: *decreased production*, *increased consumption*, and *destruction*.
- In horses, decreased production can be seen with disorders of the bone marrow associated with drug administration or neoplasia, increased consumption secondary to prolonged/severe bleeding or DIC, or destruction most commonly related to immune-mediated disease that can be primary or secondary to drug administration, infectious disease or neoplasia.
- *Hereditary thrombocytopathias* that have been reported in horses include Glanzmann thrombasthenia and a platelet fibrinogen binding deficiency.
- In addition to drugs that target platelets therapeutically (see below), hydroxyethyl starches and some NSAIDs may affect platelet function.
- Secondary hemostasis deficits that have been reported in horses included hereditary deficiencies in prekallikrein, FVIII, FIX, and FX, and consumption of toxins resulting in vitamin K deficiencies.
  - Additionally, hydroxyethyl starches can inhibit aspects of secondary hemostasis.

D   Treatment for bleeding patients

- Involves not only stopping the bleeding but also, in some cases, replacing lost blood components and volume (see section on hemotherapy).
- Local/surgical methods to stop bleeding may be used depending on the accessibility of the location of the bleeding and the stability of the patient.
- Systemic administration of pro-coagulants and antifibrinolytics have the potential to benefit a wide range of bleeding patients. In all cases, any underlying disease and/or resulting organ dysfunction will need to be addressed.
- *Local administration*/application of powders, sheets, and sponges can be used to physically stop bleeding with pressure and/or provide a surface and catalyst for coagulation.
  - Available options include oxidized regenerated cellulose, purified gelatin sponge, microfibrillar collage agents, polysaccharide hemostatic agents, thrombin products, and fibrin-based sealants.
  - Evaluation of these products in horses is extremely limited.
- *Systemic pro-coagulants* that can be considered include Yunnan Baiyao (4 g PO q6 hours can also be used topically) and *estrogen* (0.05 mg/kg).
  - Platelet-rich plasma or fresh whole blood can provide additional platelets and fresh or fresh frozen plasma and whole blood can provide additional coagulation proteins.
  - In cases of vitamin K deficiency, supplemental vitamin K (0.5–2.5 mg/kg IV, IM, SC) is required for the liver to synthesis factors II, VII, IX, and X.

- Systemic anti-fibrinolytics that can be used in horses are:
  - *ε-aminocaproic acid* (20–40 mg/kg in 1 l 0.9% NaCl IV q6 hours or 3.5 mg/kg/min for 15 minutes then 0.25 mg/kg/min CRI; can also be used topically).
  - *Tranexamic acid* (5–25 mg/kg IV, IM, SC q12 hours).
- *Naloxone* (0.2 mg/kg, IV) has been proposed as an adjunctive therapy in cases of hemorrhagic shock to reverse endogenous opioid induced vasodilation.

## E   Thrombosis

- Can be the result of increased primary or secondary hemostasis (hypercoagulation) or decreased fibrinolysis or anticoagulant activity.
- Clinical signs of thrombosis are primarily related to the size, location, and type of vessel affected. Decreased delivery of oxygen or removal of waste from the region or organ can result in *pain* and *dysfunction*.
  - Venous thrombosis can result in edema associated with increased hydrostatic pressure.
  - Arterial thrombosis can result in the area becoming cold.
- Inflammation affects multiple aspects of hemostasis, resulting in promotion of clot formation and a decrease in fibrinolysis. This can contribute to pathologic thrombosis.

*Therapy*

- Most often, therapy for thrombotic disease focuses on limiting the expansion of clots that are present and preventing the formation of additional clots.
- *Heparins* potentiate AT to increase its inhibition of activated clotting factors (unfractionated heparin 40–60 IU/kg IV, SC q8–12 hours: low molecular weight heparin – *daltaperin*. Adult, 50 IU/kg SC q12–24 hours; Foal, 100 IU/kg SC q24 hours, or *enoxaparin* adult 40 IU/kg SC q24 hours).
- Local treatment for an isolated and accessible thrombus may be considered.
- Thrombectomy has been reported for a limited number of horses with aortoiliac thrombosis. Local administration of a fibrinolytic agent (i.e. tPA) could be considered but has not been reported in horses.
- In all cases, any underlying disease and/or resulting organ dysfunction will need to be addressed.

## F   DIC

- Occurs when there is a widespread activation of coagulation secondary to a systemic disease.
- Due to the connection between inflammation and coagulation, many of these diseases have an inflammatory component like strangulating and inflammatory GI disease, and sepsis in foals.
- DIC initially results in widespread formation of microthrombi and can progress to bleeding with consumption of platelets and coagulation factors. Large vein thrombosis is also possible.

*Clinical signs*

- Clinical signs of DIC depend on the severity of the process and whether thrombosis or bleeding is predominant.
- In horses, DIC is often subclinical meaning, that the horse has an appropriate underlying disease and abnormalities on a coagulation panel.
- If microthrobi are diffuse and affect multiple organs, signs will be related to the organs affected.
- Increased bleeding tendency may be seen, but life-threatening hemorrhage is rare.

*Treatment*

    ○ Treatment of DIC should focus on the identification and treatment of the underlying cause.

    ○ Additionally, any end-organ dysfunction will need to be treated.

    ○ The use of therapeutics directed at coagulation is controversial and should be done with consideration of the current coagulation status of the patient (thrombotic vs. bleeding).

## Hemotherapy

*Kira L. Epstein*

## I Indications for hemotherapy

- Hemotherapy, or administration of blood products, is indicated when blood or blood components have been lost, destroyed, consumed, or not produced appropriately resulting in dysfunction of oxygen-carrying capacity, colloid osmotic pressure, coagulation, or the immune system. These abnormalities illustrate the main roles of blood in oxygen delivery, hemostasis, and immunity.

- Under anesthesia, acute blood loss is likely to be the most commonly encountered indication of blood-product administration, but it is important to be aware of other indications.

### A Oxygen delivery ($DO_2$)

    ○ Understanding the role of blood in $DO_2$ requires an understanding of the physiology behind $DO_2$.

      – $DO_2$ is the product of cardiac output (Q) and arterial oxygen content ($C_aO_2$).

      – $DO_2 = Q \times C_aO_2$

      – Q is the product of heart rate (HR) and stroke volume (SV).

       $Q = HR \times SV$

      – The main determinants of SV are preload and contractility on the positive side and afterload on the negative side.

    ○ Oxygen is carried in the blood as a dissolved gas, measured as $P_aO_2$, and bound to hemoglobin (Hb).

    ○ The amount of oxygen bound to Hb is determined by the percent of hemoglobin that is saturated with oxygen ($S_aO_2$) multiplied by the concentration of Hb ([Hb]).

$$C_aO_2 = 1.36 \times S_aO_2 \times [Hb] + 0.003 \times P_aO_2.$$

    ○ From this equation, it is clear that bound oxygen is the predominate form and, thus, adequate numbers of red blood cells ([RBC]) containing Hb are key to maintaining arterial oxygen content ($C_aO_2$). However, the role of adequate oxygen uptake through the respiratory system should not be forgotten as it determines not only the dissolved oxygen ($P_aO_2$) but also the $S_aO_2$ that is so important to the amount that is bound to Hb.

B   Preload

- Blood volume is a key determinant to preload and, thus, SV and $DO_2$.
- In a patient with acute blood loss, volume loss resulting in hypovolemia is likely to play an important role in the ensuing shock.
- *Clinical and clinicopathologic* parameters that are consistent with hypovolemic shock may include tachycardia, tachypnea, prolonged jugular refill, abnormalities of capillary refill time, poor pulse quality, cool extremities, hypotension, and increased blood lactate concentrations.
- In horses under general anesthesia, many of these signs may not be as consistent and interpretation may be more difficult due to the effects of the anesthetic agents and circulatory (fluids, inotropes, and/or vasopressors) and respiratory (mechanical ventilation) support the horse is receiving. Additionally, it is important to recognize that many of these abnormalities (e.g. tachycardia, tachypnea, increased blood lactate) are not unique to hypovolemic shock and there is significant overlap with metabolic shock due to decreased [RBC]/[Hb].
- Due to the importance of hypovolemia and the rarity of having blood products immediately available, replacement/resuscitation frequently begins with crystalloids.
- However, blood products (either whole blood or components) may be indicated depending on estimated percent volume blood loss and clinical and laboratory parameters related to decreased RBC and/or plasma components (see below).

*Colloid osmotic pressure* (COP)

- The COP of blood plays a role in maintaining fluid in the intravascular space which is important for maintaining circulating volume (preload and, thus, SV and $DO_2$) and preventing excessive leakage into the interstitial space (edema formation).
- Examples of disease processes that can result in low COP include loss through the GI or urinary tract (protein losing enteropathy or nephropathy) or hemorrhage and decreased production due to malnutrition or liver failure.
- Although the mechanism is not completely understood, COP also decreases consistently in horses under general anesthesia which may confound other pathologies.
- Specific cutoffs for laboratory values for initiation of supplementation of COP are not well established and may be different depending on the age of the horse, rapidity of change (acute versus chronic), and if horses are awake or under general anesthesia. In awake adult horses with an acute decrease, administration of colloid support has been suggested for horses with total protein (TP) < 4.0 g/dl, albumin < 2.0 g/dl, and/or COP < 14 mmHg.

C   Diseases resulting in low [RBC]/[Hb] include

- Acute or chronic hemorrhage.
- Destruction/hemolysis associated with immune-mediated processes (e.g. neonatal isoerythrolysis).
- Infectious (e.g. piroplasmosis).
- Toxic mechanisms (e.g. red maple leaf).
- Decreased production related to bone marrow suppression or iron deficiency.

D   Transfusion triggers

- Specific cutoffs for clinical and laboratory values to serve as *"Transfusion triggers"* have not been established in horses.

- ○ When determining whether transfusion is indicated and the type of blood product to use, the duration and cause of the anemia must be taken into consideration.
- ○ Clinical and clinicopathologic parameter changes that may indicate decreased $C_aO_2$ requiring transfusion include tachycardia, tachypnea, pale mucus membranes, decreased packed cell volume (PCV), decreased TP as a result of acute blood loss (see below), increased blood lactate, and increased oxygen extraction ratio (OER).

$$OER = [(S_aO_2\text{-}S_vO_2)/S_aO_2]\, x100$$

### Acute blood loss

- ○ Horses that have lost >30% of their blood volume are likely to require a transfusion.
- ○ In these cases, the transfusion will replace both volume (preload) and RBC ($C_aO_2$).
- ○ During surgery, collecting blood and/or blood-soaked sponges can help estimate percent blood volume loss.
  - – However, it is important to take into consideration lavage fluids as well as the effects of IV fluids and volume loading.

### Clinical signs of hypovolemic shock

- ○ Signs including sweating, colic, and lethargy can be used to determine the need for transfusion in awake horses.
- ○ Additionally, it should be recognized that changes in PCV and TP require redistribution and/or replacement of intravascular fluid making them more difficult to use to guide therapy.
- ○ TP will decrease faster than PCV due to the effects of splenic contraction, and changes will be more rapid in cases receiving IV fluid replacement.
- ○ As with signs of hypovolemic shock, effects of anesthetic drugs and cardiovascular and respiratory support may complicate interpretation of some of these signs.
  - – For example, heart rate and PCV have been noted to be quite stable in horses with blood loss under anesthesia.
  - – Horses with PCV < 20–25% and OER > 40% following acute blood loss are likely to require transfusion.

### Chronic anemia

- ○ Transfusion is indicated if there are abnormalities in clinical and clinicopathological parameters indicative of decreased $C_aO_2$.
- ○ A PCV < 12–15% indicates the need for transfusion.
- ○ Administration of blood products may be indicated for the prevention and/or treatment of coagulopathy, most frequently excessive bleeding.
- ○ In horses with known diseases predisposing to bleeding such as hereditary thrombocytopathies and clotting factor deficiencies or liver failure, blood products may be indicated prior to medical or surgical procedures.
- ○ In horses with excessive hemorrhage, treatment with blood products may be indicated to restore soluble proteins and platelets lost during bleeding in addition to restoring $DO_2$ as discussed.
- ○ In horses with DIC, blood products may be useful in re-establishing the balance in the hemostatic system and replacing lost components. While the use of blood products for horses in DIC has been described, the timing and benefit in these cases remains unknown.
- ○ For disease affecting primary hemostasis, a blood product containing *platelets* will be required. While there is no agreed upon cutoff for supplementation of platelets, administration to horses with a platelet count of <20 000/uL at risk for bleeding or showing signs of bleeding is likely indicated.

    ○ For diseases affecting secondary hemostasis and fibrinolysis, blood products containing the soluble pro-coagulant, anti-coagulant, pro-fibrinolytic, and anti-fibrinolytic proteins will be required.

*Immunoglobulins*

    ○ Administration of blood products containing immunoglobulins (IgG) can be used for the treatment and prevention of some infectious and inflammatory diseases.

    ○ Many of the plasma products used for this purpose are harvested from donors that have been hyperimmunized to infectious agents (bacterial and/or viral).

    ○ One of the most common indications for IgG administration is partial (IgG 400–800 mg/dl) or complete (IgG < 400 mg/dl) failure of passive transfer (FPT) in foals >12 hours of age due to inadequate quantity or quality of colostrum consumption.

    ○ The optimal source (local vs. commercial) and type (hyperimmunized or not; pathogen[s] hyperimmunized to) of plasma remains unknown.

## II  Types of blood products

    ● Blood products can be separated or classified based on which components of blood they contain and how they are stored. The choice of which blood product to administer is based on the needs of the recipient and the availability of products.

    ● Whole blood (WB) transfusions are indicated when recipients need all components of blood, most commonly for replacement following blood loss.

    ○ WB can be given soon after collection or stored with refrigeration for up to 21 days (citrate–phosphate-dextrose-adenosine solution).

    ○ While RBC and most plasma protein components maintain activity during refrigerated storage, for platelets to be viable WB must be used within eight hours of collection and kept at room temperature.

*Whole blood*

    ○ Should be stored in a blood-banking dedicated refrigerator with an alarm at 1–6 °C.

    ○ Clear and appropriate labelling is vital in cases of blood storage.

      – It is generally impractical for equine practices to maintain a bank of stored WB due to relatively limited need, but commercial sources of whole blood are available.

      – For horses having planned procedures with expected significant blood loss, pre-operative autologous blood donation may be a good alternative.

*Autotransfusion*

    ○ In cases of hemorrhage into a body cavity, collection and autotransfusion of blood can be considered. Commercially available devices for collection, washing, and filtering exist, or blood can be collected into a bag with anti-coagulant (lower ratio-1 : 7 to 1 : 20 citrate) and administered through a filter.

    ○ This should not be considered in cases with underlying infection or neoplasia.

*Plasma products*

    ○ Plasma products are indicated when recipients require colloid (albumin), platelets, coagulation proteins, and/or immunoglobulins.

    ○ Plasma can be harvested from WB through sedimentation or centrifugation or by plasmapheresis. When available, plasmapheresis may provide larger quantities more rapidly and result in less RBC and WBC contamination of the plasma.

○ Plasma can be categorized as fresh, fresh frozen (FFP), or frozen (FP) and products are chosen depending on the needs of the patient. Further processing (or potentially specific collection) is generally required to treat patients requiring platelets.

*Fresh plasma*

○ Fresh plasma is plasma used within eight hours of collection and kept at room temperature. Fresh plasma will contain active platelets as well as all protein components.

*Fresh frozen plasma*

○ FFP is plasma that is frozen within eight hours of collection. FFP must be stored at or below $-18°$ C (less than $-70°$ C for optimal coagulation protein preservation). FFP should be used within one year to maintain activity of all clotting factors. One study indicated that refreezing thawed plasma within one hour did not result in loss of clotting factor activity.

*Frozen plasma*

○ FP is plasma that is frozen greater than eight hours after collection or stored at or below $-18°$ C for more than one year. The main difference between FFP and FP will be the loss of labile clotting factors (i.e. FV and FVIII). For administration of IgG, hyperimmune plasma (USDA regulated) has efficacy for two to three years.

*Platelets*

○ In cases requiring platelet replacement (thrombocytopenia or thrombocytopathia with bleeding or undergoing a procedure with risk of bleeding) plasma with a higher concentration of platelets is generally used. These products can be obtained by processing fresh plasma, or, although not described in clinical cases, platelets could be obtained with plateletpheresis.

○ Centrifugation of fresh plasma can be performed to create platelet-rich plasma (PRP – single "soft-spin") or platelet concentrate (PC – additional centrifugation).

○ PC will contain active platelets for five to seven days at room temperature.

*Packed red blood cells (pRBC)*

○ Are indicated for the treatment of anemic horses with normal volume, platelet concentration, and/or plasma protein concentrations/activity.

○ Most commonly, this would occur in horses with hemolytic anemias or decreased RBC production but may also be appropriate for cases of chronic blood loss where volume overload is considered a risk and plasma protein concentration is not considered a problem.

○ pRBC can be produced by sedimentation or centrifugation.

○ In horses, sedimentation occurs rapidly, and, with monitoring, WB can be administered to primarily give the sedimented RBC (pRBC). Alternatively, the pRBC and plasma can be separated.

○ Centrifugation to separate pRBC from plasma is performed at $4°$ C at 5000 g for five minutes. After separating off the plasma, the pRBC can be washed with saline to removed plasma proteins (generally three times). Washed pRBC from the mare are recommended for the treatment of foals with neonatal isoerythrolysis.

○ pRBC can be stored for 35 days in saline-adenine-glucose-mannitol solution.

## III   Collecting blood products

• A blood donor needs to be able to donate an effective volume of high-quality blood product, free of transmissible infectious agents, and have minimal risk of initiating a transfusion reaction.

- The volume of whole blood that a horse is able to give is based on their weight and breed. It is recommended that blood donors are >500 kg.

*Note*: Blood volume varies between 6 and 10% of body mass in horses; lower range in draft horses and higher range in Thoroughbreds; therefore, this volume can be adjusted to the breed used as a donor. Horses can generally safely donate 20% of their blood volume.

*Example*: Horse 500 kg:
Blood volume @ 8% of body mass
$$= 40\,l\,(0.08 \times 500)$$
Blood volume collected $= 20\%$ of $40\,l = 8\,l = 16\,ml/kg$

## A   Donors

- o Donor horses should also have a PCV of at least 35% to minimize their risk of significant anemia post-donation and to provide adequate RBC amounts.
- o Donors should be vaccinated as recommended (generally including eastern and western equine encephalitis, West Nile virus, tetanus, rabies, and likely, equine herpes virus 1 and 4 and equine influenza in the United States).
  - – Donors of hyperimmune plasma are often vaccinated for additional pathogens and/or more frequently.
- o Donors should be tested to ensure that they are free of transmissible infectious diseases including regular screening for equine infectious anemia and equine parvovirus hepatitis, which has been implicated as being associated with the development of serum hepatitis, or *Theiler's* disease. Screening for piroplasmosis, dourine, glanders, and brucellosis is required for horses that will be used for USDA-licensed plasma products.
- o Donors should be selected to minimize the likelihood of incompatibility between donor RBC and plasma and recipient plasma and RBC. Testing that can be performed includes blood typing and antibody screening for donors and possibly recipients and crossmatching recipients with potential donors.
- o Horses have a large number (7) of blood groups and factors associated with the groups resulting in so many potential combinations that development of a herd of blood donors that will match all recipients is impossible. Fortunately, alloantibodies are uncommon and, when present, target antigens with minimal effect.

## B   Blood typing of donors

- o Blood typing of donors should be performed.
- o Donors that are Aa and/or Qa antigen positive should be avoided as these antigens appear to be more immunogenic and have been implicated in neonatal isoerythrolysis and transfusion reactions.
- o Horses of the same breed as the recipient may be more likely to have similar blood types and, therefore, may be preferable for use as a donor.
- o While alloantibodies are relatively uncommon, development of antibodies after exposure to blood and/or blood products through breeding/pregnancy or blood product administration is possible.
- o For this reason, geldings without a history of receiving blood products are usually selected because they have a lesser chance of being sensitized to RBC related to breeding and/or pregnancy.
- o Mares that have had foals should be avoided.

- Donkeys (and mules) have a unique RBC antigen (donkey factor). Donkeys (and mules) should *not* be used as donors for horses to avoid development of anti-donkey factor antibodies. Horses should be screened for anti-donkey factor antibodies before being used as a donor for a donkey (or mule) recipient.
- For *foals* with neonatal *isoerythrolysis*, washed RBC from the mare are a good choice for transfusion. Washing removes the plasma with antibodies to the foal's RBC and the mare's RBC will not be targeted by the IgG from the mare's colostrum.

## C Recipient

- Blood typing and antibody screening for recipients is often impractical prior to transfusion. In horses that are expected to require more than one transfusion, additional testing may be valuable.
- Rapid blood typing kits for horses are being developed and may become commercially available in the future.
- Antibody screening for broodmares can be used to predict development of neonatal isoerythrolysis in their foals. Those foals can then be stopped from consuming colostrum and administered colostrum from a compatible mare or hyperimmunized plasma to avoid clinical disease.

## D Crossmatching

- Can be performed to detect agglutination, and less commonly hemolytic, reactions between donor and recipient blood.
- Crossmatching for agglutination can be performed relatively quickly. Rouleaux formation can make interpretation more difficult in horses and autoagglutination can make interpretation more difficult in cases of immune-mediated hemolytic anemia.
- Major crossmatches involve mixing donor RBC with recipient plasma and minor crossmatches involve mixing recipient RBC with donor plasma. Washed donor pRBC can be used in cases where major crossmatch indicates compatibility but the minor crossmatch indicates incompatibility.
- Compatibility based on crossmatch does not eliminate the possibility of transfusion reactions but should minimize it. Experimental horses receiving incompatible blood had increased febrile reactions to transfusion.
- Crossmatch compatibility is also likely to improve RBC survival time following transfusion.
- Crossmatches may detect more incompatible pairs than blood typing and antibody screening.

## E Emergency transfusions

- Are often performed immediately without testing with little risk of serious transfusion reaction.
- Risk is low because alloantibodies are uncommon.
- Testing for compatibility is also often impractical as tests are not consistently available and take time, and access to large numbers of screened donors to choose from is uncommon.
- Risk should be lowest in horses that have not received blood products in the past. Horses with previous blood and/or blood product exposure can develop antibodies and are likely at increased risk for transfusion reactions if transfusion is performed without testing. Horses can develop antibodies within one week of transfusion, but a recent study suggested the rate of anti-RBC development in horses following blood transfusion with crossmatch incompatible blood was fairly low at 30 days (1/18 horses).

○ Several studies have reported RBC half-life following transfusion with variable results. RBC from autologous blood transfusions have a half-life of nearly 50 days when fresh and approximately 30 days after 28 days of storage. RBC from compatible allogenic blood transfusions have a half-life of 20–33.5 days. RBC from incompatible allogenic blood transfusions appear to have a half-life less than a week.

*Blood collection*

○ Blood is collected from a donor directly through a needle or using a catheter in the jugular vein. The jugular vein selected should be clipped and prepared aseptically and the needle or catheter should be placed in sterile fashion. Collection speed may be increased by using a larger diameter catheter (10 or 12 gauge rather than 14 gauge), directing the catheter toward the head during placement, placement of a catheter in both jugular veins, and occluding the jugular veins.

  – Donors should be monitored during blood donation for any significant changes in heart rate, respiratory rate and attitude. Any changes should be normalized within an hour of donation. Horses that donate more than 10–15% of their blood volume should receive replacement isotonic crystalloid fluids IV.

○ Blood should be collected into collection bags with anti-coagulant (3.2% citrate 1:9 or acid-citrate-dextrose solution if blood will be used immediately or citrate–phosphate-dextrose ± adenosine for storage of whole blood).

○ Glass bottles can be used with a vacuum to speed the collection but are *not* recommended because the vacuum can induce RBC damage and the glass inactivates platelets.

○ Bags are also preferable for centrifugation and sterile transfer to satellite bags.

## IV  Administering blood products

- For stored blood products, improper warming or thawing can damage the cells and proteins.
- For refrigerated RBC, the cells may be damaged by rewarming and giving the product directly may be best for the RBC. However, if the recipient is going to receive large volumes or is hypothermic, warming to at least room temperature is preferred. Blood products should not be warmed to greater than body temperature. Ideally a circulating, temperature controlled (30–37 °C) water bath should be used to thaw frozen plasma products.
- Products should not have visual evidence of abnormalities like clotting, hemolysis, or other discoloration, and care should be taken to avoid contamination of the blood product during connection to the recipient.

  ○ Blood products should be *administered* via a catheter placed in aseptic fashion through a commercial blood administration line containing a filter (170–260 μm).

   – Blood administration sets should be changed after 2–4 units.

  ○ *Monitoring* of the recipient is necessary to identify adverse reactions as well as to determine if clinical improvement is being achieved.

   – Monitoring during the transfusion should be performed at least every 15 minutes including heart rate, respiratory rate, and temperature. Patients should be observed very closely particularly during the first 15 minutes of the transfusion and as the rate is increased.

   – As noted previously, heart rate and respiratory rate may be difficult to use for assessment in anesthetized patients.

   – The reported incidence of *adverse reactions* in horses receiving plasma is 0–10% and for those receiving blood is 16% (1/44 fatal anaphylaxis). Adverse reactions to transfusions can be acute or delayed and non-hemolytic or hemolytic.

*Non-hemolytic reactions*

- ○ Are most common and can be caused by an immune response to the blood product (allergic) or inflammatory components within the product (leukocytes and/or cytokines – particularly with storage).
- ○ Serum sickness/hepatitis, or *Theiler's* disease, had been thought to be an immune mediated disease. More recently, evidence is mounting that the disease is an infection related to the transmission of the equine parvovirus hepatitis.
    - – In addition to fever, allergic reactions may cause clinical signs such as piloerection, sweating, muscle fasciculation, urticaria, and anaphylaxis. Most allergic reactions occur early on during the transfusion.
    - – If reactions are mild, simply slowing the administration of the product frequently resolves the signs.
    - – If reactions are more severe, the transfusion should be stopped immediately.
    - – Treatment with *corticosteroids* and/or *antihistamines* is required for some cases and *epinephrine* is indicated for severe anaphylaxis.

*Hemolytic reactions*

- ○ Acute hemolytic reactions generally occur during the transfusion or shortly after completion, while delayed occur more than 24 hours after the transfusion.
- ○ With hemolytic reactions, clinicopathologic evidence of hemolysis such as hemoglobinemia, hemoglobinuria, hyperbilirubinemia (delayed), and decreasing/not increasing PCV will occur. If a crossmatch has not been performed or if the reaction is delayed, a crossmatch may help confirm the reaction.
- ○ Acute hemolytic reactions are highly inflammatory and can lead to severe systemic signs including systemic inflammatory response, DIC, shock, and death. The more product that is given, the worse the reaction will be.
- ○ When large volumes of blood products are infused, the amount of citrate administered may lead to *hypocalcemia* (and/or hypomagnesemia) and the volume may overload the circulatory system.
- ○ Volume overload is more likely at higher volumes and rates and in smaller patients such as foals or those with cardiac (rates should be limited to 2–4 ml/kg/hr) or renal disease.
- ○ When administering large volumes of blood, storage lesions (damage of the RBC, accumulation of potassium and lactate, and depletion of 2,3-DPG) in stored products may become clinically significant and fresh products may be preferred.
- ○ Recipients should also be monitored for improvement in clinical signs (physical examination) and clinicopathologic abnormalities (e.g. abnormalities in PCV, TP, lactate, OER, IgG, coagulation test) in response to blood product administration.
- ○ The *rate of administration* for the first 10–20 minutes should be slow (~ 0.3 ml/kg during that time), but may be gradually increased if monitoring does not indicate any adverse reactions to up to 20–40 ml/kg/hr.
    - – Administration should be completed within four hours to avoid bacterial contamination and ensure platelets are viable (if fresh whole blood).
- ○ Determining the volume of blood product to use will depend on the problem being treated.
    - – *For replacement of RBC*, the volume to administer depends on the cause of the anemia.
    - – In cases of normovolemic anemia (ex: chronic blood loss or hemolytic anemia), the following formula (see Box 10.1) can be used to estimate the volume of blood required to increase the PCV of a recipient to a desired level.

---

**Box 10.1    Blood Volume for Transfusion**

*Assume blood volume is 8% of body mass.*
Blood required (L) = Body wt. (kg) × 0.08 × [(desired PCV-recipient PCV)/donor PCV]
E.g. Recipient: A 500 kg horse. PCV =15%. Desired PCV = 25%. Donor PCV = 40%.

Volume (L) for transfusion = 500 × 0.08 × [(25 − 15)/40)]
$$= 40 × 0.25$$
$$= 10\,l \text{ (i.e. 20 ml/kg)}$$

---

- – The desired PCV should not be "normal" or it will slow the body's response to replace the RBC.
- ○ In cases of acute hemorrhage, the delay in the change to PCV following hemorrhage does not allow for this type of calculation. Instead, administration of 25–50% of the estimated blood loss is recommended.
- ○ In cases of internal hemorrhage, up to 75% of RBC will return to the circulation within three days, so the need for replacement RBC and volume of blood required should be somewhat lower.

*Replacement of TP/albumin*
- ○ The following formula can be used to estimate the volume of plasma required to increase the TP/albumin of a recipient to a desired level (see Box 10.2).
- ○ The desired TP/albumin should not return the COP to "normal" or it will slow the body's response to replace TP or albumin.

*Note:* Some authors have suggested that much higher volumes of plasma are required than predicted by the above formula and recommend 8–10 l to achieve a 1 g/dl increase in TP in a 450 kg horse. This would amount to a plasma volume of at least 16–20 l in the above example.

- ○ Administering such large volumes of plasma is generally cost prohibitive. For this reason, the volume is selected based on clinical response in many cases.
  - – For replacement of coagulation factors, a volume of 4–5 ml/kg is recommended to start, with repeat coagulation testing to guide further administration.
  - – For replacement of IgG, 20 ml/kg should increase the IgG concentration by 200–300 mg/dl. This dose is approximately 1 l for most foals, which is conveniently the volume in most bags of equine hyperimmune plasma. Repeat IgG concentration testing should be performed to guide further administration.

---

**Box 10.2    Plasma Volume for Transfusion in Hypoproteinemia**

Volume required (L) = Body wt. (kg) × 0.045 l/kg × [(desired TP or albumin – recipient TP or albumin)/donor TP or albumin]
E.g. Recipient: A 500 kg horse. TP = 3.0 g/dl. Desired TP = 5.0 g/dl. Donor TP = 7.0 g/dl.

Plasma volume for transfusion = 500 × 0.045 × [(5.0 − 3.0)/7.0
$$= 22.5 × 0.29$$
$$= 6.25\,l \text{ (i.e. 1.25 ml/kg)}$$

## Suggested Reading

Fielding, C.L. and Magdesian, K.G. (2015). *Equine Fluid Therapy*. Oxford, UK: Wiley Blackwell Publishing.

Hurcombe, S.D., Mudge, M.C., and Hinchcliff, K.W. (2007). Clinical and clinicopathologic variables in adult horses receiving blood transfusions: 31 cases (1999-2005). *J. Am. Vet. Med. Assoc.* 231 (2): 267–274.

Mudge, M.C. (2014). Acute hemorrhage and blood transfusion in horses. *Vet. Clin. North Am. Equine Pract.* 30 (2): 427–436.

Tomlinson, J.E., Taberner, E., Boston, R.C. et al. (2015). Survival time of cross-match incompatible red blood cells in adult horses. *J. Vet. Intern. Med.* 29: 1683–1688.

# 11

# Thermoregulation
*Chiara E. Hampton*

## I  Introduction

- All physiologic, cellular, and tissue functions are temperature-dependent to some extent. Neuraxial and general anesthesia alter normal thermoregulation by several mechanisms.
- This chapter provides a focus on thermoregulatory mechanisms of the adult horse and the young foal, as they differ somewhat from those of other homeothermic species.

## II  Physics principles applied to thermoregulation

- According to the first law of thermodynamics, heat is a form of energy which can neither be created nor destroyed.
- This means that the heat produced by the body through metabolic processes must be transferred to another system, until an equilibrium is reached, which is implied in the second law of thermodynamics.

## III  Mechanisms of heat transfer

- There are four main routes of heat transfer:

### A  Conduction

- Heat transfers from the horse's body to the surface with which the skin is in direct contact.
- The rate of heat transfer depends on:
  - The temperature gradient ($\Delta T$) between the skin and the surface.
  - The skin area contacting that surface.
  - The nature of that surface (metals are good conductors; therefore, heat will transfer to a metal surface more readily than to materials that are poor conductors).

*Manual of Equine Anesthesia and Analgesia*, Second Edition. Edited by Tom Doherty, Alex Valverde, and Rachel A. Reed.
© 2022 John Wiley & Sons, Inc. Published 2022 by John Wiley & Sons, Inc.

*Clinical example*
  ○ Conduction is one of the reasons heat loss in horses is exacerbated by having horses lie on the non-padded floor of the recovery stall.

## B  Convection

  ○ Convection is the transfer of heat by the movement of fluids (i.e. liquid or gas).
  ○ The rate of convection depends on:
    – The $\Delta T$ between the skin and fluid.
    – The surface area of the skin.

*Clinical examples*
  ○ The air surrounding the horse's body is warmed via conduction and, as air expands when heated, it rises upward away from the body, creating an air current due to convection, which decreases the temperature of the air now surrounding the horse.
  ○ Another clinically relevant example is the cooling produced by the administration of cold intravenous (IV) fluids. Heat is transferred from the vessel walls to the fluid molecules that move away when heated and are replaced by cold ones through a convective movement.
    – In human beings, each 1l of IV fluid administered at room temperature (25 °C) decreases core temperature by 0.25 °C. Fluids to be administered intravenously should be warmed to 37 °C.

## C  Evaporation

  ○ Heat transfers from a body surface (i.e. skin, upper airways, open abdominal cavity) to the environment through the conversion of a liquid (e.g. sweat) into vapor.
  ○ Heat loss from the skin due to evaporation results from the loss of the latent heat of vaporization of moisture on the skin or solutions applied to the skin.
  ○ The rate of heat dissipation through evaporation depends on:
    – The wind speed (rate of air movement across the surface).
    – Ambient temperature.
    – Ambient humidity, and therefore by its difference with water vapor pressure on the surface.
    – Body mass-to-surface area ratio is small in horses, thus the surface area for evaporation is relatively small.

*Clinical example*
  ○ In the exercising horse, evaporative losses occur via respiration and sweating. An exercising horse may breathe fast and hard as if panting, but horses do not open mouth breathe as they are obligate nasal breathers.
  ○ Heat losses via breathing account for 15–25% of total heat loss, whereas those from evaporation through sweating contribute as much as 65%.
  ○ The amount of heat generated by exercise (i.e. due to increased metabolism) in horses can be massive, and it requires an equally efficient method to dissipate this heat.
  ○ Evaporative heat losses in horses are extremely efficient and effective due to the presence of *latherin,* a protein in the sweat. Latherin reduces water surface tension and therefore, acts as a wetting agent that promotes body cooling via evaporation.

## D Radiation

- Heat in the form of electromagnetic rays is transferred from the hottest object to the coldest one. The rate of transfer depends on:
  - The ΔT between these objects.
  - The distance between the objects.
  - The characteristics of the objects' surfaces.

*Clinical example*

- Foil blankets decrease radiant heat losses; therefore, they are useful as a passive method for prevention of hypothermia.
- Under general anesthesia, minimizing areas of exposure (i.e. skin, abdominal cavity, etc.) will minimize heat loss by radiation.

## IV Homeostasis of body temperature

- Horses are homeothermic mammals. By definition, they maintain a nearly constant body temperature, regardless of the environment temperature, by a tight regulatory system.
- Normothermia in the adult horse ranges from 99.5 to 101 °F (37.5 to 38.3 °C), and from 99 to 102 °F (37.2 to 38.9 °C) in the foal (measured as rectal temperature).
- The main source of internal heat production is metabolism derived from muscular activity and digestion, whereas the main routes of heat loss in the conscious horse are through rapid breathing and sweating.
- Derangements in body temperature outside the physiologic range are an indication of exhaustion of the regulatory processes for maintenance of body temperature.
- It is postulated that *the guttural pouches* are involved in *cooling the brain* by decreasing the temperature of the blood in the internal carotid arteries as they transverse the guttural pouch.
- In *horses,* rectal temperature is a good estimate of *core* temperature.

## V Control of body temperature

- Body temperature is controlled via a loop feedback system composed of *afferent, central,* and *efferent* mechanisms (non-specific to horses).

## A Afferent mechanism

- Thermal information is transduced by transient receptor potential (TRP) vanilloid (V) and menthol (M) receptors on the skin surface and in the dorsal root ganglia.
- Thermal signals from peripheral and central tissues travel to the processing center, the hypothalamus, after significant modulation in the spinal cord.
- The main afferent nerve fibers involved are:
  - Aδ fibers transmitting *cold* signals.
  - Unmyelinated C-fibers transmitting *warm* signals.
- Exclusive afferent pathways have not been identified, although the *spinothalamic* tracts in the anterior spinal cord seem to play a significant role in conveying thermal information.

## B   Central mechanism

- ○ Modulation of afferent information occurs in the brain stem before reaching the preoptic nucleus of the anterior hypothalamus, where inputs from thermoreceptors of the skin, deep tissues, and the spinal cord are integrated.
- ○ In the conscious horse, two temperature-controlling mechanisms are present.

*Autonomic control*
- – Occurring at the anterior hypothalamus.
- – 80% of inputs controlling autonomic responses arise from core structures (these remain intact during anesthesia).

*Behavioral control*
- – Occurring in the posterior hypothalamus.
- – 50% of inputs controlling behavioral responses arise from the skin (these are abolished under general anesthesia due to loss of consciousness).

- ○ The "set-point" theory, according to which the body's efferent response is turned off and on according to the hypothalamic temperature, does not adequately describe the complexity of the mechanisms regulating homeostasis of body temperature.
- ○ A *thermoregulatory* model, in which autonomic and behavioral responses are constantly activated and deactivated in response to the average temperature of several sites (e.g. the skin, deep tissues, and the spinal cord), constitutes a more comprehensive model.
  - – In this model, the spinal cord, brain stem and hypothalamus work in conjunction to integrate afferent inputs which will elicit individual responses if a threshold temperature is reached.
  - – *Inter-threshold range*: It is defined as the core temperature that does not elicit a thermoregulatory response. Its lower limit is the *vasoconstriction* threshold, and its upper limit is the *sweating* threshold. The inter-threshold range is 0.2–0.4 °C in humans, and it is postulated to be of similar magnitude in horses.

## C   Effector mechanism

- ○ The body temperature difference from the individual's specific threshold (thermal perturbation) will elicit an effector response, which will result in an appropriate increase in heat losses, or in an increase of heat production via an augmented metabolic rate.
- ○ Effector responses to heat originate in the *anterior* hypothalamus, whereas effector responses to cold originate in the *posterior* hypothalamus.
- ○ There are two main effector responses, *autonomic* and *behavioral*, for effective thermoregulation.

*Autonomic responses*
- ○ The autonomic response consists of the following processes.

*Piloerection*
- ○ This mechanism increases air trapping among the hairs of the animal's coat, which leads to the formation of a thermal barrier that transiently insulates it from the surrounding environment in response to cold.

*Vasomotion*
○ A mechanism by which heat loss from the skin surface is augmented (vasodilatation) or diminished (vasoconstriction) via α-adrenergic control of the arterio-venous shunts present in the skin.
○ Furthermore, distribution of cardiac output also influences thermoregulation, as when less blood flow is directed to the skin, there is a slower rate of heat dissipation through convective and evaporative processes at the body surface, and vice versa.

*Non-shivering thermogenesis*
○ Is a mechanism by which $\beta_2$-adrenergic stimulation promotes catabolism of brown adipose tissue.
  – However, this mechanism has minimal to no importance in horses, including neonates, in which brown fat deposits are negligible.

*Shivering*
○ Is a mechanism for which metabolic heat production is augmented up to 400% in adult humans by increasing muscular activity in response to cold temperature. It can range from very fine contractions to more generalized and intense tremors of the trunk or limbs.
○ Since the shivering threshold is about 1 °C lower than the vasoconstrictive threshold, shivering occurs as the *in extremis* response to severe cold.
○ This mechanism originates in the posterior hypothalamus, and occurs in conscious, sedated, or lightly anesthetized horses.
  – This event is most commonly witnessed in horses during *recovery* from general anesthesia.
○ While shivering can be very effective in restoring body temperature, it substantially increases metabolic oxygen consumption, which can have detrimental effects on the overall balance between delivery and consumption of oxygen in the body.

*Sweating*
○ A mechanism by which the body is able to dissipate heat in an environment that is exceeding core temperature.
○ Horses differ from other mammalians, including human beings, in which sweating is a *cholinergic*-mediated event.
○ In equids, sweat glands are apocrine and innervated by *adrenergic* fibers.
○ They present two mechanisms for control of sweating:
  – *Humoral*, via adrenergic agonists (i.e. epinephrine and norepinephrine) secreted by adrenal medulla.
  – *Nervous,* via autonomic adrenergic nerves. The main control mechanism is *neural,* with the *humoral* becoming active during exercise. Sweating occurs exclusively through $\beta_2$-adrenergic receptor stimulation. Agonism of the receptor induces a conformational change of the α subunit of the G protein receptor, activating adenylate cyclase and catalyzing the formation of cAMP, leading to protein kinase A formation and phosphorylation, which produces the biologic effect of sweat production.

*Behavioral responses*
○ These are the most powerful thermoregulatory effectors, and consist of behavioral changes aimed to mitigate the effect of environmental temperature on the body.
○ They can manifest as moving from direct sunlight into shade, rolling in mud, wading into water, etc., when horses are hot, and assuming a huddled posture, group aggregation, or seeking shelter in response to cold.
○ Behavioral changes require a *conscious* perception of body temperature; therefore, they are abolished during general anesthesia.

## VI    General considerations regarding thermoregulation during anesthesia

- In horses undergoing general anesthesia, body temperature decreases mainly due to:
  - *Immobility* (i.e. decreased metabolic rate).
  - *Evaporative losses* (e.g. fresh gas flows, open abdominal cavity).
- Several effects caused by tranquilizers, sedatives, and anesthetics are responsible for peri-anesthetic thermal perturbations.
  - Cold-response thresholds are decreased.
  - Warm-response thresholds are slightly increased (with a consequent widening of the inter-threshold).
  - Autonomic defenses are the only active mechanisms for thermoregulation because:
    - Behavioral responses are abolished.
    - Metabolic heat production is greatly reduced.
- General anesthesia influences thermoregulation by impairing all three levels of the feedback control system (*afferent*, *central*, and e*fferent*).
  - Regional anesthesia only seems to impair the afferent and efferent levels.
- General and neuraxial anesthesia predispose to a greater degree of heat loss in humans. No data are currently available for horses.
- Hypothermia is one of the most common complications during general anesthesia of small and large animals, although it has been widely underestimated in horses due to their small body surface area to body mass ratio.
  - However, in some temporal studies reporting data on body temperature, hypothermia is a common complication of general anesthesia in horses.
- Hypothermia is more common than hyperthermia. However, body temperature can rise under general anesthesia if the environmental temperature is high, and if closed circuit anesthesia is used. There have been reports of hyperthermia in horses during the recovery period.

### A    Effects of individual drugs on thermoregulation

- General anesthetics and opioids have little influence on sweating, but profoundly reduce the vasoconstriction and shivering thresholds. The result is a ten to twentyfold increase in the inter-threshold range.
- *Opioids* alter thermoregulation by resetting the threshold point controlled by the hypothalamus, which typically causes panting after their administration to dogs. This effect has not been described in horses.
- *Acepromazine*, *propofol*, and *inhalational* anesthetics cause vasodilatation that can worsen convective, radiant, and evaporative losses.
- Inhalational anesthetics widen the inter-threshold range and lower the patient's threshold response to hypothermia in a non-linear fashion.

## VII    Physiologic consequences of hypothermia

### A    Central nervous system

- Decreased cerebral metabolic oxygen consumption.
- Depression.

    ○ Prolonged recovery.
    ○ Sympathetic activation (stress response).
    ○ Decreased MAC.

## B Cardiovascular system

    ○ Increased incidence of arrhythmias.
    ○ Bradycardia.
    ○ Decreased cardiac output.
    ○ Hypotension.
    ○ Loss of ability to vasoconstrict.
    ○ Increased myocardial oxygen consumption.

## C Respiratory

    ○ Hypoventilation.
    ○ Hypoxemia.
    ○ Left shift of oxyhemoglobin dissociation curve.
    ○ Respiratory acidosis.

## D Miscellaneous

    ○ Decreased perfusion leading to delayed wound healing.
    ○ Increased shivering leading to increased myocardial oxygen consumption.
    ○ Decreased GI motility and increased incidence of ileus.
    ○ Platelet dysfunction.
    ○ Impaired immune function.
    ○ Cold discomfort.

# VIII Classification of hypothermia

## A Etiology-based

    ○ Primary hypothermia
       – Due to patient's exposure to a cold environment.
    ○ Secondary hypothermia
       – Due to the effect of drugs, illness (i.e. alteration in thermoregulation itself).

## B Temperature-based

    ○ Mild hypothermia (95.0–99.5 °F; 35.0–37.5 °C)
       – Not associated with major physiologic effects.
    ○ Moderate hypothermia (89.6–95 °F; 32–35 °C)
       – Triggers a two to sevenfold increase in release of catecholamines, resulting in vasoconstriction, tachycardia, and hypertension.
    ○ Severe hypothermia (86.0–89.6 °F; 30–32 °C).
       – Associated with increased risk of atrial fibrillation.

○ Critical hypothermia (<86 °F; <30 °C).
  – Induces refractory ventricular fibrillation and death.

## IX   Hypothermia in the foal

- Hypothermia is probably the most common complication observed during general anesthesia in foals.
- Neonatal and pediatric subjects are more prone to hypothermia due to:
  ○ The lack of reliable and long-lasting energy stores (i.e. glycogen stored in the liver and muscles of neonatal foals sustains normal thermoregulation for less than one hour).
  ○ Their higher metabolic rate compared to adult horses.
  ○ Less body insulation.
  ○ Higher surface area to body mass ratio.
  ○ Furthermore, autonomic regulation is an immature mechanism in the foal, yielding a less effective thermoregulatory response.
  ○ Shivering thermogenesis is the main mechanism to increase heat production in the foal, as foals have little to *no brown fat* to use in non-shivering thermogenesis.
  ○ Therefore, monitoring body temperature, and the use of external heat sources to promote normothermia during general anesthesia is of great importance.

## X   Hypothermia in the adult horse

- Among adult equids, geriatric subjects, miniature horses, and donkeys are most prone to developing hypothermia in the peri-operative period.
- Horses under general anesthesia not provided with any type of warming device, suffer a temperature loss of 0.4 °C per hour. Mean body temperature decreases below baseline body temperature after 75 minutes of general anesthesia with inhalational anesthetics.
- The decrease in body temperature under general anesthesia in most mammalians is triphasic.
  ○ An initial redistribution of heat due to vasodilatation.
  ○ A linear decrease in which heat loss outweighs production.
  ○ Vasoconstriction and retention of heat.
    *Note*: Horses seem to lack the initial redistribution of heat from core compartment to peripheral tissues; therefore, their decrease in body temperature is considered *biphasic*.
- A plateau in body temperature is observed only after about 200 minutes of general anesthesia.
- Body temperature decreases linearly during the first 145 minutes of general anesthesia with isoflurane or halothane, and then plateaus (data available up to 235 minutes of general anesthesia), with no significant difference between the two inhalants or between the sexes.
- Room temperature is significantly correlated with core temperature after 75 minutes of anesthesia, particularly in horses that have been wetted with lavages. The recommended operating room temperature is 78.8 °F (26 °C).
- Bradycardia was observed in horses anesthetized for an average of 270 minutes who did not receive external heating support during general anesthesia with sevoflurane. The temperature nadir was as low as 90.3 °F (32.4 °C) at 300 minutes of anesthesia.

- Hypothermia prolongs standing time in adult horses during recovery from general anesthesia.
- Temperature nadir of 95.5 °F (35.3 °C) under general anesthesia in adult horses is a significant predictor of time to standing in an unassisted recovery. Therefore, active warming may speed standing time.

## XI  Prevention and treatment of hypothermia

- Temperature management should be initiated in foals immediately after induction of general anesthesia with active heating devices (see below).
- Even large animals should receive thermal support during general anesthesia and recovery.

### A  Proactive heat management

- Management of body temperature should be focused on preventing hypothermia rather than in reaction to hypothermia.

*Methods of preventing hypothermia include:*
- Use of low fresh gas flows.
  - This is of more importance in foals.
- Insulating the animal to control radiant and convective losses will reduce heat loss.
- Reduce contact with cold surfaces and surgical scrub solutions.
- Active warming should start when body temperature is 99.5 °F (37.5 °C).
- Use of "internal" *warming devices* (core-to-skin, e.g. warm IV fluids, warm abdominal lavages).
- Use of "external" *warming devices* (skin-to-core, e.g. circulating hot water blankets, resistive electric blankets, forced-air warming devices).

### B  Warming Devices

*Passive*
- Blankets or towels.
- Reflective foil blankets.
- Leg wraps.

*Active*
- Forced-air warming devices (see Figure 11.1).
  - Suitable for foals, miniature horses, donkeys, and adult horses.
  - Warmed air circulated within a purpose-designed blanket (reusable or disposable) of different sizes. Heat is transferred via *convection*.
  - Reduce heat loss from 0.4 °C/hour to 0.2 °C/hour in adult horses under general anesthesia.
  - A device set at 43 °C is effective in preventing hypothermia in horses undergoing long-standing sedation procedures, and its use reduced body temperature decrease by half.
- Resistive polymer electric heating pads (see Figure 11.2).
  - Suitable for use in foals, miniature horses, and donkeys.
  - Heat is produced by electrical resistance and distributed evenly through the pad and transferred to the patient via conduction.

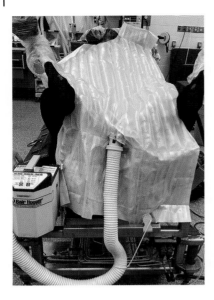

Figure 11.1   Bair Hugger™. A convective heating device.

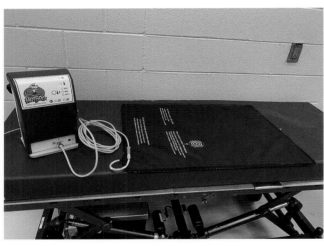

Figure 11.2   HotDog®. A resistive polymer heating device.

- Although *thermal* injuries are a potential complication of the use of these devices, the presence of a temperature sensor on the pad adds a layer of safety that is not present on other electric pad systems.
  ○ Circulating warm water blankets
    - Suitable for use in foals, miniature horses, and donkeys.
    - Heat is provided by warmed water that circulates within two layers of plastic and is transferred to the patient via convection.

*Other considerations*
  ○ A *medetomidine* continuous rate infusion (CRI) during general anesthesia can decrease heat loss in horses. Presumably, this effect would be similar for other alpha$_2$ agonists.
  ○ Radiant heat sources above the patient and surgical field may be helpful, but can lead to overheating.
  ○ Use warmed IV and irrigation fluids rather than room temperature fluids to prevent decreases in body temperature.

○ Less practical methods include warming and humidifying inspired anesthetic gases, and increasing operating room and recovery area ambient temperatures.

## XII Hyperthermia

- Hyperthermia occurs when heat production exceeds heat loss.
- Intraoperative hyperthermia in horses is most commonly associated with an episode of hyperkalemic periodic paralysis (HYPP) (see Chapter 38) and although less common, malignant hyperthermia should be ruled out.
- Disruption of physiologic processes by drugs may lead to abnormal heat dissipation, and hyperthermia.
- Cellular damage occurs at temperatures above 107.6 °F (42 °C).
- Hyperthermia causes increased oxygen consumption which may not be matched by oxygen delivery if hyperthermia is sustained, leading to metabolic derangements and anaerobic metabolism.

### A Clinical signs of hyperthermia include

○ Tachypnea.
○ Tachycardia.
○ Fatigue and central nervous system dysfunction.
○ Increased muscle tone.
○ Increased $PaCO_2$.

### B Treatment of horses with hyperthermia

*Note:* If HYPP is the cause of hyperthermia, efforts may initially have to be directed toward resolving hyperkalemia and cardiac arrhythmias (see Chapter 38).

○ Discontinuation of active and passive heating support measures.
○ Increase fresh gas flow.
○ Place fan in the direction of the patient.
○ Apply ice packs over major blood vessel in the neck and groin.
○ Wet skin with cold solutions (i.e. water, alcohol).
○ Administer room temperature IV fluids.
○ Lavage cavity with sterile fluids at room temperature.
○ Cooling measures should be discontinued when the rectal temperature has reached 101 °F (38.3 °C).

## Suggested Reading

Hubert, J.D., Beadle, R.E., and Norwood, G. (2002). Equine anhidrosis. *Vet. Clin. North Am. Equine Pract.* 18: 355–369.

Sessler, D.I. (2008). Temperature monitoring and perioperative thermoregulation. *Anesthesiology* 109: 318–338.

Tomasic, M. (1999). Temporal changes in core body temperature in anesthetized adult horses. *Am. J. Vet. Res.* 60: 556–562.

## 12

## Pharmacology of Drugs Used in Equine Anesthesia

### Phenothiazines

*Alicia Skelding*

- Phenothiazines, although still used in equine anesthesia, have largely been replaced by $\alpha_2$ agonists.
- Phenothiazines have activity at a wide variety of receptors (adrenergic, dopaminergic, histamine, muscarinic, and serotonergic).
  *Acepromazine*
    ○ *Acepromazine* is the most commonly used phenothiazine in the domestic horse.

## I  Mechanism of action of acepromazine

- *Acepromazine* interacts with a variety of receptors, displaying a number of effects in the central nervous system (CNS).
- The predominant sites of action appear to be *extrapyramidal*, and involve the basal ganglia, limbic system and brain stem.
- *Acepromazine* mediates its sedative effects via dopamine ($D_2$) receptor antagonism in the basal ganglia.
  ○ Dopamine has an important role in motor activity.
  ○ Activation of dopamine in the input nuclei causes an increase in excitatory impulses reaching the cortex.

## II  Physiologic effects

*Central nervous system*
    ○ Dose-dependent sedation, tranquilization.
        – Sedative effects can last up to two hours post administration.
    ○ Antipyretic effect.
*Cardiovascular system*
    ○ The $\alpha_1$ antagonist effect of *acepromazine* decreases systemic vascular resistance (SVR).

*Manual of Equine Anesthesia and Analgesia*, Second Edition. Edited by Tom Doherty,
Alex Valverde, and Rachel A. Reed.
© 2022 John Wiley & Sons, Inc. Published 2022 by John Wiley & Sons, Inc.

- Results in decreased arterial blood pressure (*hypotension*) in awake and anesthetized horses. However, this is only likely to be of clinical importance in hypovolemic horses.
  ○ No negative effects on cardiac function.
    - Cardiac output is generally not decreased.
  ○ Decreased hematocrit secondary to *splenic relaxation* and increased erythrocyte storage.
  ○ Its anti-arrhythmogenic properties increases the dose of *epinephrine* required to induce ventricular arrhythmias.

*Respiratory system*
  ○ Minimal effect on pulmonary function.
    - No changes in respiratory rate or tidal volume.
  ○ When combined with *romifidine + butorphanol* premedication, *acepromazine* administration improved arterial oxygenation.

*Gastrointestinal system*
  ○ Transient decrease in gastrointestinal (GI) motility.
  ○ Spasmolytic effect on intestinal tract.

*Miscellaneous*
  ○ Penile prolapse.
    - Within 10–15 minutes of administration.
  ○ Decreased *histamine* release from mast cells.

## III   Clinical use of acepromazine

### A   Standing sedation

○ Clinical doses of 0.02–0.05 mg/kg, intravenously (IV) or intramuscularly (IM).
○ Studies have used doses of up to 0.1 mg/kg; however, lower doses are advised.
○ Onset of action varies between 5 and 20 minutes following IV administration.
○ Sedative effects are not always obvious, but if effective, can last up to two hours.
○ Increasing the dose does not produce a better sedative effect.
○ Lack of analgesia limits its use to non-painful procedures when used as the sole agent.
○ Combining acepromazine with an *opioid* or *α₂ agonist* provides more reliable sedation.

### B   Premedication prior to general anesthesia

○ The administration of *acepromazine* as part of the premedication has a number of benefits including reduced risk of intraoperative fatality, minimum alveolar concentration (MAC) reduction, and improved recovery quality.

*Reduced risk of death intraoperatively*
  ○ The exact reason is undetermined, but may be related to the following factors:
    - Decreasing the MAC reduces the negative cardiovascular effects (arrhythmias, myocardial depression, cardiac arrest) of volatile anesthetics.
    - Afterload reduction leading to a decrease in myocardial wall stress.
  ○ The reduced risk of intraoperative fatality was found in association with *halothane* anesthesia, the associated benefit with more commonly used inhalant (*isoflurane, sevoflurane*) anesthetics is unknown.

*MAC reduction*
- ○ Dose-dependent effect on MAC.
- ○ *Acerpomazine* (0.05 mg/kg, IV) decreased the MAC of *halothane* by ~37%.

*Improved quality of recovery*
- ○ Administration of *acepromazine* (0.02 mg/kg, IV) improves the quality of recovery from inhalant anesthesia.
- ○ May simply be due to *acepromazine's* tranquilizing effect, increasing the time before the first attempt to stand.
- ○ May result from improved cardiovascular function of MAC reduction and consequent improvement in muscle perfusion, leading to improved muscle strength at standing.

## C Contraindications

- ○ Can cause priapism (reported in stallions and geldings). Although *rare* (≤1 in 10 000), the condition can lead to serious consequences if it persists for a few hours or is left untreated. (see Chapter 38)
  - – The onset of penile edema makes retraction of the penis difficult or impossible.
  - – Strong consideration should be given to alternatives in valuable breeding stallions.
- ○ Hypovolemia or shock are other contraindications for the use of *acepromazine*, as the $\alpha_1$ antagonism may result in severe hypotension in these cases.
- ○ Detection of *acepromazine* for up to 72 hours (depending on route of administration) has important considerations for violations of certain regulatory bodies in performance animals.
- ○ Minimum 72-hour withdrawal period has been advised.

## Suggested Reading

Doherty, T.J., Geiser, D.R., and Rohrbach, B.W. (1997). Effect of acepromazine and butorphanol on halothane minimum alveolar concentration in ponies. *Equine Vet. J.* 29: 274–276.

Driessen, B., Zarucco, L., Kalir, B., and Bertolotti, L. (2011). Contemporary use of acepromazine in the anaesthetic management of male horses and ponies: a retrospective study and opinion poll. *Equine Vet. J.* 43: 88–98.

Knych, H.K., Seminoff, K., McKemie, D.S., and Kass, P.H. (2018). Pharmacokinetics, pharmacodynamics, and metabolism of acepromazine following intravenous, oral, and sublingual administration to exercised thoroughbred horses. *J. Vet. Pharmacol. Ther.* 41: 522–535.

## Butyrophenones
*Alicia Skelding*

- • Butyrophenone tranquilizers are rarely used in the domestic horse.
- • These agents are mainly used in combination with other drugs to provide immobilization of *feral* and *wild* equine species.

*Azaperone*
- ○ *Azaperone* is a neuroleptic drug that fails to produce anesthesia, analgesia, or reliable sedation when used alone in equids.

# I  Mechanism of action

- *Azaperone* interacts with a number of receptors in the CNS.
  - ○ Sedative effects are a result of dopamine ($D_2$) receptor antagonism.
- It also has *antihistaminic* and *anticholinergic* effects.

# II  Physiologic effects

*Central nervous system*
  - ○ In horses, IM administration resulted in *unreliable* sedation.
    - – Eliciting good to excellent effect in just 71% of ponies.
  - ○ Onset of action was 10 minutes.
  - ○ Duration of effect was ~two hours.

*Cardiovascular system*
  - ○ Hypotension mediated by $\alpha_1$ antagonism.
  - ○ May also cause an increase in heart rate and cardiac output.
  - ○ These effects last longer than the sedative effects (>4 hours).

*Respiratory system*
  - ○ Minimal effect on respiratory function.
  - ○ No significant changes in arterial blood gas values (pH, $PaCO_2$, $PaO_2$).

# III  Clinical use of azaperone

- Predominately used for *neurolept* (tranquilizer + analgesic) anesthesia and immobilization in *wild* equids.
- Routinely combined with *etorphine* for immobilization of wild zebras.
  - ○ Recently marketed as "BAM™".
    - – A combination of *butorphanol*, *azaperone*, and *medetomidine* for wildlife immobilization.
    - – In the author's experience, BAM provides effective immobilization in feral equids (Przewalski's horses, zebras).
    - – Better quality of immobilization than *etorphine*-based protocols.

# IV  Contraindications

- IV administration has been advised against in horses due to the high percentage of horses (>50%) exhibiting paradoxical excitement.

## Suggested Reading

Bogan, J.A., MacKenzie, G., and Snow, D.H. (1978). An evaluation of tranquillisers for use with etorphine as neuroleptanalgesic agents in the horse. *Vet. Rec.* 103: 471–472.

Chui, Y.C., Esaw, B., and Laviolette, B. (1994). Investigation of the metabolism of azaperone in the horse. *J. Chromatogr.* 652: 23–33.

Dodman, N.H. and Waterman, A.E. (1979). Paradoxical excitement following the intravenous administration of azaperone in the horse. *Equine Vet. J.* 11: 33–35.

Serrano, L. and Lees, P. (1976). The applied pharmacology of azaperone in horses. *Res. Vet. Sci.* 20: 316–323.

## $\alpha_2$-Adrenergic Agonists

*Alicia Skelding*

- Due to the reliable sedation, analgesia and muscle relaxation associated with their administration, $\alpha_2$ agonists are of great importance in equine anesthesia.
- The effects of $\alpha_2$ agonists can be reliably reversed with selective $\alpha_2$ antagonist drugs.

## I  $\alpha_2$-receptor subtypes

- $\alpha_2$ receptors are present at diverse sites in the central (locus coeruleus and rostroventral lateral medulla in the brainstem; substantia gelatinosa in the dorsal horn) and peripheral (most organs, extra-synaptically in vascular tissue, platelets) nervous system.
- Three subtypes ($\alpha_{2A}$, $\alpha_{2B}$, $\alpha_{2C}$) of $\alpha_2$ receptors have been described.
  - A fourth subtype ($\alpha_{2D}$) has also been described in the literature; however, it seems to be a variant of the $\alpha_{2A}$ subtype, and therefore is not described here.

### A  $\alpha_{2A}$ subtype

- Located in the cerebral cortex and the brainstem.
- Stimulation of this receptor subtype in the CNS mediates *sedation*, *supraspinal analgesia* and *sympatholytic* effects.
- Causes centrally mediated *bradycardia* and *hypotension*.
- It is responsible for the MAC-sparing effects of $\alpha_2$ agonists.
- Associated with alterations in *behavior*.
- Inhibits *dopamine* release in the basal ganglia.
- Inhibits *serotonin* release in the hippocampus and cortex.
- Peripherally, the prejunctional location of these receptor subtypes results in *vasodilation*.
- It inhibits *insulin* release from pancreatic islets cells by decreasing cyclic adenosine monophosphate (cAMP).
  - Results in hyperglycemia.
- It causes a decrease in GI motility.

### B  $\alpha_{2B}$-subtype

- Located in the spinal cord and vascular endothelium.
- Mediates spinal analgesia.
- Mediates some antinociceptive actions of $N_2O$.
  - Activation of endorphin release in periaqueductal gray (PAG) by $N_2O$ stimulates a descending pathway, which releases norepinephrine and affects $\alpha_{2B}$ receptors in the dorsal horn.

○ Mediates peripheral vasoconstriction.
○ Responsible for initial hypertension following systemic administration of $\alpha_2$ agonists.
  – Baroreceptor-mediated bradycardia occurs secondary to increased vascular resistance.

C  $\alpha_{2C}$-subtype

○ Located in the spinal cord and peripherally.
○ Modulate spinal analgesia.
○ Regulates *epinephrine* release from adrenal medulla.
○ Modulates behavior.
○ Similar effects on *dopamine* and *serotonin* release as $\alpha_{2A}$ subtype.
○ Also inhibits *insulin* release.

## II  Mechanism of action

- $\alpha_2$ receptors are coupled to an inhibitory G protein ($G\alpha_i$), which inhibits adenylyl cyclase (AC). This decreases the synthesis of cAMP from adenosine triphosphate (ATP) and inhibits voltage gated calcium ($Ca^{2+}$) channels.
- In general, the prejunctional $\alpha_2$ receptors inhibit the release of *norepinephrine* because inhibition of voltage gated $Ca^{2+}$ channels prevents docking of presynaptic vesicles that contain norepinephrine.
- Postsynaptic $\alpha_2$ receptors stimulate smooth-muscle contraction (*vasoconstriction*) by increasing intracellular $Ca^{2+}$ through the inositol triphosphate ($IP_3$) pathway. They indirectly cause contraction by inhibition of AC, causing a reduction in intracellular cAMP, which normally inhibits myosin kinase, resulting in smooth-muscle relaxation (vasodilation).

## III  Physiological effects

*Central nervous system*
○ Sedation, anxiolysis (presynaptic; $\alpha_{2A}$).
○ Inhibit norepinephrine release.
  – Decreased sympathetic outflow (presynaptic; $\alpha_{2A}$).
○ Supraspinal analgesia (presynaptic, postsynaptic; $\alpha_{2A}$).
○ Spinal analgesia.
  – Inhibition of release of substance P from C fibers (presynaptic; $\alpha_{2A}$, $\alpha_{2B}$, $\alpha_{2C}$).
  – Modulation of afferent input to the dorsal horn (postsynaptic; $\alpha_{2A}$, $\alpha_{2B}$, $\alpha_{2C}$).
○ Decrease MAC of volatile anesthetics (presynaptic $\alpha_{2A}$).
*Cardiovascular system*
○ Biphasic effect on blood pressure.
  – Initial hypertension via peripheral vasoconstriction (postsynaptic $\alpha_{2B}$).
  – Persistent hypotension (presynaptic $\alpha_{2C}$).
  – Decreased sympathetic outflow (presynaptic $\alpha_{2A}$).
○ Bradycardia
  – Initially, baroreceptor mediated (secondary to increased vascular resistance).

  – Persists due to decreased sympathetic outflow (presynaptic $\alpha_{2A}$) and increased vagal tone.
  – Second-degree atrioventricular block (transient) is common.
  ○ Decreased cardiac output.
  – Secondary to bradycardia.
  – Decreased sympathetic outflow (presynaptic $\alpha_{2A}$).

*Respiratory system*
  ○ Reduction in respiratory rate and minute ventilation.
  – Centrally mediated.
  – Dose-dependent.
  ○ Pale blue/Gray mucous membranes are often apparent because of:
  – Prolonged capillary transit time.
  – Increased oxygen extraction increases the amount of deoxygenated hemoglobin present.

*Gastrointestinal system*
  ○ Decreased intestinal motility (presynaptic $\alpha_{2A}$).
  ○ Inhibition of acetylcholine release in myenteric plexus.

*Urinary system*
  ○ Promote diuresis due to:
  – Decreased release of *antidiuretic hormone* from pituitary.
  – Decreased *renin* concentrations.
  – Increased release of *atrial natriuretic peptide*.

*Endocrine system*
  ○ Transient hyperglycemia.
  – Inhibits insulin release (presynaptic $\alpha_{2A}$, $\alpha_{2C}$).
  ○ Suppression of the stress response.
  – Decreased circulating catecholamines.

*Miscellaneous*
  ○ Thermoregulation is inhibited.
  ○ Sweating (especially under the mane and forelock) is common.

# IV   Clinical use of $\alpha_2$ agonists

## A   Standing sedation

  ○ Under $\alpha_2$-agonist sedation, the horse's head will become lowered, facilitating its ability to balance on the fore limbs and kick violently with both rear limbs. For this reason, the head should be raised, especially when examining/working around the pelvic limbs.
  ○ Equipotent IV doses of $\alpha_2$ agonists are listed in Box 12.1.
  ○ Onset of action following IV administration of equipotent doses is: *xylazine > detomidine > dexmedetomidine > romifidine*.
  ○ The IM dose is two to three times the IV dose and takes 15–30 minutes for peak effect.
  ○ Ataxia is dose-related, and more severe with *detomidine, dexmedetomidine*, and *xylazine* than with *romifidine*.
  ○ Duration of action (equipotent doses): *romifidine ≥ detomidine > dexmedetomidine > xylazine*.

---

**Box 12.1**   *Equipotent IV doses* of $\alpha_2$ Agonists

| | |
|---|---|
| *Xylazine* | 1 mg/kg |
| *Detomidine* | 20–40 µg/kg |
| *Romifidine* | 80–120 µg/kg |
| *Dexmedetomidine* | 3.5 µg/kg |
| *Medetomidine* | 5–10 µg/kg |

*Note:* results differ slightly among studies, hence the range of doses.

---

*Note:* There is a discrepancy in the literature regarding the comparative sedative effects and duration of action of *romifidine* and *detomidine*. In one study, detomidine at doses of 10, 20, and 40 µg/kg, IV was associated with more potent and longer lasting sedation than romifidine at the purportedly equipotent doses of 40, 80, and 120 µg/kg, IV. However, in another study, the sedative effect of *romifidine* at 80 µg/kg, IV was longer lasting than *detomidine* at 20 µg/kg IV.

- The degree and duration of sedation is dose- and drug-dependent.
- High doses of *detomidine/romifidine* increase the intensity and duration of sedation.
  o An infusion can be administered if prolonged standing sedation is required (see Chapter 20).
  o $\alpha_2$ agonists can be combined with *phenothiazines* or *opioids*.
    - This gives more reliable sedation.
    - The horse is also less likely to suddenly react to stimuli.

## B   Premedication prior to general anesthesia

  o $\alpha_2$ agonists provide sedation and muscle relaxation prior to induction of anesthesia.
  o The dose of $\alpha_2$ agonist will depend greatly on which drugs are being used for induction.
    - If *ketamine* (2.0–2.5 mg/kg, IV) is used alone for induction following $\alpha_2$ sedation, it is critical that the horse is heavily sedated (lowered head, droopy lip, droopy ears, wide-based stance) with the $\alpha_2$ agonist before *ketamine* is administered.
    - If *ketamine* is combined with a benzodiazepine for induction, a lower dose of the $\alpha_2$ agonist may be used because the benzodiazepine will provide additional muscle relaxation.
    - If *ketamine* is combined with *guaifenesin* for induction, the dose of $\alpha_2$ may be lowered as *guaifenesin* provides potent muscle relaxation.
  o This premedication dose serves as a loading dose for constant rate infusion (CRI) administration.
  o Decreases MAC.
  o Improves recovery quality when administered intraoperatively as a CRI and when administered for postoperative sedation.
    - Increased time spent in sternal.
    - Increased time to first attempt to stand.
    - Decreased number of attempts to stand.

C   Maintenance of anesthesia

- Infusions of $\alpha_2$ agonists can be used in conjunction with other injectable drugs, primarily *ketamine*, to maintain anesthesia (see total intravenous anesthesia (TIVA) Chapter 21).
- Infusions of $\alpha_2$ agonists can be used in conjunction with inhalant anesthetics to provide analgesia and decrease MAC (see partial intravenous anesthesia (PIVA) Chapter 21).

D   Epidural analgesia

- Analgesic effects of $\alpha_2$ agonists:
    - Increase acetylcholine concentrations in the cerebrospinal fluid (CSF).
    - Inhibition of substance P release from C fibers (presynaptic).
    - Inhibition of wide dynamic range neurons (postsynaptic).
- *Xylazine, detomidine, romifidine* have been evaluated for epidural administration.
- *Detomidine* doses of 20–40 µg/kg epidurally have been recommended for epidural administration when performing flank laparotomies; however, in the author's experience, these doses are associated with extreme ataxia and sedation. Thus, lower doses of detomidine (5–10 µg/kg) are recommended for epidural administration.
- *Xylazine* is the most common $\alpha_2$ agonist that is administered epidurally.
    - Local anesthetic-like effect.
        - It is similar in chemical structure to *lidocaine*.
        - May block A$\delta$ fibers.
    - 0.17 mg/kg provided three hours of analgesia.
    - No ataxia reported at this dose.

E   Individual drugs

- Receptor affinity of selected $\alpha_2$ agonist drugs ($\alpha_2 : \alpha_1$) is listed in Box 12.2.
- Differences in affinity are due to differences in the degree of methylation of the benzene ring and halogenation of the dihydro-imidazole ring.

*Xylazine*

- MAC reduction.
    - A 30–50% decrease in isoflurane requirements when used as a CRI alone at 0.5–1.0 mg/kg/hr. Up to 70% MAC reduction has been reported when used as a CRI in combination with other drugs (e.g. lidocaine, ketamine).
- Decreases in heart rate and cardiac index.
    - However, these values are clinically acceptable.
- Significantly improves the quality of recovery from inhalant anesthesia when administered as a bolus dose (0.1–0.5 mg/kg, IV) for recovery.

| Box 12.2   Receptor Affinity of $\alpha_2$ Agonists ($\alpha_2 : \alpha_1$) | |
| --- | --- |
| • *Xylazine* | 160 : 1 |
| • *Detomidine* | 260  1 |
| • *Romifidine* | 340 : 1 |
| • *Dexmedetomidine* | 1620 : 1 |

*Detomidine*
- MAC reduction.
  - 40% decrease in MAC when administered as a bolus dose (0.03–0.06 mg/kg, IV).
  - 18% decrease in isoflurane requirements when administered as a CRI at 10 µg/kg/hr.
  - No decrease in isoflurane requirements when administered as a CRI at 5 µg/kg/hr.
- Cardiovascular changes (decreased HR, increased SVR) typical of $\alpha_2$ agonists when administered as a CRI to isoflurane-anesthetized horses, but parameters are clinically acceptable.
- Available as an oral, *transmucosal gel.*
  - Dose ~40 µg/kg.
  - Onset of action 30–40 minutes.
  - Low bioavailability (22%).
  - Less ataxia, shorter duration of action than IV administration.
  - Can also be administered intravaginally to produce sedation.

*Romifidine*
- Inconsistent results regarding inhalant sparing effects.
  - Some studies have demonstrated a decrease in MAC when administered as a CRI, others have not.
- Cardiovascular performance remained acceptable when administered as a CRI (40 µg/kg/hr) during isoflurane anesthesia compared to isoflurane alone.
  - No significant differences in cardiac index.
- Significantly improves the quality of recovery from inhalant anesthesia when administered as an IV bolus for recovery.
  - Considered to cause less ataxia than other $\alpha_2$ agonists.
- In comparison with *xylazine* for standing sedation, the cardiovascular effects of *romifidine* (decreased heart rate and cardiac output) are more pronounced and longer lasting.
  - Longer depression of sympathetic outflow.
  - Increased peripheral vagal tone.

*Dexmedetomidine*
- MAC reduction.
  - 53% decrease in sevoflurane MAC when administered as a CRI (1.75 µg/kg/hr).
- No clinically detrimental effect on heart rate or cardiac index when administered as a CRI in isoflurane-anesthetized horses.
- Significantly improved quality of recovery from inhalant anesthesia when administered as a CRI.
  - Fewer attempts to stand.
  - Longer time spent in sternal.
  - Longer time before first attempt to stand.

## V Contraindications

- Changes in intrauterine pressure in pregnant mares are of concern, but appears to be well tolerated clinically.
  - Increased intrauterine pressure following administration of all $\alpha_2$ agonists.
  - *Xylazine > detomidine > romifidine.*

- No negative effect when *detomidine* was frequently administered to mares in the last trimester of pregnancy.
- Benefit to the mare needs to be weighed against possible negative impact on fetus.

## VI    Adrenergic antagonists

- Although it is not generally necessary to reverse $\alpha_2$ agonists in equine species, it may be desirable on some occasions. For example, if a horse had to be heavily sedated with *detomidine* for a dental procedure, and the owner needs to transport the horse from the clinic soon thereafter.
- The most commonly used agents in equine medicine are *yohimbine, tolazoline,* and *atipamezole.*
- Recently, *vatinoxan (MK-467)*, a peripherally acting $\alpha_2$ antagonist, has been evaluated in equine species.

### A    Mechanism of action

- Competitive antagonists.
- Receptor affinity ($\alpha_2 : \alpha_1$) differs among agents.

*Tolazoline*
  - A weak, competitive non-selective antagonist (4 : 1).
  - Has histaminergic and cholinergic effects.
  - Approved by the Food and Drug Administration in the United States for reversal of *xylazine* in horses.

*Yohimbine*
  - Non-selective, weak antagonist (40 : 1).

*Atipamezole*
  - Potent antagonist activity (8526 : 1).

### B    Physiologic effects

- Causes norepinephrine release from the sympathetic nerve terminals (presynaptic).
  - Can cause CNS excitation if the dose is inappropriate for the degree of wakefulness or if excessively high doses are administered.
  - Reversal of analgesia.
    - Results in a sudden increase in nociception and pain.
- IV administration can result in rapid onset of *peripheral vasodilation* resulting in *hypotension* if the animal has high SVR at the time of administration (postsynaptic; $\alpha_{2B}$).
  - Coupled with bradycardia, from the $\alpha_2$ agonist, this can cause cardiovascular collapse.

### C    Clinical use

- Reasons for reversal include:
  - Cardiopulmonary compromise or prolonged recovery from an overdose of $\alpha_2$ agonist.
  - To counter the effects of prolonged sedation from high-dose *detomidine* or *romifidine*.
  - To speed recovery in feral/wild equine species.

*Yohimbine*
- – Clinical dose 0.02–0. 075 mg/kg IV (depending on the degree of sedation), administered over five minutes.
- – Can activate dopaminergic and serotonergic receptors at high doses.

*Tolazoline*
- – The label dose is 4 mg/kg IV. However, smaller doses may be adequate depending on the degree of sedation.
- – Administer slowly IV to avoid adverse cardiovascular effects.
- – Results in a stress response (increased blood glucose, cortisol and fatty acids).

*Atipamezole*
- – Clinical dose: 0.03–0.06 µg/kg, IM, IV.
- – IM administration of these reversal agents should be considered in non-emergency situations.
- – IV doses should be titrated to achieve the desired clinical effect.

D **Adverse reactions**

- ○ Highly variable behavioral responses have been reported in horses following IV administration of a bolus dose of *yohimbine to awake horses*, with some horses exhibiting sedation and others exhibiting excitation (rearing, striking, circling, agitation).
  - – Generalized muscle fasciculations are commonly reported.
  - – Horses appear agitated and anxious in response to external stimuli at higher studied doses (0.2–0.4 mg/kg, IV bolus), which is why lower doses are recommended and the drug should be titrated to achieve the desired effect.
- ○ Sweating and hyperexcitability has been inconsistently reported in horses following the IV bolus administration of higher doses of atipamezole (0.16–0.2 mg/kg).
- ○ Idiosyncratic reactions of severe tachypnea, respiratory distress, tachycardia, collapse, and death following IV administration have been reported.

E **Vatinoxan (MK-467)**

- ○ Peripheral, selective $\alpha_2$ antagonist (105 : 1).
- ○ Poor penetration of the blood–brain barrier due to low lipophilicity.
- ○ May be of greater benefit in standing horses.
  - – Administration of *vatinoxan* (150 µg/kg, IV) 10 minutes after sedation with detomidine (10 µg/kg, IV) successfully resolved the $\alpha_2$ agonist-induced hypertension, bradycardia, and GI hypomotility.
  - – Co-administration of *vatinoxan* (200 µg/kg, IV) with romifidine (80 µg/kg, IV) resulted in higher heart rates and prevented GI hypomotility, compared with administration of romifidine alone. Similar results have been found for co-administration of *vatinoxan* with detomidine.
- ○ In anesthetized horses, co-administration of *vatinoxan* with $\alpha_2$ agonists results in significant *hypotension*.
  - – In isoflurane-anesthetized horses receiving a xylazine (1 mg/kg/hr) or dexmedetomidine (7 µg/kg/hr) CRI, an IV bolus of vatinoxan (250 µg/kg over 10 minutes) caused a 48 and 58% decrease in mean arterial blood pressure (MAP) resulting in significant hypotension (defined as MAP <50 mmHg). Similar results have been identified during medetomidine CRI.

– This may be secondary to the central effect of $\alpha_2$ agonists resulting in decreased sympathetic outflow and decreased SVR in combination with the vasodilation resulting from inhalant anesthetics.

## Suggested Reading

England, G.C., Clarke, K.W., and Goossens, L. (1992). A comparison of the sedative effects of three alpha 2-adrenoceptor agonists (romifidine, detomidine and xylazine) in the horse. *J. Vet. Pharmacol. Ther.* 15: 194–201.

Hamm, D., Turchi, P., and Jöchle, W. (1995). Sedative and analgesic effects of detomidine and romifidine in horses. *Vet. Rec.* 136: 324–327.

Hollis, A.R., Pascal, M., Dijk, J. et al. (2020). Behavioral and cardiovascular effects of medetomidine in constant rate infusion compared with detomidine for standing sedation in horses. *Vet. Anaesth. Analg.* 47: 76–81.

Schatzmann, U., Jossfck, H., Stauffer, J.L., and Goossens, L. (1994). Effects of alpha-2 agonists on intrauterine pressure and sedation in horses: comparison between detomidine, romifidine and xylazine. *Zentralbl. Veterinarmed. A* 41: 523–529.

Seddighi, R., Knych, H.K., Cox, S.K. et al. (2020). Evaluation of the sedative effects and pharmacokinetics of detomidine gel administered intravaginally to horses. *Vet. Anaesth. Analg.* 46: 772–779.

Valverde, A. (2010). Alpha-2 agonists as pain therapy in horses. *Vet. Clin. North Am. Equine Pract.* 26: 515–532.

Wittenberg-Voges, L., Kastner, S.B., Raekallio, M. et al. (2018). Effect of dexmedetomidine and xylazine followed by MK-467 on gastrointestinal microperfusion in anaesthetized horses. *Vet. Anaesth. Analg.* 45: 165–174.

## Opioids
*Alicia Skelding*

- The use of opioids in horses has been controversial due to the inability of these drugs, when used alone, to cause reliable sedation or reduce MAC.
- Opioids tend to cause CNS excitation in non-painful horses at higher doses. For this reason, they are commonly used in association with sedative agents such as $\alpha_2$ agonists.

## I Opioid receptor types

- There are three types of opioid receptors: mu ($\mu$), delta ($\delta$) and kappa ($\kappa$).
- Species variations in receptor types and locations within the CNS may explain the differences in clinical response to certain opioids.

### A Mu ($\mu$) opioid receptor (MOP, OP3)

- Centrally located in the *brain* (caudate nucleus, cerebellum, cerebral cortex, periaqueductal gray, nucleus accumbens, substantia nigra) and *spinal cord* (dorsal root ganglion).

○ Peripheral locations include *enteric neurons* of the GI tract, *adrenal gland*, *pancreas*, *synovium*, and *cartilage*.
○ Three *subtypes* have been identified:

$\mu_1$

– Distributed in the brain, spinal cord and periphery.
– Mediate supraspinal and peripheral analgesia.

$\mu_2$

– Distributed in the brain, spinal cord and periphery.
– Mediate spinal analgesia.
  ■ Modify GI transit time, causing ileus.
  ■ Responsible for respiratory depression.

$\mu_3$

– Distributed in immune cells, peripheral neural cells and amygdala.
– May play a role in immunomodulation.

B   Kappa ($\kappa$) opioid receptor (KOP, OP2)

○ Centrally located in the brain (caudate nucleus, cerebellum, cerebral cortex, periaqueductal gray, nucleus accumbens, substantia nigra) and spinal cord (dorsal root ganglion).
○ Peripherally located in the heart, lung, kidney, liver, pancreas, spleen, skeletal muscle and synovium.
○ Three subtypes have been identified:

$\kappa_1$

– Distributed in the brain (nucleus accumbens, cerebellum) and spinal cord.
– Mediates analgesia.
– Increase appetite.

$\kappa_2$

– Distributed in the brain (hippocampus, thalamus, brainstem).
– Mediates analgesia.
– Mediates diuresis (inhibits antidiuretic hormone release).

$\kappa_3$

– Distributed in the brain.
– Mediates analgesia.

C   Delta ($\delta$) opioid receptors (DOP, OP1)

○ *Centrally* located in the brain (caudate nucleus, cerebellum, cerebral cortex, periaqueductal gray, nucleus accumbens, substantia nigra) and spinal cord (dorsal root ganglion).
○ *Peripherally* located in the heart, lung, kidney, adrenal gland, pancreas, skeletal muscle, thymus, and synovium.
Two subtypes have been identified:

$\boldsymbol{\delta}_1$

– Distributed in the brain and periphery.
– Mediates analgesia.

$\boldsymbol{\delta}_2$

– Distributed in the brain and spinal cord.
– Mediates analgesia.
– May be involved in thermoregulation.

## II   Mechanism of action

- Opioid receptors are coupled to an inhibitory G protein ($G_{\alpha i}$), which inhibits the action of AC. This decreases the synthesis of cAMP from ATP and inhibits voltage gated $Ca^{2+}$ channels.
- Inhibition of $Ca^{2+}$ channels in presynaptic neurons inhibits the release of excitatory neuro-transmitters (glutamate, substance P).
- Enhancement of potassium ($K^+$) outflow in postsynaptic nociceptive neurons results in hyperpolarization and increased activation thresholds.

### A   Full agonists

- Produce maximal stimulation of the receptor.
- Include *morphine, meperidine (pethidine), methadone, hydromorphone*, and *fentanyl*.
- Full agonists are potent analgesics.

### B   Partial agonists

- Have a maximal effect at the receptor that is less than the effect of a full agonist.
  - E.g., *Buprenorphine*.

### C   Mixed agonist/antagonists

- Have agonist activity at one opioid receptor and antagonist activity at another opioid receptor.
  - For example, *Butorphanol, nalbuphine*, and *pentazocine*.

### D   Antagonists

- Produce no effect at the receptor, and inhibit the activity of the agonist.
  - For example, *Naloxone, naltrexone*, and *diprenorphine*.

## V   Physiologic effects of opioids

### A   Central nervous system

*Supraspinal analgesia* ($\mu$, $\delta$, $\kappa$).
- Binding of opioid receptors within the periaqueductal gray (PAG) region inhibits gamma aminobutyric acid (GABA).
- Inhibition of dorsal horn nociceptive pathways.
- Release of norepinephrine and serotonin in the spinal cord dorsal horn.

*Spinal analgesia*
- Decreased nociceptive transmission.
  - Inhibition of presynaptic glutamate and substance P release.
  - Hyperpolarization of postsynaptic nociceptive neurons.

*Antitussive effects* ($\mu$, $\kappa$)
- Opioids have their effect at the cough center in the medulla oblongata.

- Can facilitate standing procedures.
  - In standing horses sedated with detomidine, butorphanol (0.02 mg/kg, IV) adminis-tered 20 minutes before bronchoalveolar lavage significantly decreased the intensity of coughing during the procedure.

*Sedation*
- Less commonly seen in horses when opioids are administered alone.

*Excitement and increased locomotor activity*
- Excitation is more likely when opioids are administered in high doses to non-painful horses.
- More likely to occur following IV administration.
- Concurrent sedation with an $\alpha_2$ agonist will alleviate this effect.
- IM administration is recommended when opioids are administered alone; nevertheless, excitation may still occur depending on the dose of opioid used.

### B Cardiovascular system

- Increased heart rate in awake horses.
- Minimal changes in heart rate occur in anesthetized horses.

### C Respiratory system

- Dose-dependent respiratory depression ($\mu_2$).
  - Rarely warrants intervention in awake horses.

### D Gastrointestinal system

- Decreased GI motility (central $\mu_2$, $\kappa$, peripheral $\mu$).
  - Decreased release of acetylcholine and substance P.
- Decreased propulsive contractions.
- Increased fluid absorption.
- Decreased GI secretions.

### E Urinary system

- May cause urine retention following epidural or intrathecal administration, *although this has not been reported in horses.*
  - Decreased detrusor muscle contractility.
  - Increased tone of urinary sphincters.
  - Inhibition of micturition.
- Decreased urine production ($\mu$).
- Diuresis ($\kappa$).

### F Miscellaneous

- Hyperthermia.
  - Alteration of thermoregulatory set point in hypothalamus.
- Mydriasis.
  - Secondary to catecholamine release from the adrenal gland.
- Immunomodulation.
- Pruritus has been reported following extradural morphine administration.
  - Secondary to local *histamine* release from mast cells in the skin.

## IV Clinical use of opioids

### A Standing sedation

- ○ Not used alone for sedation, but they potentiate the effects of $\alpha_2$ agonists.
- ○ Commonly used agents include:
    - – *Butorphanol* (0.02–0.05 mg/kg, IV; 0.05–0.1 mg/kg, IM).
    - – *Morphine* (0.15 mg/kg, IV; 0.25 mg/kg, IM).
    - – *Methadone* (0.1 mg/kg, IV or IM).
    - – *Meperidine* (*pethidine*) is administered IM (1–2 mg/kg).
        - ▪ IV administration can result in *histamine* release and hypotension.
        - ▪ Hyperesthesia, muscle fasciculations and sweating are also reported after IV administration.
    - – *Hydromorphone* (0.02–0.04 mg/kg IV or IM)
        - ▪ It is less commonly used in equine practice; however, recent studies reported that it produced a relatively long-lasting analgesia in a thermal pain model.
- ○ Opioids can be utilized as a CRI in association with an $\alpha_2$ agonist.
    - – For example, *Morphine + medetomidine* CRI resulted in clinically acceptable sedation and analgesia for standing laparoscopy in horses.

### B Premedication prior to general anesthesia

- ○ The use of an opioid as part of the premedication in the anesthetic protocol for horses typically depends on the preference of the anesthetist, but it does have some benefit.
- ○ However, opioids do not decrease MAC of volatile anesthetics in horses.

*Analgesia*

- ○ Providing analgesia may be especially helpful in calming a painful horse.
- ○ *Morphine* (0.25 mg/kg, IM) approximately one hour prior to induction of anesthesia (with or without *acepromazine* 0.03–0.05 mg/kg, IM) generally has a beneficial effect.
- ○ *Morphine* administration has been demonstrated to improve recovery quality from inhalant anesthesia in horses undergoing surgical procedures.
    - – 0.1–0.2 mg/kg, IV as a single dose or followed by a CRI (0.1 mg/kg/hr).
    - – Recoveries were characterized by fewer attempts to sternal, fewer attempts to stand, but shorter times to first movement compared to horses that did not receive *morphine*.
- ○ *Morphine* may produce more stable anesthesia.
    - – Fewer supplemental doses of *ketamine* may be needed to prevent intraoperative movement.
    - – The reported incidence of adverse effects in the group that received *morphine* did not differ from control horses.

### C Epidural analgesia

- ○ Opioids can be administered epidurally, alone or in combination with other drugs, to produce analgesia in the awake horse or as an adjunct to general anesthesia.
- ○ *Morphine* (0.1 mg/kg)
    - – Onset of action is slow (~30 minutes).
    - – Duration of action 8–16 hours.
    - – Epidural *morphine* (0.1 mg/kg) was not found to have a negative effect on GI motility.
- ○ *Hydromorphone* (0.04 mg/kg)
    - – Provided perineal, lumbar, sacral, and thoracic analgesia.

    – Onset of action ~20 minutes.

    – Duration of action four hours.

  ○ *Methadone* (0.1 mg/kg).

    – Onset of action 15 minutes.

    – Duration of action five hours.

## D  Opioids and ileus

○ High doses of *morphine* (0.5 mg/kg, IV q12 hr for six days) resulted in ileus and decreased fecal production.

  – Some horses demonstrated clinical signs of abdominal discomfort.

○ Clinical doses of *morphine* (0.05 and 0.1 mg/kg, once IV or IM) resulted in decreased GI motility.

  – No clinical signs of abdominal discomfort were evident.

○ Retrospective studies demonstrate conflicting evidence with respect to an increased risk of colic (or lack thereof) associated with *morphine* administration in horses following anesthesia.

○ A single retrospective study of post-anesthetic signs of colic revealed there was no increased risk of colic signs associated with *hydromorphone* administration in horses.

## V  Individual drugs

• Opioid potency is often compared to *morphine*. (see Box 12.3)

*Morphine*

○ Full μ agonist.

○ Most commonly used μ-agonist opioid.

○ Well tolerated at clinical doses (0.1–0.2 mg/kg, IV, IM).

  – Should be co-administered with a *sedative* ($\alpha_2$ *agonist*), especially in awake non-painful horses.

○ Ideal for epidural administration due to low lipid solubility.

○ Intra-articular *morphine* (0.05 mg/kg) provides anti-inflammatory and analgesic effects.

*Hydromorphone*

○ Full μ agonist.

○ Recommended doses of 0.02–0.04 mg/kg, IV, IM.

○ Clinically relevant antinociceptive effects observed with 0.04 mg/kg, IV and IM.

  – Increased thermal threshold.

  – Duration of up to 12 hours.

| Box 12.3   Opioid Potency Compared to *Morphine* | |
| --- | --- |
| ○ *Demerol* | 1 : 10 |
| ○ *Hydromorphone* | 5 : 1 |
| ○ *Methadone* | 10 : 1 |
| ○ *Buprenorphine* | 25 : 1 |
| ○ *Fentanyl* | 100 : 1 |

- High doses (0.04–0.08 mg/kg, IV, IM) in awake horses result in notable excitation (pacing, vocalizing, rearing, kicking) and decreased number of defecations.

*Note*: Behavioral signs are less likely to be exhibited if the horse is painful.

*Fentanyl*
- Full μ agonist.
- Use may be limited in adult horses due to potential for dangerous CNS excitation.
  - Dose-dependent increases in locomotor activity.
  - Potentially injurious recoveries and hyperthermia when utilized as a CRI during inhalant anesthesia.
- Similar dose-related effects in *foals*.
  - 4 μg/kg, IV-induced sedation in foals from one to six weeks of age.
  - 8 and 16 μg/kg, IV resulted in increased locomotor activity, ataxia, muscle rigidity and head pressing.
- *Transdermal* application of fentanyl to the proximal medial or lateral antebrachium using one 10 mg patch for horses <115 kg and two 10 mg patches for horses 115–585 kg results in complete absorption (bioavailability of 96%) and rapid achievement of concentrations above 1 ng/ml, considered therapeutic in other species, and achieved within 1–14 hours and remained at those concentrations for an average of $35 \pm 15$ hours. Each 10 mg patch is designed to deliver 100 μg/hour.

*Methadone*
- Full μ agonist.
- Also has effects as an N-methyl-D-aspartate (NMDA) antagonist.
- Potentiates the antinociceptive effects of *detomidine*.
- Provides acceptable surgical conditions when administered as a CRI with *detomidine* for standing procedures.
  - 0.2 mg/kg, IV then 0.05 mg/kg/hr.

*Etorphine*
- Full μ opioid agonist.
- Highly potent opioid used for restraint of *wild* and *feral* horses.
- *Caution: Etorphine is rapidly lethal to humans.*
  - Reversal agent should be readily available and personal protective equipment (PPE) should be worn when handling the drug.
- Immobilization is characterized by:
  - Analgesia.
  - Long-lasting anesthesia but often of poor quality due to:
    - Increased muscle activity, tremors, involuntary movement.
    - Hyperthermia, sweating.
    - Profound respiratory depression, resulting in apnea and cyanosis.
    - Hypertension.
    - Tachycardia (often masked by high doses of $\alpha_2$ agonists).
    - The eyes remain open and should be protected.

*Buprenorphine*
- Partial μ opioid agonist.
- Clinically relevant effects occur within 20 minutes following IV administration; however, peak effect takes 45–90 minutes.
- Provides suitable sedation (5 μg/kg, IV) for standing procedures when combined with *detomidine*.

- – May increase ataxia.
  - ○ Antinociceptive effect in foals (10 μg/kg, IV).
    - – Increased locomotor activity and tachypnea were common adverse effects.
    - – 25% bioavailability when administered sublingually (10–20 μg/kg) in foals (<21 days old).
  - ○ Sustained-release formulation (0.1 mg/kg, IM or SC) is *not* recommended in horses due to its use being associated with severe colonic impaction and increased locomotor activity.

*Butorphanol*
  - ○ Full κ opioid agonist, μ opioid antagonist.
  - ○ Very commonly used to potentiate the sedative effects of α₂ agonists.
  - ○ Clinical dose: 0.005–0.1 mg/kg, IV, IM, SC.
  - ○ Produces increased locomotor activity and decreased GI motility, similar to other opioids.
  - ○ Minimal analgesia.

*Opioid antagonists*
  - ○ The primary indication for use of opioid antagonists is for reversal of unwanted opioid-related side effects.
  - ○ The most common used opioid antagonist is *diprenorphine*, which is used to reverse *etorphine*-induced immobilization.


# Tramadol

- *Tramadol* is a centrally acting analgesic, with two distinct sites of action.


# I   Mechanism of action

- Weak agonist activity at μ, κ and δ opioid receptors.
  - ○ Affinity at μ receptor is about 1/6000 that of *morphine*.
  - ○ Its active metabolite (O-desmethyltramadol, M1) has a higher affinity (~ 200 times) for the μ opioid receptor.
    - – However, horses make very little of this metabolite.
- Inhibition of *norepinephrine* and *serotonin* re-uptake is considered to be the other mechanism of tramadol-induced analgesia.


# II   Physiologic effects

*Central nervous system*
  - ○ Sedation has been reported in horses at a dose of 2.4 mg/kg, IV.
    - – The degree of sedation is equivalent to *xylazine* (0.3 mg/kg, IV).
  - ○ Higher doses (5 mg/kg, IV) are associated with CNS stimulation.
    - – Muscle trembling, increased noise sensitivity, head nodding, yawning.
  - ○ Does not seem to increase locomotor activity.

*Cardiovascular system*
- ○ No changes in heart rate in association with 2 mg/kg, IV.
- ○ Transient increases in heart rate following 3 mg/kg, IV; however, parameters remained within acceptable physiologic range.
- ○ No changes in NIBP following 3 mg/kg, IV.

*Respiratory system*
- ○ Transient, minimal increases in respiratory rate.

*Gastrointestinal system*
- ○ Effects on motility are less than that of other opioids.
- ○ No change in GI sounds in standing horses following 1 mg/kg, IV followed by 1 mg/kg/hr. for one hour.
- ○ No change in fecal output following 2 mg/kg, IV.

## III Clinical use

- • Numerous studies have evaluated the pharmacokinetics of tramadol in horses.
  - ○ However, findings supporting its use as an analgesic in horses are lacking.
  - ○ No increases in electrical or thermal thresholds were identified following 2 or 3 mg/kg, IV.
  - ○ No analgesia was identified following 1 mg/kg, IV then 1 mg/kg/hr. in horses with induced carpal synovitis.
  - ○ Some analgesic efficacy was associated with orally administered tramadol (10 mg/kg, q12h) in horses with chronic pain from laminitis.
- • Intraarticular injection shows evidence of *chondrotoxicity*.
  - ○ Decreased chondrocyte cell viability.
- • Thus, based on its *minimal* sedating effect and *lack* of analgesia, it appears that there is no basis for tramadol use in horses.

## Suggested Reading

Donselmann Im Sande, P., Hopster, K., and Kastner, S. (2017). Effects of morphine, butorphanol and levomethadone in different doses on thermal nociceptive thresholds in horses. *Tierarztl. Prax. Ausg. G Grosstiere Nutztiere* 45: 98–106.

Guedes, A., Knych, H., and Hood, D. (2016). Plasma concentrations, analgesic and physiological assessments in horses with chronic laminitis treated with two doses of oral tramadol. *Equine Vet. J.* 48: 528–531.

Hamamoto-Hardman, B.D., Steffey, E.P., and McKemie, D.S. (2020). Meperidine pharmacokinetics and effects on physiologic parameters and thermal threshold following intravenous administration of three doses to horses. *BMC Vet. Res.* 16: 368.

Martin-Flores, M., Campoy, L., Kinsley, M.A. et al. (2014). Analgesic and gastrointestinal effects of epidural morphine in horses after laparoscopic cryptochidectomy under general anesthesia. *Vet. Anaesth. Analg.* 41: 430–437.

Maxwell, L.K., Thomasy, S.M., Slovis, N. et al. (2003). Pharmacokinetics of fentanyl following intravenous and transdermal administration in horses. *Equine Vet. J.* 35: 484–490.

Reed, R.A., Knych, H.K., Barletta, M. et al. (2020). Pharmacokinetics and pharmacodynamics of hydromorphone after intravenous and intramuscular administration in horses. *Vet. Anaesth. Analg.* 47: 210–218.

Skrzypczak, H., Reed, R., Barletta, M. et al. (2020). A retrospective evaluation of the effect of perianesthetic hydromorphone administration on the incidence of post anesthetic signs of colic in horses. *Vet. Anaesth. Analg.* 47: 757–762.

Thomasy, S.M., Slovis, N., Maxwell, L.K. et al. (2004). Transdermal fentanyl combined with nonsteroidal anti-inflammatory drugs for analgesia in horses. *J. Vet. Intern. Med.* 18: 550–554.

## Trazadone

*Alicia Skelding*

- *Trazodone* is an atypical antidepressant that is gaining popularity for treating anxiety in veterinary patients.
- It is in the *phenylpiperazine* class of drugs, and is classified as a SARI (serotonin 2A antagonist and re-uptake inhibitor).

## I   Mechanism of action

- It antagonizes postsynaptic serotonin receptors.
  - Inhibits glutamate release.
  - Stimulates *dopamine* and *norepinephrine* release in the prefrontal cortex.
- Increases serotonin concentrations by blocking presynaptic re-uptake.
  - Resulting in a sedative-hypnotic effect.
- Antagonizes *histamine* and $\alpha_1$ *adrenergic* receptors.

## II   Physiologic effects

*Central nervous system*
  - Following *IV* administration:
    - Ataxia, whole-body tremors, sweating.
    - Excitation – exhibited by circling and head-shaking.
    - Aggression following 2 mg/kg, IV.
      - Effects persists for 35–45 minutes.
      - Horse's ears are pinned back, and it is kicking, attempting to bite, and rearing.
  - Following *oral* administration:
    - Sedation, sweating.

*Cardiovascular system*
  - Increased heart rate following IV administration.
  - Transient arrhythmias have been reported.

*Miscellaneous*
  - May cause priapism.
  - Muscle fasciculations.

## III  Clinical use

- Its use is currently prohibited in performance horses.
- Possible role in behavioral modification.
- Because of the limited reports of its use in horses, further studies are warranted before its use can be recommended.

## Suggested Reading

Davis, J.L., Schirmer, J., and Medlin, E. (2018). Pharmacokinetics, pharmacodynamics and clinical use of trazodone and active metabolite m-chlorophenylpiperazine in the horse. *J. Vet. Pharmacol. Ther.* 41: 393–401.

Knych, H.K., Mama, K.R., Steffey, E.P. et al. (2017). Pharmacokinetics and selected pharmacodynamics of trazodone following intravenous and oral administration to horses undergoing fitness training. *Am. J. Vet. Res.* 78: 1182–1192.

## Benzodiazepines

*Alicia Skelding*

- Benzodiazepines are widely used in equine anesthesia, usually in combination with *ketamine* for induction of anesthesia.
- They are not used for standing sedation in adult horses due to causing muscle relaxation and subsequent ataxia. There is also the potential for paradoxical excitement when used alone.
- In neonatal foals, benzodiazepines are good sedatives, and ataxia is less of a concern since the foal will become recumbent following administration.

## I  Mechanism of action

- Benzodiazepines potentiate the effect of (γ-aminobutyric acid) GABA in the brain.
  - They enhance the affinity of the $GABA_A$ receptor for GABA.
- The result is increased chloride ($Cl^-$) conductance through the receptor and hyperpolarization of the postsynaptic neuron.

## II  Physiologic effects

*Central nervous system*
  - Sedation was not evident after administration of midazolam (0.05 or 0.1 mg/kg, IV).
    - Midazolam administration was associated with postural sway, weakness, agitation, and recumbency. One of six horses became recumbent after administration of midazolam at 0.1 mg/kg.
  - Anticonvulsant activity.

*Cardiovascular system*
  - Minimal effect on cardiovascular function.

*Respiratory system*
- Dose-dependent respiratory depression when combined with ketamine.
  - Combinations of benzodiazepines and *ketamine* should be given slowly to neonatal foals to avoid acute respiratory depression.
- Blood gas values remain physiologically appropriate.

## III    Clinical use

- *Diazepam* and *midazolam* are the most commonly used benzodiazepines in equine anesthesia.

### A    Chemical restraint

- *Not* used for standing sedation in adult horses due to lack of sedation and ataxia.
- Routinely used for sedation in neonatal *foals*.
  - *Diazepam* 0.05–0.1 mg/kg, IV
  - *Midazolam* 0.05–0.1 mg/kg, IV

### B    Induction of anesthesia

*Adult horses*
- *Diazepam* or *midazolam* (0.02–0.1 mg/kg, IV) is commonly administered with *ketamine* (2.0–2.5 mg/kg, IV) following sedation with an $\alpha_2$ agonist.
  - This improves muscle relaxation and the quality of induction.
  - No difference was identified between *diazepam* or *midazolam* when used as co-induction agents.

*Neonatal foals*
- *Diazepam* or *midazolam* (0.05–0.1 mg/kg, IV) can be used for induction with *ketamine* (2–3 mg/kg, IV), without prior $\alpha_2$ sedation.

### C    Maintenance of anesthesia

- *Midazolam* and *climazolam* have been used as part of TIVA.
- Reversal of the benzodiazepine may be necessary after long-term administration especially when using *climazolam*.
- *Midazolam* was found to be a suitable alternative to *guaifenesin* as part of TIVA with *medetomidine* and *ketamine*.
  - Clinically comparable quality of anesthesia.
  - Recovery quality was significantly better than with guaifenesin.
- Similarly, TIVA with *midazolam-ketamine-xylazine* provided good-quality anesthesia and recoveries; however, it is important to note that the procedures were of relatively *short duration*.

### D    Individual benzodiazepine drugs

*Diazepam*
- Poorly water-soluble (highly lipid soluble).
- Supplied in an organic solvent (ethanol and propylene glycol), which is irritating to tissues.
  - Can cause pain on injection.

- ○ IM absorption is unpredictable.
- ○ Metabolized primarily in the liver.
  - – Metabolites (nordiazepam, oxazepam) are excreted in urine.
- ○ Very long elimination half-life (2.5–21.6 hr).
- ○ Sensitive to light and undergoes photo degradation.

*Midazolam*
- ○ Highly water-soluble.
- ○ Rapidly absorbed following IM administration.
- ○ Undergoes hepatic metabolism.
- ○ Much shorter elimination half-life (3.5–6.5 hr) than diazepam.

*Zolazepam*
- ○ Only available in combination with *tiletamine*.
- ○ Water-soluble.

## IV Benzodiazepine antagonists

### A Flumazenil

- ○ *Flumazenil* was introduced into clinical practice in 1987, and is the only currently available benzodiazepine antagonist.

### B Mechanism of action

- ○ Competitively antagonizes the action of benzodiazepines on the $GABA_A$ receptor.
- ○ Prevents hyperpolarization of the postsynaptic membrane.
- ○ Degree of reversal is dose-dependent.

### C Physiologic effects

*Central nervous system*
- ○ Reverses electroencephalogram (EEG) changes induced by benzodiazepines.

*Cardiovascular system*
- ○ Minimal hemodynamic effects.

*Respiratory system*
- ○ Tidal volume and minute ventilation are restored to normal.
- ○ Does not exhibit any respiratory stimulatory effects.

### D Clinical use

- ○ Primary indication is competitive reversal of benzodiazepines.
  - – Most commonly used to speed prolonged recoveries in foals.
- ○ *Flumazenil* (0.01–0.05 mg/kg, IV, IM) is usually diluted and titrated IV to effect.

## Suggested Reading

De Vries, A., Thomson, S., and Taylor, P.M. (2015). Comparison of midazolam and diazepam as co-induction agents with ketamine for anaesthesia in sedated ponies undergoing field castration. *Vet. Anaesth. Analg.* 42: 512–517.

# Guaifenesin
*Alicia Skelding*

- *Guaifenesin (glycerol guaiacolate, GG)* is primarily used in equine anesthesia for its muscle-relaxing properties.
- It has minimal or no anesthetic properties, and therefore should *only be used* to improve muscle relaxation in association with anesthetic drug regimes.
- Commonly used as part of an induction protocol or TIVA protocol.

## I   Mechanism of action

- It disrupts nerve impulse transmission at the internuncial neurons of the spinal cord, brainstem and subcortical areas of the brain.
  - This results in centrally mediated muscle relaxation.

## II   Physiologic effects

*Central nervous system*
  - Skeletal muscle relaxation.
  - *No* analgesic effect.
  - Does *not* produce unconsciousness.

*Cardiovascular system*
  - Transient tachycardia when given alone.
  - Decreased arterial blood pressure.
  - Cardiac output is unchanged.

*Respiratory system*
  - Increased respiratory rate when given alone.
  - Minute ventilation is unchanged.

*Miscellaneous*
  - 30% crosses the placental barrier.

## III   Clinical use

- Supplied as a white powder that needs to be reconstituted in 0.9% saline or 5% dextrose.
  - Precipitates at <22 °C.
- If used alone, the dose necessary to produce recumbency is $134 \pm 34$ mg/kg, IV.
  - The dose is significantly less when administered with $\alpha_2$ agonists.
- High therapeutic index.
  - 4x clinical dose before death occurs.
    - Signs of toxicity include rigidity, severe tachycardia and cardiac arrest, rarely respiratory arrest.
- Short elimination half-life (1.0–1.5 hr).

### A   To improve induction quality

  - Following sedation (e.g. *xylazine* 0.3–1.0 mg/kg, IV), *guaifenesin* can be administered alone in a pressure bag until ataxia develops, at which time a bolus of *ketamine* (1.5–2.0 mg/kg, IV) can be administered to induce unconsciousness.

○ *Guaifenesin* (90 mg/kg, IV) administered for three minutes followed by *propofol* (3 mg/kg, IV) to induce unconsciousness, prevented the adverse anesthetic induction events that occur with *propofol* alone in horses.

### B    To maintain anesthesia

○ May be infused with other anesthetic drugs ($\alpha_2$ agonist, *ketamine*) as part of a TIVA protocol.

## IV    Contraindications

- Solutions >10% cause intravascular hemolysis and aseptic thrombophlebitis.
  ○ Should *not* be used as the sole immobilizing agent.

## Suggested Reading

Brosnan, R.J., Steffey, E.P., and Escobar, A. (2011). Anesthetic induction with guaifenesin and propofol in adult horses. *Am. J. Vet. Res.* 72: 1569–1575.

Davidson, G.S. (2008). Equine anesthesia: triple drip. *Int. J. Pharm. Compd.* 12: 402–404.

Knych, H.K., Stanley, S.D., Benson, D., and Arthur, R.M. (2016). Pharmacokinetics of guaifenesin following administration of multiple doses to exercised thoroughbred horses. *J. Vet. Pharmacol. Ther.* 39: 416–419.

## Ketamine

*Alicia Skelding*

- *Ketamine* is a dissociative anesthetic that is widely used as an induction agent for horses.
  ○ It can also be used at sub-anesthetic doses for analgesia in awake horses.
- *Ketamine* is manufactured as a racemic mixture of the S (+) and R (−) enantiomers. The S (+) enantiomer is more potent in terms of anesthetic properties.

## I    Mechanism of action

- It is a non-competitive antagonist at NMDA receptors.
  ○ It prevents glutamate binding.
  ○ Inhibits excitatory synaptic transmission.
  ○ Depresses the thalamocortical, limbic, and reticular activating system activity.
- *Ketamine* also has direct actions on δ opioid receptors and augments μ opioid receptor function.

## II  Physiologic effects

*Central nervous system*
- ○ Supraspinal effects.
  - – Unconsciousness (NMDA antagonism).
  - – Dissociation between thalamocortex and limbic system.
- ○ Spinal effects.
  - – Inhibits dorsal horn wide dynamic range neurons.
- ○ Analgesia.
  - – Supraspinal and spinal blockade of NMDA receptor.
  - – Reduction in NMDA mediated "wind *up*."
- ○ Increased cerebral metabolism.
- ○ Increased cerebral blood flow.
  - – Increased intracranial pressure.
- ○ Excitatory CNS effects.
  - – Increases cerebral metabolic oxygen requirements.
- ○ The neuroprotective and neuroregenerative effects of ketamine are the subjects of recent research. The neuroprotective effects of ketamine have been demonstrated in rodents.
  - – S (+) ketamine may be more efficacious than the racemic form.

*Cardiovascular system*
- ○ Direct CNS stimulation increases sympathetic nervous system outflow.
- ○ Inhibition of norepinephrine reuptake increases circulating catecholamines.
  - – Results in increased arterial blood pressure.
  - – Increased heart rate and cardiac output.
  - ▪ Increased myocardial oxygen consumption.
  - ▪ Increased cardiac work.

*Respiratory system*
- ○ Ventilatory responses to hypoxia and hypercarbia are well maintained.
- ○ "*Apneustic*" respiratory pattern.
- ○ Decrease in airway resistance.
  - – Bronchodilation.
- ○ Pharyngeal and laryngeal reflexes remain intact.
  - – However, this does not afford protection against aspiration of pharyngeal contents.

*Miscellaneous*
- ○ Increased skeletal muscle tone.
- ○ Transient increases in intraocular pressure.
  - – Mydriasis and nystagmus.

## III  Clinical use

### A  Induction of anesthesia

*Adult horse*
- ○ Following sedation with an $\alpha_2$ agonist, *ketamine* (2.0–2.5 mg/kg, IV) can be used alone or in combination with a muscle relaxant (benzodiazepine or *guaifenesin*) to induce unconsciousness.

*Neonatal foals*

- ○ *Ketamine* (2–3 mg/kg, IV) can be used with a *benzodiazepine* for induction without prior sedation.
- ○ The duration of surgical anesthesia following a single induction dose of *ketamine* in the adult horse is short (5–10 minutes), and depends on the temperament of the horse.
- ○ Anesthesia may be prolonged by using intermittent boluses of *ketamine* and the $\alpha_2$ agonist.
  - – One-third to one-half of the initial dose of each drug can be administered as needed.
  - – Re-dosing the benzodiazepine is unnecessary and may produce ataxia in recovery.

## B Maintenance of anesthesia

- ○ *Ketamine* may be used as a component of TIVA or PIVA.
  - – Most commonly with an $\alpha_2$ agonist.
  - – May also include a *benzodiazepine* or *guaifenesin* to improve muscle relaxation.

## C MAC reduction

- ○ Ketamine decreased the MAC of halothane in a dose-dependent manner with a maximum reduction of 37%.
  - – However, the 37% reduction was achieved at ketamine plasma concentrations (mean 10.8 µg/ml) that were four to five times higher than would be achieved with a ketamine CRI of 1–2 mg/kg/hr.
- ○ Ketamine (3 mg/kg/hr) in association with lidocaine (3 mg/kg/hr) decreased the MAC of isoflurane by 49%.
  - – Assuming that the maximum expected MAC reduction with lidocaine at that CRI was ~20%, this indicates that ketamine (3 mg/kg/hr) would decrease the isoflurane MAC by ~30%.
- ○ *Ketamine* administered as CRI (1 mg/kg/hr) to isoflurane-anesthetized horses, decreased end-tidal isoflurane requirements.
- ○ *Epidurally* administered ketamine (0.8 or 1.2 mg/kg) was associated with a modest and clinically unimportant decrease in MAC of halothane in ponies, when using a noxious stimulus applied to a pelvic limb. The effect of ketamine was considered to be segmental, as no decrease in MAC occurred when the stimulus was applied to a thoracic limb.

## D Epidural analgesia

- ○ Dose-dependent analgesia was associated with administration of ketamine at doses of 0.5–2.0 mg/kg.
- ○ The duration of effect was short (30–75 minutes).
  - – Analgesia of the tail, perineum, and upper pelvic limbs resulted.
  - – No adverse behavioral effects or cardiovascular effects were reported.

## E Analgesia in the awake horse

- ○ A few studies have evaluated the effects of ketamine as part of the analgesic drug regimen in awake horses.

○ *Ketamine*, alone, can be safely infused IV at 0.4–0.8 mg/kg/hr.
○ *Ketamine* (0.2 mg/kg/hr) can be combined with *lidocaine* (3 mg/kg/hr).
  – The loading dose of both drugs [*ketamine* (1 mg/kg, IV) and *lidocaine* (2.0–2.5 mg/kg, IV)] can be combined and infused over 30 minutes.

F   **Potentiation of $\alpha_2$-induced sedation in standing horse**

○ Ketamine may be used in association with an $\alpha_2$ agonist to provide sedation that is more potent than the sedation associated with the $\alpha_2$ agonist alone.
  – However, the dose of each drug must be low to prevent extreme ataxia and perhaps recumbency.
For example, *Ketamine* (0.1–0.2 mg/kg, IV) can be given with a low dose of $\alpha_2$ agonist (e.g. *xylazine* 0.3 mg/kg, IV) to potentiate the sedation, and perhaps analgesia, from the $\alpha_2$ agonist.

## Suggested Reading

Lankveld, D.P.K., Driessen, B., Soma, L.R. et al. (2006). Pharmacodynamic effects and pharmacokinetic profile of a long-term continuous rate infusion of racemic ketamine in healthy conscious horses. *J. Vet. Pharmacol. Ther.* 29: 477–488.

Villalba, M., Santiago, I., and Gomez de Segura, I.A. (2011). Effects of a constant rate infusion of lidocaine and ketamine, with or without morphine, on isoflurane MAC in horses. *Equine Vet. J.* 43: 721–726.

## Tiletamine and Zolazepam (TZ)

*Alicia Skelding*

- *TZ* (Telazol®, Zoletil®) are commercially available as a 1 : 1 combination of 250 mg of each drug in a powder form.

## I   Mechanism of action

- *Tiletamine* is a non-competitive antagonist at NMDA receptors.
  ○ It prevents glutamate binding.
    – Inhibits excitatory synaptic transmission.
    – Depresses thalamocortical, limbic, and reticular activating system activity.
- *Zolazepam* is a benzodiazepine and thus potentiates the actions of GABA by modulating the GABA binding site on the $GABA_A$ receptor.

## II   Physiologic effects

- *Tiletamine* exerts similar physiologic effects as *ketamine*.
- *Zolazepam* is a long-acting benzodiazepine and produces effects similar to midazolam/diazepam.

## III   Clinical use

- TZ is has poor analgesic properties.
- It is *not recommended* for anesthetic induction in *unsedated* horses.
- Recovery from TZ is sometimes associated with excitement and incoordination when used alone.
  ○ Recovery quality is satisfactory if the horse is sedated with an $\alpha_2$ agonist.

### A   Induction of anesthesia

- ○ TZ (1–2 mg/kg, IV) can be used to induce anesthesia following sedation with an $\alpha_2$ agonist.
  – Induction quality is excellent following $\alpha_2$ sedation.
- ○ TZ (1.5 mg/kg, IV) has a duration of surgical anesthesia that is twice that of *ketamine* (2.2 mg/kg, IV).
- ○ TZ is particularly useful for induction, *after heavy sedation*, in young Thoroughbreds and excitable horses that are prone to awakening rapidly following the conventional doses of ketamine/midazolam.
  – In these instances, TZ (1.0–1.5 mg/kg, IV) can be combined with *ketamine* (1 mg/kg, IV) for a longer-lasting effect.

## Suggested Reading

Bouts, T., Gasthuys, F., Vlaminck, L., and Van Brangeghem, L. (2002). Comparison of romifidine-ketamine-midazolam and romifidine-tiletamine-zolazepam total intravenous anaesthesia (TIVA) for clinical anaesthesia in horses. *Vet. Anaesth. Analg.* 29: 92–93.

Muir, W.W., Gadawski, J.E., and Grosenbaugh, D.A. (1999). Cardiorespiratory effects of a tiletamine/zolazepam-ketamine-detomidine combination in horses. *Am. J. Vet. Res.* 60: 770–774.

## Alfaxalone
*Alicia Skelding*

- *Alfaxalone* has recently re-emerged onto the market, formulated in a non-cremophor (cyclodextran) vehicle (Alfaxan-CD®). Numerous studies have evaluated its use in equine anesthesia.

## I   Mechanism of action

- *Alfaxalone* binds to $GABA_A$ receptors and increases $Cl^-$ conductance.
  ○ This results in hyperpolarization of the postsynaptic membrane.
- It inhibits pathways responsible for arousal and awareness.

## II  Physiologic effects

*Central nervous system*
- ○ Unconsciousness.
- ○ *Lack of* analgesic activity.
- ○ Decreased cerebral blood flow.
  - – Decreased intracranial pressure.
- ○ Decreased metabolic oxygen consumption.

*Cardiovascular system*
- ○ Stable cardiovascular parameters.

*Respiratory system*
- ○ Dose-dependent respiratory depression.

## III  Clinical use

- • The degree of ataxia in recovery from *alfaxalone* (1 mg/kg, IV + *diazepam* 0.02 mg/kg, IV) is *greater* in comparison to *ketamine + diazepam*, in pre-medicated (*romifidine + butorphanol*) ponies undergoing field castration.

### A  Induction of anesthesia

- ○ *Alfaxalone* can be used to induce anesthesia in *horses* and *donkeys*.
- ○ *Alfaxalone* (1 mg/kg, IV) can be used to induce anesthesia following *xylazine* and *guaifenesin*.
  - – *Alfaxalone* is not an ideal induction agent, and associated *adverse* effects include *tremors* and *shaking*.
  - – Thus, it is recommended that alfaxalone be administered after the horse is sedated with an α₂ agonist to improve the quality of induction.

### B  Maintenance of anesthesia

- ○ *Alfaxalone* (2 mg/kg/hr) + *medetomidine* (5 μg/kg/hr) has been used to maintain anesthesia in horses for field castration.
  - – It was suitable for short-term anesthesia in this instance.
- ○ TIVA maintained with *alfaxalone* (1.5 mg/kg/hr), *guaifenesin* (80 mg/kg/hr) and *medetomidine* (3 μg/kg/hr), after induction of anesthesia, also provided acceptable conditions for castration.
  - – Recovery quality was good to excellent.
- ○ Higher doses of *alfaxalone* (3 mg/kg/hr) are necessary if used alone for TIVA.
  - – However, there is *no* analgesic activity associated with this method of anesthesia.
- ○ *Apnea* and *respiratory depression* are the most common adverse effects reported when *alfaxalone* is used as part of a TIVA protocol.
  - – The ability to monitor and support ventilation is important.
- ○ *Alfaxalone* can be used as part of a PIVA protocol.
  - – A CRI of (0.5 mg/kg/hr) combined with *medetomidine* (3 μg/kg/hr) decreased *sevoflurane* requirements by 26% in horses undergoing arthroscopy.
    - ▪ This regimen was associated with good cardiopulmonary function.

## Suggested Reading

Goodwin, W.A., Keates, H.L., Pasloske, K. et al. (2011). The pharmacokinetics and pharmacodynamics of the injectable anaesthetic alfaxalone in the horse. *Vet. Anaesth. Analg.* 38: 431–438.

Goodwin, W.A., Pasloske, K., Keates, H.L. et al. (2019). Alfaxalone for total intravenous anaesthesia in horses. *Vet. Anaesth. Analg.* 46: 188–199.

Wakuno, A., Aoki, M., Kushiro, A. et al. (2017). Comparison of alfaxalone, ketamine and thiopental for anaesthetic induction and recovery in thoroughbred horses premedicated with medetomidine and midazolam. *Equine Vet. J.* 49: 94–98.

## Propofol

*Alicia Skelding*

- *Propofol* is a milky, white substance formulated as variations of oil in water emulsion containing soya bean, egg lecithin and glycerol.
- Most formulations do not contain preservatives, and therefore need to be discarded by six hours after opening.
- A new formulation of *propofol,* containing *benzyl alcohol* to increase the shelf life to 28 days, has been recently introduced into the veterinary market.
- *Propofol* is not commonly used in equine anesthesia partly because of *cost*, but also because of the *large volume* needed for induction, and the *poor quality* of induction when used alone.

## I   Mechanism of action

- Enhances the $GABA_A$ $Cl^-$ current through binding of the $\beta$ subunit.
  - This facilitates inhibitory synaptic transmission.
- It inhibits acetylcholine release in the hippocampus and prefrontal cortex.
- It inhibits the NMDA receptor through modulation of sodium channel gating.
- It has a direct depressant effect on neurons in the spinal cord.
  - Decreases the excitability of spinal neurons via modulation of $GABA_A$ and glycine receptors.

## II   Physiologic effects

*Central nervous system*
- Dose-dependent sedation/hypnosis/unconsciousness.
- *No* analgesic effect.
- Decreased ICP.
- Decreased cerebral metabolic oxygen consumption.
- Maintenance of cerebral metabolic autoregulation.
- Anticonvulsant.

*Cardiovascular system*
- Dose-dependent decrease in SVR.
  - Decreased arterial blood pressure.
- Dose-dependent myocardial depression.
  - Decreased contractility.

*Respiratory system*
- Dose-dependent respiratory depression.
  - Decreased tidal volume and respiratory rate.
- Apnea is common with a rapid bolus injection.

*Miscellaneous*
- Decreased intraocular pressure.
- Myoclonus and dystonia may occur.

## III  Clinical use

- *Propofol* does not seem to be suitable for induction of anesthesia in the unsedated horse.
  - The use of *propofol* alone for induction of anesthesia in the unsedated adult horse has been associated with unpredictable excitement.
  - Excitement can be prevented with the addition of *guaifenesin* to the induction protocol.

### A  Induction of anesthesia

- Induction of anesthesia in horses with *propofol* (2 mg/kg, IV) should only be performed following routine sedation with an $\alpha_2$ agonist.
  - Nevertheless, some horses sedated with an $\alpha_2$ agonist will demonstrate excitement, myoclonus, and paddling of the limbs during induction with propofol.
- *Midazolam* (0.02 mg/kg, IV) does *not* seem to improve the quality of induction.
- *Propofol* has no advantage over *ketamine* for induction of anesthesia and, in general, the qualities of inductions are *poorer* than with *ketamine*/$\alpha_2$ agonist.
- Behavioral responses (*excitement, myoclonus*) can be modified by using lower doses of propofol and adding ketamine.

### B  Propofol as a co-induction drug with ketamine

- Propofol can be used as a co-induction drug with ketamine (2–3 mg/kg, IV).
- Propofol (0.5 mg/kg, IV) is administered to improve relaxation and the depth of anesthesia.
- However, there is probably no benefit in using propofol over a benzodiazepine as a co-induction drug with ketamine.

### C  Maintenance of anesthesia

- *Propofol* is considered a close to ideal agent for infusions due to:
  - It short context-sensitive half-life.
  - Rapid clearance.
- *Propofol* can be used as the sole agent for TIVA or as a component of TIVA or PIVA.
- Following induction of anesthesia (*xylazine/ketamine*), maintenance of anesthesia with *propofol* (3–6 mg/kg/hr) + *ketamine* (1.8 mg/kg/hr) + *xylazine* (1 mg/kg/hr) provided acceptable anesthetic conditions for surgical procedures.
  - All horse's developed $PaO_2$ values ≤80 mmHg.
  - Therefore, supplemental oxygen is recommended.
  - Recovery qualities were good to excellent.

    ○ In *sevoflurane*-anesthetized horses undergoing arthroscopic surgery, a CRI of *propofol* (3 or 6 mg/kg/hr) + *medetomidine* (3 μg/kg/hr) provided good quality anesthesia.

      – *Sevoflurane* requirements were decreased.

      – Cardiovascular function was maintained.

      – The recovery quality was considered excellent with this regimen.

## Suggested Reading

Ferreira, T.H., Brosnan, R.J., Shilo-Benjamini, Y. et al. (2013). Effects of ketamine, propofol, or thiopental administration on intraocular pressure and qualities of induction of and recovery from anesthesia in horses. *Am. J. Vet. Res.* 74: 1070–1077.

Jarrett, M.A., Bailey, K.M., and Messenger, K.M. (2018). Recovery of horses from general anesthesia after induction with propofol and ketamine versus midazolam and ketamine. *J. Am. Vet. Med. Assoc.* 253: 101–107.

Oku, K., Ohta, M., Katoh, T. et al. (2006). Cardiovascular effects of continuous propofol infusion in horses. *J. Vet. Med. Sci.* 68: 773–778.

Oku, K., Ohta, M., Yamanaka, T. et al. (2005). The minimum infusion rate (MIR) of propofol for total intravenous anesthesia after premedication with xylazine horses. *J. Vet. Med. Sci.* 67: 569–575.

## Barbiturates

### *Alicia Skelding*

- Barbiturates are rarely used in modern equine anesthesia.
- *Thiopental* (*thiopentone*), a thiobarbiturate, was the only barbiturate in common use for anesthesia of the horse.
- However, thiopental is no longer produced in North America and most other countries.
- *Pentobarbital* (*pentobarbitone*) is now primarily used for euthanasia.

## I  Receptor activity of barbiturates

- Barbiturates directly activate the GABA$_A$ receptor, thereby mediating Cl⁻ influx.

### A  Use for euthanasia

    ○ Concentrated solutions of *pentobarbital* are used for euthanasia. (see Chapter 40)

    ○ A pentobarbital overdose is the most common method of euthanasia of horses in North America.

    ○ Pentobarbital concentration in the range 240–540 mg/mL are available commercially.

    ○ Most commercial solutions of pentobarbital for euthanasia contain *phenytoin sodium* (50 mg/ml), as it potentiates phenobarbital's cardiovascular and CNS depression.

    ○ To smooth induction and reduce the stress for attendants and the horse, it is common to sedate the horse (e.g. *xylazine to effect*) prior to administration of pentobarbital.

    ○ Loss of EEG activity occurs in around 60 seconds after the administration of pentobarbital; however, electrocardiogram (ECG) activity may continue for longer but heart sounds and an arterial pulse are absent.

# Intravenous lidocaine
*Patricia Queiroz-Williams*

- In recent times, the clinical use of lidocaine has grown from its initial use as a local anesthetic to take advantage of its anti-inflammatory, systemic analgesic effects, and anti-hyperanalgesic effects. In human medicine, IV administered lidocaine has been used as an infusion and as an adjunct analgesic drug.
- IV administered *lidocaine* decreases the MAC of volatile anesthetics in horses.
- In anesthetized horses, intravenously administered lidocaine (100 µg/kg/hr) blocked the EEG changes associated with castration.
- In the awake horse, lidocaine can be used alone or in combination with drugs such as *ketamine* to provide analgesia.
- Systemically administered lidocaine ameliorates the adverse effect of *flunixin meglumine* on the recovery of ischemic equine intestine.

## I   Mode of action

- The clinical effects of lidocaine as regards to relief of pain relief in humans persist for some hours after ending the infusion. In some cases, the analgesia persists for 24 hours, and this would indicate that mechanisms other than its local anesthetic effects are responsible for analgesia.
- Based on *in vitro* studies, lidocaine has a modulating effect on:
  - Calcium channels.
  - Potassium channels.
  - NMDA receptors.
  - G-coupled protein receptors.
  - The glycinergic system.
- The anti-inflammatory effects of lidocaine may contribute to its beneficial effects in acute and chronic pain. Systemic administration of lidocaine has been associated with decreases in the concentrations of:
  - IL-1.
  - TNFα.
  - ICAM-1.
  - Mucosal COX2.
  - Plasma prostaglandin E2.
- Effect on polymorphonuclear granulocytes (PMNs).
  - PMNs have a key role in inflammation through the release of pro-inflammatory cytokines and reactive oxygen species which contribute to the migration of neutrophils.
    - Lidocaine inhibits the priming of neutrophils.
    - Lidocaine inhibits PMN adhesion and migration.
- Lidocaine suppressed polysynaptic C-fibers and wide dynamic range neurons in some animal studies. This action may, in part, be responsible for the beneficial effect of lidocaine in treating patients with neuropathic pain.

## II Clinical use of intravenous lidocaine

### A As an adjunct to general anesthetics

○ Lidocaine is used in conjunction with volatile agents to decrease MAC and improve analgesia. (see Chapter 20)
○ The decrease in MAC is dose-dependent.
  – Infusion rates of 50 μg/kg/min reduce MAC by ~20%.
  – Infusion rates of 100 μg/kg/min reduce MAC by 25–30%.
○ Lidocaine can be infused concurrently with *ketamine* or $\alpha_2$ agonists.

### B To provide analgesia in the awake horse

○ Lidocaine can be safely infused at 50 μg/kg/min for up to 72 hours.
  – A loading dose (1.5–2.0 mg/kg, IV) can be infused over five minutes.
○ A CRI of 50 μg/kg/min can be safely infused with *ketamine* (0.4 mg/kg/hr).

## III Metabolism

● *Lidocaine* is metabolized in the liver and produces active and inactive metabolites. The most important active metabolites are:
  ○ Monoethylglycinexylidide.
  ○ Glycinexylidide.
● At therapeutic plasma concentrations (2–4 μg/mL) lidocaine is highly bound to the acute phase reactant, α1acid glycoprotein.
● Metabolites and unchanged lidocaine are excreted by the kidney.
● *Plasma* concentrations of lidocaine may increase if drugs, such as *ketoconazole*, that inhibit the liver cytochrome-P450 3A4 (CYP3A4) are administered concurrently.

## IV Adverse effects

● The likelihood of systemic toxicity with IV *lidocaine* is related to its plasma concentration.
● Plasma concentrations are increased during general anesthesia in comparison to the awake state.
*Note:* However, it seems, based on a study in sheep, that general anesthesia has a protective effect against the adverse CNS and cardiovascular effects of intravenously administered lidocaine.

### A CNS effects

○ Low plasma concentrations of *lidocaine* are sedating. However, the sedative effects of lidocaine have not been well evaluated in the horse.

○ Increasing plasma concentrations result in muscle twitching (e.g. blinking) and ataxia.

○ The awake horse may become recumbent.

○ Seizures (originating in *amygdala)* occur at higher doses.

○ Administration of sedatives causes a right shift in the dose–response curve.

*Treatment of seizures*

○ Most lidocaine-induced seizures are self-limiting. However, it may be necessary to sedate (e.g. an $\alpha_2$ agonist) or administer a GABA agonist in some cases.

○ Mild seizures activity in a recumbent horse should respond to benzodiazepines (e.g. midazolam, diazepam).

○ More potent GABA agonists such as *propofol* or *thiopental* may be necessary to control more severe seizures.

○ Supportive care and oxygen administration should also be implemented as deemed necessary.

### B   Cardiovascular effects

○ Occur at higher plasma concentrations than do CNS effects.

– Thus, cardiovascular effects are likely to be accompanied by seizures or unconsciousness in the previously awake horse.

○ Hypotension and myocardial depression.

○ Result from a delay in impulse transmission by Na channel blockade. This leads to:

– Decreased myocardial contractility.

– Vasodilation.

– Cardiac arrhythmias.

*Treatment*

○ It may be necessary to attend initially to CNS effects in the awake horse.

○ Treatment of hypotension should include fluid therapy and inotropes.

### C   Methemoglobinemia

○ Is an unlikely outcome of systemic lidocaine administration.

## Suggested Reading

Copeland, S.E., Ladd, L.A., Gu, X.Q., and Mather, L.E. (2008). The effects of general anesthesia on the central nervous and cardiovascular system toxicity of local anesthetics. *Anesth. Analg.* 106: 1429–1439.

Doherty, T.J. and Frazier, D.L. (1998). Effect of intravenous lidocaine on the minimum alveolar concentration of halothane in ponies. *Equine Vet. J.* 30: 300–303.

Rezende, M.L., Wagner, A.E., Mama, K.R. et al. (2011). Effects of intravenous administration of lidocaine on the minimum alveolar concentration of sevoflurane in horses. *Am. J. Vet. Res.* 72: 446–451.

# Horse-related drug Regulations in Europe

*Regula Bettschart-Wolfensberger and Simone K. Ringer*

## I  Regulations

- Any horse in Europe might enter the food chain.
- Registered drugs can be used in all equids when relevant withholding periods are respected
- Drugs on the equid list can be used with a withholding period of six months (https://eur-lex.europa.eu/LexUriServ/LexUriServ.do?uri=OJ:L:2013:042:0001:0017:EN:PDF)
- Drugs registered for other food producing animals (e.g. ruminants, pigs) can be used in equids according to the cascade (meat withholding period 28 days).
- In horses that are not supposed to enter the food chain (identified in the horse's passport) other drugs might be used if otherwise adequate therapy not possible.
- Horses without passports are considered food producers in any case.

## II  Anesthesia-related drugs that are not allowed in food producing animals

- Dexmedetomidine
- Medetomidine
- Alfaxalone
- Desflurane
- Ropivacaine
- Rocuronium
- Sugammadex, neostigmine
- Tranexamic acid
- Phenylbutazone

## 13

## Inhalational Anesthetics
*Rachel A. Reed*

## I   Introduction

- Inhalational anesthetics are the mainstay for maintenance of general anesthesia in horses for procedures lasting longer than one hour.
- Newer agents, such as *isoflurane*, *sevoflurane*, and *desflurane*, provide reliable anesthesia with predictable adverse effects on the cardiorespiratory system that are easily managed.
- Clinical features and administration of inhaled anesthetics are largely determined by their physical characteristics, especially vapor pressure, molecular weight, and chemical classification (see Table 13.1).
- With the exception of *nitrous oxide* ($N_2O$), currently available inhalational anesthetics do not provide analgesia.

## II   Mechanism of action

- The precise mechanisms of action of inhalant anesthetics are not completely understood.
- With the historical lipid solubility based theories having fallen by the wayside, a receptor-ligand mediated mechanism of action is the most likely explanation for how these agents cause immobility and unconsciousness.
- Considering immobility and unconsciousness as two distinct outcomes of the administration of inhaled anesthetics, several receptors have been proposed as responsible for each.

*Immobility*
- Is most likely produced by the action of these agents at *glycine* and *glutamate* receptors (AMPA and NMDA) within the *ventral horn* of the spinal cord.

*Unconsciousness*
- Is currently thought to be mediated by inhibition of presynaptic neurotransmitter release via actions at *sodium* and *calcium* channels.
- Several studies isolating the anesthetic to the brain or the spinal cord have established that the brain is much more susceptible to the effects of inhalational anesthetics than is the spinal cord.
  - Thus, unconsciousness is achieved at a lower anesthetic concentration than is immobility.

*Manual of Equine Anesthesia and Analgesia*, Second Edition. Edited by Tom Doherty, Alex Valverde, and Rachel A. Reed.
© 2022 John Wiley & Sons, Inc. Published 2022 by John Wiley & Sons, Inc.

Table 13.1  Physicochemical properties of common inhalational anesthetics.

|  | Halothane | Isoflurane | Sevoflurane | Desflurane | Nitrous oxide |
|---|---|---|---|---|---|
| MAC (%) | 0.82–0.95 | 1.31 | 2.31 | 7.6 | 205 |
| Blood/gas partition coefficient | 1.66 | 0.92–1.13 | 0.47–0.65 | 0.54 | $0.47^a$ |
| $^a$Brain/blood partition coefficient | 2.9 | 2.6 | 1.7 | 1.3 | 1.1 |
| Vapor pressure (mmHg at 20 °C) | 243 | 238 | 157 | 660 | 38 770 |
| Molecular weight (D) | 197 | 185 | 200 | 168 | 44 |
| Biotransformation (%) | 20 | 0.2 | 5 | 0.02 | 0.004 |
| Chemical classification | Halogenated alkane | Halogenated ether | Halogenated ether | Halogenated ether | Gas |

D, daltons.
$^a$ human data.

## III   Minimum alveolar concentration (MAC)

- MAC is the minimum alveolar concentration at 1 Atm necessary to prevent purposeful movement in 50% of subjects in response to a supramaximal noxious stimulus.
- MAC is a measure of potency of the inhalational anesthetic agent.
- In human beings, MAC is usually determined for the population as the noxious stimulus (surgical incision) can only be applied once.
  - Thus, this traditional definition of MAC represents an $ED_{50}$, or the effective dose in 50% of the patient population.
- In animals, the MAC is usually determined for each individual as the nociceptive stimulus, electrical stimulation in the case of the horse, is repeatable without causing tissue damage.
- Clinically, a minimum 1.2 MAC is required to maintain a surgical plane of anesthesia in the absence of adjunctive injectable anesthetic agents.
- MAC values for the commonly used inhalational agents can be found in Table 13.1, and the effect of injectable drugs on MAC can be found in Table 13.2.
- MAC of an anesthetic agent is useful clinically as a guide to the anesthetic depth of the patient.

### A   MAC Derivatives

- Several derivatives of the traditional MAC have been defined.
  $MAC_{NM}$ (no movement)
- Is the MAC at 1 Atm required to prevent all movement, purposeful and non-purposeful, in response to a supramaximal noxious stimulus.
  - This derivative is probably representative of an $ED_{95}$, and is approximately 1.2 MAC.
  $MAC_{BAR}$
- Is the MAC at 1 Atm required to *blunt adrenergic responses* in 50% of patients in response to a supramaximal noxious stimulus.

Table 13.2   Effect of different injectable agents on MAC in horses.

| Class | Agent | Dose/Plasma concentration | MAC reduction (%) |
|---|---|---|---|
| Phenothiazines | Acepromazine | 0.05 mg/kg IV | 30% (halothane) |
| Alpha-2 agonists | Xylazine | 0.5–1 mg/kg IV | 30–40% (isoflurane) |
| | Detomidine[a] | 30–60 µg/kg IV | 35–45% (isoflurane) |
| | Medetomidine | 3.5 µg/kg/hr | 30% (desflurane) |
| | Dexmedetomidine | 1.75 µg/kg/hr | 53% (sevoflurane) |
| | Dexmedetomidine plus Morphine | 1.75 µg/kg/hr 0.1 mg/kg/hr | 67% (sevoflurane)[d] |
| NMDA receptor antagonists | Ketamine | 10.8 µg/ml[b] | 37% (halothane) |
| Opioids | Morphine | 0.25, 2.0 mg/kg IV | No effect (isoflurane) |
| | Fentanyl[c] | 14, 20, 24 ng/ml | No effect (isoflurane) |
| | Alfentanil[c] | 95, 171, 391 ng/mlL | No effect (halothane) |
| | Butorphanol | 0.05 mg/kg IV | No effect isoflurane/halothane |
| Benzodiazepines | Diazepam | 0.05 mg/kg IV | 30% (halothane) |
| | Temazepam | 0.044 mg/kg IV | 16% (halothane) |
| Local anesthetics | Lidocaine | 50–100 µg/kg/min | 20–30% (isoflurane, sevoflurane, halothane) |
| Gaseous anesthetics | Nitrous oxide | 25–50% inspired concentration | 12–25% (halothane) |

[a] Detomidine had no or a minimal effect on MAC in other studies.
[b] This concentration is approximately 5 × concentration achieved with a CRI of 40 µg/kg/min in horses anesthetized with a volatile anesthetic.
[c] Target controlled infusions.
[d] MAC-no movement study.

- Responses commonly studied are increases in heart rate and arterial pressure, and allowable increases in these parameters in response to the noxious stimulus are between 10 and 20% over baseline values.
- $MAC_{BAR}$ is generally about 1.4 MAC, although there is a wide variation in $MAC_{BAR}$ values as a fraction of MAC in humans and animals, and values for $MAC_{BAR}$ greater than 2 MAC are reported.
  - In contrast to the MAC dose–response curve, the dose–response curve for $MAC_{BAR}$ is relatively flat.

### $MAC_{Awake}$ and $MAC_{Memory}$

- These MAC derivatives are less relevant to equine anesthesia.
- In human anesthesia, $MAC_{awake}$ is the MAC at 1 Atm at which 50% of subjects will not respond to a verbal command, and this occurs at approximately 0.35 MAC for isoflurane, sevoflurane, and desflurane.
- Although the $MAC_{awake}$ may not seem particularly relevant to the horse, it, nevertheless, is an indicator of the point at which consciousness is returning.
- The large difference between $MAC_{awake}$ and MAC reflects the greater sensitivity of the brain than the spinal cord to the effects of inhalational anesthetics.

    ○ MAC$_{Memory}$, the MAC at 1 Atm preventing memory of a noxious stimulus in 50% of subjects, is even less than MAC$_{awake}$.

## B Factors that decrease MAC

    ○ Concurrent drug administration (e.g. sedatives, analgesics, injectable anesthetics). (see Table 13.2)
        − It is noteworthy that opioids do not decrease MAC in the horse when only the opioid and the inhalant anesthetic are administered, and this may be due to the excitatory effects of opioids. *Morphine* potentiated the effect of *dexmedetomidine* in decreasing the MAC$_{NM}$ of sevoflurane in one study, but did not potentiate the effect of *xylazine* on the MAC of halothane in another study.
    ○ Pregnancy.
    ○ Hypothermia (approximately 5% reduction in MAC per 1 °C decrease in body temperature).
    ○ Endotoxemia.
    ○ Extremes of age (very young, very old). The MAC of isoflurane in foals was determined to be 36% lower (0.84%) than in adult horses.

## C Factors that increase MAC

    ○ CNS stimulants (e.g. amphetamines).
    ○ Hyperthermia.
    ○ Age (MAC increases until adulthood and then decreases).

# IV Pharmacokinetics

- The pharmacokinetics of inhaled anesthetics describe the absorption, distribution, metabolism, and elimination of the drug from the body.

## A Absorption

    ○ Inhaled anesthetics are absorbed from the alveolus directly into the pulmonary capillary.
    ○ The partial pressure of anesthetic within the alveoli represents the balance between the *rate of delivery of anesthetic to the alveoli* and *the rate at which the anesthetic is removed from the alveoli.*
    ○ The partial pressure of inhaled anesthetic within the alveolus represents a pivotal value that determines the depth of anesthesia.
    ○ The partial pressure of inhaled anesthetic and hence the depth of anesthesia can be tightly controlled by the use of an *anesthetic agent monitor.*

## B The rate of delivery of anesthetic to the alveoli is determined by the following factors

*The inspired partial pressure of inhalant* (Pi)
    ○ The higher the Pi the more rapid the rate of delivery.

*Vaporizer setting*
    ○ A high vaporizer setting will cause a more rapid rate of rise of Pi.

○ This technique, termed *overpressuring*, is commonly employed in equine anesthesia to overcome the dilutional effects of the room air within the anesthetic circuit and the patient lungs.

*Oxygen flow rate*
○ A high oxygen flow rate results in more rapid denitrogenation of the anesthetic circuit, replacing that volume of room air with oxygen and anesthetic vapor.

*Volume of anesthetic circuit*
○ Large animal anesthetic circuits are generally 30–50 l in volume. The larger the circuit, the longer it will take for the Pi to rise.
○ Therefore, circuits with smaller volumes result in a more rapid rate of rise of Pi unless the oxygen flow rate and vaporizer are adjusted accordingly (see time constant, Chapter 17).

C   Alveolar ventilation and alveolar partial pressure ($P_A$)

○ The rate at which the inspired anesthetic reaches the alveoli is dependent upon the rate and depth of patient respirations.
○ If the patient is breathing spontaneously, minute ventilation will decrease as the patient becomes anesthetized, thereby slowing the rate of rise of $P_A$.
○ Administering intermittent positive pressure ventilation (IPPV) can speed the rate of rise in $P_A$ by ensuring a constant and adequate tidal volume, and decreasing the magnitude of atelectasis.

D   The rate at which the anesthetic is removed from the alveolus

Determined by the following three *"uptake factors"*:

*Solubility of the anesthetic in blood* (see Table 13.1).
○ Solubility for each agent is measured in terms of its blood: gas partition coefficient.
○ Agents with low blood solubility cause a more rapid anesthetic induction than agents with high blood solubility.
○ This inverse relationship between solubility and speed of induction is due to the fact that agents with lower blood solubility result in:
  – A more rapid rise in the partial pressure of anesthetic in the blood.
  – A smaller drain of the $P_A$ into solubilized states within the blood (i.e. intercalated within red blood cell membranes) that do not contribute to the partial pressure of agent within the blood.

*Cardiac output of the patient*
○ Speed of anesthetic induction is inversely associated with the cardiac output.
○ The effect of increasing cardiac output on the rate of rise of $P_A$ is similar to that of increasing agent solubility.
○ The higher the cardiac output, the greater drain on $P_A$, and the longer it takes to achieve a $P_A$ capable of producing general anesthesia.

*Alveolar-to-venous partial pressure difference*
○ This factor represents a continuum of the concentration gradient down which the anesthetic vapor moves from the alveolus into the pulmonary capillary.

    o As the patient becomes anesthetized, the venous partial pressure of the inhalant begins to rise, and the concentration gradient by which the anesthetic moves from the alveolus to the capillary becomes smaller and smaller until an equilibrium is reached.

### E Distribution

    o Inhaled anesthetics are largely distributed throughout the body in accordance with their blood: tissue partition coefficients (see Table 13.1).

    o Accumulation of these agents in the fat and muscle can contribute to longer recovery times with more soluble agents, and patients will be expiring trace amounts of inhaled anesthetic for several hours after the animal appears to be clinically recovered from anesthesia as the agent washes out of these tissues.

### F Metabolism

    o Modern inhaled anesthetics undergo minimal hepatic metabolism (see Table 13.1).

    o However, older agents, including *halothane* and *methoxyflurane*, undergo significant hepatic metabolism.

### G Elimination

    o Modern inhaled anesthetics are largely eliminated from the body via exhalation in the reverse of the process outlined above for uptake.

    o With cessation of administration of the inhaled anesthetic, $P_A$ begins to fall, and the anesthetic begins to move from the pulmonary capillary out into the alveolus, now moving down a concentration gradient in the opposite direction.

## V Pharmacodynamics

### A Cardiovascular effects

    o All inhalational anesthetics cause a dose-dependent cardiovascular depression via decreased cardiac contractility and/or decreased systemic vascular resistance, leading to a reduction in mean arterial pressure.

    o Heart rate remains relatively unchanged.

    o These adverse effects can be managed by utilizing the lowest concentration of anesthetic necessary (perhaps facilitated by partial intravenous (IV) anesthesia) and by administration of *dobutamine*, a positive inotrope.

      – Other agents used to support blood pressure, perhaps at the cost of peripheral tissue perfusion, include *ephedrine, norepinephrine, phenylephrine,* and *vasopressin* (see Anesthetic Complications, Chapter 38).

    o *Halothane*, a halogenated alkane, causes the most severe cardiovascular depression in comparison to the halogenated ethers. Furthermore, halothane predisposes the patient to development of ventricular arrhythmias in the presence of catecholamines.

B **Respiratory effects**

  ◦ Inhalational anesthetics cause dose-dependent respiratory depression, resulting in a progressive increase in the arterial partial pressure of *carbon dioxide* as the anesthetic plane deepens.
  ◦ This adverse effect can be easily managed by provision of IPPV.

C **Central nervous system effects**

  ◦ Inhalational anesthetics cause a dose-dependent increase in cerebral blood flow and intracranial pressure.
  ◦ This effect could be detrimental in patients suffering from intracranial pathology or trauma.
  ◦ In patients where this is a concern, use of *partial* or *total IV* anesthesia should be considered.

D **Renal effects**

  ◦ Inhalational anesthetics cause an overall decrease in renal blood flow which results in a decrease in glomerular filtration rate and urine production. (see Chapter 5)
  ◦ To prevent renal injury, patients should be supported with IV fluids and maintenance of normal blood pressure while under general anesthesia.

E **Hepatic effects**

  ◦ Inhalational anesthetics cause a decrease in hepatic blood flow, which will slow the metabolism and clearance of co-administered anesthetic agents.
  ◦ Horses suffering from hypoxemia under anesthesia may develop increases in aspartate transaminase (AST) and sorbitol dehydrogenase (SDH) activity as evidence of *hepatocyte* insult.

F **Analgesia**

  ◦ Modern inhaled anesthetic agents including isoflurane, sevoflurane, and desflurane do not provide analgesia.
  ◦ *Methoxyflurane*, an agent of historical interest for anesthesia, does provide analgesia via an unknown mechanism.
    – It is currently available in some countries for use as a self-administered inhaler for trauma-induced pain in human beings.

## VI Nitrous oxide

  • The gaseous anesthetic $N_2O$ can be administered as an adjunctive agent in general anesthesia.
  • With a MAC value greater than 200% in animals, $N_2O$ cannot be used as a sole agent for maintenance of anesthesia.

- Nitrous oxide can be used safely in horses at concentrations of 25–50%, affording a reduction in MAC of up to 25%. Higher concentrations of $N_2O$ should be avoided as the risk for hypoxemia becomes greater with decreasing inspired fractions of oxygen.

A   Mechanism of action

- Nitrous oxide is thought to have its effect via antagonism of NMDA receptors within the CNS. This mechanism of action affords analgesia.

B   Pharmacokinetics

- Nitrous oxide is administered and taken up by the pulmonary capillary in the same way as the vaporous inhalational anesthetics. It has low solubility in the blood, allowing for rapid equilibration in the blood and the brain.
- When administered in combination with another inhaled anesthetic (e.g. isoflurane), uptake of the second gas (isoflurane) is amplified by a "*concentrating effect*" of the agent within the alveoli, and augmentation of tracheal inflow of gas from the anesthetic circuit.
- Nitrous oxide is eliminated in the expired gas and undergoes minimal hepatic biotransformation.

C   Pharmacodynamics

- Nitrous oxide is associated with minimal cardiorespiratory depression in comparison to the other inhalational anesthetics.
- The action of $N_2O$ at the NMDA receptor affords some analgesia.
- Nitrous oxide increases the risk of development of *hypoxemia* both during the anesthetic period, due to the requisite reduction in the inspired fraction of oxygen, and in the recovery period with the risk of development of *diffusion hypoxia* as $N_2O$ displaces oxygen in the alveoli.
- Hypoxemia is best avoided by limiting the inspired $N_2O$ concentration to 50% and discontinuing $N_2O$ 15–20 minutes prior to the cessation of general anesthesia, allowing for administration of nearly 100% oxygen as the $N_2O$ is expired.
  - However, delivery of safe concentrations of $N_2O$ can only be guaranteed by the use of an airway *gas analyzer*.
- Nitrous oxide will diffuse into closed gas spaces including any distended viscus and the endotracheal tube cuff.

D   Clinical use of $N_2O$

- Despite its potential benefits, $N_2O$ is rarely used in equine anesthesia primarily because of the risk of hypoxemia secondary to decreasing the inspired oxygen fraction.
- Diligent scavenging of $N_2O$ is requisite to its use. Megaloblastic anemia can occur with chronic exposure to $N_2O$ due to inhibition of *methionine synthase*.
  *Note*: Activated charcoal passive scavenging devices (e.g. activated charcoal canisters) do *not* capture $N_2O$. Nitrous oxide must be scavenged through a system that evacuates the gas from the building. Nitrous oxide has a long half-life (>100 years) in the atmosphere and contributes to the greenhouse gas effect.

## Suggested Reading

Antognini, J. (1997). The relationship among brain, spinal cord and anesthetic requirements. *Med. Hypotheses* 48: 83–87.

Bergadano, A., Lauber, R., Zbinden, A. et al. (2003). Blood/gas partition coefficient of halothane, isoflurane and sevoflurane in horse blood. *Br. J. Anesth.* 91: 276–278.

Brosnan, R.J. (2013). Inhaled anesthetics in horses. *Vet. Clin. North Am. Equine Pract.* 29: 69–87.

Gozalo-Marcilla, M., Hopster, K., and Gasthuys, F. (2013). Effects of a constant-rate infusion of dexmedetomidine on the minimal alveolar concentration of sevoflurane in ponies. *Equine Vet. J.* 45: 204–208.

Gozalo-Marcilla, M., Gasthuys, F., and Schauvliege, S. (2014). Partial intravenous anaesthesia in the horse: a review of intravenous agents used to supplement equine inhalation anaesthesia. Part 1: lidocaine and ketamine. *Vet. Anaesth. Analg.* 41: 335–345.

Gozalo-Marcilla, M., Hopster, K., and Gasthuys, F. (2014). Minimum end-tidal sevoflurane concentration necessary to prevent movement during a constant rate infusion of morphine, or morphine plus dexmedetomidine in ponies. *Vet. Anaesth. Analg.* 41: 212–219.

Gozalo-Marcilla, M., Gasthuys, F., and Schauvliege, S. (2015). Partial intravenous anaesthesia in the horse: a review of intravenous agents used to supplement equine inhalation anaesthesia. Part 2: opioids and alpha-2 adrenoceptor agonists. *Vet. Anaesth. Analg.* 42: 1–16.

Mosing, M. and Senior, J.M. (2018). Maintenance of equine anaesthesia over the last 50 years: controlled inhalation of volatile anaesthetics and pulmonary ventilation. *Equine Vet. J.* 50: 282–291.

Shafer, M., Hendrickx, J., Flood, P. et al. (2008). Additivity versus synergy: a theoretical analysis of implications of anesthetic mechanisms. *Anesth. Analg.* 107: 507–524.

Soares, J.H., Brosnan, R.J., Fukushima, F.B. et al. (2012). Solubility of haloether anesthetics in human and animal blood. *Anesthesiology* 117: 48–55.

Testa, M., Raffe, M.R., and Robinson, E.P. (1990). Evaluation of 25%, 50%, and 67% nitrous oxide with halothane-oxygen for general anesthesia in horses. *Vet. Surg.* 19: 308–312.

# 14

## Local Anesthetics

*Catherine M. Creighton and Leigh Lamont*

- Local anesthetics reversibly block the generation and propagation of electrical impulses in nerves causing sensory and motor blockade.
- In equine practice, local anesthetics are commonly administered to produce local or regional anesthesia/analgesia via:
  - Perineural injection.
  - Intraarticular injection.
  - Epidural injection.
  - Tissue infiltration.
  - Topical (e.g. corneal) administration.
  - In addition, intravenous administration of lidocaine is used in horses to:
    - Provide systemic analgesia.
    - Reduce general anesthetic requirements.
    - Manage ventricular arrhythmias.
    - Augment intestinal motility.

## I  Mechanism of action

- Local anesthetics block neuronal action potentials via inhibition of voltage-gated sodium channels (VGSCs) (see Figure 14.1).
  - VGSCs exist in three potential conformations: resting (closed), open, and inactivated (closed).
  - When depolarization occurs, the channel transitions from the resting state to the open state (activated) and allows sodium ions to flow into the cell.
  - The channel then transitions to the inactivated state which allows repolarization to occur and a transition back to the resting state.
  - Local anesthetic molecules bind receptor sites within the α-subunit of the VGSC and inhibit sodium conduction, thereby preventing action potential generation.
  - Local anesthetic molecules bind receptor sites in both open or activated and closed or inactivated states. The receptor releases the local anesthetic when they regain hyperpolarization and reach the resting state.

*Manual of Equine Anesthesia and Analgesia*, Second Edition. Edited by Tom Doherty, Alex Valverde, and Rachel A. Reed.

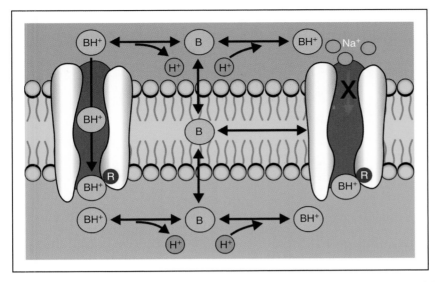

**Figure 14.1** Diagram of the cell membrane lipid bilayer with the sodium channel. Local anesthetics exist as a neutral base (B) and an ionized form (BH⁺) in equilibrium. The neutral form is lipid-soluble and easily crosses the cell membrane. The ionized form is more water-soluble and ca cross through the open channel. The neutral form can cause membrane expansion and closure of the sodium channel. The ionized form interacts with its receptor on the intracellular side of the sodium channel. (*Source:* Image credit: Wiley).

     ○ Access of local anesthetic molecules to the receptor is favored when more channels are in open and inactive states as occurs with increasing stimulation.
        – This explains why stimulation of nerve fibers facilitates onset of local anesthetic effect – a phenomenon called "use-dependent" or "frequency-dependent" block.
- Local anesthetics also modulate activity at other ion channels, receptors, and nociceptive pathways in the central nervous system (CNS), often at concentrations much less than those required for sodium channel blockade, including:
     ○ Inhibition of voltage-gated calcium and potassium channels.
     ○ Inhibition at G-protein-coupled receptors.
     ○ Activation of TRPV1 receptors.
     ○ Inhibition of N-methyl-D-aspartate (NMDA) receptors.
     ○ Inhibition of substance P binding and evoked increases in intracellular calcium.
- Local-anesthetics produce "*differential blockade*" when applied to peripheral nerves or the central neuraxis, with clinical effects appearing in the following order (see Table 14.1):
     ○ Vasodilation occurs first due to sympathetic fiber blockade.
     ○ Loss of sensation of *temperature, pain,* and *light touch* occur next due to sensory fiber blockade.
     ○ Impairment of *proprioception* and *motor function* occur last due to motor fiber blockade.

Table 14.1 Classification of nerve fibers and order of blockade.

| Classification | Diameter (µM) | Myelin | Conduction (m/sec) | Location | Function | Order of blockade |
|---|---|---|---|---|---|---|
| Aα | 15–20 | +++ | 30–120 | Afferent/efferent for muscles and joints | Motor and proprioception | 5 |
| Aβ | 5–15 | ++ | 30–70 | Efferent to muscle Afferent sensory nerve | Motor function and sensory (touch and pressure) | 4 |
| Aγ | 3–6 | ++ | 15–35 | Efferent to muscle spindle | Muscle tone | 3 |
| Aδ | 2–5 | + | 5–25 | Afferent sensory nerve | Pain (fast), touch, temperature | 2 |
| B | 1–3 | + | 3–15 | Preganglionic sympathetic | Autonomic function | 1 |
| C | 0.4–1.5 | – | 0.7–1.3 | Postganglionic sympathetic | Autonomic function, pain (slow), temperature | 2 |

*Reproduced with permission from Rioja Garcia E (2015) Veterinary Anesthesia and Analgesia, the 5th edition of Lumb and Jones, Table 17.1.*

## II Physicochemical properties

### A Chemical structure

- Local anesthetic molecules have three components:
  - *Lipophilic group* (usually an aromatic ring).
  - *Hydrophilic group* (usually a tertiary amine).
  - *Connecting intermediate chain* (including either an ester or an amide linkage).
- Local anesthetics are classified based on the connecting intermediate chain as either *aminoesters* or *aminoamides*.

### B Structure–activity relationships

*Molecular weight (*MW*)*
- Local anesthetics range in size between 220 and 288 Da.
- The ability of the drug to diffuse through tissue is inversely proportional to its MW.
  - MW may not be directly important in determining different activity profiles among different agents, but changes in MW may influence other properties such as pKa and lipid solubility.

*pKa*
- Local anesthetics are weak bases which are available commercially as salts.
- In aqueous solutions, these salts dissociate into non-ionized (neutral, *lipophilic*) and ionized (charged, *hydrophilic*) forms depending on the pH of the environment and the pKa (dissociation constant) of the drug. (see Table 14.2).
- As the local anesthetic binding site on the VGSC is located within the cell, drug in the non-ionized form is able to readily cross the cell membrane.
- Once inside the cell, a new equilibrium is established and the ionized (i.e. active) form of drug is able to interact with the VGSC receptor (see Figure 14.1).
- Local anesthetics with a low pKa (value closer to physiologic pH) have a more rapid onset of action due to less ionization at physiologic pH, while agents with a high pKa have a slower onset of action due to greater ionization at physiologic pH.

*Lipid solubility*
- The structure of the aromatic ring largely determines the agent's solubility which impacts potency, duration of action, and onset of action.
- Local anesthetics with higher solubility tend to:
  - Have higher potency.
  - Provide a longer duration of action.
  - Have a slower onset of action due to sequestration in myelin.

*Protein binding*
- The degree of protein binding determines the free fraction of drug available.
- Local anesthetics that are highly protein-bound are associated with longer durations of action because they remain at the receptor for longer.

*Stereoisomerism*
- Most local anesthetics are asymmetric molecules that exhibit two distinct spatial arrangements (mirror images) despite having the same physicochemical characteristics.
- Stereoisomers (enantiomers) may possess differing potencies, pharmacokinetic properties, and toxicities.

Table 14.2 Physiochemical properties and relative potencies of clinically used local anesthetics.

| Local Anesthetic | pKa[1] | % Ionized (at pH 7.4) | Lipid solubility[2] | % Protein binding | Relative anesthetic potency[3] | Relative potency for CNS toxicity[4] | CV/CNS ratio[5] |
|---|---|---|---|---|---|---|---|
| **Ester linked** | | | | | | | |
| Low potency, short duration | | | | | | | |
| Procaine | 8.89 | 97 | 100 | 6 | 1 | 0.3 | 3.7 |
| Chloroprocaine | 9.06 | 95 | 810 | 7 | 1 | 0.3 | 3.7 |
| High potency, long duration | | | | | | | |
| Tetracaine | 8.38 | 93 | 5822 | 94 | 8 | 2 | ND |
| **Amide linked** | | | | | | | |
| Intermediate potency and duration | | | | | | | |
| Lidocaine | 7.77 | 76 | 366 | 64 | 2 | 1 | 7.1 |
| Mepivacaine | 7.72 | 61 | 130 | 77 | 2 | 1.4 | 7.1 |
| Prilocaine | 8.02 | 76 | 129 | 55 | 2 | 1.2 | 3.1 |
| Intermediate potency, long duration | | | | | | | |
| Ropivacaine | 8.16 | 83 | 775 | 94 | 6 | 2.9 | 2 |
| High potency, long duration | | | | | | | |
| Bupivacaine | 8.1 | 83 | 3420 | 95 | 8 | 4 | 2 |
| Levobupivacaine | 8.1 | 83 | 3420 | >97 | 8 | 2.9 | 2 |
| Etidocaine | 7.87 | 66 | 7317 | 94 | 6 | 2 | 4.4 |

[1] Measured with spectrophotometric method at 36°C, except prilocaine and ropivacaine measured at 25°C.
[2] Partition coefficients expressed as relative concentrations (mol/L) in octanol and buffer at 36°C, except prilocaine and ropivacaine measured at 25°C.
[3] Potency relative to procaine.
[4] Potency relative to lidocaine.
[5] Cardiovascular to central nervous system toxicity ratio. CV denotes the disappearance of pulse and CNS denotes the onset of seizures.
*Reproduced with permission from Veterinary Anesthesia and Analgesia, the 5th edition of Lumb and Jones, 2015, Table 17.2.*

## III Pharmacokinetics

### A Absorption

- Systemic absorption of a local anesthetic is dependent on a number of factors:
  *Dose*
- The greater the dose injected, the greater the systemic absorption and peak plasma concentration ($C_{max}$).
  *Injection site*
- Administration into a highly vascular area (e.g. mucosal, pleural, or peritoneal surfaces) results in a higher $C_{max}$ and a shorter time to $C_{max}$ ($T_{max}$) compared to injection into less perfused areas (e.g. subcutaneous tissue, perineural fat).

*Lipid solubility*

○ The more potent local anesthetics with greater lipid solubility and protein binding are associated with a lower $C_{max}$ and a longer $T_{max}$.

*Vasoconstrictors*

○ Local anesthetics, except for *ropivacaine* and *levobupivacaine,* have inherent vasodilating properties.

○ The addition of a vasoconstrictor such as *epinephrine* will counteract vasodilation and decrease systemic absorption.

— The reduction in $C_{max}$ with *epinephrine* is most significant with the less-lipid soluble, less potent, shorter-acting agents (e.g. *lidocaine*).

— Vasoconstrictor-containing solutions should be avoided for blockade of areas with erratic blood supply or those lacking good collateral perfusion, due to the risk of ischemic injury.

○ With more potent, longer-acting agents (e.g. *bupivacaine*), the impact of local blood flow on systemic absorption is less significant.

## B Distribution

○ Distribution of local anesthetics is dependent on their structure:

— *Aminoesters* have a small volume of distribution (Vd) as they are rapidly hydrolyzed by plasma pseudocholinesterases and have short plasma half-lives.

— *Aminoamides* are widely distributed after intravenous (IV) administration according to a two- or three-compartment model.

*Effect of pulmonary uptake*

○ Aminoamides in the venous circulation undergo first-pass pulmonary uptake which can significantly decrease the plasma concentration of the drug temporarily.

○ This limits the amount of drug reaching the systemic circulation and the vessel-rich tissues and may limit toxicity, especially for agents with high lipid solubility and low pKa.

*Effect of hypercapnia*

○ Development of hypercapnia for any reason will increase regional cerebral blood flow and may result in increased concentrations of local anesthetic being delivered to the brain, which may increase the risk of toxicity.

## C Metabolism and excretion

○ Biotransformation of local anesthetics depends on the chemical structure of the drug.

*Aminoesters*

○ These agents are rapidly hydrolyzed in plasma (and to a lesser extent in the liver) by non-specific pseudocholinesterases.

○ The rate of hydrolysis varies with the agent but clearance is generally rapid and half-lives are measured in minutes.

○ Hydrolysis metabolites are excreted primarily in the urine.

*Aminoamides*

○ These agents are hydrolyzed by the liver cytochrome P450 enzyme system.

○ The rate of hepatic metabolism varies:

– *Lidocaine > mepivacaine > ropivacaine > bupivacaine*

○ Clearance is slower than that of the esters and half-lives are measured in hours.

- *In horses*, lidocaine undergoes hydroxylation and *N*-demethylation in the liver to monoethylglycinexylidide (MEGX) and glycinexylidide (GX) which are pharmacologically active and could contribute to toxicity during prolonged systemic infusions.
  - Factors that reduce hepatic function and/or blood flow, including inhalant anesthesia, will impact biotransformation and clearance of amide local anesthetics.
  - Metabolites are excreted primarily in urine and bile with a small portion of lidocaine excreted unchanged in equine urine.

# IV  Local anesthetic adjuvants and combinations

## A  Epinephrine

- Epinephrine (5 µg/ml) may be added to a local anesthetic solution to decrease local perfusion, delay absorption, and prolong anesthetic action.
- Due to the risk of ischemic injury, epinephrine-containing solutions should be avoided for blockade of areas with erratic blood supply or those lacking good collateral perfusion.
- When administered into the epidural or subarachnoid spaces, *epinephrine* may enhance analgesia through interaction with α-adrenergic receptors in the spinal cord and brain.

## B  α₂ agonists

*Effects on peripheral nerve blocks*

- Addition of an α₂ agonist, such as *clonidine* or *dexmedetomidine*, potentiates peripheral nerve blocks with local anesthetics in human patients and in experimental studies in animals including horses.
- This effect of alpha₂ adrenergic agonists in prolongating the effect of local anesthetics is *not* mediated by their α-adrenergic actions as it is not blocked by either *prazosin*, an alpha₁ antagonist, or *idazoxan* an α₂ antagonist.
- It is now established that α₂ agonists potentiate the effect of local anesthetics by blocking the $I_h$ current produced by hyperpolarization-activated cyclic nucleotide-gated (HCN) channels.
  - HCN channels are a subfamily of membrane proteins in the superfamily of pore-loop cationic channels.
  - HCN channels are widely expressed in the nervous system and heart.
- The current through the HCN channel is termed $I_h$. The $I_h$ current is a mixed cationic current conducted by $Na^+$ and $K^+$. It is initiated during the hyperpolarization phase of the action potential, and it functions to reset the nerve for subsequent action potentials.
- Thus, blocking the $I_h$ current precludes the development of subsequent action potentials by potentiating hyperpolarization.

*Effects on epidural anesthesia*

- Adding *xylazine* to *lidocaine* potentiates and prolongs anesthesia when administered into the caudal epidural space in horses.
  - Synergism was presumed to be due to activation of α₂ adrenergic receptors in the spinal cord dorsal horn which inhibits release of substance P and hyperpolarizes nociceptive projection neurons.
  - However, it is most likely due to the aforementioned activity at the HCN channel.
  - This combination is used commonly in clinical equine practice for caudal epidural anesthesia.

C  **Bicarbonate**

    ○ 1 mEq/10 ml added to a local anesthetic solution to increase the pH increases the amount of nonionized drug available to diffuse across membranes.

    ○ This *may* accelerate onset of the block, increase intensity and duration, and decrease pain on injection.

        – Clinical benefits of this practice remain debatable in any species and data in horses are lacking.

D  **Hyaluronidase**

    ○ This enzyme may be added to a local anesthetic solution to break down hyaluronic acid which functions as mesenchymal tissue cement.

        – In theory, this may improve diffusion of the local anesthetic.

E  **Carbon dioxide**

    ○ Carbonation of local anesthetic solutions causes local intracellular acidosis which, in theory, increases the amount of intracellular ionized drug available to bind sodium channel receptors and accelerates the onset of action.

        – This practice does not appear to significantly improve block quality in equine patients.

F  **Combinations of local anesthetics**

    ○ The combination of a quick onset, short-acting local anesthetic with a slow onset, long-acting local anesthetic has theoretical merit.

        – There is currently no evidence to suggest that this practice is clinically beneficial.

## V  Local anesthetic toxicity

    • When used correctly, local anesthetics have proven to be safe, and adverse effects are not common.

    • Toxicities can be divided into three categories: systemic, local tissue toxicity, and allergic.

A  **Systemic toxicity**

    *CNS*

    ○ In most species, the relative CNS toxicity of various local anesthetics is proportional to their potencies.

        – In horses, *procaine* is an exception with a low anesthetic potency but a high probability of CNS stimulation in this species.

    ○ In conscious horses, initial signs of *lidocaine*-induced CNS toxicity include blinking, nystagmus, muscle fasciculation, agitation, disorientation, and ataxia.

        – Some horses may assume sternal recumbency or show signs of visual impairment.

        – Rapid bolus dosages exceeding 2 mg/kg IV commonly produce these signs and are associated with mean plasma lidocaine concentrations of approximately 3 µg/ml.

        – Early signs of toxicity typically resolve after termination of the infusion but treatment with a sedative, such as *xylazine*, or an anticonvulsant, such as *diazepam*, may be indicated.

- o With higher plasma *lidocaine* concentrations, progression to seizures, unconsciousness, coma, and respiratory arrest will occur.
    - − Seizures should be treated immediately.
    - − In addition to sedatives and anticonvulsants, induction, and maintenance of general anesthesia with injectable and/or inhalant agents may be necessary.
    - − Endotracheal intubation, oxygen supplementation and hyperventilation to counteract hypoxemia, hypercarbia and acidosis are indicated.

*Cardiovascular system (CVS)*

- o At low plasma concentrations, most local anesthetics have an anti-arrhythmogenic effect.
- o At higher concentrations, greater than those that induce early signs of CNS toxicity, CVS toxicity characterized by *myocardial depression, hypotension,* and refractory *cardiac arrhythmias* is evident.
    - − Shorter-acting, less lipid soluble agents, such as *lidocaine* and *mepivacaine,* are less arrhythmogenic.
    - − Longer-acting, more lipid soluble agents, such as *bupivacaine*, are more arrhythmogenic.
    - − One of the mechanisms by which *bupivacaine* exhibits its CVS toxicity is through its inhibition of *carnitine-acylcarnitine transferase* (CACT). CACT has a vital role in cell metabolism; it transports fatty acid units into mitochondria for β-oxidation. Disruption of this process by *bupivacaine* may lead to a depletion of metabolic energy, making cardiac resuscitation techniques following local anesthetic-induced toxicity ineffective.
    - − The hypotension seen with local anesthetic-induced toxicity is caused in part by generalized *vasodilation*. This effect of vasodilation has been associated with the *nitric oxide synthase (NOS)* pathway, as less vasodilation is seen when local anesthetics are co-administered with the NOS inhibitor NG-nitro-L-arginine methyl ester (L-NAME). Nitric oxide mediates vascular smooth muscle relaxation, and is formed in a reaction catalyzed by NOS.
- o R-enantiomers have slower unbinding rates making them even more arrhythmogenic than S-enantiomers.
    - − *Levobupivacaine* and *ropivacaine* are S-enantiomers and are considered to be safer than their dextrorotatory counterparts.

*Blood*

- o *Benzocaine* and *prilocaine* have been associated with development of *methemoglobinemia*, which results from metabolic breakdown products (e.g. ortho-toluidine) capable of oxidizing the hemoglobin molecule.
- o Treatment with *methylene blue* may be indicated if oxygen-carrying capacity is compromised.

## B  Local tissue toxicity

*Neurotoxicity*

- o Direct local anesthetic-induced nerve injury is a possible but rare complication.
- o Clinically relevant concentrations of local anesthetics are considered safe for peripheral nerves but the spinal cord and nerve roots may be more prone to injury.

*Chondrotoxicity*

- o Local anesthetic-induced chondrotoxicity has been demonstrated both *in vivo* and *in vitro* and is time and concentration dependent.
- o In horses, intra-articular injection is commonly performed for diagnostic purposes, and *mepivacaine* has been shown to be less chondrotoxic compared to *lidocaine* or *bupivacaine*.

## C Allergic reactions

- ○ Allergic reactions to aminoamide local anesthetics are extremely *rare*.
- ○ Aminoester local anesthetics are metabolized to *para-aminobenzoic acid* (PABA) *derivatives* which may induce Type I hypersensitivity reactions.
- ○ Added preservatives such as *methylparaben*, which structurally resembles PABA, may also produce allergic skin reactions.

## VI Local anesthetic agents

### A Lidocaine (see Table 14.3)

- ○ The most commonly used and versatile local anesthetic in equine practice.
- ○ 2% formulations are indicated for peripheral nerve blocks, caudal epidural anesthesia, and IV administration.
- ○ Rapid onset (5–10 minutes) and intermediate duration (60–90 minutes) with local/regional administration.

### B Mepivacaine

- ○ Also commonly used in equine practice for local or regional techniques.
- ○ 2% formulations are indicated for peripheral nerve blocks or intraarticular blocks (especially for diagnostic lameness examination), and caudal epidural anesthesia.
- ○ Similar to *lidocaine* in its activity profile with a comparable onset (5–10 minutes) but a somewhat longer duration (120–180 minutes).

Table 14.3  Clinical indications and doses in horses.

| Local anesthetic | Commercial name | Indications | Doses |
|---|---|---|---|
| Lidocaine | Lidocaine HCl, Lignocaine, Xylocaine (some with epinephrine) | Infiltration, nerve blocks Epidural Intravenous (IV) | Maximum doses: 6 mg/kg Caudal epidural: 6 ml total IV infusion: 1.3–3 mg/kg loading dose; 25–100 μg/kg/min infusion |
| Mepivacaine | Carbocaine, Intra-Epicaine, Vetacaine | Infiltration, nerve blocks Epidural Intra-articular | Maximum dose: 5–6 mg/kg Caudal epidural: 6 ml total Intra-articular: 10–15 ml total |
| Bupivacaine | Marcaine | Infiltration, nerve blocks Epidural | Maximum dose: 2 mg/kg Caudal epidural: 6 ml total |
| Levobupivacaine | Chirocaine | Infiltration, nerve blocks Epidural | Maximum dose: 3 mg/kg Caudal epidural: 6 ml total |
| Ropivacaine | Naropin | Infiltration, nerve blocks Epidural | Maximum dose: 3 mg/kg Caudal epidural: 6 ml total |

## C Bupivacaine

- ○ Occasionally used in equine practice if a longer duration of action is desired (e.g. intra- or post-operative analgesia).
- ○ 0.5% formulations are indicated for peripheral nerve blocks, infiltrative anesthesia, or epidural anesthesia.
- ○ Variable onset (10–30 minutes depending on route of administration) and long duration (240–480 minutes).
- ○ More cardiotoxic than lidocaine, and IV administration is contraindicated.
- ○ Also available as a pure S-enantiomer (*levobupivacaine*) which may be associated with less systemic toxicity compared to the racemic mixture.
- ○ The sustained-release liposomal formulation of *bupivacaine* approved for periarticular administration for stifle surgery in dogs has recently been evaluated in horses. In that study, the duration of an abaxial sesamoid nerve block performed using liposomal bupivacaine was only approximately four hours.

## D Ropivacaine

- ○ Similar to bupivacaine, it is occasionally used in equine practice if a longer duration of action is desired (e.g. intra- or postoperative analgesia).
- ○ Indications, onset time and duration are comparable to bupivacaine.
- ○ Like *levobupivacaine*, *ropivacaine* is formulated as a pure S-enantiomer and may be associated with less systemic toxicity compared to racemic *bupivacaine*.

## E Proparacaine and Tetracaine

- ○ Used for topical application to desensitize the cornea for ocular examination or minor surgical procedures.
- ○ *Proparacaine* 0.5% aqueous solution has been commonly used for ocular indications in horses (~20-minute duration).
- ○ *Tetracaine* 0.5% aqueous solution or 0.5% viscous gel is similar to proparacaine but may be superior at reducing corneal sensitivity in horses (20–30 minutes duration).

## F Procaine

- ○ Rarely used for local or regional nerve blockade in horses.
- ○ IV *procaine* is a CNS stimulant in horses and has been used illegally in racehorses.
- ○ *Procaine* is commonly added to intramuscular (IM) *penicillin* formulations to prolong the duration of action. This preparation is occasionally associated with CNS stimulating effects after IM administration.
  - – Accidental IV administration may be associated with adverse effects.

# VII Clinical use

## A Local and regional techniques

- ○ Details regarding specific local and regional techniques are provided in Chapters 22–27.

- ○ *Lidocaine, mepivacaine and, less commonly, bupivacaine* is administered in equine practice for peripheral nerve blocks, infiltrative blocks, intraarticular blocks, and epidural anesthesia.
- ○ Clinical indications for these techniques include:
  - – Diagnostic lameness evaluation to localize pain.
  - – Surgical anesthesia for procedures in standing sedated horses.
  - – Adjunctive analgesia for surgical procedures in horses under general anesthesia.
  - – Post-operative analgesia.
- ○ Temporary relief of chronic pain (e.g. for laminitis).

### B   Intravenous lidocaine

- ○ Lidocaine is administered IV to awake and anesthetized horse for the purpose of analgesia, and as an adjunct to general anesthetics. The reader can find information on the proposed mechanisms of action and clinical use of IV administered lidocaine in Chapter 12.

## Suggested Reading

Brummett, C.M., Hong, E.K., Janda, A.M. et al. (2011). Perineural dexmedetomidine added to ropivacaine for sciatic nerve block in rats prolongs the duration of analgesia by blocking the hyperpolarization-activated cation current. *Anesthesiology* 115: 836–843.

Guedes, A. (2017). Pain management in horses. *Vet. Clin. North Am. Equine Pract.* 33: 181–211.

McCracken, M.J., Schumacher, J., Doherty, T.J. et al. (2020). Efficacy and duration of effect for liposomal bupivacaine when administered perineurally to the palmar digital nerves of horses. *Am. J. Vet. Res.* 81: 400–405.

Rioja Garcia, E. (2015). Local anesthetics. In: *Veterinary Anesthesia and Analgesia* (eds. K.A. Grimm, L.A. Lamont, W.J. Tranquilli, et al.), 332–354. Ames, Iowa: Wiley.

Vigani, A. and Garcia-Pereira, F.L. (2014). Anesthesia and analgesia for standing equine surgery. *Vet. Clin. North Am. Equine Pract.* 30: 1–17.

## 15

# Neuromuscular Blocking Agents in Horses
*Manuel Martin-Flores and Daniel M. Sakai*

## I Introduction

- Neuromuscular blocking agents (NMBAs) are used in balanced protocols in combination with a general anesthetic and an analgesic technique.
  - The NMBA allows lower doses of general anesthetics to be used, as the dose necessary to cause immobility is higher than the dose that produces hypnosis.
  - This minimizes anesthetic-induced cardiovascular depression.
- In the horse, the use of NMBAs is typically indicated for ophthalmologic and some orthopedic surgeries. However, the inclusion of NMBAs in the anesthetic protocols of cardiovascularly unstable animals, such as some exploratory laparotomies, can be beneficial as reducing the dose of inhalational anesthetics is of utmost importance.

## II Physiology of the neuromuscular junction

- Normal neuromuscular transmission occurs when acetylcholine (ACh) is released from pre-synaptic cells (motor nerve) at the neuromuscular junction.
- ACh binds to post-synaptic *nicotinic* ACh receptors (nAChR) and triggers a conformational change allowing the influx of $Na^+$ and $Ca^{2+}$ and the outflux of $K^+$.
- As a result, the intracellular post-synaptic membrane (sarcolemma) depolarizes.
- Voltage-gated ion channels activate, which causes a sharp, widespread multiplication of the depolarization across the sarcolemma and T tubules.
- When depolarization reaches the T tubules, intracellular channels releases $Ca^{2+}$ from the sarcoplasmic reticulum. The increased intracellular $Ca^{2+}$ activates *troponin* and promotes the interaction of *actin* and *myosin*. This mechanism of neuromuscular transmission is preserved in the whole skeletal muscle system.

*Manual of Equine Anesthesia and Analgesia*, Second Edition. Edited by Tom Doherty, Alex Valverde, and Rachel A. Reed.
© 2022 John Wiley & Sons, Inc. Published 2022 by John Wiley & Sons, Inc.

## III  Neuromuscular blocking agents

- Most NMBAs in clinical use are competitive antagonists to the nAChR.
- Upon interaction with the nicotinic receptor, NMBAs prevent the binding of ACh with the receptor; the nAChR ligated with a NMBA is therefore unable to allow an influx of $Na^+$ and $Ca^{2+}$.
  - Neuromuscular transmission and skeletal muscle contraction are thus prevented.
- This mechanism of action explains why these drugs are also referred as "*nondepolarizing*" NMBAs.
- Owing to the safety margin of the neuromuscular junction, neuromuscular transmission is affected when at least 70% of the post-synaptic nAChR are inactivated and is completely interrupted when more than 98% of the nAChR are inactivated.

### A  Pharmacology

- NMBAs have a large molecular weight and are hydrophilic, quaternary ammonium compounds.
- These characteristics prevent diffusion across biologic membranes, such as the blood–brain-barrier or placenta.
- Therefore, NMBAs do not contribute to hypnosis or analgesia, and do not affect the fetus when used at clinically relevant doses.

### B  Physiology

- All skeletal musculature will be affected by the NMBA, including the muscles that control ventilation and airway patency.
  - Thus, it is necessary to use mechanical ventilation to prevent hypercapnia, hypoxemia, and to deliver inhalant anesthesia to horses.
- Some components used to evaluate anesthetic depth in anesthetized horses, such as eye globe position, nystagmus, and palpebral reflexes will be abolished with the use of a NMBA.
  - It is important to administer an adequate dose of anesthetic to promote hypnosis and prevent awareness under anesthesia.
- The lack of central nervous system (CNS) effects implies that NMBAs do not produce sedation, hypnosis, or analgesia.
  - Thus, it is an inhumane practice to perform surgical procedures utilizing a NMBA without maintaining general anesthesia.
- Subsequent doses of a NMBA used to prolong the paralysis are lower than the initial dose. Due to the safety margin, up to 70% of the nAChR might already be occupied by the NMBA, even if full neuromuscular recovery is detected by neuromuscular monitoring.

## III  Individual NMBAs

### A  Benzylisoquinolones

- *Atracurium* and *cisatracurium* are the benzylisoquinolones used in clinical practice (Table 15.1). They do not depend on organ metabolism to be eliminated from the circulation.

*Atracurium*

- ○ Atracurium spontaneously degrades at body temperature and pH via a process called *Hofmann* elimination.
  - – Therefore, it is stored under refrigeration and at a low pH to maintain stability.
  - – A secondary route of elimination is via *enzymatic hydrolysis* through plasma *esterases*.
- ○ These combined mechanisms afford predictable clearance of atracurium, even in cases where organ function is altered.
- ○ The degradation of atracurium produces *laudanosine*. This byproduct crosses the blood–brain-barrier and is a central nervous system (CNS) stimulant.
- ○ At clinical doses, insufficient *laudanosine* accumulates to cause CNS stimulation.
- ○ Also, at clinical doses, atracurium is devoid of any relevant, direct, autonomic effects; however, indirect cardiovascular effects such as vasodilation, hypotension and tachycardia can be observed due to *histamine* release, especially when high doses are used.

*Cisatracurium*

- ○ Cisatracurium is an isomer of atracurium.
- ○ Because the solution does not contain the other nine isomers of atracurium, it has a higher potency (smaller doses are used) and the likelihood of histamine release is substantially lower.
  - – The production of *laudanosine* is also greatly reduced in comparison with atracurium at equipotent doses.

## B    Neurosteroids

- ○ The elimination of steroidal NMBAs occurs with the excretion of the parent drug or its metabolites by the liver or kidneys.
- ○ They are generally characterized by cardiovascular stability and they do not promote the release of *histamine*.

*Vecuronium*

- ○ Vecuronium is primarily eliminated by the liver. Most of the molecules are excreted intact via the biliary system and a smaller fraction is biotransformed to 3-OH.
  - – The kidney has a secondary role in the elimination of vecuronium.
- ○ The metabolite 3-OH has neuromuscular blocking activity and can extend the duration of the paralysis with prolonged administration of vecuronium.
- ○ Hepatic and liver dysfunction can also increase the duration of the block. A small study in horses concluded that doses required to produce complete block also resulted in a long duration of action.
- ○ Moreover, reversal of the neuromuscular block (NMB) from vecuronium was regarded as challenging. As a result, vecuronium may *not* be the most suitable agent for clinical use in horses.

*Rocuronium*

- ○ The parent compound is eliminated primarily by the liver and secondarily by the kidneys.
  - – Thus, accumulation is possible with hepatic dysfunction.
  - – Renal disease affects elimination to a lesser degree.
- ○ It does not have active metabolites nor releases histamine. Rocuronium has been used extensively in horses without any of the issues observed with vecuronium (Table 15.1).

## C Residual NMB

- Residual NMB is the inadvertent presence of partial block; that is, an incomplete recovery of neuromuscular function. If undetected it can negatively affect the recovery period, and its consequences may go beyond the obvious muscular weakness.
- In humans, residual block is a common complication, and it interferes with the expected respiratory response to hypoxia.
- Subjective assessment of neuromuscular function, including the observation of evoked responses to train-of-four (TOF) stimulation, is an insensitive method to detect partial block. Only objective methods such as acceleromyography have been shown to predictably reduce the incidence of residual block and limit its associated negative events during recovery (see Chapter 19, Principles of Monitoring Neuromuscular Function).
- Unfortunately, there is no study addressing the incidence or consequences of residual block in horses. Until proven otherwise, the authors' opinion is that every effort should be made to avoid residual block during recovery from anesthesia.

## IV Pharmacologic reversal of NMB

### A Acetylcholinesterase inhibitors

- Reversal of NMB can usually be accelerated by the administration of acetylcholinesterase inhibitor agents, such as *edrophonium* or *neostigmine.*
- These drugs decrease the activity of the acetylcholinesterase enzyme. As a result, ACh accumulates in the neuromuscular junction.
- The increased concentration of ACh displaces the NMBA from nAChR binding sites and accelerates the return of normal neuromuscular function.
- Reversal with these agents is indirect and hence has some important clinical implications.

*Clinical implications*:

- First, this process of reversal takes time, and several minutes should be allowed before the full effect can be appreciated.
- Second, the maximal amount of ACh that can accumulate in the neuromuscular junction depends on the rate of production and release of that molecule from the presynaptic cell. This process has a limit, and this *"ceiling effect"* to the amount of ACh available is incapable of competing with high doses of NMBAs.
- Thus, complete neuromuscular block cannot be effectively reversed with acetylcholinesterase inhibitors.
- The use of a peripheral nerve stimulator is therefore necessary not only to assess recovery, but also to evaluate whether reversal with these agents can be attempted. It is commonly recommended that 1–2 twitches in response to TOF should be observed before reversal agents are administered.
- As a general rule, the deeper the level of block, the slower and less reliable reversal will be.

### B Reversal drugs

- *Neostigmine* and *edrophonium* have been used clinically in horses (Table 15.2).
- Both drugs can produce varying levels of systemic effects resulting from the *"spillover"* of ACh to the systemic circulation and stimulation of *muscarinic* receptors, which may result in *bradycardia.*

- ○ However, both agents have been used successfully in horses without the need for *atropine*.
- ○ Diluting the acetylcholinesterase inhibitor and administering it *slowly* may help prevent severe *bradycardia*.
- ○ If required, *atropine* (0.05–0.01 mg/kg) or *glycopyrrolate* (0.0025–0.005 mg/kg) should be administered IV.

  *Note*: Because reversal with these agents cannot always guarantee that normal neuromuscular transmission will be recovered quickly, objective monitoring is still recommended even after reversal has been performed.

## C Selective relaxant binding agents

- ○ *Sugammadex* is the first agent in this class that has become available for clinical practice.
- ○ This cyclodextrin encapsulates *rocuronium* producing a complex devoid of neuromuscular blocking effects.
- ○ The bond is permanent, and it effectively reduces the concentration of free rocuronium almost instantly. As a result, neuromuscular function is restored promptly and completely.
- ○ Even deep levels of block can be antagonized, as this mechanism does not depend on the production or release of ACh.
- ○ Sugammadex has been used successfully to restore function from complete block with rocuronium in ponies. Although the agent is not yet used routinely in equine anesthesia, it offers several advantages over the use of edrophonium or neostigmine.
- ○ Sugammadex can accelerate recovery from deep rocuronium block (TOF ratio = 0).
- ○ Recovery with sugammadex is faster and more predictable than recovery with neostigmine or edrophonium.
- ○ Sugammadex administration is *not* associated with muscarinic effects (Tables 15.1 and 15.2).

Table 15.1   Characteristics of neuromuscular blocking agents commonly used in horses.

|  | Dose (mg/kg) | Duration (min) | References |
|---|---|---|---|
| Atracurium | 0.07–0.15 | 40–100 | (Hildebrand & Arpin 1988; Martin-Flores et al. 2012) |
| Cisatracurium | 0.075–0.1 | 45–60 | (Tutunaru et al. 2019) |
| Rocuronium | 0.3–0.4 | 35–80 | (Auer et al. 2007; Auer & Moens 2011) |

Table 15.2   Acetylcholinesterase inhibitors used for reversal of neuromuscular blockade in horses.

| Drug | Dose (mg/kg, IV) | References |
|---|---|---|
| Neostigmine | 0.007–0.04 | (Hildebrand & Howitt 1984; Auer & Moens 2011) |
| Edrophonium | 0.5–1.0 | (Hildebrand & Howitt 1984) |

## Suggested Reading

Auer, U. and Moens, Y. (2011). Neuromuscular blockade with rocuronium bromide for ophthalmic surgery in horses. *Vet. Ophthalmol.* 14: 244–247.

Auer, U., Uray, C., and Mosing, M. (2007). Observations on the muscle relaxant rocuronium bromide in the horse-a dose-response study. *Vet. Anaesth. Analg.* 34: 75–81.

Brull, S.J., Ehrenwerth, J., and Silverman, D.G. (1990). Stimulation with submaximal current for train-of-four monitoring. *Anesthesiology* 72: 629–632.

Eriksson, L.I. (1996). Reduced hypoxic chemosensitivity in partially paralysed man. A new property of muscle relaxants? *Acta Anaesthiol Scand* 40: 520–523.

Eriksson, L.I., Lennmarken, C., Wyon, N. et al. (1992). Attenuated ventilatory response to hypoxaemia at vecuronium-induced partial neuromuscular block. *Acta Anaesthesiol. Scand.* 36: 710–715.

Eriksson, L.I., Sato, M., and Severinghaus, J.W. (1993). Effect of a vecuronium-induced partial neuromuscular block on hypoxic ventilatory response. *Anesthesiology* 78: 693–699.

Hildebrand, S.V. and Arpin, D. (1988). Neuromuscular and cardiovascular effects of atracurium administered to healthy horses anesthetized with halothane. *Am. J. Vet. Res.* 49: 1066–1071.

Hildebrand, S.V. and Hill, T. (1994). Interaction of gentamycin and atracurium in anaesthetised horses. *Equine Vet. J.* 26: 209–211.

Hildebrand, S.V. and Howitt, G.A. (1984). Antagonism of pancuronium neuromuscular blockade in halothane-anesthetized ponies using neostigmine and edrophonium. *Am. J. Vet. Res.* 45: 2276–2280.

Hildebrand, S.V., Howitt, G.A., and Arpin, D. (1986). Neuromuscular and cardiovascular effects of atracurium in ponies anesthetized with halothane. *Am. J. Vet. Res.* 47: 1096–1100.

Martin-Flores, M., Pare, M.D., Adams, W. et al. (2012). Observations of the potency and duration of vecuronium in isoflurane-anesthetized horses. *Vet. Anaesth. Analg.* 39: 385–389.

Murphy, G.S., Szokol, J.W., Marymont, J.H. et al. (2008). Residual neuromuscular blockade and critical respiratory events in the postanesthesia care unit. *Anesth. Analg.* 107: 130–137.

Murphy, G.S., Szokol, J.W., Marymont, J.H. et al. (2008b). Intraoperative acceleromyographic monitoring reduces the risk of residual neuromuscular blockade and adverse respiratory events in the postanesthesia care unit. *Anesthesiology* 109: 389–398.

Stoelting, R.K., Longnecker, D.E., and Eger, E.I. (1970). Minimum alveolar concentrations in man on awakening from methoxyflurane, halothane, ether and fluroxene anesthesia: MAC awake. *Anesthesiology* 33: 5–9.

Tutunaru, A., Dupont, J., Gougnard, A. et al. (2019). Retrospective evaluation of clinical use of cis-atracurium in horses. *PLoS One* 14: e0221196.

## 16

# Non-steroidal Anti-Inflammatory Drugs and Corticosteroids

## Non-steroidal Anti-Inflammatory Drugs
*Stephanie Kleine*

- Non-steroidal anti-inflammatory drugs (NSAIDs), an extract of the Willow spp., were originally used in 400 BCE by Hippocrates.
- Currently, NSAIDs remain a mainstay in equine analgesia.
- These drugs are efficacious in the treatment of inflammation, musculoskeletal, gastrointestinal (GI), and perioperative pain by blocking the production of prostaglandins.

## I  Arachidonic acid cascade

- Arachidonic acid (AA) is the precursor to the production of eicosanoids, such as prostaglandins, leukotrienes, and lipoxins (see Figure 16.1).
- AA is a ω-6 polyunsaturated fatty acid that is present in cell membrane phospholipids.
- AA is liberated from the cell membrane subsequent to membrane damage.
- AA is also released by phospholipase $A_2$ ($PLA_2$), which is activated by bacterial components (i.e. LPS), cytokine (e.g. tumor necrosis factor-α; [TNF-α]), through activation of purinergic receptors, and numerous other inflammatory stimuli.
- AA is metabolized via cyclooxygenase (COX) or lipoxygenase (LOX) to prostaglandins and leukotrienes, respectively.
  - The actions of COX to form prostaglandins represents the rate-limiting step within the cascade.

### A  Isoenzymes of COX

- There are three reported isoenzymes of COX: COX-1, COX-2, and COX-3.
- COX-1 is *constitutively* expressed in most tissue types and is important in homeostatic functions.
- COX-2 expression was originally thought to be *induced* only during times of inflammation. It is now known that COX-2 is *constitutively* expressed in low levels in most tissues but upregulated during periods of inflammation.

*Manual of Equine Anesthesia and Analgesia*, Second Edition. Edited by Tom Doherty, Alex Valverde, and Rachel A. Reed.
© 2022 John Wiley & Sons, Inc. Published 2022 by John Wiley & Sons, Inc.

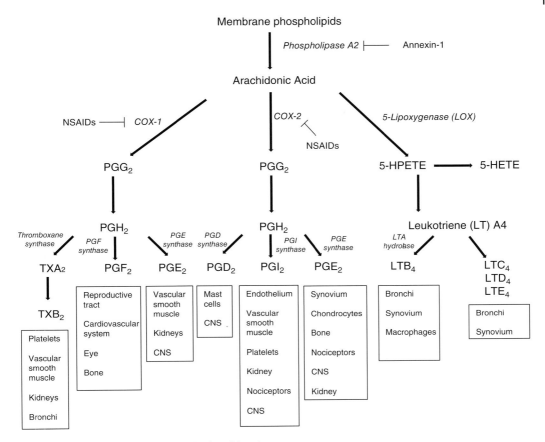

**Figure 16.1** Diagram of the arachidonic acid pathway.

- Importantly, COX-2 is involved in *renal* homeostatic functions.
- It is also expressed in *smooth muscle cells*, *lung*, the *GI tract, chondrocytes, monocytes,* and *macrophages* under basal conditions.
- COX-2 is rapidly induced during times of cellular injury or inflammation. It is implicated in physiologic and pathologic inflammation.
  - COX-3 is a variant of the COX-1 isoenzyme and is unlikely to be clinically relevant in the horse.

**B  Synthesis of prostaglandins**

- The synthesis of prostaglandin $G_2$ (PGG$_2$) and prostaglandin H2 (PGH$_2$) via COX enzymes occurs through reduction and oxidation reactions.
- PGG$_2$ is formed first by both COX enzymes, and is an unstable intermediary that is rapidly converted to PGH$_2$.
- PGH$_2$ is converted via various synthases to thromboxane A2 (TxA$_2$), prostaglandin $D_2$ (PGD$_2$), prostaglandin $E_2$ (PGE$_2$), prostaglandin $F_2$ (PGF$_2$), and prostaglandin $I_2$ (PGI$_2$).
  - COX-1 preferentially forms TxA$_2$, PGF$_2$, PGI$_2$, and PGE$_2$.
  - COX-2 preferentially forms PGE$_2$ and PGI$_2$.
  - Despite the preferential prostaglandin formation between COX enzymes, there is significant overlap in the formation of prostaglandins.

## C Role of prostaglandins

- Prostaglandins are present at peripheral and central sites and they promote nociception and inflammation.
- COX-2 expression in the spinal cord is up-regulated during periods of peripheral inflammation.
- $PGE_2$ receptors (EP1, EP2, EP3, EP4) are expressed in sensory ganglia and the dorsal horn of the spinal cord (see Table 16.1).
- Centrally, $PGE_2$ and $PGI_2$ dilate arterioles and sensitize nociceptors to the action of other mediators (e.g. bradykinin).
- PGs evoke central hyperalgesia with $PGE_2$ and $PGI_2$ being the most potent.

## II Mechanism of action of NSAIDs

- Traditional NSAIDs act by blocking the COX enzymes and the subsequent production of prostaglandins.
- Many of the original NSAIDs blocked both COX-1 and COX-2.
- NSAIDs block prostaglandin synthesis centrally and peripherally, which results in analgesic and anti-hyperanalgesic effects.
  - NSAIDs decrease the release of excitatory amino acids (i.e. *glutamate*) in sensory neurons.
  - NSAIDs have also been proposed to interact with the *endogenous opioid* system.
- *Grapiprant*, a newer NSAID, works by blocking the $PGE_2$ receptors, specifically the EP4 receptor.
- The adverse effects (i.e. GI and renal) have been attributed to inhibition of COX-1, which led to the development of COX-1 sparing (COX-2 selective) drugs.
  - In theory, use of a more COX-2 selective drug should allow for maintenance of homeostasis while inhibiting the pro-inflammatory cascade.
- However, COX-2 has been shown to be constitutively expressed in the kidneys and the potential for renal adverse effects still exists.
  - Additionally, if a COX-2 drug is overdosed the COX selectivity decreases.
- COX selectivity is measured by the ratio of inhibition of COX-1 to the inhibition of COX-2 in whole blood.

Table 16.1 Function of the four $PGE_2$ receptor subtypes.

| EP1 | EP2 | EP3 | EP4 |
|---|---|---|---|
| Contact hypersensitivity | Peripheral hyperalgesia | Suppresses allergic sensitization | Prevents irritable bowel disease |
| | Spinal inflammatory hyperalgesia | Mediates fever generation | Promotes Langerhans cell migration |
| | Facilitates joint inflammation | Suppresses allergic inflammation | Facilitates joint inflammation of arthritis |
| | | | Promotes immune inflammation |

Table 16.2    Reported COX -1: COX-2 Selectivity in horses utilizing either $IC_{50}$ or $IC_{80}$ COX ratios.

| Drug | $IC_{50}$ | $IC_{80}$ |
| --- | --- | --- |
| Flunixin meglumine | 0.336 | 0.436 |
| Phenylbutazone | 0.302 | 0.708 |
| Carprofen | 1.996 | 1.738 |
| Firocoxib | | 200 |
| Meloxicam | 3.806 | 2.239 |
| Robenacoxib | 61.01 | |
| Deracoxib | 25.67 | 22.06 |

- Some authors use the half-maximal inhibitory concentration ($IC_{50}$) while others use $IC_{80}$ or $IC_{95}$.
- The COX-1:COX-2 ratio is used to determine selectivity with higher ratios being more selective.
- The *analyte* for determination of COX-1 activity is $TxA_2$ and $PGE_2$ is used to assess COX-2 function.
- It is important to note that selectivity of all NSAIDs varies among species.
- Commonly used non-selective drugs include flunixin meglumine and phenylbutazone (see Table 16.2).
- However, coxib drugs (e.g. firocoxib) are COX-2 selective.

*Note:* Coxibs contain a tricyclic ring or sulfone/sulfonamide group which limits their ability to bind to COX-1.

- *Firocoxib* is the only coxib drug labeled for horses in the U.S.A.

## III   Clinical uses of NSAIDs

### A   Musculoskeletal analgesia

- NSAIDs are the mainstay of treatment for musculoskeletal injuries.
- They are effective at reducing inflammation and providing analgesia in both acute and chronic musculoskeletal disease.
- In a 2019 study, phenylbutazone was the most commonly prescribed NSAID for musculoskeletal analgesia in horses.
- Although phenylbutazone is more commonly used, firocoxib has been shown to be at least as effective as phenylbutazone for attenuating lameness.
- In addition to the effects on lameness scores, NSAIDs have been demonstrated to increase peak vertical force utilizing force plate measurements.

### B   Use in gastrointestinal (GI) disease

- NSAIDs are commonly utilized in veterinary practice for visceral analgesia and for the anti-endotoxin effects.

○ *Flunixin meglumine* was demonstrated to be the most commonly prescribed NSAID for equine colic; however, *phenylbutazone* has been also administered to horses with colic, despite being labeled for musculoskeletal injury only.

○ While NSAIDs are used commonly in equine GI disease, there is some evidence that NSAIDs inhibit intestinal repair mechanisms and reduce GI motility.

### C  Anti-endotoxin effects

○ Both selective and non-selective NSAIDs mitigate the clinical signs associated with endotoxemia.

○ Despite the effects on clinical signs, NSAIDs do not completely mitigate the inflammatory response in endotoxemia, as these drugs block prostanoid production and not the other important mediators (e.g. interleukin-1β or TNF-α).

○ Flunixin meglumine may increase mucosal permeability to lipopolysaccharide, while firocoxib does not.

○ Similar findings have been reported for deracoxib, but this NSAID is currently licensed only for use in dogs.

### D  Perioperative analgesia

○ NSAIDs are used as peri-operative analgesic adjuncts in routine soft tissue surgery.

○ There is some evidence that the analgesia afforded by phenylbutazone is as effective as butorphanol during equine castration.

○ Ideally, NSAIDs should be administered in the pre-operative period, as there is evidence that pre-emptive administration results in more profound analgesia.

## IV  Specific NSAIDs used in equine practice

### A  Flunixin meglumine

○ Flunixin meglumine is a non-selective COX inhibitor.

○ It is licensed in the USA for treatment of pain and inflammation associated with musculoskeletal disease. It is also labeled in the USA for alleviation of visceral pain associated with colic.

○ The equine IV dosage is 1.1 mg/kg once daily or for up to five days.
  - While flunixin meglumine is labeled for intramuscular (IM) use, IM use is associated with *Clostridial myonecrosis* and is therefore not recommended.
  - The onset of action following intravenous (IV) administration occurs at approximately 15 minutes post injection.

○ Flunixin meglumine is also available in oral paste and granule formulations. Oral administration of flunixin meglumine has been reported to have good bioavailability (approximately 72–86% based on the formulation).

○ Oral administration of injectable flunixin displays good bioavailability (71.9%) and may be suitable for oral administration to horses.

B   Phenylbutazone

- Phenylbutazone is a non-selective COX inhibitor.
- It is licensed in the USA for treatment of musculoskeletal disease.
- Recommended dosage is 4.4 mg/kg PO or IV once a day. Intravenous injections should be limited to five consecutive days. This may be followed by oral administration.
- Phenylbutazone is supplied as parenteral and oral formulations. The oral formulation is available as a paste or a powder.
- Prolonged administration of phenylbutazone has been associated with *ulcerative cystitis* in two horses.

C   Diclofenac

- Diclofenac is a non-selective COX inhibitor.
- It is supplied and utilized in equine medicine as a 1% liposomal cream (*Surpass*).
- *The potential benefit of administration of topical diclofenac is to provide analgesia while limiting systemic absorption and subsequent side effects.*
- In neonatal foals, topical administration resulted in low plasma concentrations and minimal side effects likely due to low systemic absorption. Despite the lack of data evaluating clinical efficacy, topical diclofenac may be useful when concern for side effects is high.
- It reduces lameness associated with osteoarthritis in horses.
- Additionally, it has been used topically to treat *jugular vein thrombosis*.
- The recommended topical application method is to apply a 5″ ribbon over the affected joint q12 hours for 10 days. The mean dose applied using this methodology is 73 mg.
- It is important for all people administering topical diclofenac to wear gloves during application, as the drug can be absorbed through human skin.

D   Firocoxib

- As a member of the COXIB class of drugs, firocoxib is a COX-2 selective NSAID.
- Firocoxib is licensed in the USA for use in the management of osteoarthritis-associated pain and inflammation in horses.
- In one study, *firocoxib* was as effective as *phenylbutazone* for clinical improvement of pain associated with osteoarthritis.
- Recommended dosage is 0.1 mg/kg, PO q24 hours.
  - It is supplied as 57 mg tablets and as an oral paste (*Equioxx*®).
  - A parenteral formulation is available for intravenous use for up to five days.

E   Meloxicam

- Meloxicam (*Inflacam*) is labeled for use in the horse in the U.K. It is licensed for the alleviation of acute and chronic musculoskeletal pain.
- It is supplied as a sachet of 330 mg formulated as granules.
- The recommended dose is one sachet (330 mg) PO q24 hours or 0.6 mg/kg PO q24 hours.
- Other formulations exist, such as parenteral, however these are not labeled for use in the USA.

### F Grapiprant

- o Grapiprant (*Galliprant*\*) is a newer NSAID that acts by inhibiting one of four $PGE_2$ receptors, specifically the EP4 receptor.
- o It is currently only labeled for use in dogs.
- o Pharmacokinetic and pharmacodynamic data in horses are lacking and further research is needed before routine use of grapiprant can be recommended.

## V Adverse effects of NSAIDs

### A Gastrointestinal tract

- o COX-1 and COX-2 enzymes are constitutively expressed in the GI tract.

*Stomach and Duodenum*

- o $PGE_2$ and $PGI_2$ play a role in decreasing HCl production and increasing mucosal bicarbonate concentration.
- o $PGE_2$ and $PGI_2$ are also important in mucus production and maintenance of gastric blood flow.
- o Finally, aspirin-triggered lipoxins (ATLs) are produced following COX-2 activation and have a protective effect on the gastric mucosa.
- o Gastric and duodenal *ulceration* are common adverse effects of NSAID use in many species, including the horse.
- o Additionally, NSAIDs are weak acids and can directly *irritate* the GI mucosa.
- o As NSAIDs are secreted in the bile, a high drug concentration is achieved within the GI tract, which may contribute to toxicity.
- o The use of COX-2 selective NSAIDs has reduced the incidence of ulceration in man; however, it has not decreased the incidence of NSAID-induced enteropathy.
- o In healthy horses, *phenylbutazone* and *firocoxib* can induce squamous ulceration. However, the ulceration was less severe in horses treated with firocoxib (COX-2 selective) compared to phenylbutazone (non-selective COX inhibitor).
- o Equine gastric ulcer syndrome can cause signs of intermittent, mild colic. These signs are often treated with an NSAID, which may exacerbate the gastric ulceration.
- o Originally, exercise and high-level performance was implicated in the development in NSAID-induced gastric ulcers; however, numerous studies have been unable to identify exercise as a risk factor for NSAID-induced GI ulceration.
- o COX-2 is up-regulated in healing GI tissue and is important in increasing *angiogenesis*, through $PGE_2$ and vascular endothelial growth factor (VEGF) production.
- o Inhibition of COX-2 may delay healing of damaged GI tissue.
- o This should be thoroughly considered prior to administration of NSAIDs to horses with colic.

*NSAID-induced enteropathy*

- o NSAID-induced enteropathy in humans is disease of the small intestine, distal to the duodenum.
- o In horses, this mainly manifests as *right dorsal colitis*.

- NSAID-induced right dorsal colitis is evidenced by disturbances in the mucosal microcirculation, inflammatory responses characterized by neutrophil infiltration, and subsequent mucosal ulceration.
- This condition leads to a break down in the intestinal mucosal barrier and results in a protein-losing enteropathy and subsequent hypoproteinemia.
- Clinical signs of acute right dorsal colitis include diarrhea, colic, endotoxemia, dehydration, and death. Signs of chronic right dorsal colitis are mild, intermittent colic, weight loss, and diarrhea.
- Interestingly, in human beings the development of COX-2 selective NSAIDs has decreased the incidence of gastric lesions associated with NSAID administration. However, the use of COX-2 selective NSAIDs has not decreased the incidence of NSAID enteropathy, indicating that COX-2 is likely to be constitutively expressed in the intestines.
- While the exact mechanism for the occurrence of enteropathy, specifically of the right dorsal colon, is unknown, there is some evidence that *GI dysbiosis* occurs with both non-selective COX inhibitors and COX-2 specific NSAIDs. This dysbiosis may play a role in NSAID enteropathy.

## B  Renal effects

- COX enzymes are constitutively expressed in the kidneys.
- Both $PGE_2$ and $PGI_2$ are important in sodium secretion and chloride transport within the kidney.
  - Inhibition of COX enzymes may result in decreased sodium excretion through the kidneys.
  - They are also integral in maintenance of glomerular filtration rate and total renal blood flow by stimulating the release of renin.
  - During episodes of *hypotension* or *hypovolemia*, this allows for maintenance of renal blood flow by causing vasodilation.
- In healthy, euvolemic patients, the effects of NSAIDs on renal blood flow and glomerular filtration are minimal.
- Administration of NSAIDs to hypovolemic patients results in renal vasoconstriction of the afferent arteriole, which decreases renal blood flow.
  - Ultimately, there is blood flow redistribution to the renal cortex resulting in decreased perfusion of the renal medulla.
  - Because of the blood flow redistribution, *renal papillary necrosis* is the lesion seen with NSAID-induced nephrotoxicity.
  - Therefore, restoration of vascular volume should be attempted in hypovolemic patients prior to the administration of an NSAID.

## C  Hematologic

- Thromboxane $A_2$ (TXA2) is primarily produced through the actions of COX-1 and results in platelet aggregation and vasoconstriction.
  - Therefore, COX-1 inhibition should produce an anticoagulant effect.
- In contrast, $PGI_2$ primarily produces COX-2 activation resulting in vasodilation and inhibition of platelet aggregation.

- In some species, effects of NSAIDs on coagulation have been reported. In fact, *aspirin*, which inhibits COX-1, results in irreversible inhibition of platelet aggregation. It is used in small animals to prevent thromboembolism.
- However, at least two studies in horses have shown that none of the commonly used NSAIDs, aspirin, flunixin meglumine, phenylbutazone, and firocoxib, inhibit platelet aggregation.
- With the development of COX-2 selective drugs, the incidence of myocardial infarction and stroke have increased in people.
  - This is due to the attenuation of $PGI_2$, which is important in inhibition of platelet aggregation. However, the pro-coagulant effects of COX-1 remain uninhibited.
  - While no studies have been undertaken in veterinary medicine, this is unlikely to occur in horses treated with NSAIDs.

## D  Risk factors for NSAID related adverse effects

- Co-administration of different NSAIDs or a NSAID and a corticosteroid may increase the risk for adverse effects.
  - For example, simultaneous administration of phenylbutazone and firocoxib for 10 days increases serum creatinine concentration.
- Horses with pre-existing disease may be at increased risk for delayed GI mucosal healing and further GI lesions.
- Risk factors for development of renal injury have not been fully determined in horses. However, in other species, *hypovolemia*, *hypotension*, and *anesthesia* appear to be risk factors for development of renal injury.

# Corticosteroids
*Stephanie Kleine*

- In the nineteenth century, Thomas Addison found that adrenal extracts were useful in the treatment of people suffering from chronic fatigue, weight loss, muscle degeneration, and skin darkening, later known as Addison's disease.
- It was not until the 1940s that the steroid hormones were isolated within the adrenal gland.
- Since the 1940s, the knowledge of endogenous and exogenous glucocorticoids has evolved significantly.
- Today, glucocorticoids are used in the management of numerous conditions.

## I Mechanism of action of glucocorticoids

- Endogenous glucocorticoids are produced and released from the adrenal cortex through the actions of the hypothalamic–pituitary–adrenal axis (HPAA).
  - Corticotropin-releasing hormone is released from the hypothalamus. This results in adrenocorticotrophic hormone (ACTH) release from the pituitary gland.
  - *Cortisol* is released from the adrenal cortex under the control of ACTH.
  - When glucocorticoid concentrations are high, there is an endogenous negative feedback mechanism that causes inhibition of the release of both corticotropin- releasing hormone and ACTH.
- The glucocorticoids are small lipophilic molecules, which allows them to diffuse through cell membranes and bind cytosolic glucocorticoid receptors.
- They are then transported to the nucleus where they alter transcription and gene expression.
- These molecules are important in metabolic functions.
  - They promote gluconeogenesis, glycogen synthesis, and lipogenesis.
  - They have catabolic effects on skeletal muscle, skin, peripheral fat, and connective tissue.
  - In addition, they are important in aiding in water and salt balance within the kidneys.
- The glucocorticoids exhibit anti-inflammatory effects through induction of *annexin-1* (formerly *lipocortin*) and attenuation of cytokine production. Annexin-1 results in direct inhibition of phospholipase $A_2$ and subsequent inhibition of arachidonic acid release. (see Figure 16.1)
- It is important to note that glucocorticoids not only block the COX enzymes but also the LOX pathway and inhibit production of prostaglandins and leukotrienes.

## II Clinical uses of glucocorticoids

### A Musculoskeletal injuries

- Intra-articular injection for the management of osteoarthritis.
- Intra-articular administration of corticosteroids has been shown in some studies to decrease lameness associated with both acute synovitis and chronic musculoskeletal conditions, such as osteoarthritis and those with osteochondral fragments.

- In a retrospective report, the combination of an intra-articular glucocorticoid and a systemic NSAID decreased owner-perceived lameness.
  - However, intra-articular administration of glucocorticoids can result in detectable plasma concentrations of the medication.
  - Glucocorticoids in combination with a systemic NSAID can increase the incidence of adverse events; however, the incidence of adverse events with this combination is unknown.
  - Despite the potential benefits on lameness, there is some evidence that intra-articular glucocorticoids may adversely affect cartilage and have cytotoxic effects on chondrocytes.

### B  Noninfectious inflammatory airway disease

- Equine inflammatory airway diseases include mild equine asthma, recurrent airway obstruction, and summer pasture-associated obstructive airway disease.
- Glucocorticoids are important anti-inflammatory and immunosuppressive therapeutic tools in equine inflammatory airway disease.
- Oral, parenteral, and inhaled corticosteroids improve lung function and decrease airway hyper responsiveness in horses with this condition.
  - Despite this evidence, there is no evidence that glucocorticoids decreased neutrophil accumulation in bronchoalveolar lavage fluid, a prominent finding in equine inflammatory airway disease.
- Systemic administration of corticosteroids is useful to rapidly obtain control of the clinical signs associated with this condition.
- Inhaled glucocorticoids are thought to be useful in decreasing the adverse effects of systemic glucocorticoid administration.
  - However, glucocorticoids have been detected in the plasma following inhalation.
  - Ultimately, the evidence for the decrease in adverse effects associated with inhaled corticosteroids is weak.

### C  Immunosuppression

- At high doses, glucocorticoids exhibit immunosuppressive effects.
- They alter leukocyte trafficking by decreasing neutrophil adherence to the endothelium. This is through the effects of glucocorticoids on expression of adherence molecules.
- This results in decreased extravasation and a subsequent *neutrophilia*. It also limits the initial cellular response at sites of infection.
- In addition, glucocorticoids result in a *lymphopenia*, which may be due to re-localization of lymphocytes to the reticuloendothelial system. This primarily affects the T lymphocytes. However, there is some evidence in people that immunoglobulin G may decrease by up to 20% with corticosteroid administration.
- Finally, these medications can decrease the transcription of cytokines and chemokines.
- Most commonly, glucocorticoids are used for their immunosuppressive effects in inflammatory airway disease, as discussed previously.
- Corticosteroids have been employed in the management of vasculitis, immune-mediated dermatologic conditions, inflammatory bowel disease, recurrent uveitis, immune-mediated keratitis, anemia, and thrombocytopenia.

D   Topical administration

- Administration of topical glucocorticoids has been reported for ophthalmic and dermal conditions in horses.
- Corticosteroid-containing creams, ointments, sprays, and conditioners (*Resicort*) are available for treatment of pruritic skin lesions.
  - There is some evidence that dermally applied *dexamethasone* is absorbed systemically and results in measurable plasma concentrations.
  - In addition, dermal application can result in decreased plasma cortisol and thyroid hormones, specifically $T_3$ and $T_4$.
- Ophthalmic preparations of *dexamethasone* HCl and *prednisolone acetate* are used frequently for the treatment of uveitis, immune-mediated keratitis, and eosinophilic keratitis.
  - Administration of ophthalmic corticosteroids causes low but detectable plasma concentrations.

E   Mating-induced endometritis

- In mares, an inflammatory response to spermatozoa maybe a normal mechanism to clear the spermatozoa and debris from the uterus.
- However, some mares are unable to clear the inflammation associated fluid from the uterus and inflammation persists.
- Prednisolone and dexamethasone have been used to modulate post-mating inflammation.
- While this treatment is effective, *prednisolone* (0.5 mg/kg, PO q12 hours) and *dexamethasone* (0.05 mg/kg, IV q12 hours) administered for five days, resulted in failed ovulation.
  - This may be due to direct effects of the corticosteroids on the ovary or to suppression of GnRH from the hypothalamus.
  - The results of that study recommended utilizing corticosteroids for only one to two days in the management of persistent mating-induced endometritis.

## III   Specific glucocorticoids used in equine practice

A   Dexamethasone

- Dexamethasone has been used for the management of numerous inflammatory and immune-mediated conditions including, non-infectious equine inflammatory airway disease, neurologic, dermatologic, and reproductive conditions.
- The published dose range is 0.04–0.16 mg/kg, IV, IM, or PO q24 hours.

B   Prednisone

- Unlike in some other species, prednisone is *not* used in equine medicine.
- In horses, prednisone has little clinical effect as there is minimal metabolism to prednisolone.

C   Prednisolone

- Prednisolone is used for a wide-variety of inflammatory or immune-mediated conditions, including but not limited to dermatologic, neurologic, respiratory, reproductive, vascular, intestinal, and hepatic disease states.

- *Equisolon* is licensed in Europe for use in the horse. It is supplied in 3 g sachets of oral powder. The recommended dose is 1 mg/kg.
- The published dose for equine inflammatory airway disease is 1–2 mg/kg, PO, q24 hours.

### D Betamethasone

- Betamethasone (*BetaVet*) is FDA licensed for intra-articular administration in horses with osteoarthritis.
- It is supplied as betamethasone sodium phosphate (3.15 mg/ml), which is reported to have a short onset of action, and betamethasone acetate (2.85 mg/ml, which is less soluble and has a longer duration of action.
- The dosing recommendation is 1.5 ml (9 mg betamethasone) injected intra-articularly per joint. Only two joints should be injected concurrently.
- It is supplied as a single use vial and should be used immediately after opening.

### E Triamcinolone

- Triamcinolone (*Vetalog*) is licensed for use in horses for the relief of pain and reduction of inflammation and swelling.
- It can be administered via intramuscular or intra-synovial injection.
- It has reported use in a wide variety of inflammatory and immune mediated conditions.
- The recommended IM dosage is 0.01–0.02 mg/kg as a single action.
- For intra-synovial injection, 6–18 mg. The injection may be repeated after three to four days.

### F Isoflupredone

- Isoflupredone has been evaluated in horses with equine inflammatory airway disease.
- It was determined to be at least as effective as dexamethasone at improving lung function.
- Administration of *isoflupredone* was associated with *hypokalemia*, although not all horses in the study developed this abnormality.
- The dose is 0.03 mg/kg IM.

## IV  Inhaled corticosteroids

- Two common glucocorticoids for equine inhalational therapy include *fluticasone* and *beclomethasone*.
- The goal of inhalational administration of these medications is to provide effective relief of clinical signs while limiting systemic side effects. Despite this goal, there is some evidence that these medications may be detected in the plasma after aerosol administration.
- Both glucocorticoids are supplied in a metered dose inhaler that can be used with various equine inhaler systems (e.g. *AeroHippus*, *Equine Haler*, *Flexineb*).

A Fluticasone

- ○ Fluticasone is utilized in the management of equine inflammatory airway disease, in conjunction with environmental modulation.
- ○ It has been shown to be as effective of systemic dexamethasone for inflammatory airway disease. However, the onset of action of systemic corticosteroids appears to be more rapid than inhaled fluticasone.
- ○ After aerosol administration, a metabolite of fluticasone has been detected in the plasma and urine of horses.
- ○ Flutide/Flixotide are supplied as 250 g/actuation.
- ○ The recommended dose is 1–6 g/kg q12 hours.

B Beclomethasone

- ○ *Beclomethason*e has also been used in the management of equine inflammatory airway disease.
- ○ In human beings, beclomethasone is thought to be less potent and less effective than fluticasone for asthma. However, there is no direct comparison in horses.
- ○ There is evidence that inhaled beclomethasone causes adrenocortical suppression.
- ○ The dose is 1–8 g/kg q12 hours.

## V   Adverse effects of glucocorticoids

A Musculoskeletal system

- ○ Glucocorticoids, particularly with chronic use, can result in skeletal muscle catabolism and muscle atrophy.
- ○ Six-month-old foals, treated with dexamethasone for eight weeks displayed abnormal growth. This was due to growth cartilage that was deficient in collagen and glycosaminoglycans.
- ○ Previously, glucocorticoids were thought to increase the incidence of *laminitis*.
  - – The proposed mechanism for this effect is vasoconstriction of lamellar veins, lamellar weakening, catabolic effects on protein, insufficient glucose supply to keratinocytes, and glucocorticoid-induced metabolic changes such as mild hyperglycemia and insulin dysregulation.
  - – There is no evidence to suggest a causal link between glucocorticoid administration and *laminitis* in horses.
  - – It is recommended to dose triamcinolone at up to 20 mg despite the lack of evidence for iatrogenic *laminitis*.

B Gastrointestinal Tract

- ○ Due to the inhibition of prostaglandin synthesis, glucocorticoids may induce or exacerbate GI ulceration.
- ○ The mechanism of GI adverse effects of glucocorticoid GI ulceration is similar to that of NSAIDs.

**C Metabolic effects**

- ○ Glucocorticoids can cause increases in blood glucose, insulin, triglycerides, and blood lactate concentrations.
- ○ Corticosteroid administration can result in polyuria, polydipsia, and fat redistribution.

**D Coagulation**

- ○ In human beings, administration of corticosteroids can increase the peripheral concentration of several coagulation factors and fibrinogen. Additionally, in dogs, corticosteroids can increase coagulation.
- ○ Despite the evidence of pro-coagulant effects in other species, there is no evidence to support this in horses. In fact, one study reported no change in coagulation with the administration of glucocorticoids.

**E Hepatic**

- ○ Increases in aspartate aminotransferase (AST) and gamma-glutamyl transferase (GGT) activity may occur with prolonged use of corticosteroids.
  - – This may be due to hepatic fat infiltration or altered glucose metabolism.
  - – In dogs, hepatic glycogen storage leads to increased liver enzymes activity and hepatomegaly.
  - – Horses, however, are relatively refractory to steroid-induced hepatopathy compared to dogs.

**F Suppression of HPAA**

- ○ Administration of exogenous glucocorticoids can activate the negative feedback loop of the HPAA.
- ○ The negative feedback loop results in decreased ACTH production and a subsequent decrease in the levels of endogenous cortisol.
- ○ As corticosteroids are detected within the plasma after intra-articular administration, several studies have shown that this route of administration can also depress endogenous hydrocortisone release.
- ○ Adrenocortical insufficiency is poorly described in the horse. However, there are anecdotal reports of lethargy, anorexia, and poor performance after cessation of long-term corticosteroids in horses.
- ○ Despite this, adrenocortical insufficiency should be considered during treatment with glucocorticoids. Abrupt cessation of these medications should be avoided to limit potential adrenocortical insufficiency.

**G Immunosuppression**

- ○ At high doses, glucocorticoids can exhibit an immunosuppressive effect.
  - – The mechanism of this finding is discussed above.
  - – This may increase patient susceptibility to infection or exacerbate a clinical or subclinical infection.

## H   Wound healing

- ○ Due to inhibition of the inflammatory response, glucocorticoids may inhibit wound healing.
- ○ The decreased inflammatory profile results in decreased angiogenesis, fibroblast proliferation, and synthesis of the extracellular matrix.
- ○ Despite the potential negative effects on wound healing, topical corticosteroids have shown to have a beneficial effect in the management of exuberant granulation tissue.

## Suggested Reading

Bailey, S.R. (2010). Corticosteroid-associated laminitis. *Vet. Clin. North Am. Equine Pract.* 26: 277–285.

Cox, S., Sommardahl, C., Fortner, C. et al. (2020). Determination of grapiprant plasma and urine concentrations in horses. *Vet. Anaesth. Analg.* 47: 705–709.

Doucet, M.Y., Bertone, A.L., Hendrickson, D. et al. (2008). Comparison of efficacy and safety of paste formulations of firocoxib and phenylbutazone in horses with naturally occurring osteoarthritis. *J. Am. Vet. Med. Assoc.* 232: 91–97.

Knych, H.K. (2017). Nonsteroidal anti-inflammatory drug use in horses. *Vet. Clin. North Am. Equine Pract.* 33: 1–15.

Marshall, J.F. and Blikslager, A.T. (2011). The effect of nonsteroidal anti-inflammatory drugs on the equine intestine. *Equine Vet. J.* 43 (S39): 140–144.

Mazan, M.R. (2015). Update on noninfectious inflammatory diseases of the lower airway. *Vet. Clin. North Am. Equine Pract.* 31: 159–185.

McIlwraith, C.W. (2010). The use of intra-articular corticosteroids in the horse: what is known on a scientific basis? *Equine Vet. J.* 42: 563–571.

Potter, K., Stevens, K., and Menzies-Gow, N. (2019). Prevalence and risk factors for acute laminitis in horses treated with corticosteroids. *Vet. Rec.* 185: 82.

Richardson, L.M., Whitfield-Cargile, C.M., Cohen, N.D. et al. (2018). Effect of selective versus nonselective cyclooxygenase inhibitors on gastric ulceration scores and intestinal inflammation in horses. *Vet. Surg.* 47: 784–791.

Ziegler, A., Fogle, C., and Blikslager, A. (2017). Updated on the use of cyclooxygenase 2-selective nonsteroidal anti-inflammatory drugs in horses. *J. Am. Vet. Med. Assoc.* 250: 1271–1274.

# 17

# Anesthetic Machines and Equipment
*Rachel A. Reed*

## I Introduction

- The anesthesia machine can be divided into three different systems based on the pressure of the gas within the component:
  - High pressure system (from >60 and up to 2200 psig).
  - Intermediate-pressure system (35–55 psig).
  - Low-pressure system (just above ambient pressure).

> psig = pounds/in$^2$. It indicates that the pressure is measured relative to atmospheric pressure.

## II High-pressure system

- The high-pressure system represents the primary storage location for oxygen or other gases (e.g. medical air, nitrous oxide).
- There are three different mechanisms for supplying oxygen to the anesthesia machine:
  - Cylinders (oxygen, nitrous oxide, medical air).
  - Liquid oxygen.
  - Oxygen concentrators.

### A Cylinder storage of oxygen

  - The most common means of storing oxygen for the anesthetic machine in veterinary hospitals.
  - There are a variety of cylinder sizes available for storage of oxygen (see Table 17.1). In the US, oxygen cylinders are color-coded green, while the International Organization for Standardization requires them to be white.
  - Gas cylinders should be handled with care, as damage to the cylinder could result in the cylinder becoming a dangerous projectile. Cylinders should be stored securely in a rack or fastened to the wall with chains to avoid inadvertent damage to the cylinder.

*Manual of Equine Anesthesia and Analgesia*, Second Edition. Edited by Tom Doherty, Alex Valverde, and Rachel A. Reed.
© 2022 John Wiley & Sons, Inc. Published 2022 by John Wiley & Sons, Inc.

Table 17.1 Characteristics of varying sizes of oxygen cylinder.

| Size | Capacity (L) | Pressure when full, 20 °C (psig) | Empty weight[a] (lbs.) |
|------|--------------|----------------------------------|------------------------|
| E | 660 | 1900–2200 | 14 |
| G | 3400 | 1900–2200 | 97 |
| H | 6600 | 2200 | 119 |

[a] May vary depending on the metal used in the cylinder construction.

○ As the pressure within the cylinder is directly proportional to the volume of gas present within it, the volume of oxygen remaining in the cylinder can be calculated according to Boyle's law for an ideal gas, which states that at a fixed temperature (room temperature), the pressure (P) is inversely proportional to volume (V). Therefore, pressure times volume is equal to a constant and can be expressed as:

P1 x V2 = P2 x V1, which can be rearranged as :

V2 = P2 x V1 / P1

– V2 the volume remaining in the cylinder at P2.
– P1 is the maximum pressure in the cylinder when full.
– V1 is the volume stored at maximum P1.
– P2 is the current pressure in the cylinder,

*Example:* For an H cylinder
Volume in cylinder (V2) = [Current pressure (P2)/pressure when full (P1)] x volume of full cylinder (V1)
If the current pressure in the cylinder is 1000 psig, then:

$$V = (1000/2200) \times 6600$$
$$= 3000 \, L.$$

*Note*: *Full H cylinders range between 6600 and 7080 psig.*

*Conversion factor* (see Box 17.1)
○ The volume in a cylinder can also be rapidly estimated using conversion factors.
○ The conversion factor is determined by dividing the full volume capacity by the maximum pressure achieved by the cylinder.
○ Therefore, for an H cylinder:
*Conversion factor* = V1/P1
$$= 6600 \, l/2200$$
$$\approx 3.14$$

---

**Box 17.1   Oxygen Cylinder Conversion Factors**

E = 0.28
H/K = 3.14
G = 2.41
• Liters of oxygen in cylinder = Pressure in cylinder × Conversion factor
• e.g. H cylinder, 1500 psig = 1500 × 3.14 = 4710 Liters of $O_2$ in cylinder

## B   Pressure regulators

○ A regulator (see Figure 17.1) affixed to the cylinder stem reduces the pressure of the gas leaving the cylinder to a lower, more constant pressure within the intermediate-pressure zone. This constant pressure is adjustable, and most regulators are set to maintain a constant pressure of 35–55 psig. Without the regulator, the pressure of the gas entering the intermediate-pressure zone would be far too high and would decrease over time as the cylinder empties.

○ Some anesthesia machines have second-stage regulators that further reduce the pressure of the gas prior to entering the flowmeter (see intermediate-pressure system).

○ Large cylinders (e.g. size G or H) generally attach to the regulator via a threaded diameter index safety system (DISS) (see Figure 17.2) connection to ensure connection of the correct gas to the pipeline.

○ Smaller cylinders (e.g. size E) are mounted on a hanger yoke that utilizes a pin index safety system (PISS) (see Figure 17.3) to ensure connection of the correct gas. Hanger yokes orient and support the cylinder, providing a path for unidirectional flow of gas. The yoke consists of several components including:

    – The body, which forms the main structure of the yoke.

    – The retaining screw, which secures the cylinder.

    – The index pins as part of the PISS.

    – A washer (*Bodok* seal) to ensure a leak proof seal.

    – A filter.

    – The nipple that receives gas from the cylinder.

    – A check valve to ensure unidirectional flow of gas.

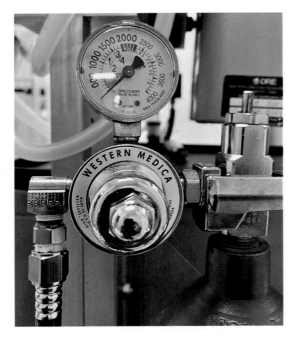

**Figure 17.1**   A pressure regulator which receives gas from the high-pressure zone and reduces it to a lower, more constant pressure.

Figure 17.2    Diameter index safety system which is used to ensure connection of correct hose to gas source.

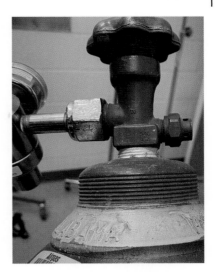

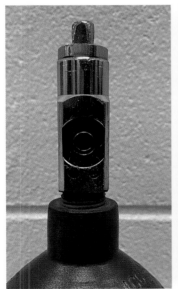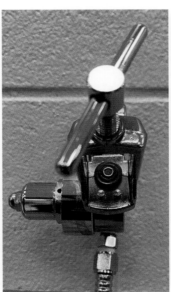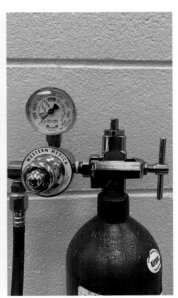

Figure 17.3    Pin index safety system which is used to ensure connection of the correct gas to the hanger yoke.

## C    Liquid oxygen storage

- ○ Can be more economical for hospitals with a larger anesthetic caseload (see Figure 17.4).
- ○ Liquid oxygen is stored at approximately 100–120 psig and between −150 and −180 °C.
- ○ Critical temperature of oxygen is −119 °C, which is the temperature at which a gas becomes a vapor and can be compressed to a liquid.
- ○ One liter of liquid oxygen converts to 860 l of gaseous oxygen at standard ambient temperature and pressure.

Figure 17.4   Liquid oxygen storage.

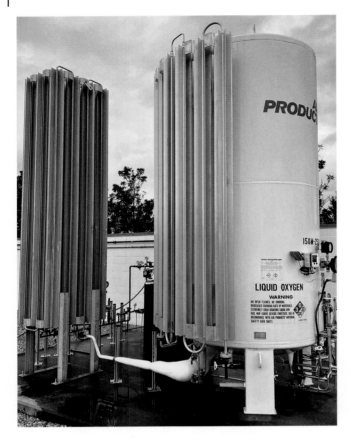

D   **Oxygen concentrators**

- ○ Are not commonly used for anesthesia of small animal patients, and have little use in equine anesthesia (see Figure 17.5)
- ○ These units are sieves that serve to filter the oxygen from the air, delivering 90–95% oxygen to the anesthetic machine.
- ○ However, oxygen concentrators are unable to deliver high flow rates of oxygen, and most units are limited to approximately 4 l/min.
- ○ Additionally, most units are unable to generate the necessary pressure to drive a ventilator.

## III   Intermediate-pressure system

- Gas exiting the regulator enters the intermediate-pressure system. The intermediate-pressure system serves to transport gas from the cylinder to the flowmeter.
- The oxygen flush valve is also included in this system and delivers high oxygen flows (40–70 l/min) at the common gas outlet to the breathing circuit, bypassing the vaporizer.

Figure 17.5 Oxygen concentrator unit.

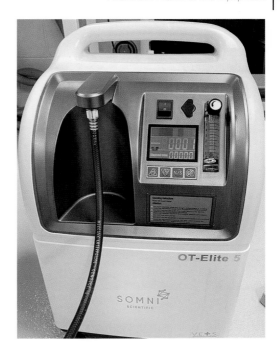

Figure 17.6 Comparison of diameter index safety system connection versus quick-connect system.

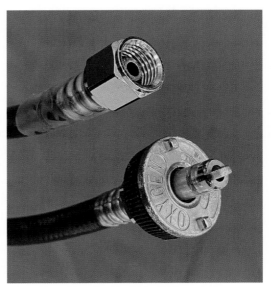

- Larger hospitals may have in-house pipeline systems carrying oxygen from a central bank of cylinders to several locations within the hospital. This is generally a copper pipe with labeling at regular intervals within the wall. Access to these pipelines is generally achieved with quick-connect or DISS connections (see Figure 17.6). Gas is then transported to the anesthetic machine via color-coded hosing (see Figure 17.7).
- Alternatively, hoses may carry the oxygen directly from the cylinder regulator to the anesthetic machine where it enters the flowmeter.

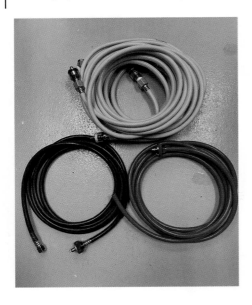

**Figure 17.7**  Color-coded hosing for gas in the intermediate-pressure zone.

## IV   Low-pressure system

- The low-pressure system includes all components of the anesthetic machine from the flowmeter to the anesthetic circuit.

### A   Flowmeter

- ○ It receives the gas from the intermediate-pressure system and supplies it to the anesthetic circuit at a specified flow rate (see Figure 17.8).
- ○ Flowmeters are designed as tapered tubes (*Thorpe* tubes) with knobs that control an adjustable orifice allowing gas into the tapered tube from the intermediate-pressure zone. An increase in the size of the orifice results in an increase in flow rate of oxygen. As gas enters the tube, a *float* or *bobbin* within the tube rises to indicate the flow rate of gas through the tube in l/minute.
- ○ Flow through the tube is dictated by the physical properties of the gas.
  - – *Viscosity* is the primarily factor affecting flow at low flow rates.
  - – *Density* is the primary factor affecting flow at high flow rates.
- ○ Flowmeters are agent specific and calibrated at 20 °C and 760 mmHg atmospheric pressure. If one component of the flowmeter fails, the entire flowmeter should be replaced.
  - – Use of a flowmeter at altitude will result in greater output from the vaporizer than indicated by the float/bobbin.
- ○ Flowmeters are color coded based on the gas for which they are designed. Many anesthetic machines have flowmeters for oxygen, medical air, and/or nitrous oxide.
- ○ The *oxygen* flowmeter is always positioned farthest *downstream* on the flowmeter manifold in order to avoid administration of a hypoxic gas mixture.
- ○ Flowmeters deliver a precise flow of gas with only about a 5% variation in standard single-taper flowmeters. Newer machines utilize dual-taper flowmeters or two flowmeters in series to allow for even more precise delivery and reducing the variability to just 2.5%.

Figure 17.8    Flowmeter manifold.

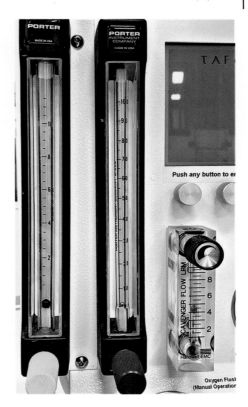

## B    The anesthetic vaporizer

- The vaporizer receives gas exiting the flowmeter manifold and stores the liquid anesthetic, and delivers precise amounts of anesthetic vapor to the breathing circuit (see Figure 17.9).
- Modern inhalant anesthetic vaporizers are agent specific, concentration calibrated, temperature and backpressure compensated, and designed to be used outside of the patient breathing circuit.
- Isoflurane and sevoflurane vaporizers are termed *variable bypass vaporizers*, meaning that gas entering the vaporizer is split into carrier and bypass gas channels based on the saturated vapor pressure of the agent and the dial setting of the vaporizer.
- Carrier gas passes over the liquid anesthetic agent becoming fully saturated with anesthetic (e.g. 240 mmHg for isoflurane) and then rejoins the bypass gas which dilutes the partial pressure of the anesthetic to achieve the partial pressure dictated by the percent concentration set on the vaporizer dial.
- Vaporizers are calibrated at sea level, and their use at altitude will result in an output of anesthetic that represents a greater percent concentration of barometric pressure. However, as the partial pressure output of the vaporizer is unchanged, the vaporizer can be used in the same way as it would at sea level.
- Inhalant anesthetics produce approximately 200 ml of vapor per ml of liquid anesthetic at ambient temperature. The volume of liquid anesthetic used per unit of time can be estimated using the following equation:

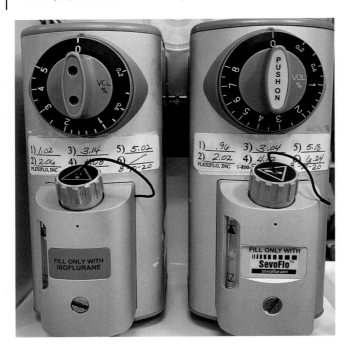

**Figure 17.9** Inhalant anesthetic vaporizers.

$$\text{mL of anesthetic used} = \frac{\left(\text{dialed}\% \div 100\right) \times \text{Fresh gas flow} \left(\text{mL} / \text{min}\right) \times \text{minutes}}{200 \text{ mL vapor} / \text{mL liquid}}$$

○ Or simplified using the following equation):

$$\text{mL of anesthetic used} = 3 \times \text{dialed }\% \times \text{Fresh gas flow (l/min)} \times \text{hours}$$

(3 is a factor used to correct for time and volume units; $\left[ \dfrac{\dfrac{1}{100} \times 1000 \times 60}{200} \right]$ )

*Note*: *Desflurane* has unique physical properties that preclude passive vaporization. A heated and pressurized vaporizer is necessary to have controlled vaporization. Desflurane vaporizers differ from variable bypass vaporizes in that they are *injection type* vaporizers that deliver a set percent of desflurane directly to the fresh gas flow. Desflurane has a high saturated vapor pressure that is close to atmospheric pressure (700 mmHg at 20 °C) and liquid desflurane has a boiling point of 23.5 °C, a temperature that might be achieved in some hospital settings. Thus, desflurane vaporizers are pressurized in order to keep desflurane in the liquid phase. This pressure is achieved by increasing the temperature to 39 °C in the sump of the vaporizer which increases the vapor pressure of desflurane to approximately 2 ATM (1520 mmHg). Heating is also necessary to compensate for the cooling that occurs as desflurane vaporizes, due to its high latent heat of vaporization. Cooling would result in large variations in temperature of the liquid desflurane.

These vaporizers are calibrated at sea level and use of this style vaporizer at *altitude* will result in a lower partial pressure of anesthetic being delivered for a given dial setting. Therefore, use of desflurane vaporizers at altitude will require higher dial settings to maintain anesthesia than would be required at sea level.

**C   The common gas outlet**

- It serves to deliver gas to the anesthesia breathing circuit.
- Gas exiting the vaporizer, which consists of oxygen and whatever fraction of inhalant anesthetic has been added by the vaporizer, moves to the common gas outlet and into the breathing circuit.

**D   Breathing circuits**

- There are two types of anesthesia breathing circuit – *rebreathing* and *non-rebreathing*.
- *Non-rebreathing* circuits are designed for small patients and are not used in equine anesthesia as the gas flow rate required to prevent rebreathing of expired gas is too high (>130 ml/kg/min).
- Only rebreathing circuits will be discussed here.
- The most common rebreathing circuit is the "*circle system*" which is essentially a circle in which gas moves in one direction in order to continuously supply oxygen and inhalant anesthetic to the patient while simultaneously removing carbon dioxide.

*Note*: The *to-and-fro anesthesia circuit* (see Figure 17.10) is a less commonly used rebreathing circuit in equine anesthesia is. Although this circuit is a rebreathing circuit, it is not a circle circuit. Expired gas from the patient moves through a $CO_2$ absorbent, into a reservoir bag, and back through the $CO_2$ absorbent and into the patient airway on inspiration. The common gas outlet inters the circuit at the patient connection and an adjustable pressure limiting (APL) valve vents circuit gas to the scavenge. This circuit does not have one-way-valves and the volume of this circuit is much smaller than the typical circle circuit.

**Figure 17.10**   To-and-fro anesthesia circuit
*Source:* Courtesy of Bonnie Gatson.

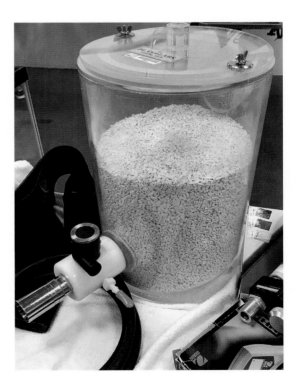

## E    Components of the circle system

*One-way valves*
- ○ Inspiratory and expiratory one-way valves ensure unidirectional flow of gas in the circuit (see Figure 17.11).
- ○ The valves (discs) can become incompetent if they do not return to their normal position on the annular seat and the disc remains displaced into the valve body, which allows for rebreathing of $CO_2$. This can be common with excessive condensation that makes the valve sticky and causes improper orientation.

*Breathing circuit*
- ○ Corrugated tubing that completes the circuit between the inspiratory and expiratory one-way valves and provides the Y-piece that serves to connect the patient endotracheal tube to the circuit (see Figure 17.12).
- ○ Large animal anesthesia circuits have an internal diameter of 50 mm.

(a)                                                                                                       (b)

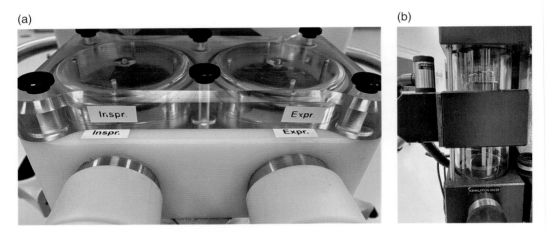

Figure 17.11    One-way valves from Tafonius (a) and Anesco (b) large animal anesthesia machines.

Figure 17.12    Large animal anesthetic breathing circuit.

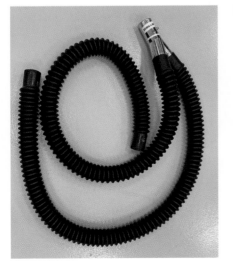

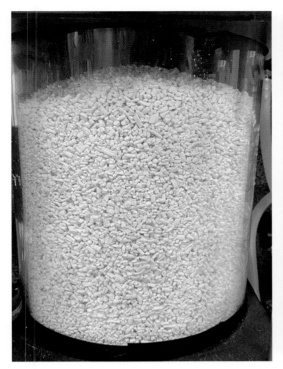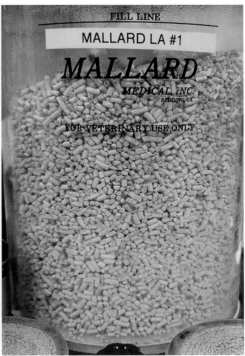

Figure 17.13  Carbon dioxide absorbent in canister. Fresh unused (left) and exhausted with color change (right).

*Carbon dioxide (CO₂) absorbent*
- Serves to remove $CO_2$ from the expired gas (see Figure 17.13).
- Within the absorbent, $CO_2$ is a removed by a chemical reaction of a base neutralizing an acid with heat and water produced as byproducts of this reaction.

*Reaction of CO₂ with soda lime*

$$CO_2 + H_2O \rightarrow H_2CO_3$$
$$H_2CO_3 + 2\,NaOH\,(KOH) \rightarrow Na_2CO_3\,(K_2CO_3) + 2H_2O + Heat$$
$$Na_2CO_3\,(K_2CO_3) + Ca(OH)_2 \rightarrow CaCO_3 + 2NaOH(KOH)$$

- pH sensitive indicators (e.g. ethyl violet) are incorporated into the absorbent to aid in determining when the absorbent has become exhausted (see Figure 17.13).

*Reservoir bag*
- Serves as a reservoir for airway gas (see Figure 17.14).
- This component is commonly replaced by a ventilator bellows in large animal anesthesia machines.

*Adjustable pressure limiting (APL) valve ("pop-off valve")*
- It vents circuit gas to the scavenge when pressure within the circuit exceeds $1$–$2\,cmH_2O$.
- This valve is closed in equine anesthesia machines when a ventilator is in use.

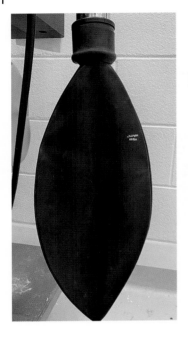

**Figure 17.14** Large animal anesthetic breathing circuit reservoir bag.

## V Time constant for anesthesia circuit ($\tau$)

- Large animal rebreathing circuits have a relatively large volume (~50 l), and therefore it can take a significant amount of time for nitrogen to be flushed out of the circuit, and for the concentration of oxygen and anesthetic to rise.
- The time to reach equilibrium (i.e. the time constant) can be calculated based on the volume (L) of the machine and the fresh gas flow (l/min).
- The time constant, tau ($\tau$), can be defined as the time required for flow through a system to reach the capacity of the system.
  - $\tau$ *(min) = Volume of circuit/flowmeter setting.*
  - $\tau = 63\%, 2\,\tau = 86\%, 3\,\tau = 95\%, 4\,\tau = 98.2\%.$

*Meaning it will take one time constant for 63% of the inspired concentration change to be achieved in the system, and three time constants for a 95% concentration change to be achieved.*

*Example:* A machine with a volume of 50 l and an $O_2$ flow of 5 l/min.
  - $\tau = 50\,l/5\,l = 10\,minutes$
  - It will take approximately 40 minutes to approach complete denitrogenation of the circuit (i.e. 4 $\tau$).
    - In order to overcome this time delay, a higher $O_2$ flow rate can be used to reduce $\tau$.
    - Also increasing the vaporizer setting initially to a value in excess of MAC for the agent being used will decrease the time required to achieve an effective partial pressure of anesthetic within the circuit. This is termed "*overpressuring*".
    - Therefore, in equine anesthesia, it is common to use initially high flow rates (up to 10 l/min of oxygen) in combination with a high vaporizer setting (e.g. 3–5% isoflurane) and adjust these settings as the inspired and expired concentration of agent reach their target.

## VI  Scavenging system

- Gas exiting the breathing circuit via the APL valve enters the scavenge system (see Figure 17.15).
- The scavenge serves to collect waste anesthetic gases and vent them to the outside or to collect the anesthetic gas via an absorbent (e.g. activated charcoal). These units can be active (suction applied to scavenge) or passive (gas is directed to the outside and moves passively). Scavenge units typically consist of five components:

*Collection mechanism*
  ○ This is generally the APL valve.

*Connection to interface*
  ○ Consists of a 19 mm internal diameter corrugated tube carrying waste gas to the interface or absorbent canister.

*Interface*
  ○ Serves as a positive pressure relief to the system when a large volume of gas is vented through the APL valve.
  ○ Also has a negative pressure relief to protect the patient from negative pressure generated by active scavenge systems.

*Connection to elimination system*
  ○ This is generally a smaller, less compliant tube that connects the interface to house waste anesthetic suction (active scavenge) or directs the gas to the exterior of the building.

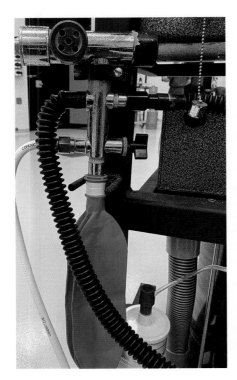

Figure 17.15    Waste gas scavenge system interface.

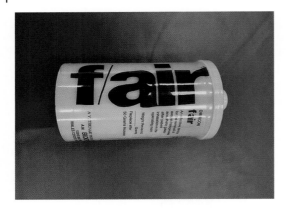

Figure 17.16   Absorbent canister designed to remove inhalant anesthetic from gas leaving the scavenge.

*Elimination system*
- Gases are vented to either the exterior of the building or absorbent canister.
- Absorbent canisters (e.g. F/air canisters) (see Figure 17.16) are weighed routinely to determine when they should be discarded. Most systems recommend discarding after the unit gains 50 g. Due to their limited capacity, these are infrequently used in equine anesthesia. Additionally, these absorbents collect anesthetic vapors (e.g. isoflurane, sevoflurane, halothane) only, and do *not* collect gaseous anesthetics such as nitrous oxide.
- Scavenging systems can be *open* or *closed*.

*Open* scavenging systems have a funnel that the waste gas suction draws anesthetic gasses from while simultaneously suctioning room air.

*Closed* scavenging systems are completely sealed to prevent escape of anesthetic gases, and incorporate a negative pressure relief valve to protect the patient airway from the negative pressure. Passive scavenging systems are generally closed. Active scavenging systems can be open or closed.

# VII   Ventilators

- Ventilators are commonly utilized in equine anesthesia to ensure adequate ventilation and reduce the development of atelectasis and hypoxemia. Most large animal anesthesia machines have built in ventilator systems.

## A   Mallard Large Animal Anesthesia Ventilator System

- A traditional anesthesia machine with dual circuit ventilator (see Figure 17.17)
- Available in electrically powered and pneumatically powered varieties.
- Features time-cycled, pressure-controlled mechanism, with ascending ventilator bellows, and adjustable positive end expiratory pressure (PEEP) valve (some models).

## B   Drager/Anesco

- Similar anesthesia machines with dual circuit ventilator (see Figure 17.18).
- Available in electrically powered and pneumatically powered varieties.
- Features time-cycled, pressure-controlled mechanism, with descending ventilator bellows.

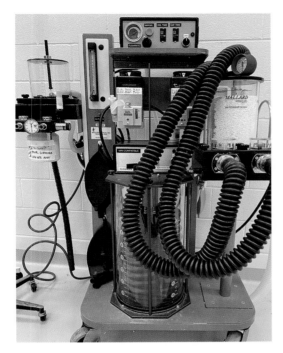

Figure 17.17   Mallard large animal anesthesia machine.

(a)                                           (b)

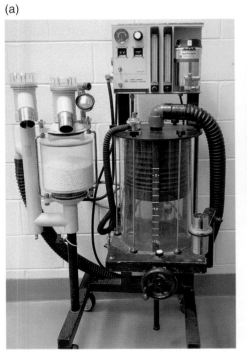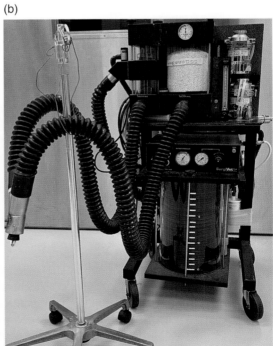

Figure 17.18   Drager (a) and Anesco (b) large animal anesthesia machines.

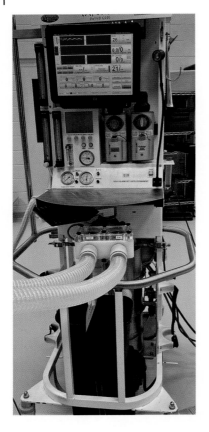

Figure 17.19   Tafonius large animal anesthesia workstation.

C   Tafonius

- A traditional anesthesia machine built into a computerized ventilator that is electrically and battery powered (see Figure 17.19).
- Features time-cycled, pressure-controlled mechanism, with piston bellows, and variable PEEP application.
- The Tafonius is a complete anesthesia workstation with monitoring system allowing for computerized measurement of tidal volume, peak inspiratory pressure, and PEEP (see Figure 17.20).
- There is no reservoir bag, but the patient can breathe spontaneously from a piston bellows system.

D   Bird mark respirator

- The Bird mark was originally designed as a single-circuit ventilator for use in human beings (see Figure 17.21). However, it can be attached to a bellows system and used as the driving gas in a dual circuit ventilator design (*"bag-in-a-barrel"*).
- This is a pneumatically driven, pressure-cycled, and pressure-controlled ventilator.
- Can be used in control, assist, or assist-control modes.
- Although the Bird Mark Respirator is no longer manufactured, they are still in use in many veterinary hospitals.

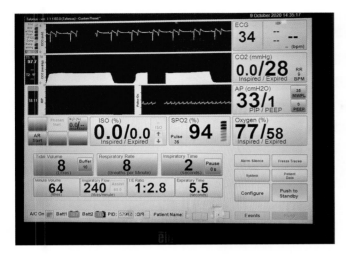

Figure 17.20    The Tafonius large animal anesthesia monitoring system screen.

(a)                                                        (b)

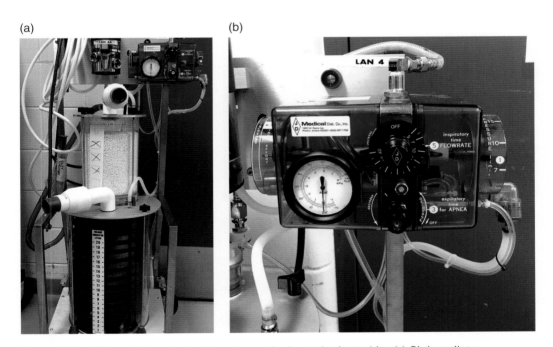

Figure 17.21    Bird ventilator attached to a large animal anesthesia machine (a). Bird ventilator control panel (b).

## VIII    Endotracheal tubes

- Large animal endotracheal tubes are generally made out of silicone with a cuff and pilot balloon (see Figure 17.22). Murphy eyes are variably present at the patient end of the endotracheal tube.

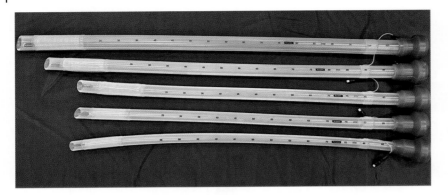

Figure 17.22 Large animal endotracheal tubes.

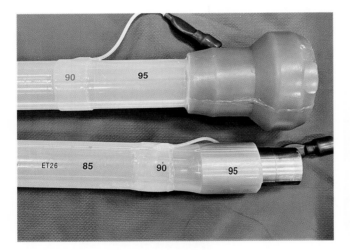

Figure 17.23 Large animal endotracheal tube connector types: bell type and metal Bivona insert type.

- Endotracheal tubes used in equine anesthesia range in size from 14 to 30 mm internal diameter.
- The trachea of an average size adult horse will typically accommodate a 26 mm endotracheal tube.
- Smaller tubes will be required for smaller horses, foals, or when nasotracheal intubation is planned.
- Large animal endotracheal tube circuit connectors come in two different varieties (see Figure 17.23).
  - Bell type connection.
  - Bivona type connection.

*Bell-type connection*: It has the benefit of maintaining a large internal diameter throughout the length of the connection.

*Bivona-type connection*: It has the benefit of a less bulky connection. Use of the Bivona type connection requires that a Bivona insert be present in the Y-piece of the breathing circuit to receive the connection (see Figure 17.24).

**Figure 17.24** Large animal breathing circuit with Bivona insert to facilitate connection to endotracheal tube.

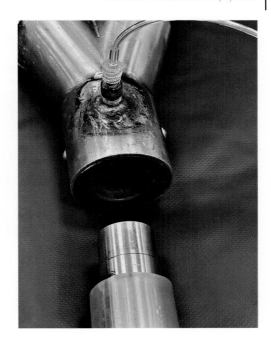

## A   Cleaning endotracheal tubes

- ○ The endotracheal tube should be thoroughly cleaned and disinfected after use.
- ○ Inflate the cuff and rinse the tube, inside and out, removing gross debris and any residual lubricant or airway mucus.
- ○ With the cuff still inflated, the tube should be placed in a disinfectant solution, per manufacturers guidelines for time and disinfecting agent.
  *Note*: *Glutaraldehyde disinfectant products should be avoided.*
- ○ The tube should be thoroughly rinsed of disinfectant and allowed to dry completely before subsequent use.

## IX   Demand valves

- Although not part of the anesthetic machine, demand valves are commonly used in equine anesthesia in situations where an anesthesia machine and ventilator are not available (see Figure 17.25).
- Demand valve units connect directly to the intermediate-pressure system and can be applied directly to the patient airway.
- The demand can be activated by either:
  - ○ Pressing a button on the valve.
  - ○ Negative pressure applied to the valve in the form of inspiratory effort made by the patient.
- The flow rate of oxygen from the valve is dependent on the pressure within the intermediate-pressure system, and can be as high as 160 l/min.

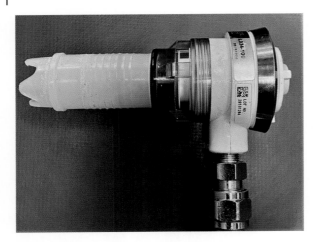

Figure 17.25    Oxygen demand valve.

## Suggested Reading

Ehrenwerth and Eisenkraft (1993) *Anesthesia Equipment: Principles and Applications*, by Jan
    Ehrenwerth and James B. Eisenkraft. Elsevier
Dorsch, J. and Dorsch, S. (2008). *Understanding Anesthesia Equipment*, 5e. Philadelphia, PA:
    Lippincott Williams and Wilkins.

# 18

## Positioning the Anesthetized Horse
*Hui Chu Lin*

## I   Introduction

- Normal horses spend most of their time standing.
- Horses normally spend only short periods (~30 minutes) in recumbency.
  - Recumbency probably becomes uncomfortable due to pressure on muscles and the skeletal system.
  - The large body mass of the horse means that dependent structures undergo a tremendous amount of pressure.
  - Horses do not normally spend time in dorsal recumbency.
- Every effort must be made to ensure that the effects of posture are minimized in the anesthetized horse, and the head, limb, and pressure points (e.g. shoulder, hip) are positioned appropriately on the surgical table.
- In addition to proper positioning and padding, it is of utmost importance that an adequate *arterial blood pressure* be maintained in the anesthetized horse in order to guarantee muscle perfusion and tissue oxygenation, with the goal of minimizing the likelihood of the horse developing myopathy.
  - A minimum mean arterial pressure of 70 mmHg is generally recommended to decrease the incidence of myopathy.

## II   Problems associated with recumbency

- Recumbency may impose significant *cardiovascular* and *pulmonary* changes, particularly over prolonged periods.
- *Myopathy* can result from ischemia.
  - Arterial blood flow is compromised and venous drainage decreased due to compression of blood vessels in dependent muscles.
  - Compressed or obstructed veins reduces tissue drainage causing an increase in tissue pressure, and this may eventually lead to a decrease in arterial perfusion.
  - Ischemia in the laterally recumbent horse usually manifests as unilateral forelimb lameness (*triceps myopathy*).

- ○ Bilateral hindlimb lameness may occur following dorsal recumbency.
- ○ Myopathy is more likely to develop in heavy, muscular horses in the presence of a low arterial blood pressure.
- *Neuropathy*, especially of peripheral nerves, can result from pressure on the nerve or stretching the nerve.

## III    Preventing complications in lateral recumbency

### A    Padding

- ○ A thick *foam* pad works well, but *water* or *air* cushions may also be used to reduce pressure at any point of the horse's body.
  - – Foam padding should be about 10–12 in. (25–30 cm) thick and covered with a waterproof material (see Figure 18.1).
  - – Air cushions should be inflated to the point that the horse is just lifted off the table allowing the horse's body to sink in; otherwise, no reduction in pressure is achieved.
  - – Air and water cushions have the disadvantage of creating an unsteady platform, and water cushions in particular create a "rocking" movement.
- ○ Covering the pad with a blanket or towels absorbs sweat and fluids which may accumulate during surgery and helps to keep the horse dry.

### B    Positioning

- ○ It is imperative that the *entire body* is situated on the padding and the body weight is evenly distributed.
- ○ Avoid having the extremities too close to or over the edge of the mat.
- ○ The *head* should be placed in a neutral position, avoiding overflexion or overextension to prevent recurrent laryngeal nerve paralysis.

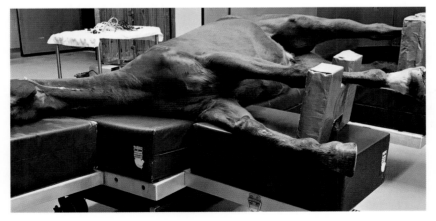

Figure 18.1    Horse positioned in lateral recumbency on a thick pad. Notice that the dependent thoracic limb is pulled forward and that the upper limbs are supported by H-shaped pads. H-shaped pads are used to prevent placing the pads on the recumbent limb.

- ○ Halters should be removed to prevent pressure-induced trauma, especially to the facial nerve and the masseter muscle, and especially in lateral recumbency.
- ○ The *eyes*, especially the lower eye, should be protected.
  - – The lids on the lower eye should be closed, and care should be taken to protect the eye and avoid "dragging" the head along the mat during positioning.
  - – Sterile lubricant should be placed on the eyes and re-applied, as necessary, during long procedures.
- ○ The *tongue* should be placed so as to prevent pressure damage.
  - – This usually involves placing the tongue uppermost and withdrawing it from the mouth.
  - – The tongue should be covered with moist towels to prevent drying.
- ○ Check that the dependent *pinna* is not trapped under the head.
- ○ The *limbs* need special attention (see Figure 18.1).
  - – The *lower thoracic* limb should be pulled forward to protect the triceps muscles, brachial vessels, and nerves from the pressure of the chest wall.
  - – Avoid pulling the lower thoracic limb backwards.
  - – The *upper limbs* should be supported in a position parallel to the tabletop, using either specific leg attachments, designed for the table, or padding.
    - ▪ It is preferable *not* to have support pads for the upper limbs resting on the lower limb. The use of an H-shaped pad avoids this.
  - – A space should be left between the adductors of the *pelvic limbs* to avoid muscle damage resulting from compression.
- ○ Check that the *penis* is not trapped under the body or hanging off the table.
- ○ Check that the bony part of the *tail* is not placed under the body.

  Tilting the laterally recumbent horse (by raising the limbs with hobbles and a hoist) to reduce pressure on the lowermost musculature is likely to transfer pressure to the hip and shoulder regions and is *not* recommended.

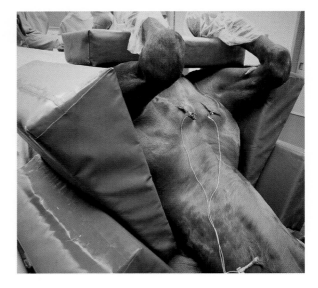

**Figure 18.2**   Horse positioned in dorsal recumbency. The horse is supported by wedge-shaped pads to distribute pressure evenly.

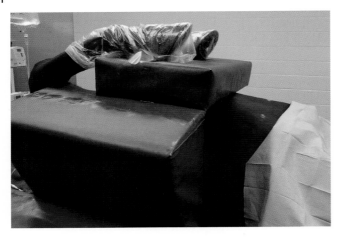

Figure 18.3   Side view of a horse positioned in dorsal recumbency with the forelimbs supported by a pad to prevent placing pressure directly on the sternal area.

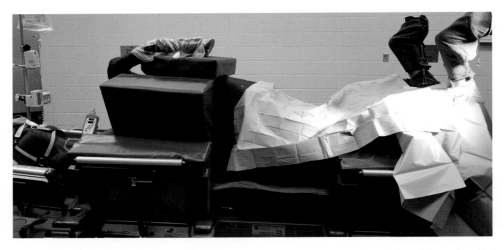

Figure 18.4   Side view of horse positioned in dorsal recumbency. The sides of the table are in a V-shape, and wedge-shaped pads support the shoulder area.

## IV   Preventing complications in dorsal recumbency

### A   Padding

- o The thickness of the padding will be dictated by the design of the surgical table.
  - – With many surgical tables, it is only possible to use a 3–5 in. (7.5–12.5 cm) pad.
- o The thickness of the pad is less critical for dorsal recumbency, provided that the horse is positioned squarely on its back.
- o Supporting the horse by hobbles and an overhead hoist to keep the horse from leaning allows use of a thicker pad.

Figure 18.5 View from behind a horse positioned in dorsal recumbency. It is important that the horse be positioned squarely and that the croup is completely on the pad.

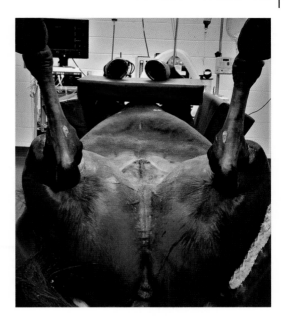

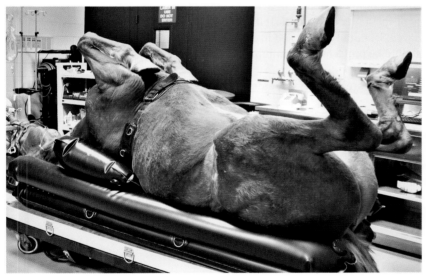

Figure 18.6 Horse positioned in dorsal recumbency. With this type of table, there is minimal lateral support and the horse is supported by a belt around the thorax.

B **Positioning** (see Figures 18.2–18.6)

- The horse should be placed squarely on its back with the body weight evenly distributed on the pad.
- Avoid having the *croup* overhang the padding.
- The horse can be maintained in dorsal recumbency either by the use of hobbles and an overhead hoist or, more commonly, from a "V" support formed by folding the table (see Figure 18.2).

- The *shoulder* area should be well padded, and a *wedge-shaped* pad works best to distribute the pressure evenly.
- The *thoracic limbs* may be allowed to rest on the sternal area if not supported from overhead, but some padding may be needed on the sternum especially if the horse has heavy shoes (see Figure 18.3).
- The *pelvic limbs* may be allowed to relax in the flexed position if not supported from overhead, depending on the facilities and the surgery in question.
  - It is important to *avoid long periods with the pelvic limbs in extension* as this is thought to increase the likelihood of *femoral nerve* damage and/or gluteal myopathy, which may lead to severe hindlimb lameness and recovery problems.
  - Horses may not be able to stand if both hindlimbs are affected, in which case the prognosis will be very poor.
- The bony part of the *tail* should not be placed under the body of the horse or between a rear limb and the padding.
- The *head* should be aligned with the body, and padding should be placed under the pole.
  - However, overextension of the head and neck should be avoided by placing a wedge-shaped pad under the nasal bones to facilitate venous drainage, minimize severe nasal congestion, and prevent upper airway obstruction following removal of the endotracheal tube during recovery.
  - Overextension of the neck may increase the risk of *recurrent laryngeal nerve* damage.
  - Removal of the halter is less critical if the horse is in dorsal recumbency; however, if not removed, it should be checked to ensure that it is not too tight.
- The *eyes* should be protected from trauma, which may occur if a "V" shaped head support is used.
- Check that the *ears* are not trapped under the pole.

## V  Dorsal recumbency with head-down position (Trendelenburg)

- Horses are usually only placed in this position for laparoscopic procedures and assisted vaginal delivery under anesthesia. (see Figure 34.3)
- Because of extreme changes in position and the need to insufflate the abdomen (e.g. with $CO_2$), significant alterations in cardiorespiratory function can occur.

### A  Circulatory changes

- Generally, the cardiac index does not seem to differ between the head-up (reverse Trendelenburg) and head-down positions at an angle of 7° for either position. However, arterial blood pressure measured in the facial artery is higher in the head-down position.
- Arterial blood pressure is also higher compared to horizontal when the Trendelenburg is established at 35°.
- Capnoperitoneum may augment the cardiac index by facilitating venous return as reflected by increases in right atrial pressure.
- However, the effects of capnoperitoneum are variable, and this variability may be affected to a large degree by the resulting intra-abdominal pressures.
  - Insufflation with an intra-abdominal pressure > 12 mmHg may impose greater effects on cardiovascular function than lower insufflation pressures.

B    **Ventilatory changes**

    ○ A variety of changes in ventilation occur when a horse is in a head-down position with or without capnoperitoneum. These include:

        – A significant decrease in $PaO_2$.

        – Increased airway pressure.

        – Increased $PaCO_2$.

        – Increased $PaCO_2$ to $ETCO_2$ difference.

        – Increased calculated $V_D/V_T$, and $Q_S/Q_T$ ratios.

        – Increased V/Q mismatch.

    ○ These changes occur earlier when capnoperitoneum is instituted.

## Suggested Reading

Binetti, A., Mosing, M., Sacks, M. et al. (2018). Impact of Trendelenburg (head down) and reverse Trendelenburg (head up) position on respiratory and cardiovascular function in anesthetized horses. *Vet. Anaesth. Analg.* 45: 760–771.

Hofmeister, E., Peroni, J.F., and Fisher, A.T. (2008). Effects of carbon dioxide insufflation and body position on blood gas values in horses anesthetized for laparoscopy. *J. Equine Vet. Sci.* 28: 549–553.

Schauvliege, S., Binetti, A., Duchateau, L. et al. (2018). Cardiorespiratory effects of a 7° reverse Trendelenburg position in anaesthetized horses: a randomized clinical trial. *Vet. Anaesth. Analg.* 45: 648–657.

# 19

## Monitoring the Anesthetized Horse

## Monitoring the Central Nervous System

*Joanna C. Murrell*

- General anesthesia can be defined as a reversible state of depression of the central nervous system (CNS) to such a degree that consciousness is lost and that on recovery nothing relating to the period of anesthesia is recalled.
- CNS monitoring is an inherent part of anesthetic monitoring and is intricately linked to monitoring the depth of anesthesia.
- The need to quantify the depth of anesthesia in man, to prevent overdose, was identified in 1848 by John Snow.
  ○ This system was later modified to produce a more sophisticated assessment of anesthetic depth.
- Attention has focussed on the electroencephalogram (EEG) as a monitor of anesthetic depth in the horse.
  ○ This interest in EEG studies probably reflects the relatively high anesthetic mortality rate in horses and the dose-dependent cardiovascular and respiratory effects of anesthetic agents.

## I Awareness during anesthesia

- In the early days of anesthesia, patient awareness during surgery was uncommon. Rather, morbidity and mortality during anesthesia were more likely due to the patient being "*too deeply*" anesthetized.
- The introduction of muscle relaxants into human clinical practice in 1942 created the potential for the patient to be inadequately anesthetized or conscious during surgery.
- This problem led to the extensive investigation of the EEG as a tool to monitor the CNS during anesthesia.
  ○ The EEG has a major advantage compared to techniques that measure changes in cardiovascular and respiratory variables, because it provides *direct* information about the functional integrity of the nervous system.

*Manual of Equine Anesthesia and Analgesia*, Second Edition. Edited by Tom Doherty, Alex Valverde, and Rachel A. Reed.
© 2022 John Wiley & Sons, Inc. Published 2022 by John Wiley & Sons, Inc.

## II  Monitoring the depth of anesthesia

- Anesthetists collate information based on clinical measurements and monitoring equipment to make an overall assessment of anesthetic depth.
  - A *single parameter* of anesthetic depth has yet to be described.
- The aim is to maintain the patient at an adequate depth of anesthesia for the surgical procedure without conscious awareness intra-operatively.

## III  Methods of monitoring the depth of anesthesia

### A  Evaluation of the eye

*Position*
  - The position of the eyes is not always symmetrical, and this is particularly noticeable when using balanced anesthesia. It is sometimes noticeable in dorsal recumbency that one eye rotates ventrally and medially, while the other eye remains central. This positioning shifts between eyes over time, and the lighter the plane the more frequent.
  - As anesthesia deepens, the eye returns to the center of the globe and there is no shifting in position.

*Nystagmus*
  - Lateral nystagmus is frequently observed during light anesthesia but disappears as anesthesia deepens.

*Lacrimation*
  - Is common during light anesthesia, reduced or absent at a surgical plane of anesthesia.

*Palpebral reflex*
  - Elicited by gently stroking the eyelashes along the upper and lower eyelids.
  - The palpebral response is progressively depressed as anesthesia deepens. It is generally present, but slow and sluggish, at surgical planes of anesthesia.

*Corneal reflex*
  - Closure of the eyelids elicited by gentle pressure to the cornea.
  - The corneal reflex should be present during anesthesia, absence indicates excessive anesthetic induced depression of the CNS.
  - *Touching the cornea carries the risk of corneal damage and routinely eliciting a corneal reflex is not recommended.*
  - Repeated stimulation of the eye reflexes may result in reflex depression and reduced usefulness.

*Effects of Ketamine or Tiletamine*
  - Eye evaluation is of limited value following the administration of *ketamine* or *tiletamine* due to the following responses:
    - Voluntary blinking.
    - Lateral nystagmus.
    - Central eye position.
    - Lacrimation.

### B   Movement

- ○ Movement indicates an inadequate plane of anesthesia.

### C   Anal tone

- ○ Stimulation of the anus should cause reflex contraction of the anal sphincter.
- ○ This is an imprecise method to assess anesthetic depth but may be useful when access to the patient's head is limited.
- ○ Absence of anal tone indicates too deep an anesthesia plane.

### D   Physiologic parameters

- ○ An increasing depth of anesthesia is commonly associated with reductions in heart and respiration rates, blood pressure, and cardiac output (CO).
  - – However, these parameters are subject to multiple influences (particularly the effects of anesthetic drugs) during anesthesia and health status of the patient, which limits their reliability as guides to depth of anesthesia.
  - – Additionally, heart rate tends to remain remarkably stable in horses.
- ○ Increases in arterial blood pressure indicate a decrease in anesthetic depth.

### E   Concentrations of inhalational anesthetic in expired gases

- ○ End-tidal concentrations (expired) reflect brain concentrations following an equilibration period.
- ○ The dose of inhalational anesthetics administered is based on the minimum alveolar concentration (MAC).
- ○ A movement response to a noxious stimulus may occur at 1 MAC.

### F   Quantitative EEG (See Section IV below)

## IV   EEG

- Electrical activity of the brain results from ionic currents generated by biochemical processes occurring at the cellular level.
- The principal generators of the EEG are thought to be dipole layers of *pyramidal neurons* in the cortical gray matter.
  - ○ These cells are orientated in the same direction, so that summation of current flow originating from adjacent neurones occurs, generating electrical activity which can be recorded at the scalp surface.
- The potential for the EEG to be a measure of depth of anesthesia was recognized in the late 1930's.
- Fast Fourier Transformation (FFT) is now utilized to quantify information contained within the raw EEG signal and to facilitate interpretation of the data.
  - ○ FFT transforms EEG data from the time to the frequency domain, producing a distribution of pure sine waves of varying frequencies which constitute the signal, described as a *power spectrum* (see Figure 19.1).

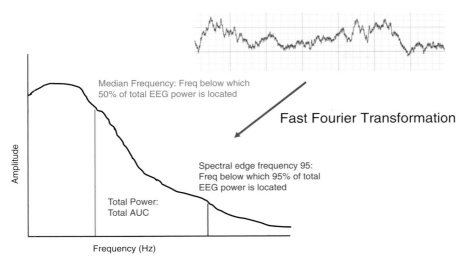

Median Frequency: Freq below which
50% of total EEG power is located

Fast Fourier Transformation

Spectral edge frequency 95:
Freq below which 95% of total
EEG power is located

Total Power:
Total AUC

Amplitude

Frequency (Hz)

**Figure 19.1** Diagram showing the power spectrum for one epoch (e.g. 1 second) of raw EEG data. The terms median frequency, spectral edge frequency and total power are indicated on the diagram.

- A number of simple descriptors of the EEG signal can be derived from the power spectrum produced by FFT.
- These include *median* and *spectral edge frequencies*, *total power* and power in the different frequency bands.
  - *Median frequency:* frequency below which 50% of the total power of the EEG is located.
  - *Spectral edge frequency* (95%): frequency below which 95% of the total power of the EEG is located.
  - *Total power:* Total area under the power spectrum curve.
  - Changes in these variables have been used to assess depth of anesthesia.

## A   EEG findings in the horse

- EEG monitoring is not currently used in the clinical setting to measure depth of anesthesia.
- However, a number of studies have investigated EEG changes during surgical stimulation (see Figure 19.2).
  - An increase in median frequency (demonstrating a shift toward high frequency activity) associated with the surgical stimulus of castration has been identified in *halothane*-anesthetized horses.
  - Across species, there are discrepancies in the results of EEG studies of nociception, but this may be accounted for, in part, by a failure to use a standard surgical stimulus.
  - EEG changes in *ponies* anesthetized with *halothane* in combination with different classes of intravenous (IV) drugs, found that only those with recognized antinociceptive efficacy reduced median frequency to a greater extent than spectral edge frequency 95%.
- These studies suggest that changes in median frequency are associated with the antinociceptive efficacy of a drug. A good correlation has been demonstrated between EEG changes and drug concentration when each drug is administered as a single agent.
- EEG changes associated with nociceptive stimulation have also been identified.
  - However, when anesthesia is maintained with multiple drugs and the patient is subjected to intraoperative stimulation of varying intensity, robust EEG changes specifically associated with depth of anesthesia are less easy to identify.

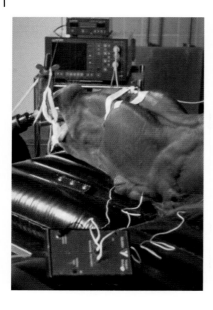

Figure 19.2 Photograph showing a set up for recording the EEG of a horse. The front box is the pre-amplifier to which the EEG electrodes are attached. The pre-amplifier is connected to a personal computer to record the raw EEG signal.

*EEG recording in the horse*

- ○ Subcutaneous needle or self-adhesive silver chloride electrodes are used to record the equine EEG (see Figure 19.3).
- ○ A 3-electrode configuration is usually adopted (see Figure 19.4):
  - – Reference electrode – parietal suture rostral to the divergence of the temporalis muscles.
  - – Active electrode – right zygomatic process.
  - – Ground electrode – caudal to the poll.

## B  Auditory evoked potentials (AEP)

- ○ The AEP is the response in the EEG to a *sound* stimulus.
- ○ It is extracted from the EEG by averaging the response to a number of stimuli so that the background noise of the underlying signal is eliminated.
- ○ The transient AEP consists of a series of positive and negative waves that represent the process of transmission and processing of auditory information from the cochlea to the brainstem, the primary auditory and frontal cortex.
- ○ The waveform can be divided into *three parts*, depending on the latency of the appearance of the wave relative to the time of the auditory stimulus.
- ○ The use of middle latency auditory evoked potential (MLAEP) waves as an indicator of depth of anesthesia during EEG studies of IV drugs is of limited value.

## C  Bispectral index (BIS)

- ○ BIS is a signal-processing technique that decomposes the EEG signal to quantify the level of synchronization, in addition to amplitude and frequency variables, thus providing a more complex description of EEG pattern.
- ○ The output from the bispectral monitor is digital, making interpretation less complex than EEG data.

Figure 19.3   Subcutaneous needle electrodes used for EEG recording.

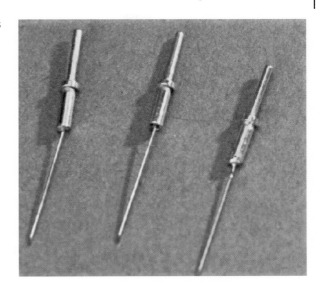

Figure 19.4   A 3-electrode configuration often used for EEG recording in the horse.

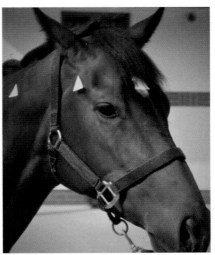

○ Studies in man have shown good correlation between adequacy of anesthesia and the BIS, although the finding is not universal.
  – In an awake unpremedicated human being, BIS is typically >90.
  – A BIS < 60 is a strong indicator of unconsciousness.

*BIS in the Horse*
  ○ BIS has been evaluated as an indicator of the degree of CNS depression in *isoflurane*-anesthetized horses.
    – The BIS is significantly *less* in sedated and anesthetized horses compared to awake horses; however, BIS is *not* significantly different between sedated and anesthetized horses.
    – This suggests that BIS may *not* be a useful technique for monitoring anesthetic depth during *isoflurane* anesthesia.
      ▪ The BIS is an index, empirically derived from algorithms of human data.

○ Published studies investigating BIS in other animals are limited, but BIS has been found to be unreliable as a guide to CNS depression in *propofol* or *sevoflurane* anesthetized pigs.
○ The simplicity of BIS data interpretation makes an attractive clinical tool to measure anesthetic depth in animals; however, the derivation of the monitor from human data may make it less reliable for veterinary application.

## Suggested Reading

Haga, H. and Dolvik, N. (2002). Evaluation of the bispectral index as an indicator of degree of central nervous depression in isoflurane-anaesthetized horses. *Am. J. Vet. Res.* 63: 438–442.

Johnson C (1996) Some effects of anesthesia on the electrical activity of the equine brain. PhD Thesis, University of Cambridge.

Martin-Cancho, M.F., Carrasco-Jiminez, M.S., Lima, J.R. et al. (2004). Assessments of the relationship of bispectral index values, haemodynamic changes, and recovery times associated with sevoflurane or propofol anesthesia in pigs. *Am. J. Vet. Res.* 65: 409–416.

Murrell, J.C., Johnson, C.B., White, K.L. et al. (2003). Changes in the EEG during castration in horses and ponies anesthetized with halothane. *Vet. Anaesth. Analg.* 30: 138–146.

Schultz, A., Siedenberg, M., Grouven, U. et al. (2008). Comparison of narcotrend index, bispectral index, spectral and entropy parameters during induction of propofol-remifentanil anesthesia. *J. Clin. Monit. Comput.* 22: 103–111.

## Cardiovascular Monitoring

*Alanna N. Johnson*

- Monitoring the cardiovascular system of anesthetized horses is important to ensure adequate oxygen delivery to the periphery in the face of the cardiovascular depressant effects of anesthetics drugs, which predispose equine patients to intraoperative hypotension and reduced CO.
- In addition to the usual concerns of cardiovascular depression and its effect on organ systems, horses are also prone to musculoskeletal and neurologic complications.
  ○ Skeletal muscle does not undergo blood flow autoregulation and therefore depends upon adequate perfusion pressure to maintain oxygen delivery. The large size of adult horses puts them at risk of muscle hypoperfusion, potentially leading to *myopathy*. Myopathy may lead to difficulty in recovery, and increased patient morbidity and mortality. Severe cases of myopathy may result in rhabdomyolysis, potentially leading to renal damage due to the effects of myoglobinuria. (*see* Chapter 38)
  ○ Unlike smaller patients, in which the lower limit of tolerated mean arterial pressure is 60 mmHg, adult horses should ideally maintain a mean arterial pressure greater than or equal to 70 mmHg in order to maintain adequate neuromuscular perfusion.
- Many methods of cardiovascular monitoring exist, and the anesthetist should be familiar with several of these methods in order to get a more complete picture of the patient's cardiovascular status.
  ○ At a minimum, arterial pulse palpation should be performed to ensure the presence of cardiovascular activity.

- More advanced monitoring should occur in most anesthetic events, with the minimum being the use of an electrocardiogram (ECG) to detect heart rate and rhythm and blood pressure measurement, preferably via direct arterial access.
- Cardiac output monitoring provides further information on the cardiovascular status of the patient, but this is not routinely measured in clinical situations due to the potentially invasive and specialized nature of the methods used to measure this parameter.

## I   Direct palpation of arterial pulse

- Manual palpation of the arterial pulse is a simple, yet useful technique for checking heart rate and circulatory status.
  - Common sites for palpation include the facial, transverse facial, metatarsal, coccygeal, and digital arteries.
  - It is wise to check the pulse periodically in this way, especially prior to placing monitoring equipment or after removing it in preparation for recovery.
  - In field anesthesia, or short elective procedures with minimal monitoring, heart rate may be monitored by palpating a peripheral pulse. Along with monitoring respiratory rate, this is the bare minimum of patient monitoring that should always be performed.
- It is important to note that the strength of the palpated pulse does not indicate the blood pressure itself, but rather the arterial pulse pressure difference.
  - This pulse pressure is the difference between systolic and diastolic arterial pressures, so one may perceive a similar pulse pressure in a normotensive and a hypotensive patient, if this difference in values is the same. For this reason, it is important to measure arterial blood pressure in anesthetized patients, even if the pulse quality feels adequate.

## II   ECG

- Use of the ECG should be routine in patients under general anesthesia, as it provides useful information about the conduction activity of the heart. For a more detailed review of the equine ECG and arrhythmias see Chapter 3.
  - The ECG records the electrical activity of the heart. It records the heart rate and detects arrhythmias. It does not provide information on the mechanical function of the heart, and the ECG may appear normal for a period after the heart stops pumping. Thus, emphasizing the importance of monitoring blood pressure.
  - The most common arrhythmia in anesthetized horses is second-degree atrioventricular block, which is considered normal, especially after the patient has received an alpha$_2$ agonist. The most common pathologic arrhythmia observed is atrial fibrillation, although premature ventricular beats and ventricular tachycardia can also occur.
- The ECG can sometimes miscalculate the heart rate, due to the monitor counting additional waves, other than the R wave, as a ventricular depolarization.
  - In these cases, the heart rate displayed is usually double the actual heart rate. Thus, it is important to confirm the heart rate with the pulse oximeter and, ideally, the direct arterial pressure waveform.
  - Additional artifacts may arise on the ECG due to patient movement, lead dislodgement/loosening, and the use of cautery.

## III Blood pressure monitoring

- Monitoring of arterial blood pressure during anesthesia is important, as it provides information about patient perfusion.
- Mean arterial blood pressure (MAP) is the product of the patient's CO and systemic vascular resistance (SVR), both of which may be altered by anesthetic drugs.

$$MAP = CO \times SVR$$

- In particular, MAP provides useful information about vital organ perfusion.
  - For all mammalian species, vital organs such as the brain, heart, and kidneys undergo autoregulation of blood flow. Autoregulation is controlled by the autonomic nervous system and responds to numerous stimuli, one of which is blood pressure.
  - The efferent and afferent blood supply to these organs will adjust based on the MAP, and within the range of 60–160 mmHg these organs can maintain an appropriate level of perfusion. Outside of this range, hypo- or hyper-perfusion can occur, which may result in organ dysfunction.

### A Non-invasive (indirect) arterial blood pressure measurement

*Doppler method* (see Figure 19.5)
  - This method utilizes high frequency sound waves to detect the patient's pulse.
  - The sending crystal in the Doppler probe transmits sound waves into the tissue. Some of these waves bounce off red blood cells pulsing through the arteries and come back to the receiving crystal. An audible pulse is heard via the Doppler unit's speakers.
  - Systolic arterial pressure can be detected using the Doppler probe, a blood pressure cuff, and a sphygmomanometer.
  - The Doppler probe is placed over a peripheral artery (usually coccygeal artery, or digital artery) and an audible arterial pulse is detected.

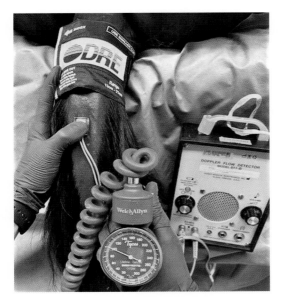

Figure 19.5   Non-invasive Doppler blood pressure measurement.

- An appropriately-sized blood pressure cuff is placed proximal to this artery. The blood pressure cuff's width should be approximately 25–40% of the limb/tail circumference.
- The blood pressure cuff is attached to a sphygmomanometer (or aneroid manometer) and inflated until the pulse can no longer be heard on the Doppler. The pressure in the cuff is then slowly deflated until the pulse is audible again. This pressure at which the pulse becomes audible is the *systolic* arterial pressure.
- *Diastolic* pressure may be identified as the change in character of sounds to more muffled and softer-sounding, but this change is less reliably detected using a Doppler, versus using a stethoscope.
- *Advantages:*
  - The system is inexpensive relative to methods of measuring direct blood pressure.
  - It is non-invasive.
  - It gives a continuous audible signal of blood flow when the cuff is deflated.
- *Disadvantages:*
  - This technique is significantly less accurate than direct arterial blood pressure measurement especially if the cuff is inappropriately sized or in extremes of hypotension, hypertension, bradycardia, and vasoconstriction.
  - Also, in very ill or vasoconstricted animals, obtaining an audible pulse signal on the Doppler may be difficult or impossible.
- The need for placement of a blood pressure cuff proximal to the Doppler probe limits the use of this technique to arteries on the limbs or tail. It is really only practical for measurement of coccygeal artery pressure; thus, access to the horse's tail is necessary and this may not always be feasible.
- A >20 mmHg error range was demonstrated in 5% of horses in dorsal recumbency, compared to direct systolic arterial blood pressure measurements.

*Oscillometric technique*

- In this technique, vibrations/oscillations in the cuff from the patient's pulse are used to determine arterial blood pressure.
- Oscillometric machines inflate the cuff until the pulse is occluded then slowly deflate until the oscillations return, become maximal, and fade again. The systolic pressure is the pressure at which the oscillations return, the MAP is the pressure at which the oscillations are maximal, and the diastolic pressure is calculated based on proprietary algorithms that vary depending upon the monitor.
- The patient's heart rate is also detected, and this may be used to assess if the blood pressure reading is reliable; because if the heart rate is incorrect, the blood pressure reading is likely inaccurate.
- Similar to the Doppler technique, the blood pressure cuff's width should be approximately 25–40% of the circumference of the limb or tail. Cuff sizes that are too large will cause falsely low readings, and cuff sizes that are too small will cause falsely high readings.
- The low heart rates of adult horses do not usually work well with oscillometric devices, as these devices are usually designed for humans or small animal patients. For this reason, and because arterial access is usually attainable, the oscillometric technique is not usually utilized in adult horses. However, this technique may be more accurate and therefore more useful in foals.

**B  Invasive (direct) arterial blood pressure measurement**

- This is the gold standard for measuring arterial blood pressure (see Figure 19.6)
- Arterial cannulation is usually achieved using small gauge (22 or 20 G) peripheral, over-the-needle catheters.
  - The most commonly used arteries are the: *facial, transverse facial, metatarsal,* and *coccygeal.*
- Once the arterial cannula is placed, it is attached to a pressure transducer and non-compressible extension tubing that is pre-primed with sterile, heparinized saline.
  - A heparinized saline syringe or pressurized fluid bag are also attached to the transducer to allow for flushing of the arterial line.
  - The transducer must be zeroed to atmospheric pressure at the level of the right atrium (usually estimated as being at the point of the shoulder).
- Once zeroed, the transducer will receive the mechanical signal of the patient's pulse, thereby deforming the strain gauge inside, converting it to an electrical signal, which then uses a Wheatstone bridge circuit to determine the pressure magnitude and display the resulting waveform on the monitor.
  - Real-time assessment of systolic, mean, and diastolic pressure is then available (see Figure 19.7).
- An additional advantage to arterial waveform analysis is the ability to assess pulse pressure variation (PPV).
  - If there is significant PPV, in which the pulse pressure (Systolic arterial pressure – Diastolic arterial pressure) is altered from beat-to-beat in a mechanically-ventilated patient, this could indicate that the patient is fluid-responsive.
  - When considering hypotensive patients, some are hypovolemic and require extra preload (i.e., they are fluid responsive), whereas others may have issues with SVR and/or contractility (e.g. septic patients).
  - Being able to assess PPV allows the anesthetist to narrow down what the best method of treatment would be, as a fluid-responsive patient should receive intravascular bolus resuscitation, whereas a hypotensive patient without PPV is more likely to need positive inotropes and/or vasopressors.

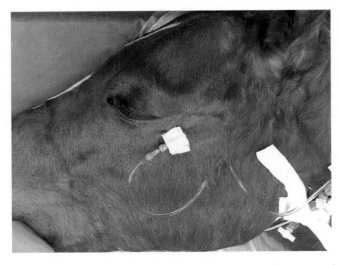

Figure 19.6  Invasive blood pressure measurement using an arterial catheter.

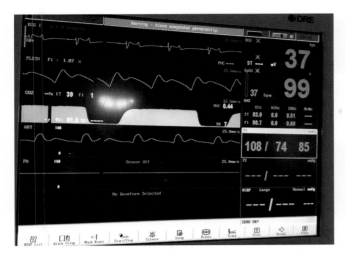

Figure 19.7  Systolic, diastolic, and mean arterial pressure, with waveform.

*Inaccuracies in measurement*

- It is important to note that *inaccuracies* in measurements are possible. Some of the most common issues causing inaccuracies are:
  - Clot formation in the catheter.
  - Air bubbles in the line.
  - Tubing that is too flexible or too long.
  - The transducer not being at the level of the heart.
  - *Over-dampening* of the arterial waveform (see Figure 19.8) is common, resulting in falsely decreased pulse pressure readings, but with minimal effect on MAP readings. Over-dampening may be caused by clot formation, air bubbles, tubing that is too flexible, or loose connections in the line. Flushing the catheter to remove clots and bubbles will usually resolve these issues, and if not, check that non-compressible tubing has been used for the connection between the catheter and the transducer.
  - *Under-dampening* may also occur (see Figure 19.9), which results in over-estimation of the systolic pressure with concomitant under-estimation of the diastolic pressure, but little effect on the MAP. Under-dampening may occur with tubing that is too stiff or too long, and in cases of increased SVR.

*Complications of arterial catheterization*

- The complication rate from *short-term* arterial catheterization seems to be low but potential complications include:
  - Hematoma formation.
  - Hemorrhage.
  - The catheter breaking and lodging in the artery.
  - Occlusion of blood flow distal to the site. This is most likely to occur in small arteries.
  - Air embolus.
  - Infection of joints close to the location of the catheter insertion has been reported on rare occasions.
  - The risk of inadvertent injection of a drug into the arterial system exists.

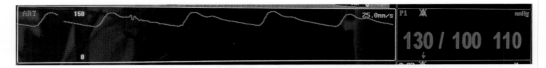

Figure 19.8   Over-dampened arterial waveform.

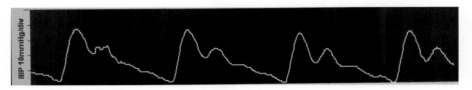

Figure 19.9   Under-dampened arterial waveform.

## IV   Cardiac output monitoring

- Cardiac output (CO) monitoring provides more accurate information on oxygen delivery and general hemodynamic status than can be garnered from measurement of blood pressure.
- Cardiac output is the product of heart rate and stroke volume, and each of these variables may be altered by several different physiologic mechanisms.
  - Anesthetic drugs and fluctuations in sympathetic/parasympathetic tone may alter heart rate and stroke volume.
  - Since stroke volume is the difference between end-diastolic volume and end-systolic volume, it may be affected by changes in preload, afterload, or cardiac contractility.
- Due to its specialized and usually invasive nature, CO measurement is typically reserved for research purposes.
  - Cardiac output measurements may be classified generally as:
  - Indicator-based methods.
  - Fick-based methods.
  - Imaging-based methods.

*Indicator-based methods*

  - Indicator-based methods of CO measurement utilize soluble, inert substances that are injected into the circulation, and their dilution in the cardiovascular system over time is used to determine the CO, in accordance with the modified Stewart-Hamilton equation.
  - Generally speaking, a known amount of indicator is injected into the circulation, where it is carried and mixed in the blood. The detector downstream measures the concentration change of the indicator in the circulation over time.
  - The two most commonly used indicator methods are pulmonary artery *thermodilution* and *lithium dilution*.
  
  Modified Stewart-Hamilton Equation:

  $$CO = \frac{\text{amount of indicator}}{\text{area under concentration curve}}$$

**A Thermodilution**

- This method utilizes the change in blood temperature in the pulmonary artery, subsequent to an injection of cooled injectate, to determine CO.
- This method requires a thermistor-tipped pulmonary artery (Swan-Ganz) catheter, advanced via the jugular vein.
- A known volume of cold saline, of a known temperature, is injected into the right atrium, and the temperature is then measured by the thermistor in the pulmonary artery.

*Note*: Due to the size of the horse's heart, if the distal port of the Swan-Ganz catheter (110 cm) is in the pulmonary artery the proximal port will be in the right ventricle. Thus, it is generally necessary to pass a separate length of tubing into the right atrium to inject the indicator when using a 110 cm catheter. Alternatively, longer, custom made catheters can be used in horses.

- Introduction of the pulmonary artery catheter carries several risks including:
  - Cardiac arrhythmias.
  - Endothelial damage/infection.
  - Pulmonary thromboembolism.
  - Pulmonary artery rupture.
  - Kinking or knotting of the catheter.

**B Lithium dilution**

- This indicator method is less invasive than thermodilution, as it does not require a pulmonary artery catheter.
- Lithium dilution technique correlates well with thermodilution CO measurements in animal models. It is among the most widely studied methods of CO determination in foals, and has been used to measure CO during rest and exercise in adult horses.

*Technique*

- A known amount of *lithium chloride* is injected into a central vein. A sensor, which is attached to a peripheral arterial catheter, then detects the concentration change of the lithium via arterial sample drawbacks.

*Disadvantages*:

- Excessive blood loss due to arterial blood draws (more concerning in small patients, such as foals).
- Cross-reaction of the lithium sensor due to the presence of certain drugs.
  - *Xylazine* and some *neuromuscular blocking agents* (NMBAs) may react with the lithium sensor and cause unreliable readings.
- This method alone does not allow for determination of systemic or pulmonary vascular resistance.

**C Fick method**

- This method of CO determination, utilizing the *Fick* principle, is one of the most historic methods used to calculate CO.
- The Fick principle simply states that the oxygen uptake by the blood is the product of the CO and the difference between the arterial and central venous oxygen content, provided there is no significant cardiac or pulmonary shunting.

Fick Equation

$$VO_2 = CO(CaO_2 - CvO_2)$$
$$CO = \frac{VO_2}{(CaO_2 - CvO_2)}$$
$$VO_2 = V_E \times (FIO_2 - FEO_2)$$
$$CaO_2 = [Hb] \times 1.36 \times SaO_2 + 0.003 \times PaO_2$$
$$CvO_2 = [Hb] \times 1.36 \times SvO_2 + 0.003 \times PvO_2$$

- In order to determine $V_E$ (expired tidal volume) accurately, spirometry must be employed. An oxygen analyzer is able to detect inspired and expired oxygen fraction ($FIO_2$ and $FEO_2$, respectively).

*Disadvantages:*
- The main drawback to this method is that a pulmonary arterial catheter must be placed in order to collect the central venous sample for $CvO_2$ determination.
- Additionally, the hemodynamic status of the patient can vastly affect the measurements, via the changes to $VO_2$, so if the patient is hemodynamically unstable, the reading will be less accurate.
    - In order to eliminate the need for pulmonary arterial catheterization, an *indirect* Fick technique has also been used, in which partial rebreathing and elimination of $CO_2$ replaces the measurement of $VO_2$.

D   Imaging methods

- Less invasive imaging modalities that may be used to determine CO include:
    - Pulse contour analysis.
    - Echocardiographic techniques.
    - Thoracic impedance (bioimpedance) techniques.

*Pulse contour analysis*
- Multiple CO monitors are currently available which utilize pulse contour analysis.
- The arterial pressure waveform is used to assess stroke volume, utilizing the area under the arterial curve before the *dicrotic notch*. However, considering that the arterial waveform may be altered by several outside factors, most of these monitors require a secondary calibration method (usually thermodilution or lithium dilution) to retain the accuracy of their readings.
- Some monitors are available that do not require this secondary calibration reading; instead, they use proprietary algorithms based on data from healthy human beings, which is less useful for veterinary species. Some of these monitors have been used successfully in foals, but the utility becomes less reliable in patients that have significant cardiovascular derangements (arrhythmias, hypovolemia, excessive, or deficient vascular resistance).

*Echocardiography*

- o *Echocardiographic* derivations of CO involve using the ultrasound to estimate stroke volume. This determination of stroke volume may be accomplished in Doppler-based methods or non-Doppler based methods.
- o Doppler-based methods require the determination of *aortic flow velocity* and *aortic diameter*.
- o Non-Doppler based methods measure the left ventricular diameter at its widest point and use mathematical modeling (usually *Simpson's* method) to calculate the volume of the left ventricle, thereby estimating stroke volume.
- o In human beings and smaller veterinary species, *transesophageal* echocardiography is frequently employed, but *transthoracic* echocardiographic techniques have also been described.
- o *Advantages:*
  - These types of techniques are minimally invasive.
  - They also provide useful information about cardiac contractility and preload.
- o *Disadvantages:*
  - These techniques require expensive equipment and highly-trained personnel who can acquire these images.
  - Additionally, while commercially available equipment will work for foals, adult horses require custom-made equipment to allow for transesophageal images.
  - Transthoracic approaches may also be challenging in adults, especially if the horse is anesthetized and in a recumbent position.

*Transthoracic bioimpedance*

- o This method uses the alterations in thoracic conductivity due to changes in fluid flow to assess stroke volume.
- o A series of electrodes is placed on the patient's thorax, a small (imperceivable) current is emitted, and the changes in conductivity over time are measured. These readings are utilized in proprietary algorithms to calculate the stroke volume.
- o This method of CO measurement has been documented in human beings, but has not had much data collection in veterinary patients. More data exist on using bioimpedance to assess pulmonary function than to assess CO, so its clinical utility is limited.

## Suggested Reading

Duke-Novakoski, T., Ambros, B., Feng, C. et al. (2017). The effect of anesthetic drug choice on accuracy of high-definition oscillometry in laterally recumbent horses. *Vet. Anaesth. Analg.* 44: 589–593.

Shih, A.C. (2013). Cardiac output monitoring in horses. *Vet. Clin. North Am. Equine Pract.* 29: 255–167.

Shih, A.C. (2019). Cardiac monitoring in horses. *Vet. Clin. North Am. Equine Pract.* 35: 205–215.

Wilson, K.A., Raisis, A.L., Drynan, E.A. et al. (2018). Agreement between invasive blood pressure measured centrally and peripherally in anaesthetized horses. *Vet. Anaesth. Analg.* 45: 467–476.

# Respiratory Monitoring

*Alanna N. Johnson*

- Due to the large body size and anatomy of adult horses, the physiologic changes resulting from general anesthesia and recumbency frequently result in significant respiratory dysfunction. Physiologic derangements associated with ventilation and oxygen delivery are common and may be severe enough to result in patient morbidity and mortality if left unaddressed.
- The goals of monitoring respiratory function in anesthetized patients include:
  - Ensuring appropriate ventilation (elimination of carbon dioxide).
  - Ensuring adequate arterial oxygen content (appropriate arterial oxygen saturation, hemoglobin content, and partial pressure of arterial oxygen).
- Monitoring respiratory function in anesthetized horses is imperative, as ventilation-perfusion (V/Q) mismatching is common, even in healthy patients. Venous admixture contributes to systemic hypoxemia, and increased dead space ventilation causes more accumulation of carbon dioxide.
- The American College of Veterinary Anesthesia and Analgesia (ACVAA) guidelines on equine anesthesia recommend monitoring respiratory rate and character, pulse oximetry, capnography, and arterial blood gas analysis. Assisted or controlled ventilation is recommended if hypoventilation occurs. Additionally, oxygen supplementation should be administered to anesthetized horses whenever possible, although this may not be feasible in field anesthesia scenarios.
- Additional respiratory monitoring may include spirometry/ventilometry (inspired and expired tidal volume), pressure-volume loops (compliance assessment), and flow-volume loops (resistance assessment).

## I  Monitoring respiratory rate and tidal volume

### A  Spontaneous ventilation

- Equine patients should be allowed to spontaneously ventilate *only* for routine procedures that are short in duration (less than one hour), and oxygen supplementation should be provided if at all possible.
- If the patient will be anesthetized for longer, or if they have systemic disease, controlled or assisted ventilation should be performed.
- If using inhaled anesthetics, variations in tidal volume and respiratory rate (as occur in spontaneous ventilation) may result in alterations in anesthetic uptake and thereby could cause rapid changes in anesthetic depth. If a patient is significantly hypoventilating for example, inhalant uptake will decrease, possibly resulting in patient movement.
- During spontaneous ventilation, respiratory rate and character should be constantly monitored to ensure apnea does not occur and that breathing is not labored. Ideally, the end-tidal carbon dioxide ($ETCO_2$) and/or arterial partial pressure of carbon dioxide ($PaCO_2$) should also be monitored.
- In situations where no multi-parameter monitoring is available, respiratory rate and character (along with pulse rate) should still be consistently checked by someone trained to do so. Alterations in respiratory rate may indicate changing anesthetic depth, as a light patient may have a trend of increasing respiratory rate.

- Anesthetized horses are also prone to altered respiratory patterns, such as Cheyne-Stokes breathing (cyclical hyperventilation and hypoventilation) and apneustic breathing (inspiratory hold pattern, associated with dissociative anesthetics).
- In situations where injectable anesthesia is being employed, oxygen demand valves are frequently used to supplement and assist ventilation in patients that are breathing spontaneously.

## B  Controlled ventilation

- In most cases of equine general anesthesia, controlled ventilation should be performed. Without positive-pressure ventilation, hypoventilation is common, which could also affect anesthetic depth. The method of ventilation varies depending upon the equipment available but, generally speaking, ventilation may be volume or pressure-controlled.
    - For both of these methods, respiratory rates are usually set to 5–7 breaths per minute for adult horses and 10–30 breaths per minute for foals.
- *Ventilation modes*:
    - Most large animal ventilators are *volume-controlled*, which means that the tidal volume is the variable set by the anesthetist. Usually, tidal volume will be in the range of 10–20 ml/kg, with the recommendation to start at the lower end and titrate up, as needed to achieve eucapnia. In this type of ventilation, the airway pressure may change depending upon alterations in compliance, but the volume delivered is the same.
    - In *pressure-controlled* ventilation, the peak inspiratory pressure is set, and this is what determines the tidal volume. For horses, this peak airway pressure is usually set to a range of 20–35 cmH$_2$O, again starting at the lower end and titrating up to attain eucapnia. If alterations in compliance occur, tidal volume will change. For example, colic patients frequently have decreased compliance due to the pressure of distended abdominal viscera on the diaphragm. Ventilation of these patients requires high-peak inspiratory pressures (30 cmH$_2$O or more) prior to the abdomen being open, thus relieving the pressure on the diaphragm. With pressure-controlled ventilation, the tidal volume would change significantly after the abdomen is open, while in volume-controlled, it would remain the same.
- All modern large animal anesthesia machines have *manometers* which measure the pressure of the patient circuit. Ventilation volumes may also be measured by some machines. Inspiratory and expiratory tidal volumes may be measured, and significant difference between these two parameters indicate a leak in the system. However, ventilometry cannot differentiate how much tidal volume goes to dead space ventilation (anatomic and physiologic) versus alveolar ventilation.
- Faster, shallower breathing results in more dead-space ventilation when compared to slow, deep breathing. Physiologic dead-space ventilation ($V_D/V_T$) ranges between 30 and 50% in awake large animal patients and is increased in anesthetized patients. The Bohr-Enghoff equation may be used to assess dead-space ventilation in anesthetized patients, where $V_D/V_T$ is dead-space ventilation, PaCO$_2$ is the partial pressure of arterial carbon dioxide, and PECO$_2$ is the end-tidal carbon dioxide partial pressure:

$$\frac{VD}{VT} = \frac{\left(PaCO_2 - PECO_2\right)}{PaCO_2}$$

*Pressure-volume and flow-volume loops*
- These may be used to assess real-time changes in compliance and ventilation.
    - In a *pressure-volume loop*, the change in the slope of the line through the loop indicates changes in respiratory compliance. If compliance is decreased, for example a patient

experiencing colic, the slope will be increased. However, in this same patient, if the abdomen is opened, thus improving the compliance, the slope of the curve will decrease. The pressure-volume loop may also be used to calculate the work of breathing.
  – *Flow-volume loops* can demonstrate respiratory resistance, and will be flattened due to obstructive and/or restrictive alterations.
  – Some newer large animal anesthesia machines, such as the *Tafonius*, provide these respiratory dynamics within the constructs of the monitor.

## II  Monitoring carbon dioxide

- Methods of monitoring carbon dioxide in anesthetized patients assess alveolar ventilation and serve to inform the anesthetist of the $PaCO_2$. Normal $PaCO_2$ values range between 35 and 45 mmHg.
- Due to significant dead-space ventilation, anesthetized large animals frequently have much higher $PaCO_2$ than $PECO_2$ readings (6–12 mmHg).
- $PaCO_2 > 60$ mmHg usually represent significant respiratory acidosis. In contrast, a $PaCO_2 < 20$ mmHg causes respiratory alkalosis and cerebral vasoconstriction, which may lead to cerebral ischemia.
- Carbon dioxide monitoring is essential in equine patients, due to the likelihood of hypoventilation and carbon dioxide accumulation. Many anesthetic agents have respiratory depressant effects, making animals less responsive to high concentrations of carbon dioxide, which is the normal stimulant for ventilation.
- Recumbent positions (particularly dorsal) can also make it more difficult to ventilate patients, especially if the gastrointestinal tract is distended. Additionally, anesthetized patients have increased physiologic dead space, which increases the $PaCO_2$ to $PECO_2$ gradient (as seen in the Bohr-Enghoff equation).
  ○ Regardless of the cause, hypercapnia may result in respiratory acidosis. If severe and untreated, acidosis impairs oxidative phosphorylation and other metabolic enzymatic processes.

### A  Minute ventilation ($V_E$)

- Is defined as the volume the patient breathes per minute.
- It is dependent upon two variables, respiratory rate ($f$) and tidal volume ($V_T$).

$$VE = f \times VT$$

- If a patient's ventilation must be adjusted, these variables affecting minute ventilation are what must be altered. For example, if a patient is hypoventilating, the $V_T, f$, or both must be increased to correct the hypoventilation.

### B  Alveolar ventilation (VA)

- Is defined as the volume of gas that is involved in gas exchange at the alveolus.
- It is inversely proportional to arterial carbon dioxide partial pressure ($PaCO_2$); therefore, halving alveolar ventilation will double the $PaCO_2$. Thus, any changes in alveolar ventilation will have significant effects on the retention of carbon dioxide by the patient.

$$PaCO_2 \propto \frac{1}{VA}$$

- $PaCO_2$ may be measured by laboratory blood gas analyzers or point-of-care machines.
- $PECO_2$ monitoring should ideally be employed in any intubated patient. These monitors are easy to use and can provide information not only on ventilatory status, but also on circulatory status and airway integrity. Most capnometers utilize infrared analysis to detect $CO_2$ concentrations. Carbon dioxide absorbs infrared light at a wavelength of 4.3 μm. This wavelength is significant when using $N_2O$, as this gas is absorbed at a wavelength of 4.5 μm. For monitors that do not use narrow-field infrared detection, the reading of these two gases could overlap (*collision broadening*), causing a falsely high reading of the $PECO_2$.

## III  Types of capnographs and capnometers

### A  Time capnography

- Is the plot of expired carbon dioxide partial pressure (*y*-axis) vs. time (*x*-axis) and is the most common type of capnography used in clinical patients.
- The advantages of this type of capnography are the ease of set-up and the information it provides about both the expiratory and inspiratory phases of ventilation.

### B  Volume capnography

- Is the plot of expired carbon dioxide partial pressure (y-axis) versus expired volume (x-axis).
- Although not used very often clinically, they provide more accurate information about ventilation/perfusion status and potential presence of atelectasis than a time capnogram.
- However, volume capnograms *do not* provide information about the inspiratory phase, as it is non-existent in this type of capnography.

## IV  Types of gas $CO_2$ analyzers

### A  Sidestream capnometers

- In this system, a sample of the respiratory gas is diverted from the breathing circuit via a sampling port, usually at the Y-piece, to a sensor in the housing unit of a multi-parameter monitor.
- The pump that aspirates the sample operates at a constant rate that varies depending upon the monitor (rates are usually between 50 and 200 ml/min), and some monitors allow adjustment of this rate.

*Advantages:*
- The advantage of side-stream capnography is that analysis is done in the monitor itself, so if the sample tubing or water trap are damaged or need to be replaced, this may be done with little cost.
- Also, the sample tubing is easily integrated into large animal anesthesia circuits via connectors built into the Y-piece or by introducing a needle into the machine end of the endotracheal tube. (see Figure 17.24)

*Disadvantages:*
- The disadvantages of this type of monitor include long warm-up times (it is best to turn the monitor on prior to bringing the horse up for induction to allow this warm-up and assure functionality) and the possibility of occlusion of the sampling line.

– Occlusion will show up as an occlusion alarm on the capnometer, and no capnogram will be displayed.
– Adult horses produce such large amounts of condensation in their expired respiratory gases, that the sampling lines may become so severely clogged that the pump is unable to deliver this liquid into the water trap. In these cases, replacement of the sampling line is indicated. If reusing sampling lines, it is also recommended to dry them out between anesthetic events.

### B  Mainstream capnometers

- In this system, the expired gas is analyzed at the machine end of the endotracheal tube.
- The probe is typically placed between the endotracheal tube and the Y-piece.
- Mainstream capnometers are typically reserved for use in foals, as the analyzers only fit conventionally-sized (15 mm outer diameter) endotracheal tube connectors.

*Advantages:*

○ The advantages of a mainstream capnometer are that no gas is diverted from the patient (this can be significant in small patients) and that no sampling line and water trap apparatus are required.

*Disadvantages:*

○ The main disadvantage of this type of capnometer lies in the fact that the analyzer is attached to the patient. This location makes dropping and breakage of the unit much more likely, which would require full replacement of the capnometer.
○ It is not suitable for used in adult horses.

## V  Normal time capnogram (see Figure 19.10)

### A  Phase I

- Occurs during the first part of exhalation.
- In this initial phase the $PECO_2$ will be zero, as the $CO_2$-free gas from the respiratory dead space passes through the monitor.

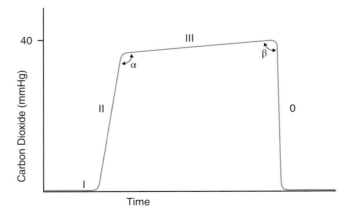

**Figure 19.10**  Normal time vs. partial pressure of carbon dioxide capnogram.

**B   Phase II**

- During this phase, the $CO_2$ concentration starts to rise as exhalation continues and alveolar recruitment is occurring.

**C   Phase III**

- This mostly horizontal phase of the capnogram is the alveolar plateau, where $CO_2$ from the lungs is being exhaled.
- The angle between phase II and phase III is referred to as the *α angle*. A slight upward slope exists in this phase, with the terminal peak being the $PECO_2$. The reasons that the upward slope exists are that more dependent, late-emptying alveoli tend to have more $CO_2$ and also gas exchange continues to occur throughout expiration, as the heart delivers more blood to the lungs with each heartbeat.

**D   Phase 0**

- Inspiration is occurring.
- The capnogram should sweep sharply downward, creating a sharp angle, referred to as the *β angle*, between phase III and phase 0.

## VI   Abnormal PECO$_2$ values and waveforms

**A   Absence of PECO$_2$ waveform**

- This could occur due to disconnection of the monitor, occlusion of the sampling line (for sidestream capnometers), complete occlusion of the endotracheal tube, cardiac arrest, or monitor malfunction.
- In some capnographs, the waveform may also transiently disappear during self-recalibration.

**B   Cardiogenic oscillations**

- These appear as small, heart-rate matching waveforms in the alveolar plateau of the capnogram. (see Figure 19.11)
- It was originally thought that cardiogenic oscillations resulted from the beating of the heart in contact with the lungs, and may have been an indication that atelectasis was present and causing the mechanical effects of the cardiac cycle on the lungs to become more apparent. However, evidence now supports the theory that the volume of pulmonary blood flow, rather than contact between the heart and lungs, is the primary factor determining the amplitude of cardiogenic oscillations. In support of this, cardiogenic oscillations disappeared when pulmonary blood flow was occluded in experimental animals.

**C   Widened α angle**

- A widened α angle may occur when there is partial obstruction of the endotracheal tube. (see Figure 19.12)

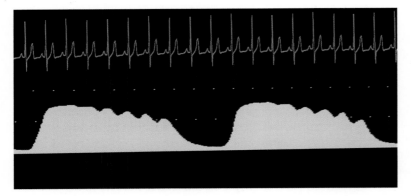

Figure 19.11    Cardiogenic oscillations on capnogram waveform. (*Source:* Courtesy of Bonnie Johnson, RVT).

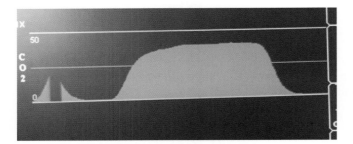

Figure 19.12    Widened α angle due to a resistance to expiration.

- This could be due to mechanical forces bending the tube, or secretions plugging the tube. Internal obstruction of the endotracheal tube is more likely in smaller patients, where a small internal diameter endotracheal tube must be used.
- In these cases, one must be careful not to bend endotracheal tubes, and if copious secretions are present, the tube may have to be exchanged for a clean one.

**D    Widened β angle**

- A widened β angle usually indicates a leak in the endotracheal tube, as the terminal phase of expiration is allowing some expired gas to leak out around the tube, escaping detection by the capnometer. (see Figure 19.13)
- To address this issue, the cuff should be inflated to correct the leak, or the endotracheal tube may have to be replaced if the cuff is faulty.

**E    Elevated baseline**

- An elevated baseline ($PECO_2$ not returning to zero value) shows that rebreathing of $CO_2$ is occurring. (see Figure 19.14)
- This situation may be noted in cases where there is excessive mechanical dead space (such as too many connectors or an endotracheal tube that is too long), a stuck one-way expiratory valve, or exhaustion of the $CO_2$ absorbent.
- These causes should all be investigated and corrected if an elevated baseline is observed.

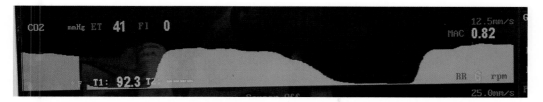

Figure 19.13    Widened β angle likely due to a leak around the endotracheal tube cuff.

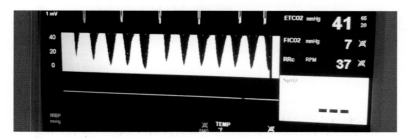

Figure 19.14    Elevated baseline indicating inspiration of carbon dioxide. *Source:* Courtesy of Dr. Nicole Trenholme, DACVECC.

## F    Hypoventilation

- Capnograms of a hypoventilating patient will usually appear as larger waveforms, with elevated $PECO_2$ readings and possibly with a decreased respiratory rate if ventilating spontaneously. (see Figure 19.15)
- However, patients may also hypoventilate while the capnograph appears normal or decreased if insufficient tidal volume is being delivered. For this reason, it is important for to note the tidal volume and the peak airway pressure, to ensure that adequate alveolar recruitment is occurring during ventilation.
- Reasons for hypoventilation may include inappropriate ventilator settings, anesthetic drugs, and increased intra-abdominal pressure (as occurs in horses with distended bowel due to colic).

## G    Hyperventilation

- Hyperventilated patients will have a capnogram consisting of shorter waves, a lower $PECO_2$ reading, and likely an increased respiratory rate. (see Figure 19.16)
- Reasons for hyperventilation under anesthesia may include being too lightly anesthetized, insufficient analgesia, and hypoxemia.

## H    Resisting the ventilator

- A patient who is resisting, or "*bucking*" the ventilator will have extra capnogram waveforms that appear when the ventilator is not firing.
- The patient's chest excursions may be noticeable during these extra waves to confirm suspicions of bucking the ventilator.

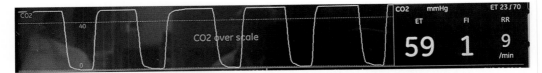

Figure 19.15   Hypoventilation, as indicated by elevated end tidal carbon dioxide.

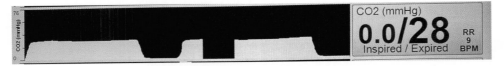

Figure 19.16   Hyperventilation, as indicated by low end-tidal carbon dioxide.

- Usually, when a patient is resisting the ventilator, it means they are either too light, or they are extremely hypoxemic and experiencing a hypoxic drive to breathe.

### I   Cardiac arrest

- During cardiac arrest capnograms may either completely disappear, or they may slowly decrease to very low levels of $PECO_2$ (<10 mmHg), depending on the speed of onset of the arrest.
- Even if the patient is being ventilated, the $PECO_2$ will be non-existent due to the lack of CO. One may also notice the effects of CO on the capnogram, even outside of arrest situations, noting that successfully treating severe hypotension results in an increase in the $PECO_2$, even without adjusting any other parameters.

## VII   Monitoring the inspired oxygen concentration

- Monitoring of oxygenation is important to prevent delivering a hypoxic mixture to the patient. (see Figure 19.17)
    - It is especially important to monitor the inspired $O_2$ if $N_2O$ is being administered.
    - It is also important to monitor the inspired $O_2$ if low-flow anesthesia is being practiced.
- The inspired and expired oxygen percentage in the patient breathing system is usually determined using an oxygen analyzer located in a multipurpose monitor.
- Gas samples are generally obtained using sidestream technology.
- Factors affecting hypoxemia and hypoxia are discussed in greater detail in Chapter 38.
*Technology*
    - A *Clark* electrode is an example of the technology used to measure oxygen.

## VIII   Pulse oximetry

- Pulse oximetry measures the oxygen saturation of hemoglobin ($SpO_2$).
- Pulse oximetry can be regarded as an indirect measure of $PaO_2$, although the relationship between the two is non-linear (see oxyhemoglobin dissociation curve Chapter 4).
- The normal $SpO_2$ is 95–100%.

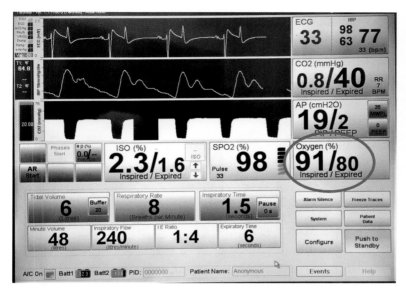

Figure 19.17   Airway oxygen analyzer indicating percent inspired and expired oxygen.

- Some pulse oximeter units contain a plethysmograph which can reflect changes in blood volume in the periphery.

## A   Types of pulse oximeters

- *Transmission* probes and *reflectance* probe are used clinically.

*Transmission probe* (see Figure 19.18a)
- o This is the most common type of pulse oximeter included with anesthesia monitors.
- o Most commonly, the probe is placed on the tongue, but other locations may be used.
  - – If unpigmented, the lips, vulva, nostril, ear, and prepuce may be used.

*Reflectance probes* (see Figure 19.18b)
- o It is less commonly used that the transmission probe.
- o The probe may be placed on the base of the tail in cases where there is no access to the head, such as in ophthalmic surgeries under general anesthesia.

*Co-oximetry*
- o Some pulse oximeters are also capable of co-oximetry, which means they can detect abnormal hemoglobin species, such as *methemoglobin* and *carboxyhemoglobin*.

## B   Technology

- Pulse oximeters work using the principle of the *Beer–Lambert Law* and spectrophotometric analysis. The *Beer–Lambert* law states that the concentration of a given solute in a solvent is determined by the amount of light that is absorbed by the solute at a specific wavelength.

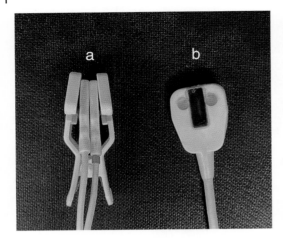

Figure 19.18 (a) Transmission design pulse oximetry probe. (b) Reflectance design pulse oximetry probe.

*Transmission* pulse oximetry
- ○ LEDs send out a wavelength of red light, usually 660 nm, and a wavelength of infrared light, usually 940 nm. Both wavelengths cross the vascular bed to a sensor.
- ○ The light received is measured by a photodetector which measures the amount of light which is not absorbed at each wavelength. This information is relayed to a microprocessor.
- ○ Oxyhemoglobin absorbs more infrared light than does reduced hemoglobin, and the latter absorbs more red light.

*Reflection* pulse oximetry
- ○ The photodetector is located on the same side of the vascular bed as the LEDs.
- ○ The light transmitted from the LEDs is reflected back to the photodetector.

C   **Factors that may affect accuracy**

- Pulse oximeters may read inaccurately due to the following:
  - Skin pigmentation.
  - Vasoconstriction.
  - Patient movement.
  - Interference from instruments and ambient light.
- Pulse oximeters frequently exhibit falsely low values, especially if pigmentation and vasoconstriction are present.
- $\alpha_2$ agonists cause peripheral vasoconstriction, making it difficult sometimes to obtain reliable pulse oximeter readings. One may try to moisten the tongue with warm water to promote vasodilation and transmission of light, but this may not be efficacious, depending upon the circumstances.
- The presence of large amounts of *methemoglob*in will cause the pulse oximeter to read a saturation of 85%, regardless of the actual $PaO_2$.
- The presence of large amounts of *carboxyhemoglobin* will cause the rare occurrence of making the pulse oximeter reading falsely high. The monitor will read a saturation of 100%, but this will be for *carboxyhemoglobin*, not *oxyhemoglobin*. The patient in this case will actually be severely hypoxemic.
- In *cyanide* poisoning the pulse oximeter will report a normal reading as the patient is not hypoxemic, but will be experiencing tissue hypoxia. Hypoxia results from the effects of cyanide on oxidative phosphorylation, rendering the cells incapable of using oxygen.

D   Advantages of pulse oximetry

- The advantage of using pulse oximetry is that the probes are easily placed and, if functioning properly, yield results quickly.
- In most cases, pulse oximeters will not read falsely high, so if there is a strong signal and a normal reading (>95%), it can be presumed with relative confidence that the hemoglobin saturation is adequate. However, a normal reading does not rule out a relative hypoxemia ($PaO_2$:$FiO_2$ ratio of <400).

E   Disadvantages

- Disadvantages to the use of pulse oximeters are due to their potential for falsely low readings as described above, along with potential interference from equipment and other outside sources (listed above).

## IX   Arterial blood gas analysis

- Because equine patients are at a high risk of hypoxemia and hypoventilation, monitoring blood gases can aid in early intervention to correct issues that would otherwise have been undetected until significant derangements were present.
- Arterial blood gases are extremely useful in monitoring acid–base parameters (respiratory and metabolic) in anesthetized horses, as this is the *gold standard* for these assessments.
- Due to the large size of most equine patients, arterial access is easily gained, providing the ability to readily monitor blood gases. The most common sites for arterial cannulation are the facial, transverse facial, coccygeal, and metatarsal arteries.
- Venous blood gases may be used for metabolic assessment, sometimes for ventilatory assessment (due to the low arterial-to-venous gradient of $CO_2$), but not generally for oxygenation assessment.
- Arterial blood gases provide information on:
  - Oxygenation.
  - Ventilation status.
  - Acid–base status (For a detailed description of acid–base physiology see Chapter 9).
- The availability of *Point-of-care* analyzers make respiratory monitoring much more accessible nowadays.

A   Arterial oxygen partial pressure ($PaO_2$)

- The $PaO_2$ is a measure of the efficiency of oxygen exchange in the lungs.
- In the standing, healthy horse, the $PaO_2$, at sea level, should be 90–100 mmHg.
- In order to interpret a patient's $PaO_2$ it is necessary to be able to estimate what the value should be under different circumstances. This can be done using the alveolar gas equation which calculates the alveolar partial pressure of oxygen ($PAO_2$).
- The $PaO_2$ is approximately 10 mmHg less than the $PAO_2$ in the standing healthy horse.

$$PAO_2 = FiO_2\left(PB - PH_2O\right) - \frac{PaCO_2}{R}$$

- $FIO_2$ = Inspired oxygen fraction. 21% = Percent oxygen in atmospheric air.
- *Note*: The normal $PaO_2$:$FiO_2$ ratio is ≥400 (*Horowitz* index).
- PB = Atmospheric pressure (760 mmHg at sea level).
- $PH_2O$ = Water vapor pressure (mmHg) in airway (~ 50 mmHg at body temp of horse).
- $PaCO_2$ = Normal 35–45 mmHg.
- R = Respiratory gas exchange ratio ($CO_2$ production to $O_2$ consumption; ~ 0.8).

**Example 1**: Expected $PAO_2$ and $PaO_2$ in a standing, healthy horse at sea level. Assume a $PaCO_2$ of 40 mmHg.

$$PAO_2 = 0.21\left[(760-50)\right] - 40/0.8$$
$$= (0.21 \times 710) - 50$$
$$= 149 - 50$$
$$= 99 \text{ mmHg}$$

Since the $PaO_2$ is about 10 mmHg less than the $PAO_2$, hence the expected $PaO_2$ would be ~90 mmHg.

*Comment*: Based on the Alveolar Gas Equation, the $PAO_2$ can be increased primarily by increasing the $FIO_2$ because the relationship between the two variables is direct; but the $PAO_2$ can also be increased to a lesser extent by decreasing the $PaCO_2$.

**Example 2**: An anesthetized horse has a $PaO_2 = 120$ mmHg and a $PaCO_2 = 50$ mmHg. $FIO_2$ = 90%, PB = 750 mmHg. Assume R = 0.8.

Expected $PAO_2$ **based** on the Alveolar gas equation:

$$\text{Expected } PAO_2 = \left[0.9(750-50)\right] - 50/0.8$$
$$= 0.9(700)] - 62$$
$$= 630 - 62$$
$$\text{Expected } PAO_2 = 568 \text{ mmHg}$$

*Comment*: Under ideal circumstances the $PaO_2$ should be closer in value to the $PAO_2$. The large difference between the expected and actual $PaO_2$ is most likely due to V/Q mismatch, and is not an unexpected finding in horses under general anesthesia. (For further information, see hypoxemia Chapter 38).

## B   Arterial carbon dioxide partial pressure ($PaCO_2$)

- $PaCO_2$ is inversely proportional to $V_A$; thus, an increase in $PaCO_2$ indicates *hypoventilation*.
- Normal values in the unsedated, standing horse are 35–45 mmHg.
- Respiratory acidosis (low pH with a high $PaCO_2$) is the most common blood-gas derangement in equine patients under general anesthesia.
  - In this circumstance, the condition will resolve with controlled ventilation.
  - Nevertheless, clinicians differ in their approach to dealing with hypoventilation, and some tolerate a $PaCO_2$ up to 70 mmHg before instituting controlled ventilation.
- Severe hypercarbia ($PaCO_2 > 75$ mmHg) is associated with an increase in CO and mean arterial pressure in horses (see Hypercarbia Chapter 38).
- The $PaCO_2$ will also increase in hypermetabolic states such as during an HYPP episode. In this case, severe life-threatening increases in serum $[K^+]$ need to be addressed promptly (see HYPP Chapter 38).

## Suggested Reading

Ambrisko, T.D., Lammer, V., and Schramel, J.P. (2014). in vitro and in vivo evaluation of a new large animal spirometry device using mainstream $CO_2$ flow sensors. *Equine Vet. J.* 46: 507–511.

Mosing, M., Bohm, S., Rasis, A. et al. (2018). Physiologic factors influencing the arterial-to-end-tidal $CO_2$ difference and the alveolar dead space fraction in spontaneously breathing anesthetized horses. *Front. Vet. Sci.* 28 (5): 58.

Sacks, M. and Mosing, M. (2017). Volumetric capnography to diagnose venous air embolism in an anaesthetized horse. *Vet. Anaesth. Analg.* 44: 190–190.

Zoff, A., Dugdale, A.H.A., Scarabelli, S. et al. (2019). Evaluation of pulse co-oximetry to determine haemoglobin saturation with oxygen and haemoglobin concentration in anaesthetized horses: a retrospective study. *Vet. Anaesth. Analg.* 46: 452–457.

## Anesthetic Agent Monitoring

*Alanna N. Johnson*

- Monitoring end-tidal anesthetic agent concentration is extremely useful clinically, as it provides an estimate of the concentration of the anesthetic agent in the brain. This measurement is particularly useful for large species like horses, in which the volume of the circuit and patient is large, thereby increasing the time constant for the system.

$$\text{Time constant} = \frac{\text{Volume}(L)}{\text{Flow}(L / \min)}$$

- For any system, it will take three-time constants for a 95% change in the system.
  - When instituting inhalant anesthesia, it will take approximately three-time constants ($\tau$) to attain system equilibration to the concentration that is set on the vaporizer. The larger the volume of the circuit and patient, the longer the time constant.
  - Because of the large time constant of adult equine patients, most anesthetists will set the oxygen flow rate high and the vaporizer setting high for the first few minutes of anesthesia. This technique is termed "*overpressuring*." Having an anesthetic gas analyzer is helpful in this situation, as it allows the expired agent percent to be observed in real-time and to know when to turn the vaporizer and fresh gas flow rate down to a maintenance level.
- Within the patient, more soluble volatile anesthetics will take longer to equilibrate, so times will vary when using *isoflurane* (more soluble) vs. *sevoflurane* (less soluble), for example. The gas analyzer removes the guess work in seeing these changes and making appropriate adjustments.
- An additional advantage to using anesthetic gas analyzers is that it allows for titration down to the minimal level of volatile anesthetic needed, particularly in patients where a partial IV anesthetic (PIVA) technique is being used.

## I   Technology

- Most anesthetic gas analyzers utilize *infrared* technology or *mass spectrometry* to determine the anesthetic concentration.
- Anesthetic gas analyzers measure the concentration of volatile anesthetics and nitrous oxide. Values for the individual anesthetic agents are displayed on the monitor as

inspiratory and expiratory concentrations. Expired concentrations accurately reflect alveolar and brain concentrations of the anesthetic after equilibration has occurred.

- Gas analyzers are generally part of a multimodal patient monitor, although they can also be standalone units.
- Gas monitors use either sidestream or mainstream technology (see Section IV: Types of gas $CO_2$ analyzers).
  - Sidestream technology is used in association with large animal machines.
  - Mainstream technology is used in association with small animal anesthetic machines.
- A constant sampling of gas occurs, similar to sidestream capnography, usually at the machine end of the endotracheal tube. Sometimes, for research purposes, samples are obtained within the lungs via a sampling catheter which is passed down the endotracheal tube.

## A  Factors that may affect accuracy

- Many of the factors that could affect accuracy are related to the *sidestream* nature of these monitors, such as obstruction of the sampling line and oversampling in small patients.
- *Methane*, which is produced in the equine large intestine during digestive fermentation, may affect gas analyzer readings, as horses excrete some of this produced methane via the respiratory tract.
- *Methane* absorbs infrared light at a wavelength of 3.3 µm. Older gas analyzers also utilized this same wavelength, which caused methane to be read as an anesthetic gas, causing anesthetic concentrations to be falsely high, or for other anesthetic gases to falsely show on the monitor when not being used. These effects were especially relevant when using older inhalants, such as halothane.
- More recent gas analyzers usually read inhalant anesthetics at 8–13 µm, a frequency at which methane is no longer detected, regardless of which anesthetic agent is used.
- Calibration is required periodically to retain optimal accuracy. Calibration is achieved using a proprietary mixed gas (provided by the monitor company) and the calibration mode of the monitor.
- As with sidestream capnographs, anesthetic gas analyzers may have their sampling lines kinked or obstructed. Adult horses in particular produce such large amounts of condensation via the respiratory tract, that this may obstruct the sampling line. For small patients, such as newborn foals, the sampling rates for the monitors may be high enough to aspirate a significant amount of the respiratory gas, so the fresh gas flow should be high enough to overcome this rate of loss.

## Monitoring Temperature
*Chiara E. Hampton*

- As neuraxial anesthesia and general anesthesia alter thermoregulation, it is of great importance to monitor changes in body temperature occurring during the perioperative period.
- Hypothermia and hyperthermia can have dramatic consequences on the homeostasis of many of the body's physiologic functions. Therefore, temperature it is a crucial parameter to be monitored on equine patients undergoing general anesthesia, but also in horses undergoing standing sedation, and loco-regional anesthesia.
- Specific guidelines on temperature monitoring for equine patients are not outlined; therefore, a standard practice in this species is yet to be established.

# I Thermal compartments

*Core compartment*

- The core compartment of the horse includes deep thoracic, abdominal, muscular, and CNS tissues.
- This compartment exhibits a temperature that is usually about 2–4 °C higher than the tissues located in the periphery.
- The temperature of this compartment is tightly regulated by several mechanisms that compose the thermoregulatory control system (see Chapter 11).

*Peripheral compartment*

- The peripheral compartment includes superficial tissues such as the skin and extremities.
- Variations in temperature of this compartment are marked. The balance between environmental conditions, such as wind-speed, humidity, temperature, body surface exposure, and core temperatures dictate variations.
- The main mechanism of change in peripheral temperatures is vasomotion, which includes *vasodilatation* in response to heat and *vasoconstriction* in response to cold.

# II Monitoring sites

## A Core temperature

*Pulmonary artery*

- The temperature of pulmonary artery blood closely reflects the core temperature.
- It necessitates placing a catheter in the pulmonary artery via the jugular vein. The tip of the pulmonary arterial catheter is provided with a *thermistor* that reads the temperature of the blood returning from the venous circulation, which has had sufficient time to rewarm by convective mechanisms in the core of the body.
- This technique is usually reserved for research purposes as it is a costly, invasive, and technically difficult.

*Aorta*

- Sensors with telemetry technology can be implanted on the wall of the aorta.
- This technique is very invasive as it requires surgical dissection. Therefore, it is reserved for research purposes.

## B Near-Core

"*Near-core*" temperature is routinely used in human and veterinary medicine to estimate core temperature, as it is technically less challenging to measure.

*Rectum*

- The rectum provides the most accurate and precise readings during the first hour of general anesthesia in adult horses, and it is considered the best non-invasive site to monitor temperature in this species.
- Readings at this site are affected by heat producing flora, blood returning from pelvic limbs, and insulation by feces. However, they are not influenced by environmental temperatures.

*Esophagus*

- ○ Specific information on the accuracy of esophageal temperatures in horses is unavailable. However, in humans, variations of up to 4 °C, depending on placement of the probe, have been observed.
- ○ The current recommendation for temperature readings in humans is that the tip of the probe is placed in the lower third of the esophagus to reflect core temperature. Readings at this location are affected by respired gases, but it has good agreement with readings from the pulmonary artery in human beings.
- ○ In the horse, placing the probe in the lower third of the esophagus may be difficult due to coiling of the probe within the oral cavity or the pharyngeal area, and due to the limited length of the probe.

*Nasopharynx*

- ○ After equilibration of core-to-periphery temperature, this location provides the best combination of accuracy and precision after one hour of general anesthesia in horses.
- ○ This location is easy and readily available to reach in anesthetized horses, and readings are accomplished by placing the tip of the temperature probe in the nasopharynx through the ventral meatus of the nostril.

*Urinary bladder*

- ○ Readings from this location are taken by inserting an indwelling urinary catheter provided with a thermistor at its tip.
- ○ The frequency of use of this technique in horses is unknown, and it is not a practical method clinically.

### C  Peripheral

*Skin*

- ○ Temperature readings can be obtained from the skin by the use of a dedicated temperature probe.
- ○ Readings from this site, including the groin, are affected by environmental temperatures, and do not provide accurate and precise readings in the anesthetized horse.

## III  Technologies

- Temperature monitoring is generally included and available on multiparameter monitors used in human and veterinary medicine.
- Electricity-based thermometry is currently the standard of care in temperature measuring and monitoring in human and veterinary medicine. They include *thermistor*, *thermocouple*, and *infrared* thermometers.
  - ○ Clinically available *digital thermometers* are generally thermistor- or infrared-based.
- Non-electrical technologies to measure temperatures include *mercury* thermometers (discontinued due to safety concerns), and *dial* thermometers (Bourdon gauge and bimetallic strip).
  - ○ Disadvantages of the latter category include longer equilibration time and lower precision.
  - ○ They are also impractical for continuous monitoring, which is preferred over intermittent readings during general anesthesia.

- If a thermometry probe is used within the body (i.e. esophagus, nasopharynx, rectum), it must be covered by an outer insulating sheath, which needs to be intact and free from any damage to avoid thermal burns and loss of electrical current.
- The followings are the three most common technologies used in human and veterinary monitors:

*Thermistor* (see Figure 19.19)

- This technology is based on the *Wheatstone* bridge circuit, which measures the changes in resistance of the circuit in response to changes in temperature. Resistance generally decreases when temperature rises.
- Thermistors are composed of a metal (e.g. manganese, zinc, iron, cobalt, or nickel) oxide sintered into a wire or fused into a rod to which an electrical current is applied.
- The range of detected temperatures is generally between 0 and 60 °C.
- They are usually small in size, exhibit rapid response time, and are sensitive to small changes in temperature.
- One of their greatest advantages is that they can be used to provide continuous readings.
- They are integrated with most multiparameter monitors used for anesthetic monitoring, can be disposable or reusable, and probes are available for esophageal, rectal, and skin (flat surface) use.

*Thermocouple*

- This technology is based on the Seebeck effect (thermoelectric effect), which states that heating the interface between two different materials generates an electric voltage.
- A thermocouple measures the difference in electrical potential that builds up across the hot-cold interface of two dissimilar metals.
- A thermocouple is composed of two dissimilar metals welded at their ends. One of the ends of the probe is held at a constant temperature (monitor end), whereas the other end is exposed to a changing temperature (patient end).
- The thermocouple converts heat into an electrical voltage, and it is displayed on the monitor as a temperature reading. The change in electrical voltage generated at the two ends of the thermocouple is proportional to the temperature reading.
- The range of detected temperatures is generally between −50 °C and 150 °C for medical thermometers.
- They are usually small in size, exhibit rapid response time, and are sensitive to small changes in temperature. They provide continuous readings, and are usually stand-alone units that can be portable and have interchangeable probes.

**Figure 19.19** Thermistor unit with probe.

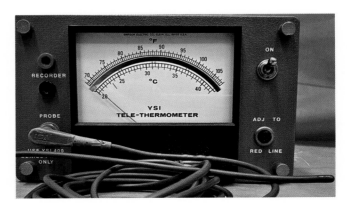

*Infra-Red*
- o This technology is based on the detection of infrared radiation arising from body surfaces.
  - – Infrared radiation is emitted by a body in proportion to its temperature.
- o Most infrared thermometers have a *pyroelectric sensor*, which reacts to the change in temperature caused by infrared radiation.
- o In human beings, infrared thermometers are designed to be used on either the tympanic membrane or the forehead. They are well tolerated because they do not require surface contact and cause no discomfort.
- o Infrared thermometers for clinical use present considerable limitations, such as intermittent readings, poor penetration of the skin layers, and less precise and accurate temperature readings compared to the other available technologies. They are also greatly affected by local vasomotion, and therefore they may not accurately reflect core temperature. The range of maximum error is 0.1–0.4 °C between temperatures of 35 and 41 °C.

## IV   Hazards of temperature monitoring

*Thermal burn*
- o Can occur if the temperature probe acts as a ground for an electrosurgical apparatus, and it is more likely to happen with damaged probes. Their use is therefore discouraged as they can also disperse electrical current if insulation is damaged.

*Probe contamination*
- o Can occur if the same temperature probe is used at different monitoring sites (e.g. a rectal probe moved to the esophagus or nasopharynx) without proper disinfection.
  - – Contamination can occur within the same patient or among patients.

*Incorrect temperature readings*
- o Can occur if the probe has been damaged, or if the tip of the probe is placed in a location that does not reflect body temperature. For example, the probe slips out of the nasopharynx or the nostrils into the oral cavity, or a probe inserted orally fails to progress into the esophagus and is measuring oral cavity temperature.

*Faulty probe*
- o Can occur if the probe or the connection with the main monitor have been damaged.

## Suggested Reading

Dorsch, J.A. (2012). *Understanding Anesthesia Equipment*, 858–870. Lippincott Williams & Wilkins.
Tomasic, M. and Nann, L. (1999). Comparison of peripheral and core temperatures in anesthetized horses. *Am. J. Vet. Res.* 60: 648–651.

## Monitoring Neuromuscular Function
### Manuel Martin-Flores and Daniel M. Sakai

- Given that NMBAs interrupt neuromuscular transmission, the principle of monitoring relies on the stimulation of a motor nerve, and the evaluation of the elicited muscular response. A peripheral nerve stimulator (PNS) is the minimum equipment necessary to monitor neuromuscular transmission.

- Methods for assessing neuromuscular function that do not rely on the use of PNS are inadequate and cannot fully represent the status of neuromuscular transmission.
- Observation of spontaneous movement, ventilation, or even measurements of tidal volume or minute ventilation, is *not* an adequate surrogate for monitoring.
- Moreover, given the normal variability in the duration of action of NMBAs, and considering that many factors can lengthen their effects (e.g. anesthetics, hypothermia, derangement in electrolyte concentrations, and other drugs such as antibiotics), relying on passage of time is an inadequate way to ensure that neuromuscular transmission is restored prior to recovery from anesthesia.

## I   Peripheral nerve stimulation

- Peripheral nerve stimulation requires an electrical stimulus delivered in close proximity to a motor nerve. The stimulus should fulfill some characteristics, in regard to current, duration of stimulation, and pattern of stimulation.

### A   Current

- The magnitude of an evoked response increases with the current delivered by the PNS.
- Typically, a *supramaximal* current, that is, a current above that which elicits a maximal response, is used.
- A supramaximal current ensures that all muscle fibers are stimulated.
- Hence, subsequent decreases in a response can be attributed to neuromuscular blockade, and not to insufficient stimulation. For this reason, a PNS should deliver *constant current* and not constant voltage; that is, the current is kept constant even if resistance through the skin changes.
- Supramaximal current can be painful. In some instance (described below), submaximal current may also be used.

### B   Duration of stimuli

- Square wave impulses of 0.1–0.3 msec are typically used during PNS.
- Stimuli of such short duration maximize the chances of stimulating the nerve but not the muscle directly.
- Direct muscle stimulation bypasses the neuromuscular junction and is not indicative of neuromuscular transmission.

### C   Pattern of stimulation

- Stimuli can be delivered in several patterns, the train-of-four (TOF) being the most commonly used.
- Other patterns (e.g. the single twitch) are reserved for research as they are difficult to implement in the clinical setting or provide no real advantages over the well-established TOF, hence, this discussion will only consider TOF.

## II  Repetitive stimulation and fade

### A  TOF

- The TOF consists of a sequence of four electrical stimuli delivered at 2 Hz (every half a second).
- In the absence of neuromuscular blockade, four equal responses (twitches) are elicited (TOF count = 4).
- Complete neuromuscular block results in zero twitches in response to TOF (TOF count = zero).
- The *onset* and *offset* of neuromuscular block are progressive processes, with a TOF count of 4 decreasing in steps to 0 and recovering in the opposite direction.
- During partial levels of neuromuscular block, a *fade* during the TOF can be observed with a TOF count of 4; that is, a progressive decrease in the magnitude of the four twitches of the train occurs. This *fade* can be quantified and is referred to as the TOF *ratio*. The TOF ratio is quantified by measuring the magnitude of the fourth twitch (T4) in reference to the first twitch (T1); that is T4 : T1.
- TOF ratio = 1.0: intact neuromuscular function.
  – The fourth twitch has the same magnitude as the first twitch.
- TOF ratio higher than 0 and lower than 0.9 = partial neuromuscular block.
  – The first twitch has higher magnitude than the fourth twitch.
- TOF ratio = 0. Full neuromuscular block.
  – All twitches disappear after each TOF stimulation.
- Fade during repeated stimulation results from the actions of the NMBA on pre-synaptic receptors.
- This interaction produces a progressive decrease in the amount of ACh that is released after each stimulation into the neuromuscular junction.

*Advantages of TOF*
- There are several practical advantages to using TOF for monitoring neuromuscular transmission.
- TOF remains one of the most sensitive indicators of residual block.
- Some evidence supports the use of *submaximal* currents when measuring the TOF ratio, as long as the current is sufficient to elicit four responses.
- *Submaximal* stimulation is better tolerated. Because the TOF ratio is measured within each train of stimuli, baseline measurements are not needed; each TOF acts as its own control.

## III  Methods to measure the evoked response

### A  Mechanomyography

- The measurement of force of contraction, is widely considered the gold standard, and is measured directly with a force transducer.
- This method, however, is cumbersome to perform, and requires a set up that prevents any movement, so that the isometric force of contraction can be measured.

### B  Alternative methods

- Surrogate methods can be applied to measure the evoked responses:

*Visual or tactile*:
- ○ Involves simple observation or palpation of the evoked twitches.
- ○ These methods have a *low sensitivity* to detect fade (partial neuromuscular blockade).

*Acceleromyography* (AMG):
- ○ Unlike mechanomyography, AMG measures the acceleration of a free moving limb, via an acceleration-sensitive crystal that can be fixed with tape to a hoof.
- ○ This technique detects the peak acceleration of the evoked contraction and is based on Newton's second law (force = mass x acceleration). It is easy to instrument and has been used extensively in many species.

*Electromyography*
- ○ Unlike the previous two methods, electromyography does not quantify movement, rather it measures the compound action potential; that is, muscular cellular activation in response to motor nerve stimulation.
- ○ The compound action potential is linearly correlated with the force of contraction.

## IV    Peripheral motor nerves used for monitoring neuromuscular blockade

- • In equines, the most commonly used nerves for monitoring neuromuscular transmission are the:
  - ○ Peroneal
  - ○ Radial
  - ○ Facial
- • The selection of the nerve to be stimulated depends on the recumbency, procedure, and accessibility.
- • The peroneal nerve is the most commonly used in the clinical setting.

*Peroneal*:
- ○ The electrodes are placed on the lateral aspect of pelvic limb, distal to the stifle. (see Figure 19.20)
- ○ The positive electrode is placed over the tibial tuberosity and the negative electrode placed ~4 cm distally, between the long and lateral extensor muscles.
- ○ Stimulation of the peroneal nerve results in extension of the hoof.

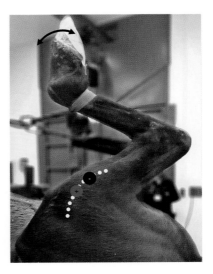

Figure 19.20    Lateral aspect of the pelvic limb. The trajectory of the peroneal nerve is sketched (dotted line). Electrodes are placed over the trajectory of the nerve, distal to the tibial tuberosity, separated by ~4 cm, with the positive electrode proximal. Alternatively, the electrodes could be placed perpendicular to the nerve so that it passes in the path of the stimulus between both electrodes. Stimulation of the peroneal nerve results in extension of the hoof.

*Radial*:

- ○ The electrodes are placed at the lateral aspect of the thoracic limbs, distal to the elbow.
- ○ The positive electrode is placed over the radial tuberosity and the negative electrode is placed ~4 cm distally between the digital lateral extensor and lateral ulnar muscles.
- ○ Stimulation of the radial nerve evokes carpal extension.

*Facial*:

- ○ The electrodes are placed caudal to the commissure of the lips, ventral to the *zygomatic* muscle.
- ○ The negative electrode is placed 3 cm cranial to the positive electrode.
- ○ Electrical stimulation evokes contraction of the lower lip.
- ○ It should be noted that resistance to block has been observed when the facial nerve was used.

## Suggested Reading

Martin-Flores, M., Campoy, L., Ludders, J.W. et al. (2008). Comparison between acceleromyography and visual assessment of train-of-four for monitoring neuromuscular blockade in horses undergoing surgery. *Vet. Anaesth. Analg.* 35: 220–227.

Martin-Flores, M., Saki, D.M., Campoy, L. et al. (2014). Recovery from neuromuscular block in dogs: restoration of spontaneous ventilation does not exclude residual blockade. *Vet. Anaesth. Analg.* https://doi.org/10.1111/vaa.12109.

Martin-Flores, M., Sakai, D.M., Tseng, C.T. et al. (2019). Can we see fade? A survey of anesthesia providers and our ability to detect partial neuromuscular block in dogs. *Vet. Anaesth. Analg.* 46: 182–187.

Mosing, M., Auer, U., Bardell, D. et al. (2010). Reversal of profound rocuronium block monitored in three muscle groups with sugammadex in ponies. *Br. J. Anaesth.* 105: 480–486.

Murphy, G.S. and Brull, S.J. (2010). Residual neuromuscular block: lessons unlearned. Part I: definitions, incidence, and adverse physiologic effects of residual neuromuscular block. *Anesth. Analg.* 111: 120–128.

# 20

## Standing Sedation
*Catherine M. Creighton*

- Standing sedation is used to facilitate the performance of diagnostic or therapeutic procedures in horses when general anesthesia is not desired or warranted.
- The goal of standing sedation is to provide a level of sedation adequate for the procedure, without excessive ataxia or response to surgical or other stimuli.
    - To achieve this, a combination of drugs and techniques is usually required including: a sedative, an analgesic, and locoregional techniques when appropriate.

## I  Indications for standing sedation

- Standing sedation is commonly used to facilitate:
    - Dental procedures such as tooth extraction, and mandibular fracture repair.
    - Laparoscopic procedures such as ovariectomy, cryptorchidectomy, and hernioplasty (see Figure 20.1).
    - Ocular examination, diagnostic and therapeutic procedures and surgery of the eye and adnexa.
    - Sinus endoscopy (sinusoscopy), sinus trephination and sinus flap surgery.
    - Nasal surgery, guttural pouch surgery, epiglottic and subepiglottic surgery, palatal surgery, and laryngeal and pharyngeal surgery.
    - Perineal procedures such as repair of cervical lacerations and perineal injuries.
- Recently, standing sedation has been described for select orthopedic procedures such as non-displaced condylar fractures, transphyseal screw implantation, implant removal and pedal osteitis or sequestration.

## II  Advantages of standing sedation over general anesthesia

- Lower complication rates compared to general anesthesia.
- The cost associated with procedures employing standing sedation is often significantly less than with general anesthesia.
- Monitoring the sedated horse is simpler than monitoring the anesthetized horse.
- Reduced time to complete the procedure in most cases.

*Manual of Equine Anesthesia and Analgesia*, Second Edition. Edited by Tom Doherty, Alex Valverde, and Rachel A. Reed.
© 2022 John Wiley & Sons, Inc. Published 2022 by John Wiley & Sons, Inc.

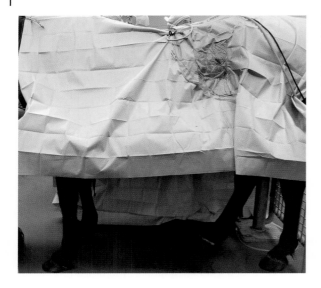

Figure 20.1   Mare sedated for a laparoscopic ovariectomy. The mare was premedicated with acepromazine (0.04 mg/kg, IM) and morphine (0.15 mg/kg, IM). Detomidine (6 µg/kg, IV) was administered 40 minutes later and a CRI of detomidine (5 µg/kg/hr) is being administered. Notice that the mare is standing fairly square.

## III   Disadvantages of standing sedation

- Surgical conditions are not always ideal as the horse may move in some fashion; however, this is usually not a problem if the horse is adequately sedated and has anesthesia of the surgical site.
- Oversedation results in excessive ataxia, which may cause stumbling, and recumbency on rare occasions.
- Access to the surgical site may not be optimal for all procedures.

## IV   Patient evaluation and preparation

- Horses not accustomed to handling, fractious or extremely painful horses may not be appropriate candidates for standing sedation.
- Patient evaluation and stabilization is performed as it would be prior to general anesthesia.
- In general, no specific preparation is required prior to standing sedation other than that required specific to the planned procedure.
  - Horses are often fasted for 24–36 hours prior to laparoscopic procedures; reduced volume of ingesta allows improved visualization of the abdomen and its contents.
- The procedure should be carried out in a quiet location with minimal external stimuli.
  - Ideally the horse is placed in a chute or stocks where it can be restrained during the procedure.
- An intravenous (IV) catheter should be placed.
  - Very few procedures can be completed with the sedation and analgesia achieved from a single IV injection.
  - Placement of an IV catheter will facilitate administration of additional sedative and analgesic drugs.

- A urinary catheter and urine collection system is recommended for procedures expected to take longer than one hour as $\alpha_2$-agonist administration is associated with increased urine production.
  - This will prevent the horse and personnel from slipping on the wet floor during the procedure.
- Have personnel available to monitor the horse during the procedure.
  - Because dosing of sedative and/or analgesic drug doses may need to be adjusted during the procedure.
- Cotton may be placed in the horse's ears to decrease response to auditory stimuli.
- The horse's head may be secured with side ties from the stocks.
- Alternatively, a support stand is placed in front of the horse to support the head and stabilize the horse, or the head can be rested on padding (see Figures 20.2 and 20.3).
  - Supporting the horse's head also prevents nasal edema and the resulting dyspnea associated with prolonged periods of decreased head height resulting from sedation. It also prevents compression of the neck if a frontal bar is present in the stocks.
  - Padding should be used around the horse's halter to prevent nerve damage (see Figure 20.3).
- Ideally, the sedated horse should stand *square* on the forelimbs. A sedated horse may not stand square on the rear limbs, and may point a foot, but will not generally be ataxic if it is standing square on the forelimbs (see Figure 20.1). This requires that sedative/analgesic drugs be titrated to effect to prevent oversedation and ataxia.
- Management of mares with a foal at their side:
  - Separating the mare and foal is generally not recommended.
  - Foals will follow the mare to the surgical area.

**Figure 20.2**  Support stand used to support head of sedated horse.

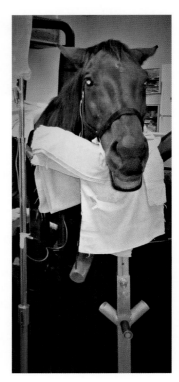

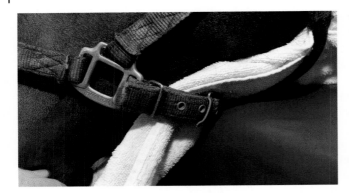

Figure 20.3  Padding around halter to prevent nerve damage. *Source:* Image supplied by Greg Hirshoren.

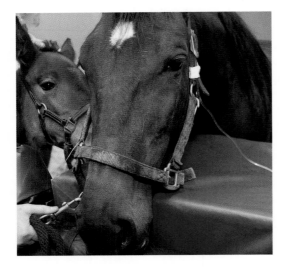

Figure 20.4  Sedated mare with foal at her side. *Source:* Image supplied by Greg Hirshoren.

- Neonatal foals may lie on a pad placed in front of the mare.
- Older foals will stand at the mare's head but will need to have a handler (see Figure 20.4).

## V  Drug administration

- Sedation is primarily based on an $\alpha_2$ agonist, and an opioid can be included to provide more analgesia and augment sedation.
- Sedative and analgesic drugs are either administered by IV bolus or constant rate infusion (CRI) techniques during the procedure.
- Horses can be premedicated intramuscularly (IM) with sedative and/or analgesics prior to being removed from the stall and placement of an IV catheter, especially for surgical procedures of longer duration.

A   Premedication with IM administered drugs

- IM sedation is often used in conjunction with a CRI of sedative/analgesic drugs.
- The IM drug(s) is administered 30–45 minutes before taking the horse out of its stall.
- The rationale behind IM sedation is to decrease the horse's stress, provide more balanced analgesia and sedation, and decrease the dose of $\alpha_2$ drugs administered as a CRI.
- Decreasing the CRI will decrease the severity of ataxia.

| Examples of IM Premedication Protocols |
| --- |
| - *Acepromazine* (0.05 mg/kg) + *Morphine* (0.1 mg/kg). <br> - *Acepromazine* (0.05 mg/kg) + *Hydromorphone* (0.04 mg/kg). <br> - *Acepromazine* (0.05 mg/kg) + *Butorphanol* (0.1 mg/kg). <br> *Note*: *Acepromazine* is contraindicated in a *nephrosplenic entrapment* procedure due to its splenic dilating effect. |

B   Bolus injections

- An IV bolus is the most common method of sedation for *short* procedures.

| Examples of IV Bolus Doses of alpha$_2$ Agonists ± an Opioid |
| --- |
| - *Xylazine* (0.5–1.0 mg/kg) ± *Butorphanol* (0.02 mg/kg) <br> - *Detomidine* (8–10 µg/kg) ± *Butorphanol* (0.02 mg/kg) <br> - *Dexmedetomidine* (3–5 µg/kg) ± *Butorphanol* (0.02 mg/kg) <br> *Morphine* or *methadone* (0.1 mg/kg) or *Hydromorphone* (0.04 mg/kg) can be used in place of butorphanol. <br> *Note*: The bolus dose(s) is generally less if the horse has had IM premedication. |

- IV bolus technique is easy and convenient but allows for swings in the degree of sedation and analgesia.

C   Continuous rate infusions (CRI)

- CRIs are usually used for *longer* procedures.
- An $\alpha_2$ agonist, most commonly *detomidine*, is infused alone or with an opioid.
- Less drug may be used over time with a CRI technique compared to repeated bolus administration.
- A loading dose (Ld) is administered initially.
  - To avoid over sedating the horse, the loading dose should be titrated to effect.

| Examples of $\alpha_2$-agonist CRIs |
| --- |
| - *Detomidine*: Ld 8–10 µg/kg, IV; CRI: 6–10 µg/kg/hr. <br> - *Dexmedetomidine*: Ld 2.0–3.5 µg/kg, IV; CRI: 1–3 µg/kg/hr. <br> - *Romifidine*: Ld 40–80 µg/kg, IV; CRI: 18–30 µg/kg/hr. <br> - *Xylazine*: Ld 0.5–1.0 mg/kg, IV; CRI: 0.6–1.5 mg/kg/hr. |

*Note*: The required Ld and CRI depends on whether the horse has been premedicated IM (e.g., *acepromazine + morphine*) or is receiving an opioid CRI (see below).

## D  Opioids as part of the CRI

| Examples of Opioid Doses (IV) When used in Conjunction with an $\alpha_2$ Agonist |
| --- |
| Butorphanol: Ld 0.02 mg/kg; CRI: 0.01–0.03 mg/kg/hr.<br>Morphine: Ld 0.05–0.1 mg/kg; CRI: 0.03–0.1 mg/kg/hr.<br>Methadone: Ld 0.1–0.2 mg/kg; CRI: 0.05 mg/kg/hr. |

- An opioid may be added to an $\alpha_2$ agonist CRI, but the dose of each drug may have to be decreased to avoid over sedation.

## E  Ketamine use in standing sedation

- Low-dose ketamine can be used in association with an alpha$_2$ agonist to potentiate sedation and analgesia.
- For example. *Ketamine*: Ld 0.1–0.2 mg/kg, IV: CRI: 0.4–0.8 mg/kg/hr.

## F  Intravenous lidocaine use in standing sedation

- Low-dose lidocaine can be infused as part of the sedation protocol.
- For example, Ld 1–2 mg/kg, IV over five minutes. CRI: 25–50 µg/kg/minute.

*Note*: Lidocaine toxicity is a possibility if a horse is being infused with IV lidocaine in addition to getting injected with large volumes of lidocaine for local anesthesia of the flanks and ovarian pedicles (e.g. as in bilateral ovariectomy).

## G  Reversal of sedation

- Reversal of alpha$_2$ mediated sedation may be desirable after standing sedation, especially if the procedure is of long duration.
- For example:
  - *Yohimbine* (0.02–0.04 mg/kg, IV).
  - *Tolazoline* (1–4 mg/kg, IV).
- The dose of the reversal agent required will depend on the degree of sedation and its impact on reversing analgesia.
- Reversal drugs should be administered slowly (over five minutes) to avoid causing hypotension.

# 21

# General Anesthesia Techniques

*Regula Bettschart-Wolfensberger and Simone K. Ringer*

- General anesthesia involves a *sedation, an induction, a maintenance, and a recovery phase.*

## I  Sedation

- It is recommended that the induction of anesthesia be preceded by deep sedation.
- However, sedation might be omitted in debilitated animals (e.g. septic foals).

### A  Reasons to sedate prior to anesthesia induction

- To reduce stress and facilitate handling.
- To smooth induction.
- To decrease the dose of induction drug(s).
- To decrease the dose of maintenance drug(s).
  - e.g. decrease the minimum alveolar concentration (MAC) of inhalational anesthetics.
- To provide analgesia (e.g. $\alpha_2$ agonists, opioids).
- To improve recovery (e.g. $\alpha_2$ agonists).

### B  Drugs used for sedation prior to induction

- $\alpha_2$ agonists alone or combined with *opioids* or *phenothiazines* (see Table 21.1).
- Most commonly, sedating drugs are administered intravenously.
- Intramuscular administration of a sedative may be necessary in some horses to facilitate placement of a jugular catheter or administration of IV drugs.
  - *Detomidine* (small injectate volume) is the most commonly used and reliable option for intramuscular administration.
  - Generally, the IM dose must be 2–3 × the IV dose to achieve the same effect.
- Benzodiazepines alone, or with opioids, may be used for sedation of neonatal foals (see Chapter 31), but they cause ataxia without sedation in older horses.

*Manual of Equine Anesthesia and Analgesia*, Second Edition. Edited by Tom Doherty, Alex Valverde, and Rachel A. Reed.

Table 21.1 Drugs used for sedation prior to induction of anesthesia. Dosages should be adapted to the character and general condition of the horse until a state of deep sedation is achieved with minimal response to external stimuli.

| Drug | Dose (IV) (mg/kg) | Comments |
|---|---|---|
| **α₂ agonists** | | |
| Xylazine | 1.0–1.5 | IM dose is 2–3×IV for all drugs. |
| Detomidine | 0.01–0.02 | 0.02–0.03 mg/kg IM. |
| Romifidine | 0.08–0.12 | |
| Medetomidine | 0.007–0.009 | Not approved for use in horses in US. |
| Dexmedetomidine | 0.003–0.007 | Not approved for use in horses in US. |
| **Phenothiazines** | | |
| Acepromazine | 0.02–0.05 | May be administered IM 30–45 minutes prior to IV sedation with an α₂ agonist. |
| | | May be administered IV at lower end of dose range. Onset of maximum effect is 10–15 minutes. |
| **Benzodiazepines** | | Not used for sedation of adult horses. Effective for sedation of neonatal foals, especially if combined with an opioid. |
| Midazolam/ Diazepam | 0.05–0.1 | Mainly used as an adjunct for anesthesia induction. |
| **Opioids** | | Only used in combination with α₂ agonists to improve quality of sedation. In foals, often combined with a benzodiazepine. |
| Butorphanol | 0.01–0.03 | |
| Methadone | 0.05–0.2 | |
| Morphine | 0.1–0.2 | Morphine is often administered IM to avoid the risk of *histamine release*. |
| Hydromorphone | 0.04 | |

## II  Induction of anesthesia

- Anesthesia should only be induced once the horse is deeply sedated.
- Preferably, induction is performed in a quiet and safe environment with well instructed personnel.

### A  Drugs used for induction of anesthesia (see Table 21.2)

- *Ketamine* alone or combined with a *benzodiazepine, propofol,* or *guaifenesin.*
  - Adjunctive drugs improve muscle relaxation.
- *Alfaxalone,* alone or combined with *guaifenesin* or a *benzodiazepine.*
- *Propofol*, alone or combined with *ketamine.*
- Inhalational anesthetics (e.g. in foals).

Table 21.2  Examples of induction regimens used in equines. Anesthesia should only be induced once the horse is deeply sedated. Recommended drug doses for sedation are reported in Table 21.1.

| Sedation | Induction Dose (mg/kg, IV) | Comments |
|---|---|---|
| $\alpha_2$ agonist | Ketamine (2.0–2.5) | Provides 5–10 minutes of general anesthesia. May be slightly longer if detomidine, romifidine, (dex) medetomidine are used for sedation. |
| $\alpha_2$ agonist | Ketamine (2.0–2.5) <br> + <br> Diazepam/midazolam (0.02–0.1) | Improved relaxation with benzodiazepine, facilitates intubation. |
| $\alpha_2$ agonist | Ketamine (2.0–2.5) <br> + <br> Guaifenesin (50–100) | Guaifenesin improves relaxation. <br> $\alpha_2$ agonist dose may be reduced, if so desired. |
| $\alpha_2$ agonist | Ketamine (2.0–2.5) <br> + <br> Propofol (0.5) | Propofol is added to improve relaxation and deepen anesthesia. It is used in place of a benzodiazepine. |
| $\alpha_2$ agonist | Tiletamine/zolazepam (1–2) | Longer duration of anesthesia (10–20 minutes) depending on dose), compared to ketamine alone. <br> Recovery quality is acceptable. |
| $\alpha_2$ agonist | Propofol (2.0) | Myoclonus, paddling may occur. <br> Short duration of anesthesia. <br> Good induction drug for foals, titratable to effect. Large volumes needed for full size horses. |
| $\alpha_2$ agonist | Alfaxalone (1.0) <br> + <br> Guaifenesin (35) or Midazolam/diazepam (0.05) | Muscle tremors are common. <br> Recoveries may not be as good as with ketamine. |
| $\alpha_2$ agonist | Thiopental (3–5) | Inductions may not be as smooth as with ketamine/benzodiazepine but are acceptable. <br> No analgesia. |
| $\alpha_2$ agonist | Thiopental (3–5) <br> + <br> Guaifenesin (50–100) | Can be mixed and infused together. <br> No analgesia. |

- ○ *Tiletamine/Zolazepam*. Has a longer duration of action than ketamine/benzodiazepine.
- ○ *Thiopental* (not presently available in North America).

## III  Maintenance of anesthesia

- Prolongation of general anesthesia, beyond the effect of the induction drugs, is frequently necessary.
- The maintenance phase of general anesthesia can be classified into *inhalational*, *total intravenous* (TIVA), or *partial intravenous anesthesia* (PIVA) depending on the drugs used.

## Inhalational Anesthesia

- Inhalational anesthetics are commonly used to maintain general anesthesia in equines, especially for longer procedures.
- With modern inhalational anesthetics the end of the anesthetic effect is practically independent of drug metabolism.
- Inhalational anesthetics can be used over prolonged time periods without the risk of metabolite accumulation and prolonged recovery.
- *Isoflurane* and *sevoflurane* are the most commonly used inhalational anesthetics for equines.

## I  Clinical use of inhalational anesthetics

- Inhalational anesthetics are routinely used to maintain anesthesia for procedures lasting >60 minutes.
- Inhalational anesthetics may be used in conjunction with *injectable* drugs.
- Injectable drugs reduce the MAC of the inhalation anesthetics and may provide analgesia (see PIVA).
- The use of inhalational anesthetics as induction agents has been recommended for foals. However, the procedure is considered by some to be more stressful than induction with an injectable drug(s), and has been associated with an increased mortality rate in one study.
  - Nevertheless, this finding of increased mortality rate was not corroborated by another study, and is not accepted by all clinicians (see Chapter 31).

## II  Potential advantages of inhalational anesthesia

- End-tidal concentrations can be monitored continuously with an end-tidal agent specific monitor.
- Anesthetic depth can be lightened relatively rapidly by flushing the anesthesia circuit with oxygen.
- Anesthesia can be rapidly deepened by administering "*top-ups*" of injectable anesthetics.
- The airway is secured and oxygen enriched gas mixtures help prevent hypoxemia.
- There is minimal metabolism and drug accumulation over time.
- Elimination of the drug is primarily via exhalation.

## III  Potential disadvantages of inhalational anesthetics

- Cardiorespiratory depression.
- Minimal analgesia.
- Narrow therapeutic index.
- Recovery can be uncoordinated if the horse tries to stand too soon.
  - Hence, the practice of sedating horses in recovery.
- Equipment is expensive as are modern inhalational drugs (e.g. sevoflurane, desflurane).
- Atmospheric pollution: inhalational anesthetics contribute to ozone depletion and greenhouse warming.
- Pollution of surgical suite if not properly scavenged.

## IV   Recovery quality

- Is negatively correlated with the duration of anesthesia.
- Use of sedatives or tranquilizers, *especially $\alpha_2$ agonists*, is recommended in the recovery period to prevent the horse from attempting to stand before the "*hang-over*" effect of the inhalational anesthetic is eliminated.
- *Morphine* (0.1–0.2 mg/kg IM before recovery) can improve the recovery quality.

## Total Intravenous Anesthesia (TIVA)

## I   Potential advantages of TIVA over inhalational anesthesia

- Less cardiorespiratory depression, depending on the injectable anesthetics used.
- Superior analgesia, depending on the injectable anesthetics used.
- Morbidity and mortality may be lower.
- Improved recoveries.
- Decreased surgical stress.
- No pollution of surgical suite.

## II   Potential disadvantages of TIVA

- Drug accumulation and a build-up of active metabolites (with elimination half-lives longer than the parent drugs (e.g. midazolam and its metabolite 1-hydroxymidazolam) with prolonged infusions.
  - ○ Drug accumulation can be reduced by decreasing the infusion rate over time.
  - ○ Therefore, to prevent metabolite accumulation, potentially with poor recoveries, it has been recommended that TIVA should be limited to 90 minutes. However, this recommendation may not apply to all drug regimens, and may not be of consequence if the infusion rate(s) are decreased over time or in the case of drugs (e.g. *propofol*) with a short context-sensitive half-time (CSHT).
- Monitoring of plasma drug concentrations is not feasible at present.
- Evaluation of anesthetic depth may be difficult depending on the drugs used.
- Decreasing the anesthetic depth takes longer than for inhalational anesthesia because is more dependent on drug metabolism and elimination, and cannot be accelerated.
  - ○ Exception exists for drugs that can be antagonized ($\alpha_2$ agonists, benzodiazepines).
- A fluid pump or syringe pump is necessary for accurate drug delivery.

## III   Methods of drug delivery

- Under ideal circumstances the amount of drug delivered, per unit time, should equal the drug's clearance ($C_L$).
- A constant rate infusion (CRI) should maintain a steady-state plasma concentration (Cp).

- A CRI is based on $C_L$ and the desired Cp, and can be expressed, in its simplest form as:

$$\text{CRI}\left(\mu g/kg/\min\right) = \text{Cp}\left(\mu g/mL\right) \times C_L\left(mL/\min/kg\right).$$

### A  Intermittent injection of drugs

- ○ This is the simplest method of drug delivery.
- ○ This method is satisfactory for maintaining anesthesia of short-duration.
- ○ However, it is not possible to maintain a steady plasma concentration using this method.

### B  Drip technique

- ○ With this technique, anesthetic drugs are added to commercial bags of isotonic fluids.
  - – Commercial fluid bags are overfilled, so this is a source of error.
- ○ The drip chamber is adjusted to give the desired flow rate.
- ○ For large volumes of injectate, it may be necessary to withdraw an equal volume of crystalloid from the fluid bag before adding the drug(s).

### C  Infusion pump

- ○ Can be programmed to deliver a specific volume of fluid in a given time.
- ○ The drugs to be infused are added to commercial bags of replacement fluids (e.g. 0.9% NaCl). (see Fig. 21.1)

### D  Syringe pump

- ○ Is an accurate method for delivering smaller volumes (maximum syringe volume is 60 ml).

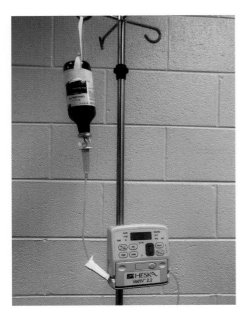

**Figure 21.1**  Use of a fluid pump to deliver a constant rate infusion of lidocaine. *Source:* Courtesy of Dr. Stephanie Kleine.

E   Computerized syringe pump

- A more sophisticated method of delivery.
- The pump delivers "*Target-Controlled Infusions*" based on drug-specific, kinetic/dynamic data incorporated into specific software programs; however, these systems have not yet been developed for equine anesthesia.

## IV   Choice of injectable drugs

- No one drug can adequately supply the basic components of balanced anesthesia in horses (sleep, relaxation, analgesia).
  - Therefore, two or more drugs are used in TIVA.
- The CSHT is an important concept to consider when infusing anesthetic drugs.
  - The CSHT is the time for the Cp to decrease by 50% following a specified time of infusion.
- For almost all drugs, the CSHT increases with infusion time.
  - The CSHT is relatively short and constant over time for *propofol,* and long for *thiopental.*
    - Therefore, prolonged infusions of *thiopental* may result in long recoveries.

## V   Drug combinations used for TIVA

- Commonly used TIVA protocols are listed in Table 21.3.
- It is important to consider the effect of premedication (e.g. *acepromazine*) on TIVA protocols.
  - *Acepromazine* administration is associated with an important clinical decrease in MAC, and thus would be expected to have an important contribution to TIVA.

Table 21.3   Commonly used TIVA protocols in equine practice. Recommended dosages for sedation are reported in Table 21.1.

| Sedation | Induction Dose (mg/kg) | Maintenance |
|---|---|---|
| **$\alpha_2$ agonist Ketamine** | | |
| Xylazine | Ketamine (2.0–2.5) ± Diazepam/midazolam (0.02–0.1) | Re-dosing: $\frac{1}{3}$-$\frac{1}{2}$ of initial dose of *xylazine* and *ketamine* every 10 minutes. |
| Detomidine/ Romifidine | Ketamine (2.0–2.5) ± Diazepam/midazolam (0.02–0.1) | Re-dosing: $\frac{1}{3}$-$\frac{1}{2}$ of initial dose ketamine every 10 minutes. $\frac{1}{3}$-$\frac{1}{2}$ of initial dose $\alpha_2$ agonist every 15–20 minutes. |
| **$\alpha_2$ agonist + Ketamine + Guaifenesin (*Triple Drip*)** | | |
| Xylazine/ Detomidine/ Romifidine | Ketamine (2.2) | Guaifenesin (5%), 0.5–1 L. Ketamine (2 g). Xylazine (500 mg)/or Detomidine (20 mg)/or Romifidine (50 mg). Infuse at a rate of ~2–3 mL/kg/hr. Dose rate needs to be adjusted to effect over time. |

**A** α₂ agonists + Ketamine

- ○ Are the most widely studied TIVA combinations.
- ○ Frequently used for short field procedures.
- ○ Anesthesia is induced with *ketamine* (or ketamine/benzodiazepine,) following sedation with the α₂ agonist.
- ○ Anesthesia is maintained with intermittent boluses (most common method in field conditions) or an infusion.
- ○ Generally limited to 45–60 minutes.

**B** α₂ agonist + Ketamine + Guaifenesin

- ○ *Ketamine, xylazine*, and *guaifenesin* is the most commonly used TIVA combination when using an infusion.
  - – Colloquially referred to as *"Triple Drip."*
- ○ Frequently used for procedures lasting up to 90 minutes.
- ○ Infusion times >90 minutes will worsen recovery quality, and this is most likely due to accumulation of *guaifenesin*.
  - – Using a lower dose of *guaifenesin* may reduce ataxia/weakness in recovery.
- ○ To reduce the potential for accumulation of *guaifenesin* and the associated bad recoveries, guaifenesin should *not* be used for induction.

**C** Propofol

- ○ Propofol is an ideal anesthetic for prolonged TIVA: it has a short CSHT leading to rapid recoveries.
- ○ However, if used alone for TIVA in horses it has the following disadvantages:
  - – Severe respiratory depression.
  - – Hypotension.
  - – No analgesia.
  - – Poor inductions.
- ○ In an attempt to improve the quality of anesthesia, propofol may be combined with one or more drugs (e.g. *α₂ agonists, ketamine, guaifenesin, opioids*), thereby allowing for a reduced dose of propofol.
- ○ Recoveries are generally good if sedative drugs are administered, but serious respiratory depression limits the clinical use of propofol.
- ○ If propofol is used alone for maintenance of anesthesia, a CRI of up to 0.3 mg/kg/min is necessary to prevent movement in response to surgical stimulation.
- ○ Lower infusion rates and better outcomes result if *propofol* is part of a multimodal drug regimen, including an α₂ agonist.
  e.g. *Propofol* (0.14–0.20 mg/kg/min) + *Ketamine* (3.0 mg/kg/hr).
  e.g. *Propofol* (0.13–0.17 mg/kg/min) + *Ketamine* (1.0 mg/kg/hr) + α₂ agonist (e.g. *Medetomidine* 1.25 µg/kg/hr or *Xylazine* 0.5 mg/kg/hr).
- ○ The high *cost* of propofol is another limiting factor.

**D** Alfaxalone

- ○ Alfaxalone has been used alone and in combination with different drugs (*medetomidine, guaifenesin, opioids*) for TIVA.

- ○ Good hemodynamic stability, but clinically important respiratory depression is associated with its use.
- ○ *Alfaxalone* does not appear to be a good drug choice for TIVA when used *alone* for long procedures.
  - – Alfaxalone administration at 3 mg/kg/hr for three hours was associated with unacceptable recovery quality in horses. The horses exhibited paddling, muscle twitches, and exaggerated responses to noise and handling.
- ○ In contrast, good anesthetic conditions and recoveries were reported when *alfaxalone* (2 mg/kg/hr) was infused with *medetomidine* (5 μg/kg/hr) for 60 minutes.
  - – However, it is important to understand that these horses were premedicated with *acepromazine* (0.03 mg/kg, IV), and *guaifenesin* (35 mg/kg) was administered at induction, and this may have had a positive influence on the recovery. In addition, the duration of alfaxalone infusion was short.
- ○ The high cost of *alfaxalone* limits its use in horses.

## Partial Intravenous Anesthesia (PIVA)

- PIVA involves the combined use of *inhalational* and *IV* anesthetics, sedatives, and analgesics to produce the desired degree of unconsciousness, analgesia, and muscle relaxation whilst maintaining good cardiopulmonary function.
- The goal of PIVA, is to achieve a state of "*balanced*" anesthesia by using two or more drugs in combination.
- By reducing the delivered concentration of inhalational anesthetics their negative cardiorespiratory effects will be reduced if IV drugs with less depressant effects replace them.

## I   Potential advantages of PIVA

- Reduced cardiorespiratory depression (lower concentration of inhalational drugs).
- Superior analgesia, reduced risk for postoperative hyperalgesia.
- More stable anesthesia.
- Decreased likelihood of intraoperative movement in response to surgical stimulation.
- Improved outcome (i.e. better recoveries, decreased morbidity and mortality).

## II   Potential disadvantages of PIVA

- Cardiopulmonary depression of inhalational drugs, although reduced, is still present.
- Need to have equipment to deliver IV and inhalational drugs if they are to be delivered accurately.
- Monitoring the plasma concentrations of IV drugs is not feasible at present.
- Accumulation of IV drugs or their active metabolites might occur during long procedures, negatively influencing recovery.
  *Note*: Drug accumulation, although generally not an issue, can be avoided by decreasing the infusion rate over time.

## III  Choice of IV drugs for PIVA

- The major goals of PIVA in horses are:
  - To provide analgesia.
  - To reduce the MAC of the inhalational drug.
  - To reduce inhalational anesthetic associated cardiopulmonary depression.
  - To facilitate a smooth recovery.
- Drugs chosen for PIVA should, at least, meet these requirements. Desirable traits include:
  - MAC reduction (e.g. *ketamine, $\alpha_2$ agonists, lidocaine*).
  - Analgesia (e.g. *ketamine, $\alpha_2$ agonists, lidocaine, opioids*).
  - Minimum effects on cardiopulmonary system (e.g. *ketamine, lidocaine*).
  - Minimal organ toxicity at appropriate doses (e.g. *ketamine, lidocaine, opioids, $\alpha_2$ agonists*).
  - Short context-sensitive half-life *(e.g. dexmedetomidine, medetomidine, xylazine, propofol)*, no clinically important accumulation of active metabolites as the duration of drug infusion increases.
  - Reduction of stress response (e.g. *$\alpha_2$ agonists*).
  - Compatibility with other drugs used for infusion.
    *Comment*: As in the case of TIVA, no drug meets all these requirements; therefore, more than one IV drug is often used in combination with inhalational anesthesia.

## IV  Drugs and drug regimens used in PIVA

A variety of injectable drugs and drug combinations can be used in PIVA (see Table 21.4). *Note:* It is assumed, that to facilitate a smooth recovery, horses will be sedated once placed in the recovery area after completion of the injectable drug(s) infusion.

### A  Lidocaine

- *Dose-dependent MAC reduction ~ 20–30% (3–6 mg/kg/hr).*
- It is generally recommended that the CRI be stopped 30 minutes before the end of anesthesia in order to decrease the incidence of ataxia in recovery. However, the plasma concentration of lidocaine and its metabolites, and hence the degree of ataxia, will decrease as the horse spends time in lateral recumbency before attempting to rise. Thus, ataxia would be expected to be of less consequence if the horse is sedated in recovery and delays attempts to stand.

### B  $\alpha_2$ agonists

- The use of an $\alpha_2$ agonist in PIVA results in better recoveries than following the use of lidocaine or ketamine in PIVA protocols.
  - This effect is to be expected based on the sedating effects of $\alpha_2$ agonists.
- $\alpha_2$ agonists cause *diuresis* and the resultant loss of fluid and electrolytes has to be accounted for when fluid infusion rate is determined.
  - A urinary catheter should be placed for longer procedures.

Table 21.4 Commonly used constant rate infusions for partial intravenous anesthesia (PIVA) in horses. PIVA consist of combining inhalation anesthetics with injectable anesthetics/adjuvants.

| Drugs | Dose rate (mg/kg/hr) | Comments |
|---|---|---|
| Medetomidine/ Dexmedetomidine/ Xylazine | 0.0035–0.005 0.00175–0.0025 0.5–1.0 | Diuresis: urinary catheter recommended when $\alpha_2$ agonists are infused. MAC decrease is 30–50% for these drugs. |
| Detomidine Romifidine | 0.010 0.018–0.040 | No MAC reduction expected. Minimal MAC reduction. |
| Lidocaine | 3–6 | A loading dose of 2–3 mg/kg is usually administered over 10–15 minutes IV, although it can be administered in 1–2 minutes without adverse effects in normotensive patients. MAC decrease 20–30%. Discontinue CRI 30 minutes before recovery. |
| Ketamine | 1–2 | MAC 15–25%. |
| Ketamine + $\alpha_2$ agonists | 1–2 + See first row | MAC decrease 50–70%. Urinary catheter recommended. |
| Lidocaine + Ketamine | 4 + 2 | Discontinue *lidocaine* CRI 30 minutes before recovery. MAC decrease 30–40%. |
| Lidocaine + Ketamine + Xylazine | 4 + 2 1 | Discontinue CRI of *lidocaine* 30 minutes before recovery. Urinary catheter recommended. MAC decrease 70–90%. |
| Lidocaine + Ketamine + Medetomidine | 4 + 2 0.0035 | Discontinue CRI of *lidocaine* 30 minutes before recovery. Urinary catheter recommended. MAC decrease 70–90%. |

*Medetomidine/Dexmedetomidine/Xylazine*
  ○ MAC reduction is dose-dependent.
*Dexmedetomidine*
  ○ Dexmedetomidine (1.75 µg/kg/hr) decreased the MAC of sevoflurane by 53%.
  ○ The addition of *morphine* (a bolus of 0.15 mg/kg IV, and a CRI of 0.1 mg/kg/hr) to dexmedetomidine (1.75 µg/kg/hr) was associated with a combined decrease of 67% in MAC.
  ○ In contrast, *morphine* did not augment the effect of *xylazine* on halothane MAC in horses. *Note*: In situations where it is not feasible to administer an infusion (e.g. lack of a syringe pump), it is efficacious to administer *dexmedetomidine* IM (2.5–3.0 µg/kg) at 45–60-minute intervals. Dexmedetomidine is injected using a 24-gauge needle superficially into the muscle. Injecting dexmedetomidine in this way slows its uptake, and is associated with only a mild increase in blood pressure, and little to no effect on CO and HR. (Editor: personal communication Dr. Bernd Driessen June 2020).

*Xylazine*
  ○ The clinical impression is that *xylazine* (1 mg/kg/hr) decreases MAC by at least 40%.

*Detomidine/Romifidine*
  ○ It is of interest that *detomidine* and *romifidine* were associated with only a modest or *no* isoflurane sparing effect in some clinical studies.
  ○ To the contrary, a large bolus of *detomidine* (0.03 or 0.06 mg/kg, IV) was associated with a decrease in the MAC of isoflurane of approximately 40% for up to 2 hrs.
  ○ *Detomidine* (0.005 mg/kg/hr) was *not* associated with a decrease in the end-tidal isoflurane concentration needed to maintain a surgical plane of anesthesia in one study.
  ○ *Detomidine* (0.01 mg/kg/hr) was associated with a decrease of just 15% in the end-tidal isoflurane concentration needed to maintain a surgical plane of anesthesia in another study. *Romifidine* (0.04 mg/kg/hr) was associated with an isoflurane sparing effect of 18% in the same study.

C   Ketamine

  ○ The MAC reduction with ketamine in horses seems to be less than with $\alpha_2$ agonists. MAC reduction is dose-dependent, and at common dose rates (1–2 mg/kg/hr) the MAC is reduced by ~20%.
  *Note*: In halothane-anesthetized horses, the maximum decrease in MAC was 37% at a plasma concentration of ~10 µg/ml, which is about four to five times greater than the plasma concentration achieved with common infusion rates.

D   Ketamine and $\alpha_2$ agonists

  ○ *Dexmedetomidine* and *xylazine* would seem to be the most appropriate $\alpha_2$ agonists for PIVA based on their MAC reducing effects.
  ○ The expected MAC reduction of the combination of *ketamine* (1–2 mg/kg/hr) with *dexmedetomidine* (1.75 µg/kg/hr) or *xylazine* (1 mg/kg/hr) is 60–70%.

E   Lidocaine + Ketamine

  ○ In one study, *lidocaine* (3 mg/kg/hr) + *ketamine* (3 mg/kg/hr) decreased the MAC of isoflurane by ~50%.
  ○ The duration of anesthesia was 166 minutes. Horses were not sedated in recovery, and made their first attempt to stand at 17 minutes.
  ○ The recovery qualities were not significantly different from the isoflurane control group but were subjectively considered to be better in the control group.
    – Presumably, the quality of recovery with this drug regimen can be improved by administering an $\alpha_2$ agonist.

## Suggested Reading

Bennett, R.C., Steffey, E.P., Kollias-Baker, C., and Sams, R. (2004). Influence of morphine sulfate on the halothane sparing effect of xylazine hydrochloride in horses. *Am. J. Vet. Res.* 65: 519–526.

Devisscher, L., Schauvliege, S., Dewulf, J., and Gasthuys, F. (2010). Romifidine as a constant rate infusion in isoflurane anaesthetized horses: a clinical study. *Vet. Anaesth. Analg.* 37: 425–433.

Goodwin, W.A., Pasloske, K., Keates, H.L. et al. (2019). Alfaxalone for total intravenous anaesthesia in horses. *Vet. Anaesth. Analg.* 46: 188–199.

Gozalo-Marcilla, M., Gasthuys, F., and Schauvliege, S. (2014). Partial intravenous anaesthesia in the horse: a review of intravenous agents used to supplement equine inhalation anaesthesia. Part 1: lidocaine and ketamine. *Vet. Anaesth. Analg.* 41: 335–345.

Gozalo-Marcilla, M., Gasthuys, F., and Schauvliege, S. (2015). Partial intravenous anaesthesia in the horse: a review of intravenous agents used to supplement equine inhalation anaesthesia. Part 2: opioids and alpha-2 adrenoceptor agonists. *Vet. Anaesth. Analg.* 42: 1–16.

Niimura Del Barrio, M.C., Bennett, R.C., and Hughes, J.M.L. (2017). Effect of detomidine or romifidine constant rate infusion on plasma lactate concentration and inhalant requirements during isoflurane anaesthesia in horses. *Vet. Anaesth. Analg.* 44: 473–482.

Schauvliege, S., Gozalo Marcilla, M., Verryken, K. et al. (2011). Effects of a constant rate infusion of detomidine on cardiovascular function, isoflurane requirements and recovery quality in horses. *Vet. Anaesth. Analg.* 38: 544–554.

Steffey, E.P. and Pascoe, P.J. (2002). Detomidine reduces isoflurane anesthetic requirement (MAC) in horses. *Vet. Anaesth. Analg.* 29: 223–227.

Umar, M.A., Fukui, S., Kawase, K. et al. (2015). Cardiovascular effects of total intravenous anesthesia using ketamine-medetomidine-propofol (KMP-TIVA) in horses undergoing surgery. *J. Vet. Med. Sci.* 77: 281–288.

Villalba, M., Santiago, I., and Gomez de Segura, I.A. (2011). Effects of constant rate infusion of lidocaine and ketamine, with or without morphine, on isoflurane MAC in horses. *Eq. Vet. J.* 43: 721–726.

# 22

## Anesthesia of the Head and Neck

### Anesthesia of the Head

*Jim Schumacher, John Schumacher, and Ray Wilhite*

- Regional nerve blocks of the head, apart from those of the eye, are most commonly performed to facilitate surgery of the dentition or paranasal sinuses.
- Regional nerve blocks can be used in the sedated horse to allow suturing of lacerations of the head.
- Administration of the regional nerve block to the head can be facilitated by applying a nose twitch to the horse.
  - Regional nerve blocks of the head are shown in Figures 22.1–22.5.

A   Infraorbital nerve block
  - Facilitates surgery of the *nose, upper lip,* or *incisors.*
  - The infraorbital nerve can be anesthetized at its point of emergence from the *infraorbital foramen* or within the infraorbital canal (see Figure 22.1).
    - When the nerve is anesthetized at its *point of emergence*, the desensitized area comprises the skin of the ipsilateral lip, nostril, and face, to the level of the foramen.
    - When the nerve is anesthetized *within the infraorbital canal*, additional desensitized structures include the ipsilateral premaxillary incisors, canine tooth, wolf tooth, cheek teeth, and associated alveoli and gingiva.
  - Adequate restraint and great care should be taken during its administration because the infraorbital block is tolerated poorly if the needle tip pierces the nerve, and this may result in permanent nerve damage.
    *Note:* It is preferable to use an *over-the-needle catheter* (2 in, 18G) rather than a hypodermic needle. In that way, the catheter instead of a needle is advanced into the canal decreasing the likelihood of piercing the nerve.
  - Instilling local anesthetic within the infraorbital canal assures that the infraorbital nerve is anesthetized.

*Manual of Equine Anesthesia and Analgesia*, Second Edition. Edited by Tom Doherty, Alex Valverde, and Rachel A. Reed.

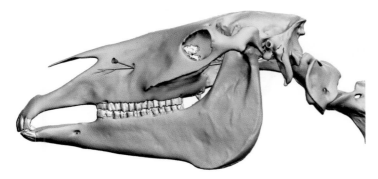

Figure 22.1    Approach to the infraorbital nerve within the infraorbital canal.

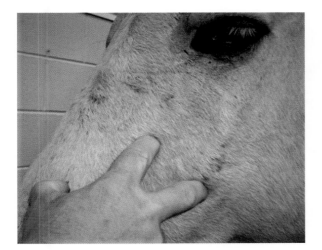

Figure 22.2    Location of the infraorbital canal between the nasoincisive notch and the facial crest.

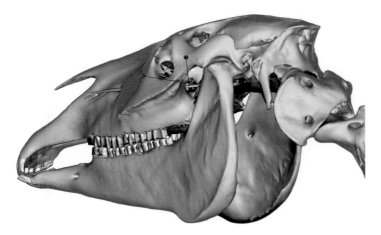

Figure 22.3    Approach to the maxillary nerve within the pterygopalatine fossa.

(a)

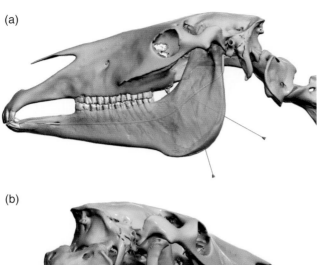

(b)

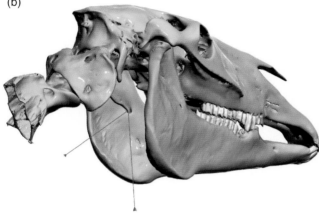

Figure 22.4    Extraoral approach to the mandibular nerve. Lateral aspect (a) and medial aspect (b).

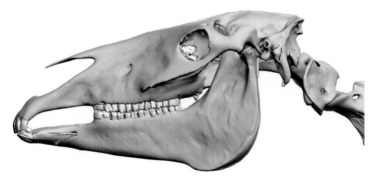

Figure 22.5    Approach to the mental nerve at the level of the mental foramen.

*Location*

o The infraorbital foramen is located by placing a thumb (or middle finger) in the notch formed by the nasal bone and premaxillae (i.e. the nasoincisive notch) and the middle finger (or thumb) on the rostral end of the facial crest.

– The foramen is located with the index finger halfway between these points and 1 to 3 cm caudal to an imaginary line connecting these points.

o The bony ridge of the foramen can be palpated beneath the ventral edge of the *levator nasolabialis* muscle (see Figure 22.2).

*Technique* (within the infraorbital canal)

    o Insert a 21- or 22-gauge, 3.81 cm (1.5 in.) needle, or preferably an *over-the-needle catheter* (2 in, 18G), through the skin about 1 cm rostral to the foramen, after pushing the ventral edge of the *levator nasolabialis* muscle dorsally.

    o Insert the needle/catheter about 2.5 cm into the canal and deposit 4–5 ml of local anesthetic solution.

## B  Maxillary nerve block

    o All the dental structures of the ipsilateral maxilla and premaxilla and most of the ipsilateral paranasal sinuses and nasal passage are desensitized

*Location*

    o The maxillary nerve is anesthetized at the *pterygopalatine fossa*, where the nerve enters the infraorbital canal to become the infraorbital nerve.

*Technique*

    o Insert the point of a 20- to 22-gauge, 8.9 cm (3.5 in.) spinal needle just ventral to the zygomatic process and dorsal to the transverse facial vessels, at the level of the caudal third of the eye.

      – Use a *Tuohy* needle or a needle with a short bevel to help avoid inadvertent venipuncture of large vessels in the vicinity of the nerve.

      – Venipuncture may result in a retrobulbar *hematoma*, causing the eye to protrude slightly, putting the horse at risk of developing a corneal ulcer.

      – The point of the needle is inserted at a 90° angle to the head so that it enters the *pterygopalatine fossa*, just caudal to the maxillary tuberosity at a depth of 6.5–7.0 cm (see Figure 22.3).

      – The horse may jerk its head in the unlikely event that the needle contacts the nerve.

      – If blood is withdrawn from the needle, the needle has been inserted too far ventrally or caudally.

    o 15–20 ml of local anesthetic is deposited near the *pterygopalatine fossa*, as the needle is withdrawn slightly.

    o A retrobulbar hematoma can be avoided by inserting the needle only 5 cm, at which point its tip should have penetrated the masseter muscle and entered an extra-periorbital body of fat. Local anesthetic injected into this fat diffuses to surround the nerve.

    o Structures innervated by the maxillary nerve are desensitized within 10–15 minutes.

## C  Mandibular alveolar (or inferior alveolar) nerve block

    o Desensitizes the ipsilateral side of the *mandible* and all its dental structures.

    o The mandibular alveolar nerve can be anesthetized where it enters the mandibular canal at the *mandibular foramen*.

*Location*

    o The mandibular foramen is located on the medial aspect of the vertical ramus of the mandible, at the intersection of an imaginary line extending along and caudal to the occlusal surface of the mandibular cheek teeth and a second imaginary line that passes perpendicular to the first line from the lateral canthus of the eye.

*Extra-oral approach*

- ○ Insert the point of a 20- to 22-gauge, 15.2–20.3 cm (6–8 in.) spinal needle at the ventral border of the mandible, near the angle of the mandible.
- ○ Advance the point of the needle 10–15 cm dorsally along the medial surface of the vertical ramus to reach the intersection of the previously described imaginary lines, and deposit 10–20 ml of local anesthetic (see Figure 22.4a and b).
  - – The stylet of the needle can be used to judge the depth of the insertion of the needle.
  - – The mandibular alveolar nerve courses toward the mandibular foramen in a dorso-caudal direction, so the nerve can be anesthetized if the tip of the needle resides caudal and dorsal to the foramen. The nerve fails to become anesthetized if the tip of the needle resides ventral or rostral to the foramen.
- ○ The *lingual nerve*, which supplies motor and sensory innervation to the tongue, arises from a common trunk with the mandibular alveolar nerve *close to the mandibular foramen*. Inadvertent anesthesia of this nerve desensitizes the tongue, which may result in self-inflicted trauma to the tongue.
  - – Feed should be withheld from the horse for at least several hours after the mandibular alveolar nerve has been anesthetized, to minimize the likelihood of the horse inflicting trauma to its desensitized tongue.
- ○ Structures innervated by the mandibular alveolar nerve are desensitized within 15–30 minutes.

*Intra-oral approach*

- ○ Equipment: A 3.81 cm (1.5 in.), 20- to 22-gauge hypodermic needle, bent in a slight curve in the direction of its bevel, attached to an extension set with a Luer-lock and secured to a rod that has a T-handle.
- ○ Introduce the rod with attached needle and extension set into the mouth, with the curve of the needle directed up.
- ○ Insert the tip of the needle into the mucosa overlying the rostral border of the vertical ramus of the mandible, just distal (caudal) to the mandibular third molar and slightly dorsal to the level of the occlusal surface of the dental arcade, staying lateral to the palatoglossal arch.
- ○ Advance the needle until the rostral edge of the ramus is encountered, and rotate the rod so that the point of the needle is oriented laterally.
- ○ Angle the rod to the contralateral side of the oral cavity and walk the tip of the needle along the medial side of the vertical ramus to a depth of 3.5 cm.
- ○ Deposit 5 ml of local anesthetic.
- ○ The likelihood of inadvertently anesthetizing the *lingual nerve* is low when using the intra-oral approach.

D   Mental nerve block

- ○ The mandibular alveolar nerve traverses the mandibular canal and emerges at the mental foramen, and at this point, it is referred to as the *mental nerve*.
- ○ Anesthetizing the mental nerve at the *mental foramen* or the mandibular alveolar nerve within the rostral end of the *mandibular canal* is referred to as the *mental nerve block*.
  - – Anesthetizing the mental nerve *as it exits the mental foramen* desensitizes the skin of the lip and chin of that side of the head.

– Anesthetizing the mental nerve *within the mandibular canal* also desensitizes the ipsilateral mandibular canine tooth, incisors, and cheek teeth and associated alveoli and gingiva.

Note: The mental nerve block is tolerated poorly because the point of the needle contacts the nerve directly. For this reason, an *over-the-needle catheter* may be a better choice than a hypodermic needle as described for the infraorbital block.

*Location*
- The mental foramen can be palpated on the lateral aspect of the horizontal ramus of the mandible at the level of the intermandibular space ventral to the commissure of the lips, after pushing the tendon of the *depressor labii inferioris* muscle dorsally.

*Technique* (within the mandibular canal)
- Insert a 21- or 22-gauge, 3.81 cm (1.5 in.) needle, or an *over-the-needle catheter* (2 in, 18G) through the skin 2 cm rostral to the mental foramen after pushing the tendon of the *depressor labii inferioris* muscle dorsally (see Figure 22.5).
- Advance the needle/catheter 2 cm into the mandibular canal and deposit 5–10 ml of local anesthetic.
  - The curvature of the mentum of the mandible, close to the site of the mandibular foramen, may inhibit inserting the needle at the requisite acute angle to the horizontal ramus of the mandible. Bending the shaft of the needle eases insertion of the needle into the mandibular canal. Due to the curvature of the mentum, it is generally easier to pass an *over-the-needle catheter* than a hypodermic needle into the mandibular canal.

## E   Ethmoidal nerve block

- The ethmoidal nerve provides sensory innervation to the caudal portion of the ipsilateral frontal sinus, dorsal nasal concha, and caudal portion of the nasal septum.

*Location*
- The site of insertion of the needle is at the rostromedial aspect of the supraorbital fossa, caudal and medial to the orbit, where the caudal aspect of the zygomatic process of the frontal bone projects from the squamous temporal bone.

*Technique*
- Insert a 6.4 cm (2.5 in.), 20-gauge spinal needle at the site of insertion, to its hub, caudodorsal to rostroventral in a sagittal plane, at an angle of 110° (measured using a protractor), and dorsolateral to ventromedial, at angle of 110°, in a transverse plane.
  - The needle can be inserted at these same angles by directing the needle parallel to the rostral edge of the vertical ramus of the ipsilateral hemi-mandible and aiming toward the contralateral angle of the mandible.
- Five ml of local anesthetic is deposited.

## Suggested Reading

Campoy, L. and Sedgwick, S.R. (2020). Standing sedation and locoregional analgesia in equine dental surgery. *Vet. Clin. North Am. Equine Pract.* 36: 477–499.

Rice, M.K. (2017). Regional nerve blocks for equine dentistry. *J. Vet. Dent.* 34: 106–109.

Tanner, R.B. and Hubbell, J.A.E. (2019). Management of complications associated with regional nerve blocks in equine dental patients. *J. Vet. Dent.* 36: 40–45.

# Maxillary Nerve Block in Donkeys
*Usama Hagag*

## I  Indications

- Desensitizing the maxillary branch of the trigeminal nerve is potentially useful for:
  - Surgical procedures of the paranasal sinuses, maxilla and premaxilla.
    - Providing anesthesia for various dental procedures on the desensitized side.
    - Providing anesthesia for surgeries involving the nasal wall, nasal diverticulum, gums, hard palate and upper lip of the corresponding side.
  - Providing adjunctive analgesia for donkeys undergoing sinus and orofacial surgeries.
  - *Note*: Deep sedation is required as a maxillary nerve block alone is not sufficient for performing standing tooth extraction or orofacial surgeries.

## II  General principles

### A  Local anesthetic drug selection and doses

- *Lidocaine HCl 2%, bupivacaine HCl 0.5% and mepivacaine HCl 2%* are commonly used local anesthetics for blocking the maxillary nerve.
- *Mepivacaine* has a fast onset, minimum tissue irritation and acts longer than *lidocaine*.
- *Bupivacaine HCl* is four times more potent and acts longer than *lidocaine* and *mepivacaine*.
- 20 ml of the local anesthetic solution is required to block the maxillary nerve.

### B  Ultrasound-guided maxillary blockade allows for:

- Visualization of regional anatomy.
- Navigation away from sensitive structures, thus reducing the risk of complications.
- Guiding the needle toward the nerve with greater accuracy and a higher success rate.
- Reducing the need for multiple needle insertions, hence reducing tissue damage.
- Decreasing the volume of anesthetic required to achieve effect.
- Minimizing block performance time (faster onset of pain control).
- Monitoring the perineural spread of local anesthetic during injection.
- Identifying flow when using color-flow Doppler, which is useful for confirming the location of blood vessels.

### C  Equipment

- Disposable or sterile gloves (preferred).
- Local anesthetic agent.
- 20 ml disposable syringes.
- Disposable needles.
  - A 25-gauge (25 mm) needle to deposit 1–2 ml of local anesthetic subcutaneously at the injection site.

- – An 18-gauge, 90 mm spinal needle to deliver the local anesthetic adjacent to the maxillary nerve.
  - ○ Ultrasound machine supplied with multi-frequency probe for ultrasound-guided maxillary block.
    - – The quality of ultrasound images depends on the quality of the machine, proper transducer frequency selection and clinician's skills.
    - – Linear or micro-convex multi-frequency transducers (5–10 MHz) are suitable to image the maxillary nerve.

*Note*: The operator should be familiar with:
- Ultrasound equipment settings to optimize images.
- Anatomy of the *pterygopalatine fossa* and appearance of each structure on the ultrasound image.

## III Patient preparation

### A Physical restraint

- ○ The donkey should be restrained in stocks to minimize risk to personnel as it may react if the needle hits or pierces the nerve during the procedure.
- ○ A lip twitch may be required to control the animal's head during needle insertion and injection of the local anesthetic.

### B Chemical restraint

- ○ Sedation is necessary to control the donkey and minimize head movement.
- ○ *Xylazine HCl* (0.8–1.2 mg/kg, IV) or *detomidine HCl* (0.01–0.02 mg/kg, IV) can be used.

### C Preparation of injection site

- ○ Shave the area ventral to the lateral canthus of the eye and caudal to the facial crest to minimize the risk of infection and define the exact site of injection.
- ○ Prepare the injection site aseptically.
- ○ Apply the *coupling gel* for ultrasound-guided blocks.

## IV General technique

- Knowledge of topographic landmarks of the injection site and recognition of anatomic structures in the *pterygopalatine fossa* (ultrasound-guided technique) are indispensable for successful maxillary block.
- Local anesthetic should be accurately deposited close to the nerve.
  - ○ Knowledge of the landmarks reduces the risk of inadvertent injury of adjacent vascular structures.
  - ○ A smaller volume of local anesthetic will be required.
  - ○ A rapid onset of action will be achieved.

## A Needle insertion

*Blind technique*

- o In the *blind* technique, the preference of the clinician determines whether the needle is introduced *perpendicular* or *oblique* to the skin surface.
- o The needle is inserted deeply until it contacts the *palatine* bone, then withdrawn a few millimeters before injection.
- o Head jerking may occur due to needle contacting the nerve.
- o Care should be taken to avoid personnel injury, needle breaking or animal injury.
- o If blood appears in the needle hub, the needle should be slightly withdrawn and redirected.

*Ultrasound guided approach*

- o In the ultrasound-guided approach, the needle path is monitored, and the needle is advanced until it is within a few millimeters (~3 mm) of the nerve.

## V Checking for desensitization

- Successful blind or ultrasound-guided technique is verified by a lack of response when a noxious stimulus (e.g. needle prick) is apply to the skin of the ipsilateral naris.
- Testing of skin sensation can be performed 15–20 minutes following local anesthetic administration, as the maxillary nerve is relatively large and some time is required for desensitization.
- Donkeys may react to stimulation by head, neck and/or trunk movement.
- Failure to block the nerve may be the result of inaccurate placement of the needle and/or inadequate exposure of the nerve to local anesthetic.

## VI Complications

- Though rare, may include:
  - o Infection at the site of injection.
  - o Inadvertent vascular puncture.
  - o Retrobulbar hematoma.
  - o Facial hematoma.
  - o Exophthalmos.
  - o Ocular muscle paralysis.
  - o Horner's syndrome.
  - o Blindness.
  - o Retrobulbar infection and meningitis.

## VII Specific techniques for maxillary block

## A Blind maxillary nerve block

- o Knowledge of regional anatomy is the key for accurate deposition of local anesthetic and avoiding injury of nearby structures.
  - – Landmarks include the facial crest, zygomatic arch, lateral canthus of eye, caudal part of maxilla, and vertical ramus of the mandible.

- Two techniques can be used for blind deposition of the local anesthetic into the pterygopalatine fossa.

*Angled approach* (see Figure 22.6)

- Insert the needle at the narrowest point of zygomatic arch (angle formed by the caudal part of maxilla and vertical ramus of mandible).
- Advance the needle (18-gauge, 90 mm spinal needle) rostromedially and ventrally in the direction of the sixth molar tooth of the contralateral maxillary arcade.

*Perpendicular approach* (see Figure 22.7)

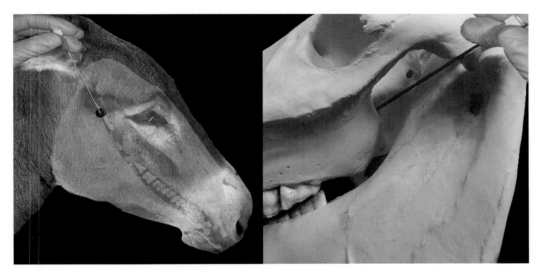

Figure 22.6   Angled, blind approach to the maxillary nerve in the donkey.

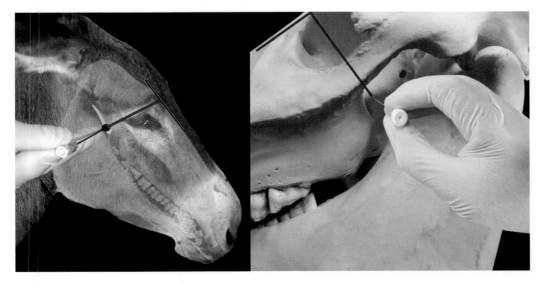

Figure 22.7   Perpendicular approach to the maxillary nerve in the donkey.

○ Follow the facial crest caudally to the point where the crest starts to deviate dorsally to become a part of zygomatic arch.
– Draw an imaginary line running perpendicular to the dorsal head contour through the lateral canthus of the eye.
– The puncture site is 2 cm ventral to the lateral canthus of the eye.
○ Insert the needle perpendicular to skin surface.

B   **Ultrasound-guided maxillary nerve block** (see Figure 22.8)

○ Place the probe caudal to the facial crest (red line) and ventral to an imaginary line connecting the medial and lateral canthi and extending beyond the facial crest (green line).
○ Direct the ultrasound beam toward the last maxillary cheek tooth of the other side.
○ Scan from dorsal to ventral to localize the maxillary foramen as a hypoechoic break of the hyperechoic palatine bone (p) (see Figure 22.9).
○ Insert the spinal needle (oblique to skin surface) 1 cm ventral to the probe in the long axis of the ultrasound beam (in-plane approach).
– This approach aims to align and move the long axis of the needle along the long axis of the ultrasound beam.
– With this approach the full needle tip and shaft are within the field of view (white arrows).
○ Advance the needle deeply toward the maxillary foramen until the maxillary nerve and its associated vascular structures (see Figure 22.9) the deep facial vein (v) and infraorbital artery (a) are recognized.
– Vascular components appear as well-differentiated oval to round hypoechogenic structures surrounded by a hyperechogenic thin rim.
– The maxillary nerve is identified as a bright hyperechogenic structure as deep as 4–5 cm of below the skin surface.

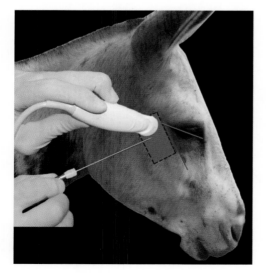

**Figure 22.8**   Ultrasound-guided approach to the maxillary nerve in the donkey.

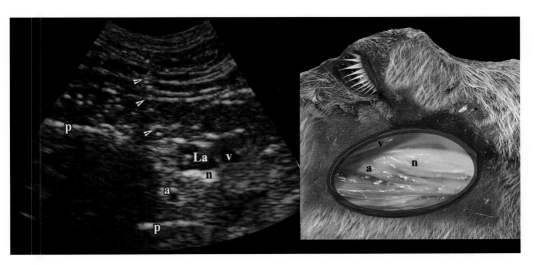

Figure 22.9   Ultrasound image of the maxillary nerve and adjacent structures in the donkey. p = palatine bone. n = maxillary nerve. v = deep facial vein. a = infraorbital artery. La = anechoic shadow around the nerve due to spread of local anesthetic from needle tip.

        ○ After negative aspiration, the local anesthetic is slowly injected.
            – It is necessary to evacuate air from the needle and syringe before injection to avoid air artifacts in the ultrasound image.
            – Spreading of local anesthetic from needle tip around the nerve can be monitored as anechoic (La) shadow.

## Cervical Plexus Block

*Luis Campoy*

## I   Introduction

- In human beings, the cervical plexus is formed by the anterior divisions of cervical spinal nerves C2–C4, and it innervates the skin and superficial structures of the cervical region.
- Procedures involving the cervical region such as thyroid and parathyroidectomies and carotid endarterectomies are commonly carried out under a superficial cervical plexus block (see Egan et al., Seidel et al.).
- An ultrasound-guided technique to block the cervical plexus (C2 and C3) to provide sufficient analgesia in horses undergoing standing prosthetic laryngoplasty has been described (see Campoy et al.). Additionally, the authors compared the use of this block with a more frequently used surgical site infiltration in horses undergoing the aforementioned surgical procedure. There was an overall improvement in the surgical field conditions associated with the block (less edema and less hemorrhage); however, surgical times were not shorter.
  - ○ The effects of this block on anesthetic requirements and quality of recovery following prosthetic laryngoplasty in horses undergoing general anesthesia with an inhalational agent were investigated (see Morris et al.).

    o Non-blocked horses were 4.7 times more likely to require additional medication during surgical manipulation, and six times more likely to receive adjunctive intravenous anesthesia.

    o Additionally, blocked horses were 25 times less likely to receive additional medication in the recovery period.

    o No differences were observed in recovery quality between groups.

## II   Indications for the block

- Prosthetic laryngoplasty under general anesthesia or procedural sedation.
- Ear surgery (in combination with additional nerve blocks).
- Skin lacerations of the base of the ear and occipital area.

## III   Contraindications

- Peripheral neuropathies.
- Skin infection close to the puncture site.

## IV   Clinical anatomy (see Figure 22.10)

- In Figure 22.10, dissection of the C1–C3 segments and immediately under the skin and subcutaneous tissues, the *splenius m., omotransversarius m., cleidomastoideus m., parotidoauricularis m., omohyoideus m., sternothyroideus m., sternocephalicus m.,* and *cutaneous colli m.* as well as the parotid gland can be observed. The external jugular vein and the linguofacial v. can also be observed.

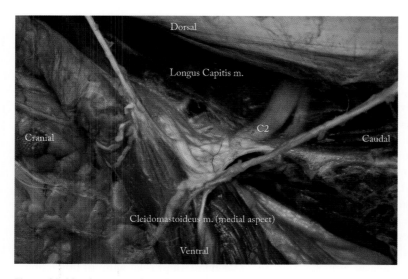

**Figure 22.10**   Anatomy of surgical site for cervical plexus block.

- Approximately 6–8 cm caudal to the wing of the atlas, the second cervical spinal nerve can be observed emerging from the intervertebral foramina running laterally.
- The components of the cervical plexus can be observed within the fascial plane ventral to the tendon of the *longissimus atlantis m.*, superficial to the *longus capitis m.*, and along the medial surface of the *cleidomastoideus m.*
- The transverse cervical nerve can be seen exiting in between the *omotransversarius* and the *cleidomastoideus* muscles and coursing the lateral surface of the cleidomastoideus m in a ventral direction toward the laryngeal area.
- The great auricular nerve branches off C2 and courses superficial to the neck muscles and over the body of C2 toward the ear from the fascial plane between the *omotransversarius m.* and *cleidomastoideus m.* It then divides into the anterior and posterior auricular branches.
  - The *occipital* nerves can also be seen coursing dorsally along the surface of the neck muscles toward the occipital area.
  - Minor cutaneous branches originating in the third cervical spinal nerve (C3) can also be identified over the *cleidomastoideus m.*, external jugular vein, *sternocephalicus m.*, *cutaneous colli m.*, *omohyoideus m.*, and *sternothyroideus m.* before being lost in the subcutaneous fascia.

## V Expected distribution of anesthesia

- A cervical plexus block will desensitize the skin over the surgical approach to the lateral larynx, as is necessary for laryngoplasty, but not the larynx itself (or some of the musculature such as the *cricopharyngeus m.*).
  - Infiltration at the level of C2 will also desensitize the great *auricular nerve* and the *occipital nerves*.
  - Blockade of the *great auricular* nerve will desensitize part of the posterior aspect of the ear as well as the skin around the base of the ear.
  - The *occipital* nerve block will also desensitize part of the posterior aspect of the ear (the posterior medial aspect as well as the skin over the occipital area).

### A Local anesthetic

  - *Mepivacaine* is commonly used by the author to provide sufficient duration to complete the surgery and to provide immediate postoperative analgesia.
    - 40 ml of a 2% is administered.
  - An additional 10 ml will be necessary to infiltrate the superficial cutaneous branches originated in C3. (see Figure 22.11)

### B Patient preparation and positioning

  - The horse should be positioned in the stocks, and it should be sedated appropriately to increase its tolerance for this procedure.
  - The head should be supported under the chin and pulled in a rostral direction so that the head and the neck are aligned (see Figure 22.12).
  - The lateral and ventral aspects of the laryngeal area and neck are clipped and surgically prepared.

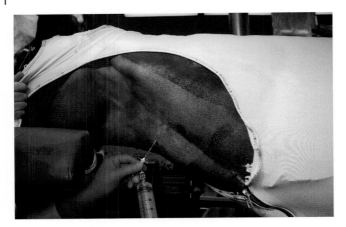

Figure 22.11    Infiltration of subcutaneous tissues caudal to the incision site. This is necessary for a complete block for prosthetic laryngoplasty surgery.

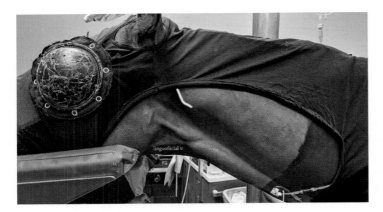

Figure 22.12    Surface anatomy and landmarks for cervical plexus block.

## VI    Step-by-step performance of the block

### A    Surface anatomy and landmarks (see Figure 22.12)

- The wing of the atlas and vertebral body of C2 should be identified as well as the *linguofacial* and *jugular* veins.
- The ultrasound transducer should be positioned ventral and approximately midway between the body of the second cervical vertebrae in a craniocaudal position, caudal to the parotid gland and ventral to the *omotransversarius muscle* in order to obtain a short axis view of C2.

### B    Ultrasound anatomy (see Figure 22.13)

- The *cleidomastoideus m.* can be observed with the *longus capitis m.* deep (medial) to it. A dense hyperechoic line formed by the fascias of both muscles can be seen separating the two muscles.

    ○ Caudal to the parotid gland and within this interfascial plane, a set of vessels can be seen in their short axis. Approximately 2 cm caudal to these vessels, C2 can be seen as a flat hyperechoic discoid/double discoid structure.

**C Needle insertion technique** (see Figure 22.14)

    ○ A 20-gauge 9 cm long (3.5 in.) Tuohy needle should be advanced in-plane toward the intermuscular plane between the *cleidomastoideus* and the *longus capitis* muscles.

    ○ Some of the local anesthetic solution can be used to hydrodissect this interfascial plane. Usually, the blood vessels tend to be attached to the cleidomastoideus m.

    ○ Once the tip of the needle is located in the proximity of C2, approximately 40 ml of local anesthetic solution can be injected (see Campoy et al. 2018).

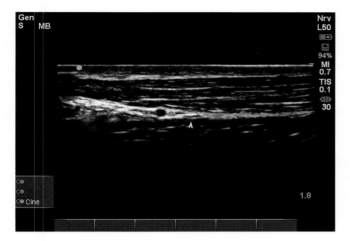

**Figure 22.13** Ultrasound image of injection site for cervical plexus block.

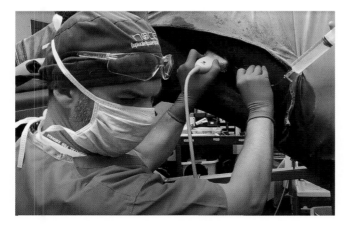

**Figure 22.14** Insertion of Tuohy using ultrasound guidance for cervical plexus block.

– An additional 10 ml of mepivacaine 2% should be infiltrated along a dorsoventral line in the subcutaneous tissue approximately 10 cm caudal to the caudal aspect of the incision site to complete the block for a prosthetic laryngoplasty (see Figure 22.11).

## VII  Complications

Potential complications include:
- ○ Transient Horner's syndrome occurs in about 25% of horses.
- ○ Transient laryngeal hemiplegia of the right arytenoid has been observed following standing prosthetic laryngoplasty.
  - – It is suspected that diffusion of additional local anesthetic infiltration resulted in blockade of the *right caudal laryngeal nerve*, resulting in altered right *cricoarytenoideus dorsalis* function and transient right arytenoid dysfunction (see Morris et al).

## Suggested Reading

Campoy, L., Morris, T.B., Ducharme, N.G. et al. (2018). Unilateral cervical plexus block for prosthetic laryngoplasty in the standing horse. *Equine Vet. J.* 50: 727–732.

Egan, R.J., Hopkins, J.C., Beamish, A.J. et al. (2013). Randomized clinical trial of intraoperative superficial cervical plexus block versus incisional local anesthesia in thyroid and parathyroid surgery. *Br. J. Surg.* 100: 1732–1738.

Morris, T.B., Lumsden, J.M., Dunlop, C.I. et al. (2020). Clinical assessment of an ipsilateral cervical spinal nerve block for prosthetic laryngoplasty in anesthetized horses. *Front. Vet. Sci.* 7: 284.

Seidel, R., Zukowski, K., Wree, A. et al. (2016). Ultrasound-guided intermediate cervical plexus block and perivascular local anesthetic infiltration for carotid endarterectomy: a randomized controlled trial. *Anaesthesist* 65: 917–924.

## 23

# Anesthesia of the Eye
*Daniel S. Ward*

Some form of sedation and local anesthesia is usually required for satisfactory ophthalmic examination in horses. In addition, these techniques are often adequate for minor diagnostic and surgical procedures.

## I Restraint

### A Intravenous sedation

- Sedation is invaluable for promoting cooperation for eye examinations and standing ocular procedures in horses.
  - *Xylazine* (0.3 mg/kg, IV) for short-term (~10 minutes) sedation.
  - *Detomidine* (0.005–0.01 mg/kg, IV) for more prolonged sedation (~20 minutes).
  - *Butorphanol* (0.01–0.02 mg/kg, IV) may be added to either *xylazine* or *detomidine* to reduce motion in fidgety horses.
    - *Butorphanol* results in mild head shaking in some horses which may complicate procedures, but tends to reduce pacing and gross body movements.
    - Thus, adding *butorphanol* to an $\alpha_2$ agonist for sedation is a compromise between these two factors.

## II Topical local anesthesia

### A Topical anesthesia

  - Is generally used to facilitate examination of a painful eye.
  - It allows the performance of minor diagnostic and surgical procedures of the cornea and conjunctiva.

### B Proparacaine and tetracaine

  - Are the most commonly used topical anesthetics.

*Manual of Equine Anesthesia and Analgesia*, Second Edition. Edited by Tom Doherty, Alex Valverde, and Rachel A. Reed.
© 2022 John Wiley & Sons, Inc. Published 2022 by John Wiley & Sons, Inc.

- ○ Onset of action is less than 1 minute, maximum effect is achieved in approximately 5 minutes, and the duration of action is approximately 15–30 minutes.
- ○ Some evidence indicates *tetracaine* is slightly more effective than *proparacaine*, and viscous *tetracaine* has a significantly longer duration of action.
- ○ Surface toxicities are more common with *tetracaine*.

### C Adverse effects of topical anesthetics

- ○ They reduce Schirmer tear test values.
- ○ They cause minor corneal epithelial damage (which can cause surface irregularities).
- ○ They suppress would healing with prolonged usage.
- ○ *Therefore, topical anesthetics should not be prescribed for pain relief.*

## III Subconjunctival anesthetic injection

### A Technique

- ○ 0.2 ml of *lidocaine*, *mepivacaine*, or *bupivacaine* is injected under the bulbar conjunctiva 5 mm posterior to the limbus, using 25-gauge needles.

### B Indication

- ○ Can serve as an adjunct to topical anesthetics to facilitate procedures, or to provide analgesia immediately after procedures.
- ○ Anesthetic effect may last up to two hours with all three topical local anesthetics.

## IV Subcutaneous injectable local anesthesia

### A Technique

- ○ Local anesthetic injections are accomplished using 25-gauge, 2.5 cm (1 in.) needles.
- ○ Injection volumes are usually 1–2 ml.

### B Local anesthetic drugs

- ○ Can be classified on the basis of duration of action:
  - – *Lidocaine*: Short to medium duration (one to two hours).
  - – *Mepivacaine*: Short to medium duration (two to four hours).
  - – *Bupivacaine*: Long duration (four to six hours).

### C Adjunctive agents

- ○ May increase the anesthetic effect and duration of the local anesthetic.

*Hyaluronidase*
- ○ Mixed with local anesthetic (1500 IU/100 ml).
- ○ Hyaluronidase breaks down ground substance, allowing better diffusion of anesthetic.
- ○ Well-documented effectiveness in retrobulbar anesthesia in humans, especially when combined with ocular compression.
- ○ Not evaluated in horses, only modestly helpful in retrobulbar blocks in cattle.

*Epinephrine*
- ○ Diluted (1 : 200000) by adding epinephrine (0.1 ml of 1 : 1000; 5 µg/ml) to 20 ml lidocaine (2%).

       ○ Resulting vasoconstriction increases anesthetic residence time in infiltrated area, as well as limiting systemic absorption of anesthetic.

*Bicarbonate*

       ○ The acidity of local anesthetics makes their injection painful.

       ○ The addition of 1 ml 8.4% sodium bicarbonate/10 ml of local anesthetic makes the injection more comfortable.

       ○ However, the clinical benefits of this method are debatable.

$\alpha_2$ *agonists*

       ○ The addition of an $\alpha_2$ agonist prolongs the effect of local anesthetics by an $\alpha_2$ independent mechanism. (see Chapter 14)

**D Methods of using injectable local anesthetics**

       ○ Injectable local anesthetics can be used for:
         – Nerve block anesthesia.
         – Field block anesthesia.
         – Infiltration anesthesia.

       ○ Specific ocular nerve blocks are either *motor* or *sensory* to the eye and adnexal structures.

       ○ The *auriculopalpebral* motor block is the most important nerve block technique, but the sensory blocks listed may be helpful in certain minor surgical procedures of the eyelids.

       ○ *Sensory* nerves are generally blocked more effectively than motor nerves.

       ○ Field blocks and infiltration anesthesia are also important, and are used primarily for sensory blockade.

## V Motor nerve blocks

**A Auriculopalpebral nerve** (see Figure 23.1 and 23.2)

       ○ Usually, the only block necessary for diagnostic evaluation of the equine eye.

       ○ Terminal branch of facial nerve (seventh cranial).

       ○ It courses over the zygomatic arch, giving off the rostral auricular branch to the auricular plexus and the zygomatic branch to the orbicularis oculi muscle.

       ○ Motor to the orbicularis oculi muscle.

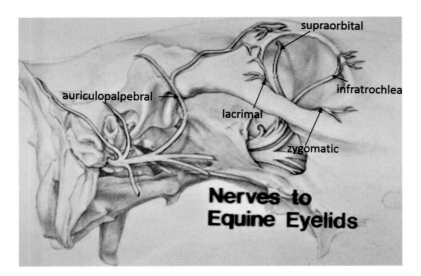

**Figure 23.1** Anatomy of the major motor and sensory nerves of the equine periocular region.

*Location*

  ○ The block is usually performed where the nerve is palpated along the dorsal edge of the zygomatic arch, just anterior to its highest point.
  ○ Can also block the auriculopalpebral nerve where the zygomatic arch meets the superotemporal aspect of the orbital rim or more caudally near the base of the ear.
  ○ A 23-gauge, 2.5 cm (1 in.) needle is used to inject 1–2 ml of local anesthetic.
  ○ Auriculopalpebral blocks diminish the blink response so artificial tear ointment should be applied following examination of the eye.

## VI  Sensory nerve blocks (see Figures 23.1–23.3)

### A  Supraorbital nerve

  ○ Terminal branch of the ophthalmic nerve (5th Cranial).
  ○ Sensory to most of the superior lid.
  ○ Arises from the frontal nerve through the supraorbital foramen along with the supraorbital artery.
  ○ Facilitates minor surgical procedures of the nasal portion of the superior lid.

*Location*

  ○ The supraorbital foramen is palpable on the superior orbital rim just as the rim starts to widen nasal to its midpoint.
  ○ Töth's law states that if the thumb and middle finger on the right hand are placed at the nasal and temporal canthi (respectively) of the left eye, the index finger will fall on or near the supraorbital foramen (see Figure 23.4).

*Technique*

  ○ Insert a 23- to 25-gauge, 1.6–2.5 cm (5/8–1 in.) needle into the foramen and after aspirating, to ensure avoidance to the supraorbital artery, inject 2–3 ml of local anesthetic as the needle is withdrawn.
  ○ As the supraorbital nerve exits its foramen, its branches intermingle with terminal branches of the auriculopalpebral nerve.
    – Anesthetic deposited at the superficial aspect of the foramen will block some of these distal auriculopalpebral twigs, and therefore have some effect on *motor* function of the orbicularis oculi muscle.
    – However, a well-placed auriculopalpebral block alone should be effective for motor blockade, and the supraorbital nerve, strictly speaking, is a sensory nerve.

### B  Lacrimal nerve

  ○ A branch of the ophthalmic nerve. It runs along the dorsal rectus muscle to ramify in the lacrimal gland and upper eyelid.
  ○ Sensory to the temporal canthus (lateral canthus) and temporal 25% of the superior lid.
  ○ It is blocked along the superior orbital rim just nasal to the temporal canthus by injecting 2–3 ml of local anesthetic with a 23-gauge, 2.5 cm (1 in.) needle.

### C  Infratrochlear nerve

  ○ A branch of the nasociliary nerve, which itself is a branch of the ophthalmic nerve.
  ○ It is sensory to the *nasal canthus* (medial canthus).
  ○ It is blocked at its location with a notch in the superior orbital rim near the nasal canthus by injecting 2–3 ml of local anesthetic with a 23-gauge, 2.5 cm (1 in.) needle.

**Figure 23.2**   Sites of equine periocular nerve blocks. 1: auriculopalpebral; 2: supraorbital; 3: lacrimal; 4: infratrochlear; 5: zygomatic.

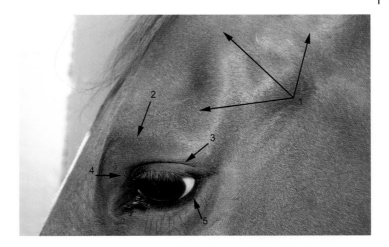

**Figure 23.3**   Approximate areas of desensitization afforded by periocular sensory nerve blocks in the horse. Blue – supraorbital. Red – infratrochlear. Black – zygomatic. Green – lacrimal.

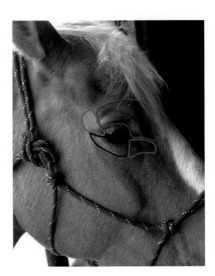

**Figure 23.4**   Locating the equine supraorbital foramen using Töth's law.

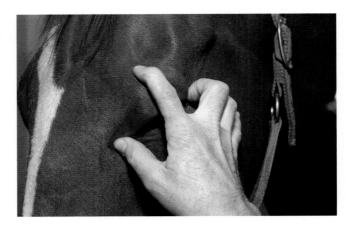

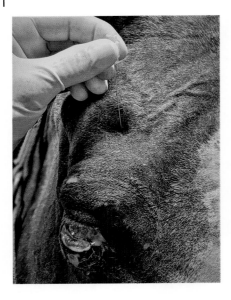

### D Zygomatic nerve

- ○ A terminal branch of the maxillary nerve.
- ○ Also derives twigs from the zygomaticotemporal and lacrimal branches of the ophthalmic nerve.
- ○ Sensory to the temporal 75% of the inferior lid.
- ○ Blocked at the inferior orbital rim adjacent to the temporal canthus by injecting 3–5 ml of local anesthetic with a 23-gauge, 2.5 cm (1 in.) needle.

## VII Deep orbital nerve blocks

### A Nerves blocked

- ○ Local blocks placed deep within the orbit provide anesthesia and akinesia of the globe by their actions on *oculomotor*, *trochlear*, *trigeminal* (ophthalmic branch), and *abducens* nerves, all of which enter the orbit near the orbital apex.

*Oculomotor nerve*
- ○ Motor to the dorsal, ventral, and medial rectus muscles, the inferior oblique muscle, the levator palpebral muscle, and the pupillary sphincter muscle.

*Trochlear nerve*
- ○ Motor to the superior oblique muscle.

*Trigeminal nerve*
- ○ Sensory to the eye and ocular adnexae.

*Abducens nerve*
- ○ Motor to the lateral rectus and retractor bulbi muscles.

### B Techniques

*Four-point block*
- ○ A 20-gauge, 8.9 cm (3.5 in.) spinal needle is inserted into the orbit at the 12 : 00, 3 : 00, 7 : 00 and 9 : 00 positions (*6 : 00 should be avoided to minimize the chance of damaging the optic nerve*).
- ○ A slight "pop" is felt as the orbital septum is penetrated; if the needle does not penetrate the septum, anesthetic may migrate subconjunctivally.

     ○ Deposit 5–10 ml of local anesthetic at each site.

*Peterson-type block*

     ○ This is a modification of the Peterson deep orbital block used in cattle.

     ○ A slightly curved 18-gauge, at least 8.9 cm (3.5 in.) needle is inserted 1 cm temporal to the temporal canthus. The needle is directed inferonasally toward the opposite nasal canthus and 15–20 mL of local anesthetic injected.

*Supraorbital fossa block* (see Figure 23.5)

     ○ This is the preferred method for retrobulbar block.

       – It requires only one injection.

       – It provides excellent anesthesia and akinesia.

       – Very low complication rate.

     ○ 20-gauge, 8.9 cm (3.5 in.) spinal needle introduced into the supraorbital fossa.

     ○ The needle is directed ventrally toward the retrobulbar muscle cone.

     ○ When the cone is encountered, resistance will be felt and subtle dorsal rotation of the globe will occur as the muscle cone is pushed down.

     ○ With additional pressure the needle will penetrate the muscle cone and the globe will return to its normal position.

     ○ 6–10 ml of local anesthetic is then injected.

**C Potential complications of deep orbital blocks**

     ○ Retrobulbar hemorrhage.

     ○ Inadvertent penetration of the globe.

     ○ Laceration of the optic nerve.

     ○ Sudden death has been reported anecdotally following deep orbital blocks in cows.

       – Presumably due to injection of anesthetic into the subarachnoid space of the optic nerve, which is contiguous with the subarachnoid space of the brain.

## VIII   Field block anesthesia of the eye

**A Line blocks**

     ○ Deposition of a line of local anesthetic along the superior and/or inferior orbital rims will effectively block all motor and sensory innervation to the eyelid(s), greatly facilitating surgical approaches and subpalpebral lavage apparatus placement.

**B Infiltration anesthesia of the eye**

     ○ Simply refers to injection of local anesthetic solution into tissues without regard for the course of nerves supplying the area of interest.

       – Motor and sensory innervation of the infiltrated area will be affected, with the sensory component usually affected to a greater extent than the motor component.

       – This technique generally requires larger volumes of anesthetic solution, and can affect the architecture of histopathology if applied overzealously.

## Suggested Reading

Labelle, A.L. and Clark-Price, S.C. (2013). Anesthesia for ophthalmic procedures in the standing horse. *Vet. Clin. North Am. Equine Pract.* 29: 179–191.

Robertson, S.A. (2004). Standing sedation and pain management for ophthalmic patients. *Vet. Clin. North Am. Equine Pract.* 20: 485–497.

# 24

## Anesthesia of the Limbs
*Jim Schumacher, John Schumacher, and Ray Wilhite*

## I Indications

- Regional anesthesia is used primarily to:
  - Localize the site of pain causing lameness.
  - Provide anesthesia for surgery performed with the horse conscious and standing.
  - Provide adjunctive analgesia for anesthetized horses undergoing surgery.
  - Provide temporary analgesia for a painful condition (e.g. for horses with laminitis).

## II General principles

### A Selection of the local anesthetic drug and dose

  - The local anesthetics most commonly used in the horse to induce regional anesthesia are *2% lidocaine* HCl and *2% mepivacaine* HCl.
  - The anesthetic effect of *lidocaine* generally lasts about 45–60 minutes.
  - The local anesthetic effect of *mepivacaine* generally lasts 90–120 minutes. Mepivacaine elicits a milder tissue reaction than lidocaine and is more reliable in producing local and regional anesthesia.
  - *Bupivacaine* HCl is longer acting than *mepivacaine* and is used when regional anesthesia is performed for palliation of pain.

### B Deposition of local anesthetic

  - When determining the site of pain causing lameness, the local anesthetic should be deposited accurately adjacent to the nerve and within the subcircumneural space (see Figure 24.1).
  - This reduces the risk of inadvertently anesthetizing nearby nerves.
  - Depositing a local anesthetic outside the circumneural sheath is likely to fail to sufficiently anesthetize the targeted nerve.
  - The *smallest volume* capable of anesthetizing the nerve should be used when regional anesthesia is performed to localize a site a pain causing lameness. A large volume may

*Manual of Equine Anesthesia and Analgesia*, Second Edition. Edited by Tom Doherty, Alex Valverde, and Rachel A. Reed.
© 2022 John Wiley & Sons, Inc. Published 2022 by John Wiley & Sons, Inc.

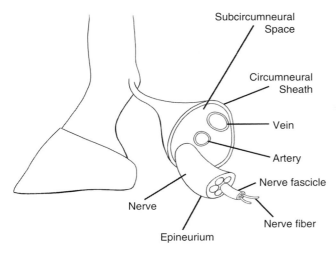

**Figure 24.1** Subcircumneural space surrounding the nerve, artery, and vein within the circumneural sheath.

travel proximally, within the subcircumneural space, resulting in inadvertent desensitization of proximal structures not intended to be desensitized.

○ A greater volume of local anesthetic solution can be deposited when regional anesthesia is used to provide analgesia for surgery or to provide temporary palliation of pain.

○ The volume of local anesthetic used to anesthetize nerves located within the proximal portion of the limb (i.e. proximal to the carpus or tarsus) is usually greater than that used to anesthetize nerves in the distal portion of the limb, because proximally located nerve trunks are thicker. Increased volume is necessary to cover multiple nodes of Ranvier, which are spaced further apart in large nerves.

○ Anesthesia of the nerves of the distal portion of the limb usually takes effect rapidly (5–10 minutes), but the larger nerves of the proximal portion of the limb may not become anesthetized for 20 minutes or more.

## C  Equipment

○ Needles and syringes should be disposable.

○ Length and bore of the needle depend on the particular nerve to be anesthetized.

○ Most nerves of the distal portion of the limb (i.e. distal to the carpus or tarsus) are anesthetized using a 25-gauge, 1.6 cm (5/8 in.) needle.

○ Longer (e.g. 3.8 cm [1.5 in.]), larger-bore needles (e.g. 22- or 20-gauge) are used to anesthetize nerves located more proximally on the limb.

○ If a relatively *large-bore* needle is to be used, subcutaneous deposition of a small amount of local anesthetic (using 25-gauge needle) may reduce resentment by the horse.

○ Syringes that lock onto the needle hub (i.e. Luer-lock syringes) should *not* be used for nerve blocks.

○ The syringe may have to be detached quickly from the needle to prevent the needle from being pulled out, bent, or broken. Luer-slip syringes can be detached quickly from the needle.

## III  Patient preparation

### A  Physical restraint

- ○ When regional anesthesia is used to determine the site of pain causing lameness, the horse is best restrained physically, rather than chemically, so that lameness can be evaluated without the influence of sedation on gait.
- ○ A person experienced in handling horses should restrain the horse.
- ○ Most horses receiving a nerve block can be controlled with a lip twitch or a lip chain.
- ○ Nerve blocks are generally performed most safely with the horse unrestrained by stocks. A fractious horse can be restrained in an equine stocks to minimize risk to personnel, but stocks reduce accessibility of many sites for injection and, therefore, may jeopardize the safety of the horse and the clinician performing the injection.
- ○ Anesthetizing nerves in the distal portion of the limb is usually easier for the clinician and safer for the horse and clinician when the horse is not restrained in stocks.

### B  Chemical restraint

- ○ Sedation may be necessary to control a fractious horse. If sedation is required to perform regional anesthesia, the horse's gait should be evaluated while the horse is sedated, before administering the nerve block.
- ○ *Xylazine* HCl (0.4 mg/kg, IV) or *acepromazine* (0.04 mg/kg, IV) can be administered without interfering substantially with assessment of gait.
- ○ If the clinician is concerned that sedation may be detrimental to evaluating lameness, the horse can be examined after the effects of sedation dissipate, provided that the local anesthetic is longer lasting than the effects of the sedative.

*Note*: Waiting until the effects of sedation dissipate, however, may confound the results of regional anesthesia, because the local anesthetic may diffuse proximally in the subcircumneural space, resulting in desensitization of structures not intended to be desensitized.

### C  Preparation of the injection site

- ○ Clipping the hair at the site of injection is not necessary, unless it aids palpation of landmarks used to determine the exact site of injection.
- ○ The site of injection should receive a brief scrub, using an antiseptic soap or wiped with alcohol.
  - – The site should be prepared more carefully if an adjacent synovial structure is at risk of being penetrated.
  - – Sterile gloves are an unnecessary precaution against inducing infection, unless penetration of a synovial structure is a risk.

## IV  General technique

- • The clinician must have good knowledge of landmarks surrounding the nerve to be desensitized.
- • The more accurate the placement of the needle, the smaller the volume of local anesthetic required.

- The block is likely to be ineffective if the anesthetic solution fails to enter the subcircum-neural space. If the nerve cannot be palpated, depositing local anesthetic solution in several different planes increases the likelihood of injecting into this space.

A   Needle insertion

- The site of injection and preference of the clinician determine whether an injection is performed with the limb bearing weight or held.
- Nerve blocks performed distal to the fetlock of a hind limb are performed most safely with the limb extended and held on the thigh of the clinician performing the block.
- The needle is inserted, without the syringe attached, with a quick thrust through the skin.
- The needle is sometimes redirected, without being withdrawn through the skin, so that the anesthetic is deposited in several tissue planes.
- If blood appears in the needle hub, the needle should be redirected slightly.

B   Localization of lameness

- When localizing the site of pain causing lameness, regional anesthesia is usually initiated distally on the limb and advanced proximally, in a stepwise manner, until the lameness is eliminated.
- If the site of pain causing lameness is quite far proximal, multiple nerve blocks must be administered before lameness is ameliorated.
- A *less common approach* to performing regional anesthesia to determine the site of pain causing lameness is to first eliminate a large portion of the limb as the site of pain by performing a regional nerve block high on the limb.
  - This can be done on a hind limb, for example, by administering a low plantar nerve block (i.e. a low, four- or six-point nerve block) to determine if the lameness is proximal or distal to the fetlock. The site of pain causing lameness of a hind limb is usually located proximal to the fetlock. If the horse remains lame, administering regional anesthesia distal to the fetlock is avoided, because negative results of the low plantar nerve block indicate that the site of pain causing lameness is proximal to the fetlock joint.
  - This approach decreases the horse's discomfort and speeds the examination, provided that lameness is caused by pain at a site proximal to the site of the regional nerve block.
  - This approach slows the lameness examination, however, if the lameness is eliminated with the first regional nerve block, because the effects of that nerve block must be allowed to dissipate before proceeding with a nerve block performed distal to the initial nerve block.

## V   Checking for desensitization

- The effectiveness of anesthesia in desensitizing the targeted region is usually determined by applying *noxious stimuli* to the dermatome of the anesthetized nerve.
- Instruments used to apply *noxious* stimulation include a ball-point pen, a key, or an unfolded paper clip.
- Some horses react to stimulation of the distal portion of the limb by *striking or kicking*.
- Noxious stimulation may be applied more safely, if the distal portion of the limb is held, or if stimulation is applied using a long, pointed instrument.

- Skin sensation can usually be first assessed at 5–10 minutes after regional anesthesia has been administered to the *distal* portion of the limb.
- The absence or presence of skin sensation *usually* provides a reasonable assessment of the efficacy of regional anesthesia.
- Pain and lameness may still be present, even though skin sensation is eliminated.
- Conversely, pain and lameness may be eliminated without the loss of skin sensation.
- The correlation between skin sensation and deep pain sensation is poor, if *lidocaine* was the local anesthetic agent administered.
- A *stoic* horse may not react to noxious stimulation of skin, even when full skin sensation is retained.
- If the results are *inconclusive*, the horse's response to the same stimulation applied to the corresponding region of the *contralateral* limb can be compared.

## VI   Complications

- Although extraordinarily rare, complications of regional anesthesia may include:
  - The shaft of a broken needle becoming lost in tissue.
  - Subcutaneous infection at the site of injection.
  - Inadvertent penetration of an adjacent synovial structure by the needle may result in infection of that structure and failure to desensitize the region innervated by the targeted nerve.
  - Conversion of a fracture from non-displaced to displaced, as a result of eliminating pain caused by a non-displaced fracture. A horse should *not* receive regional anesthesia if a non-displaced fracture is suspected.
  - False negative results resulting from the following:
    - Variations in neurologic anatomy.
    - Failure to direct the needle into the subcircumneural space.
    - Injection of the local anesthetic into an inadvertently penetrated adjacent synovial structure or blood vessel.

*Comment: The results of regional anesthesia should be interpreted with some degree of skepticism.*

## VII   Forelimb: distal aspect

### A   Palmar digital nerve block at the level of the cartilages of the foot

  - The neurovascular bundle containing the palmar digital nerve (PDN) can be palpated in the angle formed by the cartilage of the foot (lateral or collateral cartilages) and the palmar aspect of the pastern (see Figure 24.2).
    - These nerves are usually anesthetized with the limb held.
  - To anesthetize each PDN, 1.5 ml or less of anesthetic solution is deposited at the proximal margin of the cartilage of the foot using a 25-gauge, 1.6 cm (5/8 in.) needle.
    - More proximal deposition is more likely to result in desensitization of the proximal interphalangeal joint.
  - Anesthesia of both PDNs at the level of the cartilages of the foot (i.e. distal to the dorsal branches of the PDNs) desensitizes the *entire* foot except for the dorsal part of the coronary band, which is innervated by *dorsal branches* of the PDNs.

**Figure 24.2** The neurovascular bundle containing the palmar/plantar digital nerve and location of needle insertion for the palmar digital nerve block at the level of the cartilages of the foot.

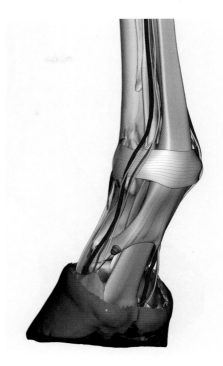

- The dorsal branches of the PDNs do not innervate the distal interphalangeal joint, and so, they need *not* be anesthetized to achieve complete desensitization of the distal interphalangeal joint.
- In some cases, anesthesia of the PDNs can result in desensitization of structures more proximal, including the proximal interphalangeal joint and even the carpometacarpal joint.

B   Midpastern semi-ring block

- Used by some clinicians when the PDN block fails to improve lameness.
- After the PDNs have been anesthetized (see above), 10 ml of local anesthetic solution is deposited subcutaneously around the dorsal half of the pastern, using a 25-gauge, 1.6 cm (5/8 in.) needle.
- The dorsal branches of the PDNs contribute little to sensation within the foot, so a semi-ring block, performed after a PDN block has failed to improve lameness, is also unlikely to improve lameness.

C   PDN block at the level of the base of the proximal sesamoid bones (abaxial sesamoid, or basisesamoid, nerve block)

- Used to desensitize the foot for *surgery* or to localize the site of pain causing lameness that has failed to improve after anesthetizing the PDNs at the level of the cartilages of the foot.
- The neurovascular bundle containing the PDNs can be easily palpated along the abaxial border of each proximal sesamoid bone (see Figure 24.3).
- The PDNs are anesthetized at this level using a 25-gauge, 1.6 cm (5/8 in.) needle.

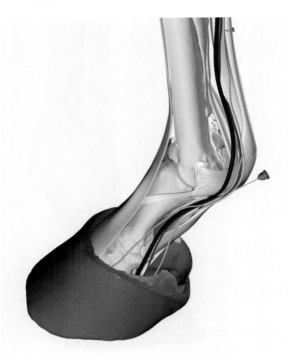

Figure 24.3   The neurovascular bundle containing the palmar/plantar digital nerve and location of needle insertion for palmar digital nerve block at the level of the proximal sesamoid bones.

- ○ A portion of the metacarpophalangeal joint is likely to become desensitized after performing an abaxial sesamoid nerve block. Taking the following precautions may decrease the area of the metacarpophalangeal joint that is desensitized:
    - – Inserting the needle so that its tip resides near the base of the proximal sesamoid bones (sometimes referred to as a basisesamoid nerve block).
    - – Using a small volume of local anesthetic solution (i.e. <2 ml).
    - – Directing the needle distally, rather than proximally.
- ○ Anesthetizing the PDNs and their dorsal branches at the level of the base of the proximal sesamoid bones (i.e. an abaxial sesamoid nerve block) desensitizes the following structures:
    - – The foot and the middle phalanx.
    - – The distopalmar aspects of the proximal phalanx and associated soft tissues.
    - – The proximal interphalangeal joint.
    - – Frequently, the palmar portion of the metacarpophalangeal joint.

**D   Low four-point nerve block (i.e. Low palmar nerve block)**

- ○ With the low four-point nerve block, the medial and lateral palmar nerves and the medial and lateral palmar metacarpal are anesthetized near the distal aspect of the third metacarpal bone.
    - – This nerve block can be performed with the limb held or with the horse bearing weight on the limb.
- ○ The lateral and medial palmar nerves course along the dorsal aspect of the deep digital flexor tendon.

**Figure 24.4** Location of needle insertion for the low four-point nerve block.

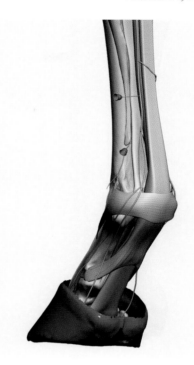

    – They are anesthetized by depositing local anesthetic (~2 ml), adjacent to the dorsal surface of the deep digital flexor tendon using a small gauge needle, such as a 25-gauge, 1.6 cm (5/8 in.) needle (see Figure 24.4).

    – Both palmar nerves should be anesthetized either above or below the easily palpated communicating branch, the *ramus communicans* (see Figure 24.5). Alternatively, this ramus can also be anesthetized with 1 ml of local anesthetic solution (i.e. a low five-point nerve block).

*Note:* Anesthetizing one palmar nerve proximal to the ramus and the other distal to the ramus allows sensory impulses to transmit through the ramus from the nerve anesthetized proximal to the ramus to the other palmar nerve anesthetized distal to the ramus.

    ○ The lateral and medial palmar metacarpal nerves lie between the palmar surface of the third metacarpal bone and the axial surface of the lateral and medial splint bone (i.e. the second and third metacarpal bones).

      – These nerves are anesthetized by depositing local anesthetic solution (~1 ml) beneath the distal end (button or tab) of each splint bone, where the nerve emerges, using a 25-gauge, 1.6 cm (5/8 in.) needle (see Figure 24.5).

    ○ The low four-point nerve block is administered to localize pain causing lameness that has not improved after anesthetizing the PDNs at the level of the proximal sesamoid bones or to desensitize the foot or pastern for surgery.

    ○ Anesthetizing these four nerves desensitizes the *fetlock* and structures distal to the fetlock.

      – Some skin sensation may remain over the dorsal aspect of the fetlock from sensory impulses transmitted through a branch of the medial cutaneous antebrachial nerve.

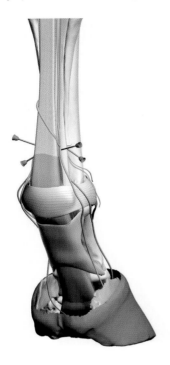

Figure 24.5 Desensitization of palmar/plantar nerves distal to the *ramus communicans*.

### E High four-point block (i.e. High palmar nerve block)

- The medial and lateral palmar and the medial and lateral palmar metacarpal nerves are anesthetized slightly distal to the carpometacarpal joint.
- To anesthetize each *palmar* nerve in this location, 2–3 ml of local anesthetic solution is deposited through a needle (25-gauge, 1.6 cm [5/8 in.]) inserted through heavy fascia to where the palmar nerve lies adjacent to the dorsal surface of the deep digital flexor tendon (see Figure 24.6).
  - The palmar nerves are usually anesthetized with the horse *bearing weight* on the limb.
- The lateral and medial *palmar metacarpal* nerves are anesthetized slightly distal to the carpometacarpal joint, at the juncture of the palmar surface of the third metacarpal bone and the axial surface of the second or forth metacarpal bone, where each nerve lies, by depositing local anesthetic solution (~2–3 ml) through a 20- to 22-gauge, 3.8 cm (1.5 in.) needle (see Figure 24.6)
  - The palmar metacarpal nerves are usually anesthetized with the limb held.
- The high four-point nerve block is sometimes the next nerve block administered to localize pain causing lameness that has failed to improve after anesthetizing the palmar and palmar metacarpal nerves at the level of the distal end of the second and forth metacarpal bones.
- A *complication* of the high four-point nerve block is anesthesia of the carpometacarpal and intercarpal (middle) joints from inadvertent penetration of a distopalmar outpouching of the carpometacarpal joint.

Figure 24.6  Location of needle insertion for four-point (high palmar) nerve block.

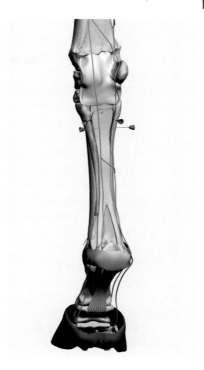

***Note***: Direct infiltration of local anesthetic solution around the proximal aspect of the suspensory ligament to desensitize this ligament also risks inadvertent anesthesia of the carpometacarpal and intercarpal joints.

- ○ Anesthetizing the lateral and medial palmar nerves alone, slightly below the level of the carpometacarpal joint, desensitizes the *flexor tendons*.
- ○ Anesthetizing the palmar metacarpal nerves alone, at this level, desensitizes the splint bones and their interosseous ligaments, but fails to completely desensitize the proximal portion of the suspensory ligament.

**F   Lateral palmar nerve block**

- ○ The lateral palmar nerve originates proximal to the carpus and is formed by the *lateral palmar branch of the median* nerve and the *palmar branch of the ulnar* nerve.
- ○ The lateral palmar nerve gives off a branch (i.e. the deep branch), about 2 cm distal to the head of the lateral splint bone. The deep branch of the lateral palmar nerve innervates the proximal portion of the *suspensory* ligament and divides into the lateral and medial palmar metacarpal nerves.
- ○ The lateral palmar nerve can be anesthetized at several sites.

**Site 1**

- ○ The origin of the suspensory ligament and the proximal portion of the second and forth metacarpal bones can be desensitized by anesthetizing the lateral palmar nerve at the level of the middle carpal joint, as it courses distal to the accessory carpal bone close to the accessoriometacarpal ligament, before it gives off the deep branch that innervates these structures.

- The *site of injection* is located on the palmar border of the accessoriometacarpal ligament, midway between the ligament's origin on the distal aspect of the accessory carpal bone and its insertion on the proximal aspect of the forth metacarpal bone.
- 5 ml of local anesthetic solution is deposited beneath the 2- to 3-mm thick flexor carpal retinaculum into the accessoriometacarpal ligament using a 20- to 22-gauge, 2.5 cm (1 in.) needle.
  - This block (sometimes referred to as the Wheat block) is usually performed with the horse *bearing weight* on the limb.
- This technique results in a high incidence of *penetration of the carpal synovial sheath*, and so could lead to an erroneous conclusion, if the amount of local anesthetic solution deposited within the carpal synovial sheath were enough to ameliorate pain associated with disease of the structures contained within this *synovial* cavity.
- Even though the site of injection is close to the distal aspect of the carpus, inadvertent infiltration of local anesthetic into the carpometacarpal or intercarpal joint using this technique is unlikely.

**Site 2**

- The lateral palmar nerve can also be anesthetized at the medial aspect of the *accessory carpal bone* (see Figure 24.7).
- At this level, the lateral palmar nerve, together with the lateral palmar vein and artery, lies adjacent to the medial aspect of the accessory carpal bone.
- The site of injection is palpated as a longitudinal groove in the fascia over the medial aspect of the accessory carpal bone, dorsal to the insertion of the flexor retinaculum that forms the palmaromedial aspect of the carpal canal.
  - This nerve block (sometimes referred to as the Castro block) is performed with the horse *bearing weight* on the limb.

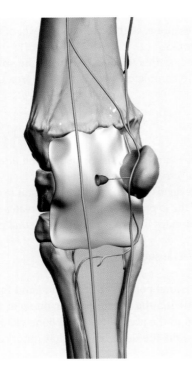

Figure 24.7 Location of needle insertion for the lateral palmar nerve block at the medial aspect of the accessory carpal bone.

- A 25-gauge, 1.6 cm (5/8 in.) needle is inserted into the distal third of the groove in a mediolateral direction, and when the point of the needle contacts the medial aspect of the accessory carpal bone, 1.5–2 ml of local anesthetic solution is injected.
- This technique of anesthetizing the lateral palmar nerve *avoids* inadvertent deposition of the local anesthetic into the *carpal synovial sheath* but may cause some horses to react violently, if the needle contacts the nerve.
- Amelioration of lameness after anesthesia of the lateral palmar nerve alone, proximal to its deep branch, incriminates the proximal portion of the suspensory ligament, or at least the proximopalmar metacarpal region, as the site of pain causing lameness, provided that more distal regions have been eliminated as a site of pain.
- Anesthetizing the medial palmar nerve at the level of the proximal aspect of the metacarpus in conjunction with anesthesia of the lateral palmar nerve (at any of the described sites), provides extensive desensitization of the distal portion of the limb (i.e. metacarpus and structures distal to it).

## VIII  Forelimb: proximal aspect

- The carpus and structures distal to it can be desensitized by anesthetizing the median, ulnar, and medial cutaneous antebrachial nerves.
- Although these nerves are sometimes anesthetized for diagnostic purposes, they are most commonly anesthetized to desensitize the distal portion of the limb for surgery.

### A  Median nerve

- The median nerve is anesthetized at the caudomedial aspect of the radius, just distal to the elbow (cubital) joint, where the ventral edge of the posterior superficial pectoral muscle inserts on the radius (see Figure 24.8).
- A 20-gauge needle is inserted to a depth of 1–2.5 cm, and 10–15 ml of local anesthetic solution is injected.
  - The needle is advanced close to the radius to avoid penetrating the median vein and artery.
- Anesthesia of the median nerve alone *partially* desensitizes the carpus, the distal aspect of the antebrachium, and the structures innervated by the medial and lateral palmar nerves.

### B  Ulnar nerve

- The ulnar nerve is anesthetized about 10 cm proximal to the accessory carpal bone, at which point it lies about 0.5–1 cm beneath the skin surface, under the superficial fascia, in the groove between the *ulnaris lateralis* and *flexor carpi ulnaris* muscles (see Figure 24.9).
- ~5 ml of local anesthetic is infused superficially and deeply, through a 20-gauge, 2.5 cm (1 in.) needle.
- Anesthetizing the ulnar nerve alone desensitizes the skin of the lateral aspect of the forelimb, from the site of injection to the fetlock.

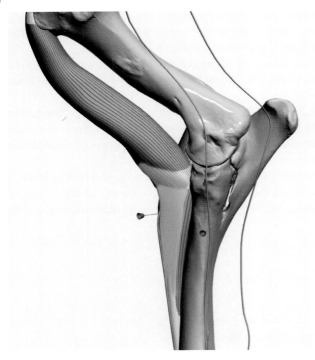

Figure 24.8   Location of needle insertion for blockade of the median nerve and the medial cutaneous antebrachial nerve at the caudomedial aspect of the radius.

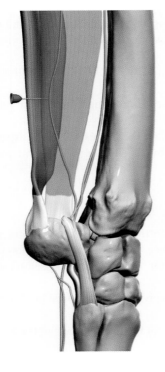

Figure 24.9   Location of needle insertion for blockade of the ulnar nerve proximal to the accessory carpal bone.

– Because little information can be gained by anesthetizing the ulnar and median nerves separately, these nerves are usually anesthetized at the same time when trying to determine the site of pain causing lameness.
- Lameness caused by lesions of the accessory carpal bone and surrounding structures, the small metacarpal bones and their interosseous ligaments, and the proximal aspect of the suspensory ligament may be *partially* ameliorated by anesthetizing the ulnar nerve.

## C  Medial cutaneous antebrachial nerve

- Anesthesia of the medial cutaneous antebrachial nerve, a branch of the musculocutaneous nerve, desensitizes skin on the dorsal and medial aspects of the metacarpus.
- The medial cutaneous antebrachial nerve can be anesthetized immediately proximal to the dorsal aspect of the elbow joint, where it can be easily palpated as it crosses the *lacertus fibrosus,* by injecting 5 ml of local anesthetic solution adjacent to it.
- Distal to the *lacertus fibrosus,* on the medial aspect of the forelimb, the medial cutaneous antebrachial nerve divides into two branches, which can be anesthetized on the medial aspect of the radius, halfway between the elbow and the carpus (i.e. about 10 cm proximal to the chestnut) (see Figure 24.8).
  – One branch lies on the cranial aspect of the cephalic vein, and the other lies on the cranial aspect of the accessory cephalic vein.
  – Because the location of these branches varies, local anesthetic solution should be infiltrated subcutaneously, cranial and caudal to the cephalic and accessory cephalic veins.
  – 5 ml of local anesthetic solution is infiltrated at each site.

# IX  Hind limb

## A  Plantar digital nerve block at the level of the cartilages of the foot

- The technique of anesthetizing the plantar digital nerves is identical to that of anesthetizing the PDNs (see Figures 24.2 and 24.3).
- Anesthesia of both plantar digital nerves at the level of the cartilages of the foot desensitizes the entire foot, except for the dorsal part of the coronary band, which is innervated by the lateral and medial dorsal metatarsal nerves, which are branches of the deep peroneal nerve.
- The medial dorsal metatarsal nerve courses along the medial side of the long digital extensor tendon, and the lateral dorsal metatarsal nerve courses distally close to the lateral splint bone and deviates dorsally in the region of the fetlock.
  – Anesthetizing the dorsal metatarsal nerves has no effect on lameness, because the nerves only innervate the skin on the dorsal aspect of the fetlock and pastern.
- The incidence of lameness caused by pain in the hind foot is much lower than that of the forefoot, and the likelihood of ameliorating lameness with a plantar digital nerve block is small.

B   **Mid-pastern ring block**

  ○ The mid-pastern ring block of the hind limb is performed in the same way as the mid-pastern ring block of the forelimb.
   – As for the forelimb, there is *little indication* for performing a mid-pastern nerve block on a hind limb.

C   **Plantar digital nerve block at the level of the base of the proximal sesamoid bones (abaxial sesamoid or basisesamoid nerve block)**

  ○ The plantar abaxial sesamoid nerve block desensitizes the same structures that are desensitized on the forelimb with the *palmar* abaxial sesamoid nerve block.
  ○ The technique of the *plantar* abaxial sesamoid nerve block at the level of the proximal sesamoid bones is identical to that of the palmar abaxial sesamoid nerve block (see Figure 24.3).
  ○ The likelihood of ameliorating lameness of a hind limb with the abaxial sesamoid nerve block is *much lower than* that of ameliorating lameness of a forelimb with the same block.

D   **Low six-point nerve block (i.e. low plantar nerve block)**

  ○ For the low plantar nerve block, the medial and lateral plantar nerves, the medial and lateral plantar metatarsal nerves, and the dorsal metatarsal nerves are anesthetized at the level of the distal end of the third metatarsal bone, distal to the anastomotic branch (*ramus communicans*) that connects the plantar nerves (see Figure 24.5).
   – The *ramus communicans* of the hind limb is more difficult to palpate than that of the forelimb and is usually absent.
   – These nerves are usually anesthetized with the horse *bearing weight* on the limb.
  ○ The *lateral and medial plantar nerves* lie at the dorsal border of the deep digital flexor tendon, and each is anesthetized by depositing ~2 ml of local anesthetic solution adjacent to the dorsolateral or dorsomedial aspect of the surface of the deep digital flexor tendon, using a 25-gauge, 1.6 cm (5/8 in.) needle, proximal to the plantar pouch of metatarsophalangeal joint.
  ○ The *lateral and medial plantar metatarsal nerves* are anesthetized by depositing local anesthetic solution (~1 ml), beneath the distal end of each small metatarsal bone (i.e. the button or tab), where the nerve emerges, using a 25-gauge, 1.6 cm (5/8 in.) needle.
  ○ The *lateral and medial dorsal metatarsal nerves* are anesthetized by depositing 2 ml of local anesthetic solution subcutaneously in a semi-ring block over the dorsal aspect of the metatarsus.
  ○ These nerves only innervate the skin on the dorsal aspect of the fetlock and pastern, *so anesthetizing these nerves has no effect on lameness caused by pain in the fetlock or digit.*
  ○ The low plantar nerve block desensitizes the fetlock and structures distal to it.
  ○ Because of the *low incidence* of lameness caused by pain at, or distal to the hind fetlock, the low six-point nerve block (or low four-point nerve block) is often administered first, to rule out lameness in the fetlock region and digit, before proceeding with diagnostic regional or intra-articular anesthesia to desensitize more proximal areas of the hind limb more likely to be the site of pain causing lameness.

**E   High six-point nerve block (i.e. high plantar nerve block)**

- ○ Anesthesia of the medial and lateral plantar nerves, the medial and lateral plantar metatarsal nerves, and the medial and lateral dorsal metatarsal nerves several centimeters distal to the proximal border of the splint bones provides complete analgesia to the distal portion of the limb (i.e. metatarsus and structures distal to it).
- ○ To anesthetize the plantar metatarsal nerves slightly distal to the level of the proximal border of the splint bones, a 22- or 20-gauge, 3.8 cm (1.5 in.) needle is inserted about 1 cm distal to the proximal border of these bones and axial to them, until its point contacts the third metatarsal bone, where it articulates with the adjacent second or third metatarsal bone. Two to 3 ml of local anesthetic solution is deposited at this location (see Figure 24.10).
  - – The high six-point nerve block is usually performed with the horse *bearing weight* on the limb.
  - – Anesthetizing both plantar metatarsal nerves alone, slightly distal to the proximal border of the splint bones, desensitizes the small metatarsal bones and their interosseous ligaments, and the most proximal portion of the suspensory ligament.
  - – Although *unlikely*, local anesthetic solution can be instilled *inadvertently* into the tarsometatarsal joint when anesthetizing the plantar metatarsal nerves slightly distal to the proximal border of the splint bones.
  - – Inadvertent administration of local anesthetic into the tarsal sheath *is likely*, however, when anesthetizing the plantar metatarsal nerves.

**Figure 24.10**   Location of needle insertion for the high plantar nerve block.

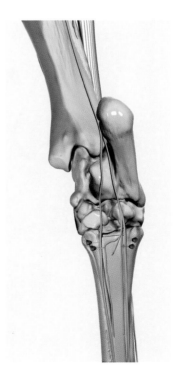

- To anesthetize the medial and lateral plantar nerves slightly distal to the proximal border of the splint bones, 3–5 ml of local anesthetic is deposited using a 25-gauge, 1.6 cm (5/8 in.) needle inserted through *heavy fascia* to where each plantar nerve lies adjacent to the dorsal surface of the deep digital flexor tendon (see Figure 24.10).
  - The medial and lateral plantar nerves are usually anesthetized with the horse bearing weight on the limb.
  - Anesthetizing the lateral plantar nerve at this level anesthetizes the deep branch of the lateral plantar nerve, which divides into the medial and lateral plantar metatarsal nerves.
  - Anesthesia of the lateral plantar nerve alone at this level, desensitizes the same structures that are desensitized by anesthesia of the medial and lateral plantar metatarsal nerves.
- All but the proximodorsal aspect of the limb distal to the level of the proximal border of the splint bones is desensitized by anesthetizing the medial and lateral plantar and plantar metatarsal nerves.
- Subcutaneous deposition of local anesthetic around the dorsal, medial, and dorsolateral aspects of the metatarsus at this level (i.e. a semi-ring block) anesthetizes the dorsal metatarsal nerves and completes the high plantar nerve block.
- To block the deep branch of the lateral plantar nerve, a 2.5 cm (1 in.), 23-gauge needle is inserted perpendicular to the skin surface on the plantarolateral surface of the metatarsus about 1.6 cm (5/8 in.) distal to the head of the fourth metatarsal bone (see Figure 24.11).
- The block is performed with the hock on the clinician's thigh with the hock and stifle flexed at a 90° angle. The adjacent lateral plantar nerve is also likely to be blocked, when blocking the deep branch of that nerve.

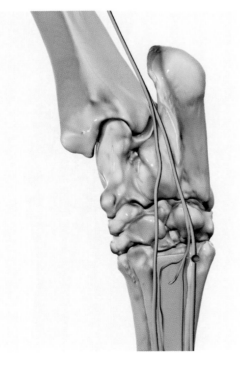

**Figure 24.11** Location of needle insertion for the deep branch of the lateral plantar nerve.

F   Tibial and peroneal (Fibular) nerve blocks

*Tibial Nerve*

- ○ The tibial nerve is anesthetized approximately 10 cm proximal to the point of the hock on the *medial* aspect of the limb where the nerve lies in thick fascia on the caudal surface of the *deep digital flexor* muscle, cranial to the Achilles tendon (see Figure 24.12).
   – To anesthetize the *tibial* nerve, 15–20 ml of local anesthetic solution is deposited at this site, in several planes, in the fascia overlying the deep digital flexor muscle, through a 20- or 22-gauge, 3.8 cm (1.5 in.) needle.
- ○ Amelioration of lameness after the tibial nerve has been anesthetized incriminates the *suspensory ligament,* or at least the proximoplantar metatarsal area, as the site of pain, provided that more distal structures of the limb have been eliminated as a source of pain by administering a low plantar nerve block.
   – The tibial nerve block is unlikely to ameliorate lameness caused by osteoarthritis in distal joints of the hock.

G   Deep and superficial peroneal nerves

- ○ The tibial nerve and the deep and superficial peroneal (fibular) nerves must be anesthetized to completely desensitize the hock and structures distal to the hock.
- ○ The *peroneal* nerves are anesthetized on the lateral aspect of the limb, about 10 cm above the point of the hock, in the groove separating the *lateral and long digital extensor muscles* (see Figure 24.13).
- ○ To anesthetize the deep peroneal nerve, a 20- to 22- gauge, 3.8–5.1 cm (1.5–2 in.) needle is inserted into the groove and directed medially, staying within the septum between the muscles, for about 3–4 cm.

**Figure 24.12**   Location of needle insertion for blockade of the tibial nerve.

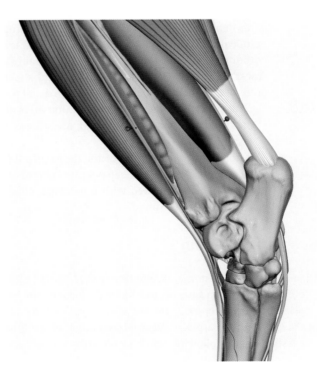

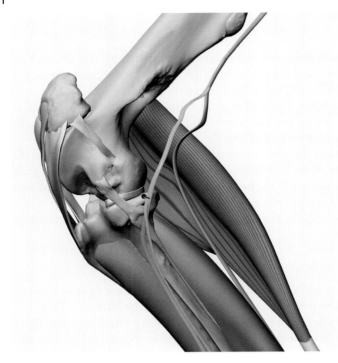

Figure 24.13    Location of needle insertion for blockade of the peroneal nerve.

  – The ability to move the tip of the needle up and down ensures that the needle has been inserted between the muscle bellies, where the nerve lies.
○ After depositing ~10 ml of local anesthetic solution at this site to anesthetize the *deep* peroneal nerve, more local anesthetic (~5 ml) is deposited superficially, as the needle is withdrawn, in three or four planes to anesthetize the *superficial* peroneal nerve.
○ Anesthetizing the tibial and the deep and superficial peroneal nerves proximal to the point of the hock desensitizes the entire distal portion of the limb.
  – The superficial peroneal nerve innervates only skin, so anesthetizing this nerve is not important when regional anesthesia is performed as part of a lameness examination.
○ The horse may *drag the toe* of the desensitized limb or *knuckle at the fetlock,* when the tibial and superficial and deep peroneal nerves are anesthetized. The distal portion of the limb should be protected with a bandage, after administering a peroneal nerve block, before the horse is trotted.

## Suggested Reading

Claunch, K.M., Eggleston, R.B., and Baxter, G.M. (2014). Effects of approach and injection volume on diffusion of mepivacaine hydrochloride during local analgesia of the deep branch of the lateral plantar nerve in horses. *J. Am. Vet. Med. Assoc.* 15: 1153–1159.

Seabaugh, K.A., Selberg, K.T., Valdes-Martinez, A. et al. (2011). Assessment of the tissue diffusion of anesthetic agent following administration of a low palmar nerve block in horses. *J. Am. Vet. Med. Assoc.* 15: 1334–1340.

Schumacher, J., Taintor, J., Schumacher, J. et al. (2013). Function of the ramus communicans of the medial and lateral palmar nerves of the horse. *Equine Vet. J.* 45: 31–35.

Van de Water, E., Oosterlinck, M., and Pille, F. (2016). The effect of perineural anaesthesia and handler position on limb loading and hoof balance and the vertical ground reaction force in sound horses. *Equine Vet. J.* 48: 608–612.

## 25

# Anesthesia of the Perineum and Testicle

## Pudendal Nerve Block – Electrostimulation Technique

*Kirsty Gallacher and Luiz Santos*

## I  Target nerves and region anesthetized

- Pudendal nerve, caudal rectal nerve and combined superficial perineal nerves.
- In geldings and stallions, blocking the pudendal and caudal rectal nerves desensitizes the anus, perineum, penis, and internal lamina of the prepuce (see Figure 25.1).
- In mares, blocking of the pudendal and caudal rectal nerves desensitizes the anus, perineum, vulva, and vestibule (see Figure 25.2).

## II  Location (see Figure 25.3)

- The tuber ischiadicum is palpated and an imaginary horizontal line depicted to create the ventral boundary of the injection site.
- The external anal sphincter along with either the dorsal vulvar lips or retractor penis muscle constituted the medial boundaries.
- The upper limit is at the ventral aspect of the external anal sphincter.
- The semimembranosus muscle indicates the lateral boundary (area marked/surrounded by red dotted line) (see Figure 25.3).

## III  Technique

*Desensitizing superficial planes*
- The rectum should be emptied of feces prior to this loco-regional block.
- Prepare the perineal area aseptically.
- Insert a 25-gauge, 2.5 cm (1 in.) needle to desensitize the skin and subcutaneous tissue.
- Infiltrate between 2 and 5 ml of 2% lidocaine at each injection point.

*Desensitizing the pudendal plexus*
- In mares, it can be helpful in some instances to insert a gloved hand into the vestibule to palpate the needle and guide its insertion path away from the rectal or vaginal wall. This is especially true when they have poor perineal conformation such as recessed anus and sloped vulva (see Figure 25.4).
- Attach a 30° bevel, 20-gauge G, 15 cm (5.9 in.) insulated needle to a peripheral nerve stimulator.

*Manual of Equine Anesthesia and Analgesia*, Second Edition. Edited by Tom Doherty, Alex Valverde, and Rachel A. Reed.
© 2022 John Wiley & Sons, Inc. Published 2022 by John Wiley & Sons, Inc.

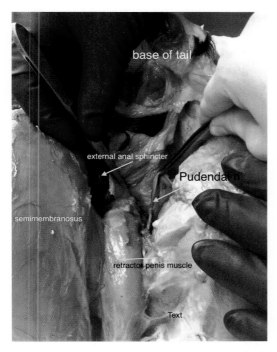

Figure 25.1   Dissection of the pelvic cavity showing the pudendal nerve stained with methylene blue after dissection in a Thoroughbred gelding. *Source:* Reprinted with permission of Gallacher et al. (2016).

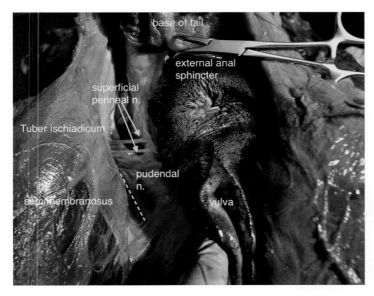

Figure 25.2   Caudal aspect of the pelvic cavity displaying the superficial perineal nerves and the pudendal nerve in a mare.

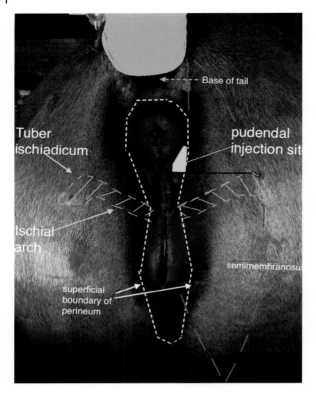

**Figure 25.3** Landmarks for the pudendal nerve block in the horse. The white dotted line indicates the boundaries of the superficial perineal region in the mare. The red dotted line indicates the area occupied by the semimembranosus muscle. The black horizontal line at the level of the tuber ischiadicum demarcates the ventral boundary of the injection site. The yellow triangle shows the needle insertion site.
*Source:* Reprinted with permission of Gallacher et al. (2016).

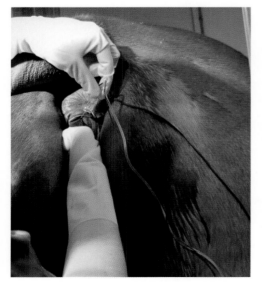

**Figure 25.4** Peripheral nerve locator needle positioning in a mare.

- Insert the insulated needle into the perineum at a point ventrolateral to the external anal sphincter at an angle of 45° to the sagittal plane (see Figure 25.4).
- The needle is advanced through the perineum toward the nerve while the peripheral nerve stimulator delivers the electrical stimuli to evoke an appropriate muscle contraction.
- A stimulation frequency of 1–2 Hz, stimulus duration of 0.1 ms, and current of 1 mA is used initially to induce a motor response. The strength of the observed contraction of both the anal sphincter and perineal muscles/vulvar lips helps to determine the optimal needle location. The current is then gradually decreased to refine the approach, indicating close proximity to the nerve. If a current reduction does not result in muscular contraction before reaching 0.4–0.6 mA, the needle should be redirected until the previous muscle response reappeared and subsequently, the anesthetic solution is injected.
- Needle depth varies between 5 and 10 cm depending on the size of the horse and perineal conformation.
- Before each injection, a small volume should be aspirated to test for intravascular puncture.
- In males, the penis usually protrudes within 5 minutes, confirming local blockade.
- Allow up to 20 minutes for the block to work.

## IV Choice and volume of anesthetic

- At least 10 ml per injection site is recommended to obtain successful blockade. Typically, 20 ml is used each side in a 500 kg horse.
- The choice of local anesthetic agent in mares includes 2% lidocaine, 2% mepivacaine, or 0.5% bupivacaine depending on the type of procedure being performed and duration of analgesia required.
- In males, we recommend using lidocaine or mepivacaine; bupivacaine is best avoided due to potential prolonged penile extrusion.
- Time to desensitization varies between 5 and 20 minutes depending upon the local anesthetic used.

## V Caution

- Risk of intravascular injection, hematoma, nerve damage and rectal puncture.

## Pudendal Nerve Block – Blind Approach

*Jim Schumacher*

- Blocking the pudendal nerves at the ischium desensitizes the penis and internal lamina of the prepuce.
- With successful blockade, the penis relaxes and can be extruded.

### A Location

- ○ The sites of injection are on the right and left sides of the anus about 2 cm dorsal to the ischial arch and an equal distance to the anus (see Figure 25.3).

### B Technique

- Insert a 21- or 22-gauge 3.8 cm (1.5 in.) needle (angled ventrally toward the midline) at each site until the point of the needle contacts the ischial arch, where the pudendal nerves course around the ischium.
- Deposit 10–20 ml of local anesthetic adjacent to each nerve.
- The penis usually protrudes within five minutes but may take up to 20 minutes.

### C Choice of anesthetic

- A short-acting local anesthetic, such as lidocaine HCl, should be used rather than mepivacaine HCl to avoid prolonged protrusion of the penis and prepuce, unless prolonged penile and preputial desensitization is required.

## Local Anesthesia for Castration

*Philip D. Jones*

## I Introduction

- It seems reasonable to assume that castration is a noxious stimulus.
- In support of this assumption, it has been demonstrated that:
  - EEG changes occurring in horses undergoing castration while anesthetized with halothane (1.2% expired) were considered to be indicative of nociception.
    - It is of interest that the EEG changes were abolished by an intravenous (IV) *lidocaine* infusion.
- Local anesthesia of the skin, cremaster, and spermatic cord is employed for castration of standing horses. Anesthesia of the spermatic cord can be achieved using an intratesticular (IT) injection of a local anesthetic or an injection of local anesthetic directly into the spermatic cord. The disadvantage of injecting directly into the spermatic cord is that it may cause a hematoma. However, an IT injection or injection into the spermatic cord is less commonly performed when horses are castrated under general anesthesia (see Figure 25.5).
- Local anesthesia of the testicle is considered by many to be the *standard of care* for equine castrations performed under general anesthesia.
  - This is in addition to perioperative administration of an NSAID.
- *Comment*: The British Equine Veterinary Association recommends that anesthetized horses be administered an IT injection of local anesthetic prior to castration, and that an NSAID be administered prior to and for three days post castration.
- Some clinicians are opposed to administering an IT local anesthetic based on the assumption that there is an increased risk of bleeding and infection; however, these assumptions have been proven to be incorrrect.
- Yet, the lack of efficacy of an IT block with *lidocaine* has been reported in some studies. In one study, IT *lidocaine* failed to completely block the increase in blood pressure in

**Figure 25.5** Intratesticular injection of 2% mepivacaine (Carbocaine®).

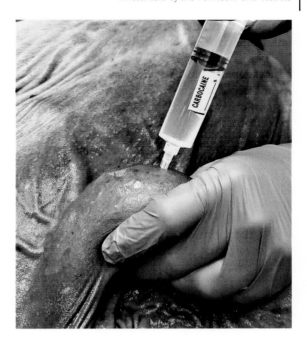

isoflurane-anesthetized horses undergoing castration. However, that study was confounded by the administration of *dobutamine* intraoperatively.
- Nevertheless, IT *lidocaine* was associated with a significant decrease in the number of supplemental doses of *ketamine* needed to prevent movement during castration.
  - But there was no benefit in regard to *cremaster muscle* relaxation.
- The reason for IT *lidocaine* being only partially effective in blunting the blood pressure response and ineffective in relaxing the cremaster muscle can be attributed to:
  - The *extensive innervation* of the scrotal skin, testicle, spermatic cord, and cremaster muscle.
  - The *poor distribution* of IT administered lidocaine to the cremaster muscle.
- *Mepivacaine* (2%), when administered IT to anesthetized horses undergoing castration was associated with:
  - Decreased postoperative pain.
  - A diminished postoperative increase in IL-6 and TNFα.
- In horses anesthetized with *xylazine/ketamine*, IT *mepivacaine* (2%), in comparison to IT *lidocaine* (2%), was associated with:
  - Increased cremaster muscle relaxation.
    - This finding is consistent with the fact that administering an IT injection of *mepivacaine* relaxes the testicle in the standing horse undergoing castration.
  - A decrease in the number of supplemental doses of *ketamine* needed to prevent movement.

## II Nerve supply

- The testicles, epididymis, and spermatic cord are innervated by *sympathetic* fibers of the autonomic nervous system.
- The cremaster muscle, scrotal skin, and spermatic fascia derive *somatic* innervation from the *genitofemoral* nerve, which originates from the lumbar plexus, and supplies sensory and motor function.

- As these fibers are *not within* the cord, it may explain why IT lidocaine is not effective in relaxing the cremaster, as lidocaine does not readily cross the parietal layer of the tunica vaginalis. However, there is no obvious answer as to why mepivacaine appears to be more efficacious than lidocaine in relaxating the cremaster muscle.
- Complete anesthesia of the surgical site for castration, as required in the non-anesthetized horse, would involve desensitizing all the aforementioned structures and the scrotal skin.
  - Nevertheless, because cutting the spermatic cord is the most noxious part of castration, anesthesia of the cord appears to adequately block noxious stimuli when used in association with sedation or general anesthesia.

## III   Uptake and distribution of IT administered drugs

- Drugs administered IT are taken up by the *lymphatic system* and are *dispersed* throughout the spermatic cord.
  - This has been demonstrated using *radiolabeled* lidocaine.
- Peak concentrations of IT-administered drugs are likely achieved in the spermatic cord within three to five minutes.
  - In one study, *methylene blue* was detected in the spermatic cord 20 cm proximal to the testicle at 1.5 minutes post IT injection.
- In contrast, IT-administered drugs are *poorly* distributed to the cremaster muscle.

## IV   Volume of IT local anesthetic

- The volume needed will vary with the size of the testicle, and the latter will vary with age and breed.
- 10 ml in each testicle is an approximate volume for full-sized adult horses.
- Another approach is to inject enough volume to make the testicle feel firmer.
  - Increasing the pressure within the testicle may also increase the rate of uptake by the lymphatic system, and result in a faster onset of the block.

## Suggested Reading

Abass, M., Picek, S., and Garz, J.F.G. (2018). Local mepivacaine before castration of horses under medetomidine isoflurane balanced anaesthesia is effective to reduce perioperative nociception and cytokine release. *Equine Vet. J.* 50: 733–738.

Bowen, M., Redpath, A., Dugdale, A. et al. (2020). BEVA primary care clinical guidelines: Analgesia. *Equine Vet. J.* 52: 13–27.

Crandall, A., Hopster, K., Grove, A., and Levine, D. (2020). Intratesticular mepivacaine versus lidocaine in anaesthetised horses undergoing Henderson castration. *Equine Vet. J.* 52: 805–810.

Gallacher, K., Santos, L.C., Campoy, L. et al. (2016). Development of a peripheral nerve stimulator guided technique for equine pudendal nerve block. *Vet. J.* 217: 72–77.

Haga, H.A., Lykkjen, S., Revold, T., and Ranheim, B. (2006). Effect of intratesticular injection of lidocaine on cardiovascular responses to castration in isoflurane-anesthetized stallions. *Am. J. Vet. Res.* 67: 403–408.

Murrell, J.C., Johnson, C.B., White, K.L. et al. (2003). Changes in the EEG during castration in horses and ponies anaesthetized with halothane. *Vet. Anaesth. Analg.* 30: 138–146.

Portier, K.G., Jaillardon, L., Leece, E.A., and Walsh, C.M. (2009). Castration of horses under total intravenous anaesthesia: analgesic effects of lidocaine. *Vet. Anaesth. Analg.* 36: 173–179.

Schumacher, J., Bratton, G.R., and Williams, J.W. (1985). Pudendal and caudal rectal nerve blocks in the horse – an anesthetic procedure for reproductive surgery. *Theriogenology* 24: 457–464.

# 26

## Anesthesia of the Abdominal Wall

### Thoracolumbar Paravertebral Block (TPVB) – Electrostimulation Technique

*Luiz Santos and Kirsty Gallacher*

- Paravertebral thoracolumbar anesthesia can be used as an alternative to infiltration anesthesia or an epidural during standing procedures when incisions of the flank are required.
- Advantages of paravertebral anesthesia over infiltration anesthesia include smaller doses of local anesthetic, a wider area of desensitization, the absence of hematomas, and the absence of any potential interference with tissue healing.
- TPVB can be used for a range of standing surgical procedures including laparoscopic surgeries, granulosa cell tumor removal, exploratory laparotomy surgeries such as colic cases and cryptorchid surgery.

### A   Location

- The first step is to mark with a surgical pen the lumbar transverse process of L3 by drawing an imaginary line [authors prefer using a 30 cm (12 in) ruler] along the most caudal extension of the last rib (2 cm) and perpendicular to the long axis of the spinal vertebrae. (see Figure 26.1)
- The distance between the caudal border of the last rib and the spinal process of L3 is around 15 cm in the adult horse.
- The distance between the injection sites (from L3 to L2 to L1 and to T18) is approximately 5–6 cm in the adult horse. (see Figures 26.2 and 26.3)

### B   Technique

*Note*: it is generally necessary to sedate the horse and place it in stocks prior to attempting the block.

*Desensitizing superficial planes*

- Insert a 21-gauge, 3.81 cm (1.5 in) needle (angled perpendicular to the skin) to desensitize the skin, subcutaneous and superficial musculature of each injection site.
- Infiltrate 5 ml of 2% lidocaine at each of the three injection points.

*Desensitizing the thoracolumbar nerves*

- Insert a long beveled, 20-gauge, 150 mm insulated needle either caudo-ventrally (see Figure 26.3) or cranio-ventrally (see Figure 26.3) at a 45° angle to the skin until it impinges on the transverse process of L3 (needle depth around 100 mm in lean body weight horses).

*Manual of Equine Anesthesia and Analgesia*, Second Edition. Edited by Tom Doherty, Alex Valverde, and Rachel A. Reed.
© 2022 John Wiley & Sons, Inc. Published 2022 by John Wiley & Sons, Inc.

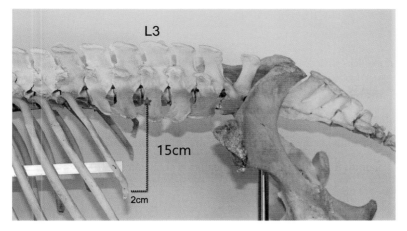

Figure 26.1 First step, localizing the transverse process of L3.

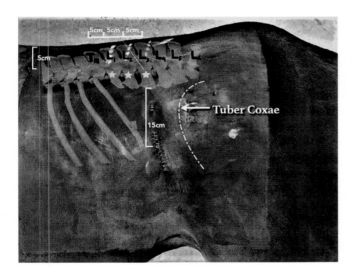

Figure 26.2 Left thoracolumbar area of a standing adult Thoroughbred horse for paravertebral block of T18, L1, and L2 nerve roots. Yellow stars represent the location of thoracolumbar nerves.

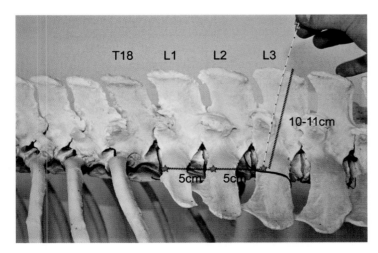

Figure 26.3 Red stars indicate location of nerve roots of T18, L1, and L2. Note the distance between the dorsal aspect of the transverse processes and the ridge of the spinous processes (±10–11 cm). This distance is relative to the horse's body score condition.

- o The needle is then *walked-off* cranially until the intertransverse ligament between L3 and L2 is penetrated. Penetration of the ligament is felt as an initial increase in resistance to the advancing needle followed by sudden loss of resistance.
- o First, aim to identify an evoked muscle contraction of the flank region using a 1 mA current. Twitching of the lumbar muscles should occur because of direct muscle stimulation, but as the needle is slowly advanced an evoked contraction of the muscles composing the flank region (external and internal oblique abdominal muscles and transverse abdominal muscle) should be seen.
- o The proximity with the nerve root of L2 is confirmed when a positive twitch of the most caudal aspect of the flank (closer to tuber coxae) is present when the current is decreased to 0.5 mA. By using a low current intensity, the unspecific direct muscular stimulation unrelated to the proximity to the paravertebral branches is avoided.
- o Infiltrate 5 ml of either 2% lidocaine, 2% mepivacaine, or 0.5% bupivacaine when at maximum positive stimulation and another 5 ml infiltrated when retracting the needle 2 cm above this point (total of 10 ml per nerve root).
- o The procedure should be repeated to desensitize nerve roots of L1 and T18 at the transverse process of L2 and L1, respectively.
- o The proximity to the root of T18 is confirmed by contraction of the most cranial aspect of the flank (closer to the last rib).
- o Adequacy of the block should be checked 15 minutes later by sensory loss of the surgical field to pinprick sensation.

*Note: Always aspirate before injecting. Avoid injection of local anesthetics if blood is seen at the hub of needle. If loss of resistance or aspiration of air is present, the needle should be withdrawn to a retroperitoneal position before the local anesthetic is deposited.*

## Paravertebral Nerve Block – Blind Technique
*Alex Valverde*

### I  Indications

- • Desensitizing the flank is potentially useful for:
  - o Surgical procedures of the abdominal cavity in the standing horse.
    - – Laparoscopic surgery for abdominal exploration, closure of the nephrosplenic space, ovariectomy, uterine torsion.
- • Adequate sedation and analgesia are required to enhance the usefulness of the block.

### A  Equipment

- o Sterile gloves (preferred).
- o Local anesthetic agent (lidocaine).
- o 20 mL disposable syringes.
- o Spinal needle.
  - – An 18-gauge 15.2-cm needle.

## II  Patient preparation

### A  Physical restraint

- The horse should be restrained in stocks to minimize the risk to personnel.

### B  Chemical restraint

- Sedation is necessary to complete the block and facilitate the surgery.
- Drugs with analgesic properties and that are less likely to cause ataxia are recommended.

### C  Preparation of injection site

- Shave the epaxial area above the flank where the surgical approach would take place and include from the 17th thoracic vertebrae to the 1st sacral vertebrae.
- Prepare the injection site aseptically.

## III  General technique

- Knowledge of topographic landmarks of the injection site and recognition of anatomic structures to locate T18, L1, and L2 nerves is indispensable for a successful block (see Figure 26.4).
- Local anesthetic should be accurately deposited close to the nerve.
  - To reduce the risk of inadvertent injection into adjacent vascular structures always aspirate before injection.

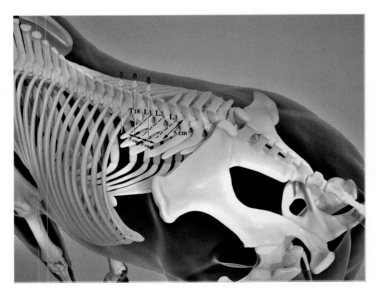

**Figure 26.4**  Anatomic location of spinal nerve roots T18, L1, L2, and L3 and location of needle insertion.

## A   Needle insertion

- ○ In an adult horse (450–600 kg), introduce the spinal needle starting at spinal nerve L2.
- ○ The ventral branch of the spinal nerve is at an average depth of $11.3 \pm 0.7$ cm from the epaxial skin. The dorsal branch is at an average depth of $9.5 \pm 0.8$ cm.
- ○ The needle is introduced *perpendicular* and 5 cm lateral to the dorsal midline, at a level in line with the most caudal point of the last rib (18th rib), which corresponds to the location of the $L_3$ transverse process. (see Figures 26.5 and 26.6)
- ○ The needle is advanced until it contacts the transverse process of L3 and is *"walked-off"* the cranial edge until it advances through the intertransverse ligament for blockade of the ventral branch of nerve L2.
- ○ Aspirate to verify for negative pressure and confirm extra-abdominal location, and for absence of blood. (see Figure 26.7)
- ○ Inject 15 ml of 2% lidocaine.

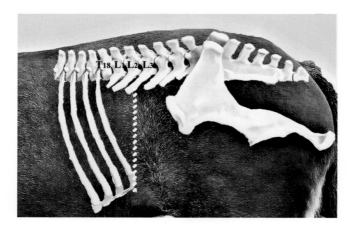

**Figure 26.5**   Use of caudal border of last rib to determine location of third lumbar transverse process.

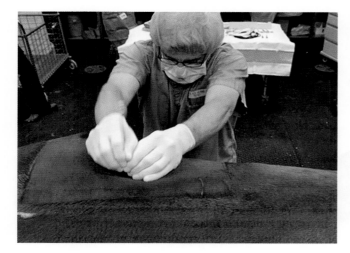

**Figure 26.6**   Insertion of needle for blind paravertebral block.

Figure 26.7 Aspirate prior to injection to ensure that the needle tip is not within a blood vessel.

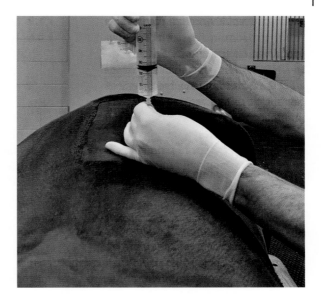

- Retract the needle to its previous location dorsal to the intertransverse ligament, where the L3 transverse process is again identified with the needle tip and inject 5 ml of 2% lidocaine for blockade of the dorsal branch of nerve L2.
- Repeat these steps and maintain a distance of 5 cm from the dorsal midline and move the needle 5–6 cm cranially from the previous site to block L1.
- Repeat the previous step by moving the needle 5–6 cm cranially from the L1 site to block T18.

## Transversus Abdominis Plane Block

*Alex Valverde and Flavio SA. Freitag*

### I   Indications

- Desensitizing the transversus abdominis plane (TAP) is potentially useful for:
  - Surgical procedures of the abdominal cavity using a median or paramedian approach in the anesthetized horse.
    - Analgesia for abdominal exploration.
    - Enhancing relaxation of the abdominal wall.

### II   Anatomy

- The lateral and ventral abdominal wall are innervated by rami from thoracic (T) spinal nerves $T_{10}$ to $T_{18}$.
- The ventral wall also receives innervation from lumbar (L) nerves $L_1$ (*iliohypogastric nerve*) and $L_2$ (*ilioinguinal nerve*).

- Blockade of these nerves provides anesthesia of the abdominal wall, including the skin, subcutaneous tissue, muscular layers and parietal peritoneum, prepuce, and mammary gland.
- The lateral abdominal wall consists of three muscles:
  - The external abdominal oblique.
  - The internal abdominal oblique.
  - The transversus abdominis.
- The ventral abdominal wall includes the same three muscles, and the *rectus abdominis*.
- $T_{10}$-$T_{18}$ spinal nerves run within the facial plane between the lateral surface of the transversus abdominis muscle and the medial surface of the internal abdominal oblique muscle and are located in a line between the umbilicus and the xiphoid cartilage, approximately midway between the ventral midline and the costal arch.

## III  TAP block

- Aseptic technique is mandatory when performing the block.
- The following blocks have been described, with information based on cadaver studies and some clinical application.

### A  Flank approach

- A descriptive study was performed with pony cadavers in dorsal recumbency using an ultrasound (US) guided technique. (see Baldo et al., Suggested reading)
  - A 6–13 MHz linear array ultrasonic probe was used.
- The study described a single-point injection technique in each hemiabdomen.

*Technique*
- The probe was placed midway between the most caudal aspect of the last rib and the most cranial aspect of the iliac crest, at a point that intersects from an imaginary line that originates from the caudal aspect of the umbilicus and runs lateral toward the placement of the US probe. (see Figure 26.8)

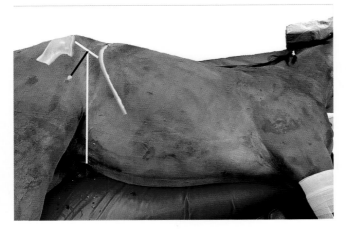

**Figure 26.8**  Transversus abdominus plane block using the flank approach.

- A 20 or 21-gauge, 3.5–4-in (8.9–10 cm) needle was inserted in the fascial plane between the internal oblique muscle and the transversus abdominis muscle, at a 20° angle using an "in-plane" approach (ventral-dorsal direction).
- *Bupivacaine* (0.5%), 0.5 ml/kg mixed with methylene blue was injected into each hemiabdomen.
  - Initially, 2–3 ml was injected to visualize hydrodissection (separation of muscle layers) for correct placement.
  - Upon correct placement, the remaining anesthetic was injected slowly, and the needle advanced periodically to optimize the spread of injectate.

*Results*
- Nerves T14 to L3 became stained with methylene blue, but not in all cases. The success rate in staining nerves T16-L2 was over 75%. Assuming that staining the nerve corresponded to blocking nervous transmission, the described technique had a success rate of ≥75% in blocking transmission in T16 to L2.

B   Intercostal ventral approach (see – Küls et al., Suggested reading)

- This study was performed initially using horse cadavers in lateral recumbency.
- The aim of the cadaver study was to establish the most appropriate injection points and injectate volume required to stain the nerves providing sensation to the ventrolateral abdominal wall and skin in horse cadavers (i.e. T9-L 2).
- The study was then performed in sedated, standing Shetland ponies (113–194 kg) using an US-guided technique.

*Technique*
- In this technique, a *three-point* injection technique was employed in each hemiabdomen (see Figure 26.9).
- Injections were administered caudal to ribs 9, 14, and 18 to block the respective thoracic spinal nerve.
- The US probe was placed 10 cm ventral to the costochondral joint of the corresponding intercostal space.

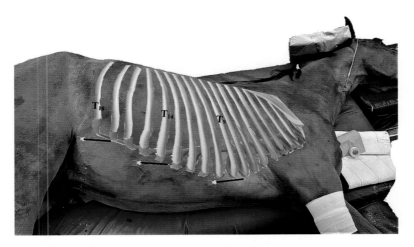

Figure 26.9   Transversus abdominus plane block using the intercostal ventral approach.

- A 20 or 21-gauge, 3.5–4-in (8.9–10 cm) needle was inserted in the fascial plane between the internal oblique muscle and the transversus abdominis muscle, at a 45° angle in an "in-plane" direction (caudocranial).
- Bupivacaine (0.125%), 0.1 ml/kg, was deposited at each injection point of both hemiabdomens (0.3 ml/kg per hemiabdomen).
  - Initially, 2–3 ml was injected to visualize hydrodissection, for correct placement.
  - Upon establishing correct placement, the remaining volume was injected slowly.

### Results
- In cadavers, this technique resulted in staining nerves $T_8$–$T_{18}$.
- In standing ponies, there was a decreased response to pinprick stimulation for nerves $T_8$–$T_{18}$, with an onset of effect at 30 minutes and a duration of up to 120 minutes for nerves $T_{12}$–$T_{17}$ and up to 180 minutes for nerves $T_8$–$T_{11}$, based on <50% response to pinprick.

### C   Subcostal approach (see Suggested reading – Freitag et al.)

- This study was performed with horse cadavers in either lateral or dorsal recumbency.
- Described as a *two-point* injection technique in each hemiabdomen (see Figure 26.10).

### Technique
- The *landmarks* used include the xiphoid cartilage, the umbilicus, and the cutaneous trunci muscle.
  - The *first* injection point was midway the xiphoid cartilage and the umbilical scar.
  - The *second* injection point was based on the imaginary division of the caudal half of the abdomen (starting on the first injection point) in three equal parts, using the line that divides the caudal and middle part as the injection site.
  - Both injections, were located ventral to the *cutaneous trunci* muscle limits.
- The US probe was placed at each of the injection points, perpendicular to the central axis.
- A 20 or 21-gauge, 3.5–4-in (8.9–10 cm) needle was inserted in the fascial plane between the *transversus abdominis* muscle and the *rectus abdominis* muscle, at a 45° angle in a "in-plane" approach (dorsoventral).

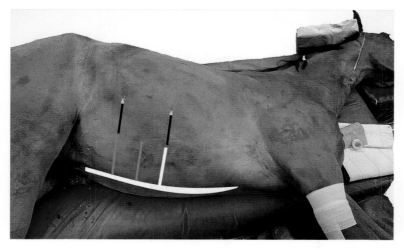

Figure 26.10   Transversus abdominus plane block using the subcostal approach.

- Bupivacaine (0.5%), 0.06–0.08 ml/kg, with methylene blue was injected into each injection point of both hemiabdomens (0.12–0.16 ml/kg per hemiabdomen).
  - Initially, 2–3 ml was injected to visualize hydrodissection, for correct placement.
  - Upon establishing correct placement, the remaining volume is injected slowly.

*Results*
- Staining of nerves $T_{10}$–$T_{16}$ with a frequency of ≥60% occurred for cadavers in lateral recumbency.
- Staining of nerves $T_{13}$–$T_{17}$ with a frequency of ≥60% occurred for cadavers in dorsal recumbency.

## Caudal Intercostal Block for Abdominal Surgery (CIBAS)
*Benjamin Gingold*

- An intercostal nerve block for desensitization of the ventral and lateral abdominal and thoracic wall has been described.
- The block includes individual desensitization of intercostal nerves $T_8$–$T_{18}$.
- The block has been described as suitable for relieving post-celiotomy incisional pain.

## I  Anatomy

- Because the ventral wall also receives innervation from lumbar (L) nerves $L_1$ (*iliohypogastric* nerve) and $L_2$ (*ilioinguinal* nerve), this block will *not* provide complete anesthesia of the ventral midline on its caudal aspect.

*Technique*
- The block can be performed with the horse standing or in dorsal recumbency.
  - The block can be performed "*blind*" as described below.
  - However, the procedure can be performed more accurately and safely with US and/or nerve stimulation guidance.
- In a line parallel to the spine at the level of the ventral aspect of the tuber coxae, the skin over ribs $T_8$-$T_{18}$ is clipped and aseptically prepared. (see Figure 26.11)
- Performing the block at the level of ventral aspect of tuber coxae is challenging in a dorsally recumbent patient but aim to inject as dorsally as possible (up to the level of the tuber coxae).
- At each of these intercostal spaces, the needle is inserted through the skin to the caudal rib edge where the *intercostal* ($T_8$–$T_{17}$) or *costoabdominal* ($T_{18}$) nerve passes. Contact is made with the rib and the needle is then "*walked*" off the back to position the needle adjacent to the nerve.
  - A 20–22 G 1–1.5-in (2.54–3.81 cm) needle is suitable for this procedure.
- Aspiration is made prior to injection to minimize risk of injection into a blood vessel.
- A volume of 6–10 ml is injected per site.
  - If unsure of the proximity of the needle to the rib, a larger volume should be injected.

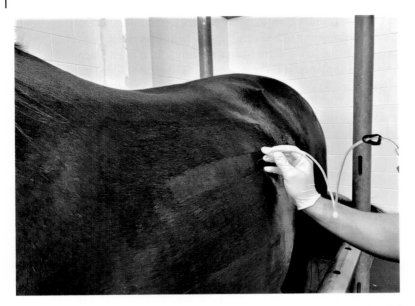

Figure 26.11    Caudal intercostal block performed in the standing horse for abdominal surgery.

- The procedure is repeated for the other side of the body wall.
- The block can be repeated as needed post-surgery.
- The duration of the block is typically 8–12 hours when *bupivacaine + dexmedetomidine + epinephrine* is injected.

*Drugs administered*
- *Bupivacaine* is the local anesthetic of choice because of its long duration of action.
  – As a rule of thumb, 160 ml of bupivacaine (0.5%) can typically be administered for horses ≥400 kg.
- Bupivacaine can be combined with an $\alpha_2$ agonist (e.g. d*exmedetomidine* or *medetomidine*) or other adjuvants to prolong the duration of the block.
  – *Dexmedetomidine* (1–2 µg) or *medetomidine* (2–4 µg) per 1 ml of bupivacaine.
  – *Epinephrine*: 5 µg/1 ml of bupivacaine. This is equivalent to adding 0.1 ml of 1 : 1000 epinephrine to 20 ml of bupivacaine (making a 1 : 200#000 mixture).
- Other adjuvants that can be added to bupivacaine include:
  – *Buprenorphine* 0.015 mg per 1 ml of bupivacaine.
  – *Dexamethasone* 0.03 mg per 1 ml of bupivacaine.

## II   Disadvantages of the CIBAS technique

- When compared to the TAP block, CIBAS:
  - It is time consuming.
  - Uses a large volume of local anesthetic.
  - Does not provide a complete block of the midline.

## Suggested Reading

Baldo, C.F., Almeida, D., Wendt-Hornickle, E. et al. (2018). Transversus abdominus plane block in ponies: a preliminary anatomical study. *Vet. Anaesth. Analg.* 45: 392–396.

Freitag, F.A.V., Amora, D.D., Muehlbauer, E. et al. (2021). Ultrasound-guided modified subcostal transversus abdominis plane block and influence of recumbency position on dye spread in equine cadavers. *Vet. Anaesth. Analg.* in press, DOI: https://doi.org/10.1016/j.vaa.2021.03.006.

Gingold, B.M.C., Hassen, K.M., Milloway, M.C. et al. (2018). Caudal intercostal block for abdominal surgery in horses. *Vet. Rec.* 183: 164–165.

Küls, N., Trujanovi, R., Otero, P.E., and Larenza-Menzies, M.P. (2020). Ultrasound-guided transversus abdominis plane block in Shetland ponies: a description of a three-point injection technique and evaluation of potential analgesic effects. *J. Equine Vet. Sci.* 90 (1–7).

## 27

# Epidural Analgesia and Anesthesia
*Alex Valverde*

- Epidural administration of drugs is an effective method of providing anesthesia and/or analgesia of the perineum in the standing horse.
  - Depending on the drug, dose, and volume used, analgesia of more rostral areas can also be achieved.
- The epidural space is accessible at the lumbosacral (L–S) joint (cranial epidural) and caudal to the sacrum (caudal epidural).
- *The caudal epidural* space (sacrococcygeal or Co1–Co2) is the preferred and most commonly used site in the horse as it is easier and safer to perform an epidural injection here than at L–S space.
  - There is no risk of dural puncture and cerebrospinal fluid (CSF) tap.
  - Less risk of motor blockade to the pelvic limbs and associated weakness, ataxia, and or immobilization.
    - However, if a large volume of injectate is administered at the caudal epidural space it can result in a cranial epidural block.
    - This will also occur with a catheter advanced rostrally toward the lumbosacral area. Rostral spread may be beneficial or detrimental depending on the drug used and the goal in question (see specific drugs below).
- *Cranial epidural* (L–S space) is less commonly used.
  - It is technically more difficult to perform, especially in heavily muscled horses.
  - The technique is used mainly for CSF collection.
    - It requires longer needles.
    - The landmarks are not so obvious.
  - There is a greater risk of motor blockade and ataxia.
  - A catheter advanced *caudally* from the L–S space to the sacral area can produce a caudal epidural block.
  - A catheter advanced *rostrally* from the L–S space to the thoracolumbar area can provide segmental analgesia of the thorax and abdomen.

*Manual of Equine Anesthesia and Analgesia*, Second Edition. Edited by Tom Doherty, Alex Valverde, and Rachel A. Reed.
© 2022 John Wiley & Sons, Inc. Published 2022 by John Wiley & Sons, Inc.

## I   Anatomy and technique for caudal epidural

### A   Location

- ○ The spinal cord extends to the level of the caudal half of the second sacral vertebra.
- ○ Epidural injection can be performed at the sacrococcygeal (S–Co) or first intercoccygeal (Co1–Co2) space, without risk of spinal injection.
- ○ Either space is located by moving the tail up and down while palpating the intervertebral space (see Figure 27.1).
  - – As a guide, the spaces are approximately 2.5–7.5 cm (1–3 in.) cranial to the first tail hairs.
  - – The depth of the space from the skin is 3.5–8 cm (1.3–3 in.).

### B   Technique

- ○ Aseptic technique is mandatory.
- ○ Superficial local anesthetic infiltration (e.g., 1 ml of 2% lidocaine, 23 or 25-gauge needle) at the site of injection facilitates insertion of the needle or catheter. (see Figure 27.2)
- ○ Sedation may be necessary in the awake horse.
  - – Oversedation should be avoided as the horse will not then stand squarely, making it more difficult to keep on the midline when inserting the needle/catheter.
- ○ Hypodermic needles, spinal needles, or epidural catheters can be used.
  - – 22-, 20-, or 18-gauge, 3.8–8.9 cm (1.5–3.5 in.) needle or spinal needle, depending on the size of the horse.
  - – 17- or 18-gauge, 7.6–8.9 cm (3–3.5 in.) *Tuohy* needle for insertion of a 19- or 20-gauge epidural catheter.

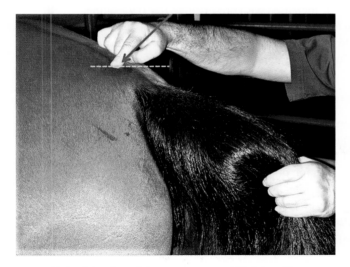

**Figure 27.1**   Palpation of the sacrococcygeal (S-Co) and intercoccygeal space (Co1-Co2) by moving the tail up and down to flex and extend the joints.

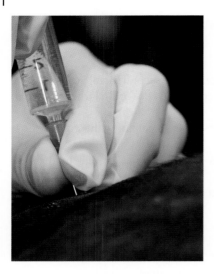

**Figure 27.2**   Superficial infiltration of local anesthetic using a 23–25-gauge needle to desensitize the area in which the spinal needle will be inserted.

- ○ Hypodermic needles and spinal needles are generally used for one-time drug administration.
- ○ Catheters are recommended for repeated drug administration and long-term use.
- ○ The needle is introduced at a 30–90° angle to the plane of the skin and advanced into the epidural space by traversing the intervertebral ligament (see Figures 27.3 and 27.4).
- ○ The volume of injection can be increased with preservative-free 0.9% saline.
    - – Volumes <10 ml can be injected over one to three minutes.
    - – Volumes >10 ml should be injected slowly (five minutes), due to mechanical compression of nerve endings in the epidural space resulting in the horse becoming recumbent.

C   Verification of needle or catheter placement

- ○ Placement is verified by one or more of the following methods:
    - – Hanging-drop technique: aspiration of a drop of fluid from the hub of the needle by the negative pressure of the epidural space.
    - – Lack of resistance upon injection of air.
    - – Lack of resistance upon injection of drugs.
    - – Ease of advancement of epidural catheter.
- ○ *Catheters* are introduced 10–30 cm into the epidural space.
    - – They should be secured to the skin with adhesive and suture material. (see Figure 27.5)
    - – Asepsis should be maintained.
    - – Epidural catheters can remain in place for weeks.

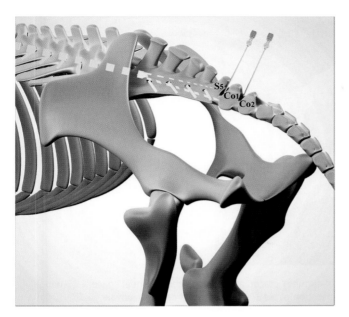

**Figure 27.3** *(epidural with spinal cord included).* A caudal epidural using the $S_5$-$Co_1$ space or first intercoccygeal space can be performed with a 22-, 20- or 18-gauge, 1.5 to 3.5 in. (2.54 to 8.89 cm) hypodermic needle or spinal needle, depending on the horse's size. The needle is introduced at 30–90° to the plane of the skin, and the angle is adjusted, as required to place the tip in the epidural space. Note the location of the caudal end of the spinal cord at the $L_6$-$S_1$ area and the projection of caudal nerves (cauda equina) in the sacrococcygeal epidural space.

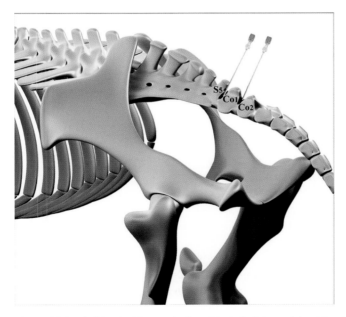

**Figure 27.4** *(epidural without spinal cord included).* A caudal epidural using the $S_5$-$Co_1$ space or first intercoccygeal space can be performed with a 22-, 20- or 18-gauge, 1.5 to 3.5 in. (2.54 to 8.89 cm) hypodermic needle or spinal needle, depending on the horse's size. The needle is introduced at 30–90° to the plane of the skin, and the angle is adjusted, as required to place the tip in the epidural space.

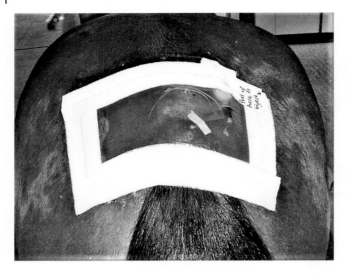

Figure 27.5 *(epidural catheter).* An epidural catheter placed at the first intercoccygeal space. A 17-gauge, 3 in. (7.62 cm) Tuohy needle was used for insertion of a 19-gauge epidural catheter, advanced 10–30 cm into the epidural space, and secured to the skin with adhesive material.

## II Indications for epidural drug administration

- Depending on the drug(s) used, epidural techniques can provide effects that range from analgesia to complete anesthesia. Therefore, indications include:
  - ○ Anesthesia of the rectum, anus, perineum, tail, urethra, bladder, vulva, vagina, penis, or inguinal region for surgery performed in the standing horse.
  - ○ Adjunct analgesia during general anesthesia for surgery of these same anatomic areas and hindlimbs.
  - ○ Pain management with opioids (e.g. *morphine*) for caudal and cranial anatomic areas.

## III Contraindications

- Skin infection at or near the site of injection.
- Spinal cord disease.
- Weak patients with an increased risk of ataxia/recumbency.

## IV Effects

### A Analgesia

- ○ Is induced by drugs that block conduction in Aδ and/or C-fibers.
  - – Local anesthetics and xylazine block both types of fibers.
  - – Opioids and $\alpha_2$ agonists (except xylazine) are more selective for C-fibers.

### B Anesthesia

- ○ Is induced by drugs that block Aδ and C-fibers.
- ○ Local anesthetics, *xylazine, ketamine*.

C   **Other spinal effects**

   o   *Proprioceptive deficits* are caused by drugs that block A$\alpha$ fibers.
      –   Local anesthetics and *xylazine*.
   o   *Motor blockade* (e.g. ataxia, recumbency) is caused by drugs that block A$\alpha$ and A$\beta$ motor fibers.
      –   Local anesthetics and $\alpha_2$ agonists (high doses).
   o   *Sympathetic blockade* is caused by drugs that block B fibers.
      –   Local anesthetics only.

D   **Systemic effects**

   o   Absorption of the drug by epidural vessels can result in different systemic effects depending on the drug injected.
      –   Sedation (e.g. $\alpha_2$ agonists).
      –   Excitement (e.g. opioids). But unlikely when opioids are administered epidurally.
      –   Ataxia (e.g. local anesthetics and $\alpha_2$ agonists).
      –   Cardiorespiratory effects including hypotension, hypertension, bradycardia can result from $\alpha_2$ agonist administration due to systemic absorption.

## V   Complications

   •   Failure to achieve analgesia and/or anesthesia can result from:
   o   Poor technique.
   o   Fibrous tissue at the site from previous injections.
   o   Anatomic abnormalities making it difficult to locate the landmarks for needle/catheter placement.
   o   Excessive ataxia and occasionally recumbency from overdose of local anesthetics, $\alpha_2$ agonists or the combination.
   o   Ataxia and weakness may not be evident while the horse is in the stocks as it may lean against the stocks for support, so it is important to evaluate the horse before attempting to move it.
      –   It may be necessary to place the horse in a sling or support the hindquarters with a tail rope until motor function returns.
      –   If recumbency results, sedation or a light plane of general anesthesia may be necessary to maintain the horse in recumbency until motor function is regained.
      –   Systemic pruritis has been reported following epidural co-administration of *morphine* and *detomidine*.

## VI   Drugs

A   **Local anesthetics**

   o   Epidurally administered local anesthetics can induce dose-related sensory, motor, and sympathetic blockade.
   o   The main indication is to produce perineal anesthesia for surgical procedures.

- ○ Higher doses and volumes can travel rostrally and block all fiber types, causing ataxia/paresis and hypotension.
- ○ Can be combined with $\alpha_2$ agonists. (see Section F below)

*Lidocaine (2%) or mepivacaine (2%)*
- ○ The most commonly used local anesthetic drugs for epidurals.
- ○ Dose: 0.2–0.25 mg/kg (1.0–1.25 ml of 2% *lidocaine* or *mepivacaine*/100 kg) for a caudal epidural.
- ○ Fast onset of complete anesthesia (6–10 minutes) and relatively short duration of action (60–90 minutes) with lidocaine. *Mepivacaine* has a similar onset time but a longer duration of effect (120–180 minutes).

*Ropivacaine* (0.5%)
- ○ Longer acting than *lidocaine*.
- ○ Dose: 0.8 mg/kg (1.6 ml of 0.5% *ropivacaine*/100 kg) for a caudal epidural.
    - – The volume of injection can be increased with preservative-free 0.9% saline, but should not exceed 10 mL (500 kg horse), to avoid rostral spread resulting in hind limb weakness or recumbency.
    - – Fast onset of complete analgesia (10 minutes) and intermediate duration of action (3 hours).
    - – Minimal ataxia and cardiorespiratory effects.

## B  Opioids

- ○ Epidurally administered opioids results in prolonged analgesic effects.
    - – Proximity of drug deposition to the spinal cord facilitates the interaction with opioid receptors.
- ○ Epidural opioids result in analgesia, but not anesthesia.
- ○ Main indication is to produce analgesia of the perineal area and hindlimbs.
    - – However, there is evidence that opioids may be effective for abdominal pain.
- ○ *Morphine* and *methadone* are the most effective opioids for epidural injection.

*Morphine* (0.1–0.2 mg/kg)
- ○ Has a slow onset (1–5 hours) and long duration (6–16 hours) of action.
- ○ Long duration of effect is due to its hydrophilic nature which results in a longer half-life in CSF than lipophilic drugs.
- ○ Systemic opioid-induced effects, such as excitement, are much less likely than with intravenous (IV) or intramuscular (IM) administration of morphine.
- ○ The volume of injection can be increased to a maximum of 30 ml in a 450 kg horse, to facilitate rostral spread of *morphine* over the spinal cord.
    - – Preservative-free 0.9% saline should be used as a diluent.
- ○ Preservative-containing *morphine* solutions are more concentrated (10 or 15 mg/ml) than preservative-free (1 mg/ml).
    - – Dilution of preservative-containing solutions with preservative-free 0.9% saline solution decreases the risk of neurotoxicity from preservatives.
    - – Large volumes of preservative-free morphine must be injected slowly (five minutes minimum) to avoid compression of nerve endings.
    - – Preservative-containing solutions are more practical and less expensive than preservative-free solutions.

*Methadone* (0.1 mg/kg)
- o Rapid onset (15 minutes) and intermediate duration (5 hours) of action.
- o Preservative-free solution is 1% (10 mg/ml) and should be diluted with preservative-free 0.9% saline solution to a maximum of 30 m in a 450 kg horse.

## C  α₂ agonists

- o Epidural administration provides analgesia of longer duration than do systemic doses.
- o Main indications are to provide intra- and postoperative analgesia of the perineum.
- o *Xylazine* can block all types of fibers, causing ataxia/paresis.
  - – α₂ agonists do not give a complete sensory block at clinical doses.
- o Systemic effects (sedation, hypertension/hypotension, bradycardia) are common.
- o *Xylazine* and *detomidine* are most commonly used.

*Xylazine* (0.17–0.22 mg/kg)
- o Intermediate onset action (15–30 minutes) and an intermediate duration of action (3.5 hours).
- o Mild sedation may be evident.
- o Analgesia of the perineal area, hindlimb, and forelimb.
- o Volume of injection in a 450 kg horse:
  - – May be diluted to a maximum of 10 ml for perineal analgesic effects.
  - – May be diluted to a maximum of 20–30 ml if rostral spread is desired for analgesic effects.

*Detomidine* (0.01–0.06 mg/kg)
- o Higher dose rates are associated with extreme sedation and ataxia.
  - – Thus, low dose rates are recommended.
- o Intermediate onset of analgesia (10–25 minutes) and intermediate duration of action (2 hours).
- o Combining with morphine (0.1–0.2 mg/kg) is recommended for intra- and postoperative pain, as well as long-term management of traumatic hindlimb accidents.
- o Volume of injection may be increased to a maximum of 20–30 ml (in a 450 kg horse), by adding 0.9% saline solution, if rostral spread is desired.

## D  Ketamine

- o Rarely used epidurally.
- o Epidural ketamine blocks N-methyl-D-aspartate (NMDA) receptors in the spinal cord.
- o Causes analgesia of the tail, perineum, and upper hindlimb.
- o Fast onset of analgesic action (10 minutes) and a short duration of action (30–75 minutes).
- o Dose: 0.5–2 mg/kg.
- o Systemic effects (e.g. sedation, ataxia) can occur with high doses.
- o Epidural injection should be diluted (10–30 ml in a 450 kg horse).

## E  Combinations

*Opioids and α₂ agonists*
- o *Morphine* can be combined with α₂ agonists.
  - – This provides a faster onset from the α₂ drugs, as well as giving the prolonged effect of morphine.
- o The full dose of each drug may be given without adverse effects.
- o Useful for long-term pain management.

- ○ α$_2$ agonists and local anesthetics.
- ○ When used in combination, careful dosing of the local anesthetic is required to avoid excessive ataxia from an additive effect.
    - − The dose of local anesthetic should be decreased by about 30%.
- ○ Useful for standing surgery.
- ○ Prolonged effect over local anesthetic alone.

## Suggested Reading

Natalini, C.C. (2010). Spinal anesthetics and analgesics in the horse. *Vet. Clin. North Am. Equine. Pract.* 26: 551–564.

Robinson, E.P. and Natalini, C.C. (2002). Epidural anesthesia and analgesia in horses. *Vet. Clin. North Am. Equine. Pract.* 18: 61–82.

# 28

## Pathophysiology of Pain
*Rachel A. Reed*

## I Introduction

### A Acute vs. chronic pain

- **Acute pain** is a physiologic response to an insult in the periphery. Acute pain is protective in nature, alerting the subject to potential or actual tissue injury.
- **Chronic pain** is a disease process in and of itself. It is the consequence of severe and sustained acute pain, which causes a cascade of events either peripherally, centrally, or both to result in a pathologic pain state in which the subject continues to feel pain beyond the expected course of the inciting insult.

### B Five general steps in the pain pathway

There are five steps in the pain pathway: *transmission, transduction, modulation, projection,* and *perception*.

*Transmission*
- The pain pathway begins in the periphery at the site of injury.
- Receptors in the periphery respond to changes in temperature, mechanical insult, or pH alterations activating "*first order neurons*," which are represented by specialized nociceptive fibers (i.e. Aδ and C fibers). Aβ fibers (touch fibers) can also potentially act as nociceptive fibers.

*Transduction*
- These first-order neurons travel from the site of insult to the dorsal horn of the spinal cord where they synapse predominantly in laminae I and II within interneurons and "*second-order neurons*" within the spinal cord.
- Second-order neurons are represented by tracts that connect the spinal cord with the thalamus (e.g. spinothalamic tract).
- Within the spinal cord, Aδ fibers predominantly activate *glutamate* receptors including alpha-amino-3-hydroxy-5-methyl-4-isoxazoleproionic acid (AMPA), kainite, and N-Methyl-ᴅ-aspartate (NMDA) at the synapse with the *second-order neuron*. C fibers predominantly release substance P to activate second-order neurons.

*Manual of Equine Anesthesia and Analgesia*, Second Edition. Edited by Tom Doherty, Alex Valverde, and Rachel A. Reed.

*Modulation*
  ○ Within the spinal cord, this nociceptive action potential can be either:
    – *Augmented*, resulting in amplification of the nociceptive impulse, or
    – *Inhibited*, resulting in diminution of the impulse.
*Projection*
  ○ Nociceptive action potentials then travel up in tracts within the spinal cord toward the brain, predominantly the thalamus and synapse with *"third-order neurons."*
*Perception*
  ○ Nociceptive impulses arrive within the cortex through third-order neurons and are perceived by the subject.
  ○ *Nociception* now becomes *pain*.

## II Ascending nociceptive pathways

- *Primary sensory afferent neurons* include Aβ, Aδ, and C fibers.
- The cell bodies of these neurons lie within the *dorsal root ganglion* (DRG) of the spinal cord with the exception of those neurons supplying sensory innervation to the face, which lie within the *trigeminal ganglion*, and some neurons supplying the viscera, which lie in the *cranial ganglia* and *nodose ganglia*.
  Trigeminal nerve fibers innervating the face enter the pons and descend to the medulla and synapse in the spinal trigeminal nucleus, and then ascend through the spinal cord as the trigeminal tract toward the thalamic area.
- These sensory afferents respond to heat, cold, chemicals, mechanical damage, or changes in pH.
  ○ They can be *monomodal* (responding to only one stimulus type) or *polymodal* (responding to more than one stimulus type).
- Activation of nociceptive fibers is caused by depolarization of axonal nerve terminals.
- Sensory afferents differ in regard to their *size*, degree of *myelination*, and *conduction velocity* (see Table 28.1).
  ○ Aδ fibers release *glutamate* as their neurotransmitter and are responsible for fast, first pain sensation due to their conduction velocity. This represents surgical/sharp pain.
  ○ C fibers predominantly release *substance P* and to a lesser extent glutamate. Their slower conduction velocity is responsible for the slow, second-pain sensation, which represents burning/inflammatory pain.
  ○ This causes a "double-pain sensation."
- Axons from these fibers extend from the periphery into the dorsal horn of the spinal cord, terminating primarily in laminae I, II, and V.
  ○ Aδ synapse in laminae I.
  ○ C fibers synapse in laminae I and II.
  ○ Aβ fibers synapse in laminae III–V.

Table 28.1 Diameter, degree of myelination, conduction velocity, and stimulus of Aβ, Aδ, and C fibers.

| Fiber | Diameter | Myelination | Conduction velocity | Sensation |
|-------|----------|-------------|---------------------|-----------|
| Aβ | Large | Thick myelination | Fast, >10 m/s | Non-painful sensation |
| Aδ | Medium | Light myelination | Medium, 2–10 m/s | Fast, sharp pain |
| C | Small | Unmyelinated | Slow, <1.5 m/s | Slow, burning pain |

- Within the spinal cord, action potentials arising from primary sensory afferents interact with *interneurons* and *secondary order neurons* within spinal tracts.
  - These neurons carry the action potential to the ventral horn completing spinal reflex pathways in addition to carrying the action potential to higher centers within the brain including the nucleus raphe magnus, locus ceruleus, and periaqueductal gray.
  - The major ascending tracts carrying nociceptive input that have identified in animals include the *spinothalamic tract*, *spinocervicothalamic tract*, and *postsynaptic dorsal column*.
- Action potentials traveling up the spinal cord are subject to *modulation*, as described above, which may augment or inhibit the impulse.

## III  Types of nociceptors

- Various types of nociceptors have been described.

*Transient receptor potential ion channels* (TRPs)
  - These receptors can be activated by:
    - Heat.
    - A decrease in pH.
    - Various peptides.
  - These receptors are present in the periphery on *first-order sensory neurons*, and within the dorsal horn on *second order nociceptive fibers*.

*Neuronal sodium channels* (NaV)
  - NaV channels are voltage-gated receptors that generate action potentials along the nociceptive afferent.
  - Nine sodium channels have been described based on the alpha subunit of the receptor.

*Acid-sensing ion channels* (ASICs)
  - These channels serve to activate nociceptive afferents in the presence of a decreasing pH.
  - Such reductions in local pH are observed with tissue injury and inflammation.
  - These receptors are most densely distributed in the *skeletal muscle* and *heart*.

*Glutamate receptors*
  - AMPA, Kainate, NMDA
  - These are cation channels within the spinal cord dorsal horn and serve to activate second-order neurons.
  - AMPA and kainate receptors are primarily involved in the conduction of day-to-day physiologic pain. NMDA receptors are unique in that they are both ligand gated and voltage gated.
  - These receptors also play a unique role in the development of *wind-up* and *chronic pain* states (see Central Sensitization below).

*Neurokinin 1 receptors* (NK-1)
  - NK-1 receptors are present within the dorsal horn and serve to activate second-order neurons primarily within laminae I of the spinal cord.
  - NK-1 receptors are activated by substance P released by the first-order neuron within the spinal cord.

*Lamellated corpuscles*
  - As described in the solar dermis of the equine hoof, these are low-threshold mechanoreceptors that activate Aδ fibers in the transmission of fast pain.
  - Naked nerve endings have also been identified within the equine hoof, and are thought to be sensitive to calcitonin gene-related peptide, substance P, neurokinin A, and peptide histidine-isoleucine.

## IV Descending modulatory pathways

- Descending pathways serve in suprasegmental modulation of the nociceptive impulses arriving from the periphery.
- These pathways, originating from the *periaqueductal gray* and *nucleus raphe magnus*, release many neurotransmitters that modulate the ascending nociceptive tracts. Endogenous *opioid* ligands such as endorphin and dynorphin are some of the most notable.
- These descending pathways play an important role as the pharmacologic targets of many of the analgesic agents used in equine medicine. Notably, opioid receptor agonists and alpha$_2$ agonists.

## V Development of chronic pain states

### A Peripheral sensitization

- Prolonged and high-intensity activation of peripheral nociceptors results in release of inflammatory mediators locally at the site of injury. These inflammatory mediators include cytokines, kinins, hydrogen ions, potassium ions, inflammatory peptides, and arachidonic acid derivatives including leukotrienes and prostaglandins.
- This *"inflammatory soup"* results in *two* primary effects at the first-order nerve terminal:
  - Existing nociceptive fiber nerve terminals lower their threshold, making them more easily activated.
  - Non-nociceptive fibers that would normally transmit non-noxious stimuli, now transmit noxious stimuli (i.e. Aβ fibers).
- These two processes result in primary *hyperalgesia* (painful stimulus is perceived as more painful than normal) and *allodynia* (non-painful stimulus is perceived as painful).
- Primary hyperalgesia and allodynia caused by peripheral sensitization is generally specific to the site of injury.

### B Central sensitization

- Central sensitization refers to processes within the central nervous system (CNS) that have resulted in chronic pain states, such as hyperalgesia or allodynia.

*NMDA receptor*

- This receptor has an important role in the development of central sensitization and hence chronic pain states.
  - The NMDA receptor is both ligand gated and voltage gated, and under normal conditions, this receptor is obstructed by a magnesium ion ($Mg^{++}$).
- Prolonged and high-intensity activation of AMPA and kainate receptors on the second-order neuron will cause significant depolarization of the second-order nerve terminal and displacement of the $Mg^{++}$ within the NMDA receptor.
  - Displacement of the $Mg^{++}$, allows binding of glutamate and glycine to the NMDA receptor, resulting in its activation.
- Activation of the NMDA receptor results in an alteration in protein synthesis within the nerve terminal, phosphorylation of existing AMPA, kainate, and NMDA receptors, and insertion of additional glutamate receptors within the nerve terminal.

- Thus, the affected second-order nerve becomes more easily activated by action potentials arriving from the periphery.
  o This process, termed "*wind up,*" results in *secondary hyperalgesia* and *allodynia*. A centrally mediated chronic pain state.
  o *Wind-up* that was originally caused by high-intensity action potentials from a very specific location (e.g. a laceration) will result in secondary hyperalgesia and allodynia to the *specific location* and the *area surrounding it*. This is due to the close proximity of multiple ascending nociceptive fibers within the dorsal horn from the same region, and the presence of wide dynamic range interneurons that can impact large areas of the dorsal horn. *Note*: It is important to recognize that although unconsciousness, as provided by inhalational anesthetics, renders the patient unaware of painful stimuli; these processes, which lead to development of chronic pain, can still take place in the anesthetized patient.
    - The only way to prevent these processes from occurring is via the provision of *preemptive analgesia*.

### C Neuropathic pain

- o Neuropathic pain is pain that is caused by direct damage to the somatosensory system, either within the CNS or to a peripheral nerve. Neuroplasticity caused by inflammatory mediators, nerve growth factor, and NMDA receptor activation is thought to occur, resulting in a lowered threshold for activation of the nerve fiber.
- o Although the exact mechanisms of the development of neuropathic pain is an area of speculation, there is significant evidence that *hyperpolarization-activated cation channels* (HCN) are involved. This conclusion is based on the presence of these receptors in the DRG neurons, upregulation of the receptors in states of neuropathic pain, and resolution of pain behavior when agents that block these receptors are administered to mice with experimentally induced neuropathic pain. Recognition of involvement of HCN channels in the development and maintenance of neuropathic pain identifies a possible mechanism for management of neuropathic pain via drugs that block the HCN channels within the DRG.
- o Nerve growth factor and neurotrophic factors can cause development of neuromas and collateral sprouting of axons. These serve as a source of ectopic action potentials (random abnormal action potential generation).
- o Ectopic action potentials are thought to be responsible for phantom limb pain phenomena.
- o This process has been identified in horses by Jones et al. using electron micrographic analysis of digital nerves harvested from horses that had developed severe laminitis (see Suggested reading).

## VI Physiologic consequences of pain

- The aforementioned processes not only cause significant discomfort but also result in several physiologic consequences including:
  o Increased sympathetic nervous system activity.
  o Increased oxygen demand.
  o Increased workload on the heart.

- ○ Increased minute ventilation to satisfy increased oxygen demand.
- ○ Increased circulating *cortisol* adversely affecting immune function and coagulation.
- ○ Overall, increased morbidity and mortality.
- Acute pain is best *treated*, and chronic pain states best *prevented*, by multi-modal analgesic approaches. Incorporation of analgesic agents that inhibit or disrupt the nociceptive pathway at multiple locations will provide the most effective analgesia.
- Techniques that are especially effective in prevention of development of chronic pain states include *local anesthetic* techniques and *drugs* that prevent activation of the NMDA receptor (e.g. *ketamine*).

## Suggested Reading

Bowen, I.M., Redpath, A., Dugdale, A. et al. (2019). BEVA primary care clinical guidelines: Analgesia. *Equine. Vet. J.* 52: 13–27.

Mair, T. (2019). *Equine. Vet. Edu. 31*: 338–391.

Jones, E., Venuela-Fernandez, I., Eager, R.A. et al. (2007). Neuropathic changes in equine laminitis pain. *Pain* 132: 321–331.

29

# Pain Recognition in Horses
*Karina B. Gleerup, Casper Lindegaard, and Pia Haubro Andersen*

## I Introduction

- Pain is an individual experience and is therefore difficult to objectify in non-verbal species. Pain evaluation is however, of cardinal importance for optimal pain treatment and essential for early detection of pain and disease.
- Historically, physiologic variables were the only measures described for evaluating pain. Heart rate (HR), respiration rate (RR), and blood pressure (BP) may convey important information about pain; however, these parameters are also altered by disease processes including endotoxemia, cardiovascular compromise and/or dehydration, and hence are not specific to pain.
- Pain research has moved more toward *composite* pain scales based on *behavioral* traits, since these have proven valuable for detecting pain in non-verbal species. Also, in human beings, facial expressions and body postures are considered to communicate pain with a high degree of specificity.
- We suggest that composite scales be used whenever possible, and recognize that a plethora of scales have been published, focusing on different types of patients. The aim of this chapter is to give a practical guide, as to how pain evaluation can be implemented in the daily routines of a hospital, and not to give a comprehensive review of the pain evaluation literature.
- For extensive reviews of the field of pain evaluation in horses, please consult *van Loon and Van Dierendonck*, and *Gleerup and Lindegaard* (see Suggested reading).

## II Steps necessary to implement pain scoring in the hospital routine

- Implementation of systematic pain evaluation in hospitalized horses requires an active and whole-hearted decision that involves all caregiving staff.
- Routines must be as clear and simple as possible.
- In the following, the steps necessary to set up systematic pain evaluation in a hospital setting are described.

*Manual of Equine Anesthesia and Analgesia*, Second Edition. Edited by Tom Doherty, Alex Valverde, and Rachel A. Reed.

## A  Select a practical and applicable pain scale

(see Table 29.1 for selected published pain scales)

- ○ A pain scale used in a hospital setting, should only be as detailed as necessary. If a scale is composed of simple descriptive scales of common pain behaviors, the resulting scale will generally show good performance regarding content validity and rater agreement.
- ○ If a number of the specific items composing the scale describes general pain behavior, good performance may also be expected across pain types.
- ○ As an example, a pain scale validated for visceral pain, also proved useful for evaluating head pain and orthopedic pain.
- ○ More comprehensive and disease-specific scales monitoring signs characteristic for specific patient types have been developed for abdominal pain and orthopedic pain. These scales may be most applicable for specialist purposes.

## B  Select a key person responsible for the procedures of clinical pain-scoring

- ○ Pain scoring may not yet be routinely used in equine hospitals, and to keep the continuity of this emerging field, it is recommended that a specific professional be appointed to this area, to take care of quality assurance and introduction of new staff.
- ○ The pain scoring routines are affected by the work situation, and it has been shown in human hospitals that pain scoring may be less prioritized when the hospital is busy.
- ○ In large equine hospitals, nurses and other technical staff often spend the most time with the horses, making the horses more comfortable in their company, which may encourage them to show a more genuine behavior.
- ○ Therefore, it is an advantage if veterinary nurses or other technical staff, are given the responsibility for pain evaluations.

## C  Develop local routines for pain scoring

- ○ Identify which horses should receive systematic pain assessments.
- ○ Make routines for preparation and management of scoring sheets.
- ○ Provide a standard-operational procedure (SOP) for when horses should be assessed and by whom.
- ○ Write protocols, detailing exactly how to carry out the pain scoring. (see Table 29.2)

**Table 29.1**  Selected pain scales published and applicable for horses.

| Patients/pain types | Pain assessment methodology |
| --- | --- |
| Hospitalized horses following orthopedic surgery | Remote observation of pain behaviors from video-surveillance. Illustrations to guide. |
| Acute colic | EQUUS-COMPASS/EQUUS-FAP<br>Direct observation and scoring of a number of defined descriptive scales |
| Clinical, acute pain | Equine Pain Scale (EPS)<br>Direct or remote observation and scoring of a number of defined descriptive scales |

Table 29.2   Example of the pain scoring sheet used for the equine pain scale for repeated measures. The sheet must be simple and easy to overlook. It should be easy to see changes over time but also a sudden extreme value in one single category. Another example of the same pain scoring scale is published in Gleerup and Lindegaard (2016).

| Category (#) | Behavior category | Name: Date: Description | Time Score |
|---|---|---|---|
| **A** (1) | Pain face | No pain face | 0 |
| | | Pain face present | 2 |
| | | Intense pain face | 3 |
| **B** (2) | Gross pain behavior | None | 0 |
| | | Occasional | 2 |
| | | Continuous | 4 |
| **C** (3) | Activity | Exploring, attention toward surroundings or resting | 0 |
| | | No movement | 1 |
| | | Restless | 3 |
| | | Depressed | 4 |
| **D** (4) | Location in the stall | At the door, watching the environment | 0 |
| | | Standing in the middle facing the door | 1 |
| | | Standing in the middle facing the sides | 2 |
| | | Standing in the middle facing the back or standing in the back | 3 |
| **E** (5) | Posture/weight bearing | Normal posture and normal weight bearing | 0 |
| | | Foot intermittent of the ground/occasional weight shift | 1 |
| | | Pinched (groove between the abdominal muscles visible) | 2 |
| | | Continuously taking one foot off the ground and trying to replace it | 3 |
| | | No weight bearing on one foot, abnormal weight distribution | 4 |
| **F** (6) | Head position | Foraging, below withers or high | 0 |
| | | Level of withers | 1 |
| | | Below withers | 2 |
| **G** (7) | Attention toward the painful area | Does not pay attention to painful area | 0 |
| | | Brief attention to the painful area (e.g. flank watching) | 2 |
| | | Biting, nudging, or looking at the painful area (e.g. flank watching) | 4 |
| **H** (8) | Interactive behavior | Looks at observer or moves to observer when approached | 0 |
| | | Look at observer when approached, does not move toward observer | 1 |
| | | Does not look at observer or moves away, avoids contact | 2 |
| | | Does not move, not reacting/introverted | 3 |
| **I** (9) | Response to food | Takes food with no hesitation | 0 |
| | | Looks at food | 1 |
| | | No response to food | 3 |
| | | | Sum |

    ○ Decide where the results should be entered and where the pain record is located.

    ○ Describe procedures if a pain scoring exceeds a certain value, i.e. communication of "*pain alarms.*"

## D  Assessment

    ○ In order to monitor pain efficiently, pain assessment sheets with a monitoring schedule should be included in the medical record.

    ○ A guideline for the chosen pain scale, (see Tables 29.1 and 29.2), should be placed on the stall door or treatment board. (see Figure 29.1)

    ○ Details and time of the assessment should be printed or written on the score sheets.

## E  Conduct training sessions for all caregiving personnel

    ○ To provide optimal patient care, caregivers must have sufficient knowledge, skills and attitudes toward the relevance of pain assessment.

    ○ However, to be able to use a pain scale, a brief education of one to two hours duration has been shown to suffice and, generally the composite scales seem to have good inter-observer reliability.

    ○ This is, however, only true for simple scales with unambiguous descriptions of each score, leaving little room for interpretational error.

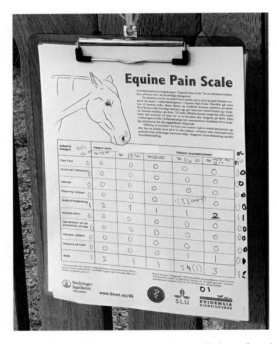

Figure 29.1   Pain scoring record on stall door of equine patient in hospital.

## III How pain scoring is performed – key points

- The pain scoring process should be short.
- Use a structured score sheet.
- Get a view of the horse as discretely as possibly, during a quiet time in the stall. If possible, use *video* surveillance.
- Approach the stall and note the change in behavior.
- Open the door and offer social contact and, if appropriate, a snack, note the response to this.
- Summarize results and file in the record.

### A Use a structured score sheet (e.g. Table 29.2)

- Changes over time in the level of pain will be reflected in the repeated pain score and these are more informative than exact score values.
- It is therefore valuable to plot pain scores on a time line to be certain to note temporal changes, as is already used in many hospitals for some physiological variables (e.g. rectal temperature).

### B View the horse, as discretely as possibly, during a quiet time in the stall

- Pain behavior is considered most genuine when the horse is undisturbed, since pain behavior may be disrupted if the horse is focused on something in the surroundings.
- It is therefore important to quietly observe the horse from a distance and discretely enter the stable.
- If there are two observers, quiet conversation may help the horse to accept that he is not the subject of interest.

### C Timing

- Timing is also important since the pain intensity may fluctuate throughout the day.
- Pain scorings performed before morning feeding or even before the morning team has arrived, may hold information about "*break through pain*" resulting from inefficient pain medication through the night. These horses may not be found to be in pain till much later in the day, if normal morning routines are carried out.
- It is, at all times, important to avoid walking directly up to any horse for a clinical evaluation or to give medication without prior evaluation from a distance. Any horse that has been subjected to anesthesia is at risk of colic but may only show subtle signs.

### D Recommended intervals for assessing pain

- Baseline assessments should be performed in all horses and preferably as soon as possible. Be aware of how stress from hospital admission might affect assessment of pain.
- *Elective and/or minor surgeries/routine cases*: Assess twice daily.

- *Acute or major surgical procedures* (traumatic wounds with or without surgery, colic horses): Assess every two to six hours depending on intervention and analgesic management.
- *Stable acute major surgeries*: Assess every six to eight hours or more frequently, depending on the analgesic regimen.
- *Horses with sudden, unexpected high pain scores*: re-assess after one hour.

*Recommendations*
- The distribution of patients, their pain levels prior to surgery, and the anesthetic and analgesic protocols, vary among clinics.
- Timeframe recommendations for re-assessment, therefore, are ideally part of the hospital policies, and should be discussed among the specialties, including the nursing staff.
- Break-through pain shows as a sudden and high rise in pain scores. This pain is often challenging to manage adequately, requiring more repeated and frequent reassessments.
- The power of repeated pain assessment is primarily to detect the potential change in the pain score observed over time.
- Any horse subjected to a painful or a pain-relieving intervention, should be monitored before and after the intervention, in order to assess the impact of the intervention. This will allow the clinician to amend the pain management accordingly.

## IV  Video assistance

*Key points*
- Recent advances in technology and development of cameras for use in agricultural and monitoring systems has created entirely new options for smart surveillance of livestock, and this trend is increasingly moving into veterinary clinics. Cameras for agricultural purposes can be used even during poor lighting conditions and during the night using infra-red technology.
- Ideally, two cameras should be placed and secured in each box stall to capture corners, floor, and the door of the box stall.
- Roof-mounted cameras will not allow interpretation of the facial expressions or subtle movements of the limbs.
- Keep recordings on hard disk for a minimum 24 hours to allow for evaluation over time.
  Video monitoring may also allow monitoring of interactions if these are performed routinely.
  - Video-based observation is often superior to direct observation, as it can provide more accurate information about the undisturbed behavior, and potentially also allow for a longer observation period.
  - Video-surveillance recordings are most efficiently screened for pain behavior, by moving fast forward over the recordings since the last pain evaluation. With experience, it will be obvious if the horse displays repetitive pain behaviors out of the normal range.
  - Horses with *stereotypic* behaviors may be difficult to evaluate, as stereotypic behaviors increase in frequency, when the horse is in pain or stressed.

     ○  As for direct observation, changes over time are most valuable and will allow, for example, monitoring of emerging cast or bandage pressure sores or wound infection.

## V  Factors that influence pain scoring

*Key points*
- Horse personality (introvert vs extrovert) and pain threshold (warm-blooded vs. cold-blooded horses).
- Fear and stress (e.g. from hospitalization).
- Medications (e.g. sedatives, anesthetics, muscle relaxant, and analgesics, especially opioids).
- Human contact (*positive* – owner, *negative* – unfamiliar persons) and other social intervention.

### A  Baseline measures or input from owner should be considered

     ○  Owners are capable of recording ordinary pain behavior, and self-explanatory schemes for monitoring of pain behavior before admission may prove valuable for historic reference and further clinical examination.

### B  Fear and stress

     ○  Fear and stress alter the interactive behavior of horses.
     ○  Therefore, it is advisable, at all times, to keep hospital environments as calm and stress free as possible. This can be achieved in many ways, e.g. reducing traffic and using stress-free handling during treatments.

### C  Medication

     ○  Medication may affect both the gross behavior and facial expression of horses.
     ○  Opioids, empirically are known to cause drowsiness or excitation in some horses.
     ○  Anesthesia will affect the behavior and facial expressions of horses as a "hang-over" effect for an unknown time period.
     ○  Medication that induces muscle relaxation, obviously also relaxes muscles involved in many pain behaviors, and therefore reduces facial muscle activity and body movement in general.
     ○  All these medical treatments may affect the pain assessment, resulting in falsely higher or lower pain scores.

### D  Owner contact and other social intervention

     ○  Social interventions or distractions and even contact with the owner or other people may reduce signs of pain.
     ○  Walking in unfamiliar surroundings may interfere with the display of pain behavior, and falsely lead the clinician to believe that the horse is not in pain.
     ○  Such reduction in pain-related behavior is a temporary event, emphasizing the need for observation of the undisturbed horse.

## VI    Interpretation of pain scores

*Key points*
- Non-painful horses may score a number of points in any pain scale. Cut-off values depend on the pain scale used and the routines applied.
- Changes in pain scores and trends for pain scores over time is more important to determine the individual patient's development.
- A single pain score depends on individual horse factors and only very high values should be used as an absolute measure of the pain intensity.
- If a horse scores an extreme value in any one category, that horse should be examined, despite the final total score.
  - Interpretation is most valuable when evaluated in combination with an exhaustive list of influencing factors.
  - Although many pain scales are based on behavioral categories which individually are not necessarily pain specific, the highest score in any category often represents extremely abnormal behavior. Further investigation is therefore warranted, regardless of the total score at that time point.
  - Regardless of the pain scale applied, any pain evaluation will have certain elements of subjectivity. However, use of a validated pain scale will ensure the best possible assessment of the actual pain level over time.

## VII    Guide on how to use the Equine Pain Scale (EPS) (see Table 29.2)

*Key points*
- Score the freely moving horse in quiet surroundings in a box stall.
- Observe from a distance without disturbing the horse – this means that routine pain scoring cannot be performed during the morning feeding routines.
- Score the first seven categories in the EPS scoring sheet before approaching the horse (the "non-interactive" parameters).
- Approach the stall and note the response from the horse as you approach and as you open the door. Score category 8 (interaction).
- Offer the horse palatable feed, if the horse is not allowed feed, you can still offer a very small amount. Score category 9.
- Reflect on the pain score before giving analgesic treatment.

### A    Detailed description of the EPS

- In the following, we describe how to use and assess data obtained by a composite scale, as for example the EPS (see Gleerup & Lindegaard, or the Lawson scale; Suggested reading).
- These scales are intended for assessing pain in horses in box stalls. The scales are composed of several simple descriptive scales, each accounting for one specific behavior commonly described to occur in horses in pain.
- The difference between the EPS and the Lawson pain scale is the inclusion of HR and respiratory rate in the latter. Both approaches may show advantages and disadvantages.

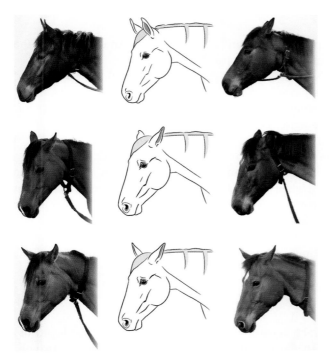

**Figure 29.2** The top row displays pictures of horses that are not in pain. They have neutral facial expressions, the horse on the left with both ears forward and the horse on the right with both ears listening backwards, to underline that ears-back does not necessarily reflect pain. In the middle, is a drawing that shows a horse with a neutral facial expression. *Source:* Photographs Karina Bech Gleerup.

The middle row displays pictures of horses with "low ears," there is an increased distance between the base of the ears. Two different horses are depicted to exemplify this type of pain face, while the middle is the standardized drawing.

The bottom row displays pictures of horses with asymmetrical ears. These horses have a changed movement pattern of the ears, as the ears does not seem to move all to forward and also here is an increased distance between the base of the ears. Two different horses are depicted to exemplify this type of pain face, while the middle is the standardized drawing.

In common for the horses in pain is seen:

- Muscle tension of the muscles surrounding the eyes (*m. levator anguli oculi medialis*)
- Changed quality of the glance (withdrawn during painful events)
- Changed shape of the nostrils (dilated medio-laterally to an edged square-like shape)
- Tension of the lips and chin.
- Increased tension of the muscles visible on the lateral aspect of the head (especially *M. zygomaticus* and the *M. caninus*)

Illustrations: Andrea Klintbjer, photographs Karina Bech Gleerup, poster Anders Rådén

○ The main strength of composite scales, is that they monitor multiple aspects of pain, and that they therefore reflect changes in pain level, increase or decrease, which is valuable information for the clinician.

○ It is our experience that the entire range of caregivers, from clinicians to nurses and other staff as well as horse owners can be instructed to score pain reliably using the EPS, after a very short educational session.

### B Pain Face, present or not

○ Horses show specific facial expressions of pain (see Figure 29.2). An evaluation of the facial expression is best performed when the horse is undisturbed.

○ Look at the horse systematically, starting with the ears, then the eyes, the lower head and finally evaluate the facial expression as a whole.

○ How do the ears move, what are the angles, how wide is the distance between the ears?

○ Are the muscles around the eyes tense? Is the glance focused or withdrawn?

○ What is the shape of the nostrils?

○ Are lips and chin tense and are the muscles on the side of the face tense?

○ Then go back to a pattern recognition mode and decide. In most cases, more than one feature of the pain face is present when a horse is in pain. Do not spend more than about 30–60 seconds, otherwise the pattern recognition will be disturbed. This parameter should be assessed according to the guidelines in Table 29.2.

○ If no obvious pain face is observed, score "0" is applied. If there is an occasional presentation of a pain face, score "2" is applied, and if the pain face is present most of the time, score "3" is given.

### C Gross pain behavior

○ Horses in severe pain often display repetitive or excessive behaviors. These behaviors may be considered "normal" behaviors, displayed in a different context in non-painful horses.

○ An example is *flehmen*, where the upper lip is curled upwards with the head raised. This behavior may be incited by a particular scent, for example from mares in estrus.

○ In painful horses, this is considered a gross pain behavior and may be displayed excessively. Gross pain behaviors are displayed repetitively, obviously with changing frequency, and may include head movements like head tossing with or without stretching and twisting the neck, tail swishing, grinding of teeth, kicking, pawing, rolling (see Figure 29.3), stretching, mouth playing (see Figure 29.4).

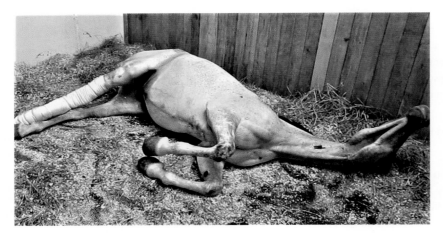

Figure 29.3 An example of low-level intensity "rolling." This horse later presented with colic after anesthesia. *Source:* Photograph Karina Bech Gleerup.

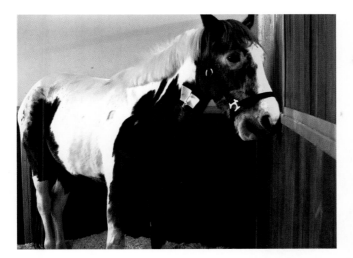

**Figure 29.4**   An example of the gross pain behavior "mouth playing." *Source:* Photograph Karina Bech Gleerup.

o Horses that display stereotypic behaviors when not in pain, may score higher on the baseline pain evaluation but they often will intensify the specific stereotypy when in pain.

o If none of these behaviors are observed, a score "0" is applied, if one or more of these behaviors is observed occasionally, a score "2" is applied, and if any of these behaviors are seen more or less continuously, a score "4" is applied.

**D   Activity**

o This category is used to assess whether the horse displays normal activity. The score "0" is applied to horses that are attentive toward the surroundings, feeding, exploring, or in a normal resting position.

o A score "1" is applied if the horse is not moving, without being in the normal resting position.

o A score "3" is applied to horses that seem restless (moving around without finding rest and without exploring for a reason).

o Horses that seem depressed and inactive but not in a typical resting position (see Figure 29.5), are given a score "4."

**E   Location in the stall**

o This category assesses the level of interest in the surroundings, by classifying where the horse positions itself within the stall.

o Generally, horses prefer to stand at the front where they can overlook the environment (see Figure 29.6), but can of course be at other places for foraging or drinking or for contact with peers.

o The score "0" is given to horses standing at the door or the front observing the environment or in any other way occupied with normal behavior (e.g. feeding) at another position.

o Horses may stand in the front of the box stall, although not alert (see Figure 29.7) this does *not* give a score "0" but rather a score "1," as this is abnormal behavior.

o A score "1" is applied to horses standing in the middle of the stall and facing the front.

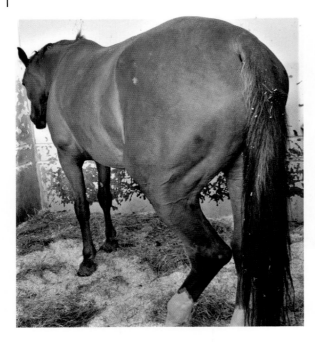

Figure 29.5 This horse is not in a normal resting position as the front limbs are not square and it looks tense in face and body. Head position in level of withers. The horse is not interested in the surroundings or in contact. Standing in the middle, facing the back. *Source:* Photograph Karina Bech Gleerup.

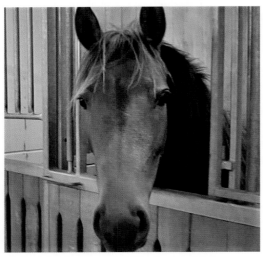

Figure 29.6 An attentive horse standing in the front of the box stall – normal behavior. *Source:* Photograph Karina Bech Gleerup.

- If the horse is standing in the middle facing the sides, the score should be "2" and if the horse stands in the middle and faces the back or stands in the back, the score should be "3."

### F   Posture/weightbearing

- This parameter weighs as a sign of orthopedic pain but also of general discomfort. Horses with normal weightbearing and posture are awarded a score "0."
- Horses that take a foot off the ground intermittently or shows occasional weight shifts should be given a score "1."

Figure 29.7 A horse, standing in the front of the box stall with no attention to the surroundings – Abnormal behavior. *Source:* Photograph Karina Bech Gleerup.

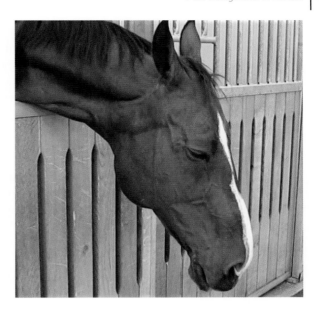

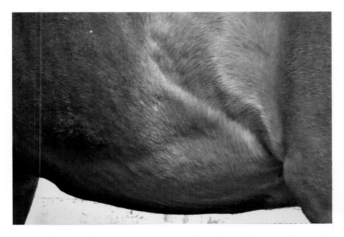

Figure 29.8 This horse is "tucked up," there is tension of the abdominal wall due to abnormal weight distribution and/or due to abdominal discomfort. *Source:* Photograph Karina Bech Gleerup.

○ Horses that show a contracted abdominal posture, looking "*tucked up*" (a grove between the abdominal muscles, see Figure 29.8) should be given a score "2." This can be a result of abnormal weight bearing or abdominal pain.

○ If the horse is continuously trying to take the foot of the ground and trying to replace it, the score should be "3" and if there is no weightbearing at all (see Figure 29.9), the score is "4."

○ In this category, it should be noted that, most often, resting horses will be relaxing one hind limb, this is obviously considered normal (score "0").

**G   Head position**

○ Horses normally hold their heads above the withers in order to overlook the surroundings or hold it low while foraging. Hence, a score of "0" is applied to horses in either of these two positions. Horses with the head level with the withers (see Figure 29.6) are given a score "1" and horses with the head below the withers (see Figure 29.7), that are *not* feeding, are given a score "2."

**H   Attention toward the painful area**

○ Horses with a painful wound (see Figure 29.10), fracture, bandage or cast (see Figure 29.11) will occasionally show more interest toward this area. This interest may sometimes only manifest itself as turning the head and looking very briefly at the painful area.

○ In more pronounced cases this may include nudging (see Figure 29.12) or mutilating the area and/or the bandage. Horses that do not show any attention toward the area are scored "0."

○ If a horse shows only brief attention toward a painful area, a score "2" is applied. It is important to be aware that the painful area might not only include the site of surgery but does always include the abdomen in horses (see Figure 29.13).

○ If the horse looks at a specific area several times during observation or if it bites or nudges a specific area, a score "4" should be applied.

**I   Interactive behavior**

○ This parameter tests the horse's interactive or social desire, which is generally high but may vary among individuals.

○ The stall is approached and the door opened and the horse is observed during the action. A score "0" is applied to horses that look at and move toward the observer when approached.

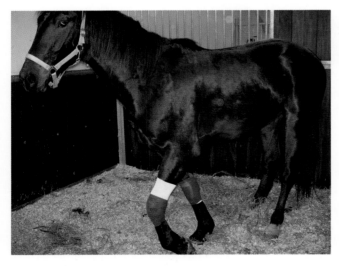

**Figure 29.9**   This horse is not weight bearing on the left front limb. Notice how the weight is shifted on the three other legs to support the left front most possible. *Source:* Photograph Karina Bech Gleerup.

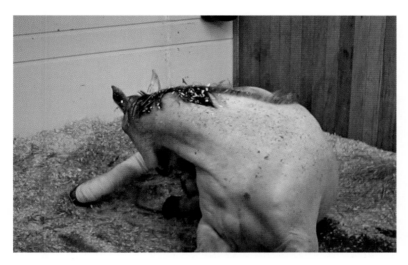

Figure 29.10 This horse had wound surgery on the right hind limb not many hours prior to this "attention toward pain." Analgesic treatment was scheduled shortly after this. *Source:* Photograph Karina Bech Gleerup.

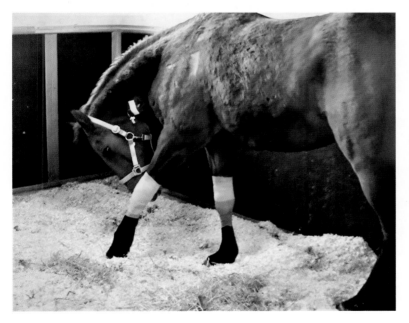

Figure 29.11 This horse shows attention toward the painful area. In this case, the pain may either arise from the bandage or from the carpal joint. *Source:* Photograph Karina Bech Gleerup.

- o Horses that only look and do not move toward the observer should be given a score "1."
- o Horses that do not look at the observer, move away or obviously avoid contact, score "2."
- o Horses that do not react at all and appear introverted or look depressed (see Figure 29.14) should be given a score "3."

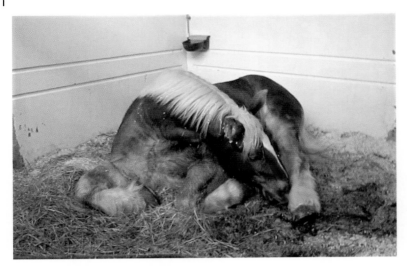

Figure 29.12 This horse was lame. The stifle was the reason for the lameness, however, left alone in the box stall, the horse started to nudge the area of the fetlock. When looking closer, the horse had pressure wounds here from excessive lying down, due to long-term lameness. This cold-blooded horse did not show a lot of pain behavior. *Source:* Photograph Karina Bech Gleerup.

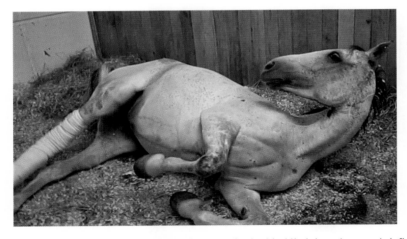

Figure 29.13 This horse had wound surgery in the hind limb but also very briefly shows attention toward the abdomen. This horse presented with colic shortly after, this attention toward pain was the only pain expression pointing toward the abdomen and not the site of surgery. *Source:* Photograph Karina Bech Gleerup.

### J Response to food

- ○ Horses should, in general, be interested in food and hence should seek available food. However, some diseases may decrease appetite without being painful (endotoxemia and fever for instance).
- ○ Sick horses and horses in an unusual environment (e.g. a hospital) may also be more selective with regards to what they eat.

**Figure 29.14** Horses in severe pain or long-term pain, may not show any interest in contact with humans. The horse on the photo had colic and was in severe pain. *Source:* Photograph Karina Bech Gleerup.

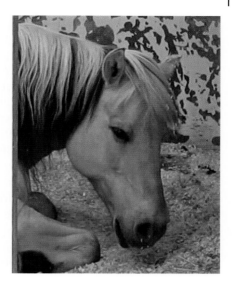

○ After evaluating interactive behavior, the horses are offered palatable food and the reaction observed.

– A score "0" is applied to horses that take food without hesitation.

– A score "1" is applied to horses that take the food with significant hesitation or only look at it, without taking it.

– Horses that do not respond to the food at all should be given a score "3."

## VIII  Interpretation and actions due to EPS Pain Scores

- After performing the pain assessment as described above, the scores from each of the nine categories are summed up to yield a final pain score.
- For the EPS, this will attain a value between 0 and 30. Horses that score below seven are generally managing pain well.
- Horses that score above 10–14 should be re-examined and considered for further drug or non-drug interventions to reduce/control pain.
- For horses that score between 7 and 14, the clinician should revisit the various categories of the pain score and interpret this carefully by comparing to the normal behavior (baseline if possible) of the specific horse. This is best done by discussing the case with the caretakers or nurses and re-assess the horse after a while.

### A  Key points – Action for score "4"

○ Any horse that scores "4" in any single category, *regardless of the obtained global pain score*, should be carefully re-evaluated for a potential need of further pain management.

○ A horse that scores the level "4" in any single category should be re-evaluated for a potential need of further analgesia. Although a single element of the EPS cannot stand alone, it is important to realize that a score "4" in one single category could be the only sign of moderate to severe pain exhibited by a *stoic* horse.

○ The power of this composite pain scale, is a high rater agreement and the fact that it reflects even small changes in pain intensity during the disease course. High rater agreement means that different raters generally agree on what is observed, and this provides reliable data for the record and repeated evaluations.

  – For example, a post-surgical colic horse that scored four and six points for the two latest days which suddenly presents with 9–12 points, is in high risk of exacerbation of disease and needs a thorough clinical examination.

  – The scale can also be used to assess the effect of a given *analgesic*. The administration of an appropriate medication should decrease the pain score according to the pharmacological properties of that drug.

  – Failure to significantly change the pain score warrants further examination and evaluation of alternative analgesic interventions. Changes in the range of 3–4 points are considered as clinically relevant, but lesser changes may be relevant after repeated scoring and evaluation of the trend over time.

## Suggested Reading

Bussieres, G., Jacques, C., Lainay, O. et al. (2008). Development of a composite orthopaedic pain scale in horses. *Res. Vet. Sci.* 85: 294–306.

van Dierendonck, M.C., Burden, F.A., Rickards, K., and van Loon, J. (2020). Monitoring acute pain in donkeys with the equine Utrecht University scale for donkeys composite pain assessment (EQUUS-DONKEY-COMPASS) and the equine Utrecht University scale for donkey facial assessment of pain (EQUUS-DONKEY-FAP). *Animals (Basel)* 10: 354. https://doi.org/10.3390/ani10020354.

Gleerup, K. and Lindegaard, C. (2016). Recognition and quantification of pain in horses: a tutorial review. *Equine Vet. Educ.* 28: 47–57.

Gleerup, K.B., Forkman, B., Lindegaard, C., and Anderson, P.H. (2014). An equine pain face. *Vet. Anaesth. Analg.* 42: 103–114.

Gleerup KB et al. (2014) Facial expressions as a tool for pain recognition in horses, in The 10th International Equitation Science Conference, Janne W. Christensen, et al., Editors. 2014, DCA – Danish Centre for Food and Agriculture 64.

Graubner, C., Gerber, V., Doherr, M., and Spadavecchia, C. (2011). Clinical application and reliability of a post abdominal surgery pain assessment scale (PASPAS) in horses. *Vet. J.* 188: 178–183.

Lawson, A., Opie, R.R., Stevens, K.B. et al. (2019). Application of an equine composite pain scale and its association with plasma adrenocorticotropic hormone concentrations and serum cortisol concentrations in horses with colic. *Equine Vet. Educ.* https://doi.org/10.1111/eve.13143.

van Loon, J. and Van Dierendonck, M.C. (2015). Monitoring acute equine visceral pain with the equine Utrecht University scale for composite pain assessment (EQUUS-COMPASS) and the equine Utrecht University scale for facial assessment of pain (EQUUS-FAP): a scale-construction study. *Vet. J.* 206: 356–364.

van Loon, J. and Van Dierendonck, M. (2018). Objective pain assessment in horses (2014–2018*). Vet. J.* 242: 1–7.

van Loon, J.P.A.M. and Van Dierendonck, M.C. (2019). Pain assessment in horses after orthopaedic surgery and with orthopaedic trauma. *Vet. J.* 246: 85–91.

Obel, N. (1948). *Studies on the Histopathology of Acute Laminitis*. Almquisst & Wiksells Boktrycker.

Regan, F.H., Hockenhull, J., Pritchard, J.C. et al. (2016). Identifying behavioural differences in working donkeys in response to analgesic administration. *Equine Vet. J.* 48: 33–38.

Sampson, F.C., O'Cathain, A., and Goodacre, S. (2020). How can pain management in the emergency department be improved? Findings from multiple case study analysis of pain management in three UK emergency departments. *Emerg. Med. J.* 37: 85–94.

Torcivia, C. and McDonnell, S. (2020). In-person caretaker visits disrupt ongoing discomfort behavior in hospitalized equine orthopedic surgical patients. *Animals (Basel)* 10: 210. https://doi.org/10.3390/ani10020210.

Van Loon, J. and Van Dierendonck, M.C. (2017). Monitoring equine head-related pain with the equine Utrecht University scale for facial assessment of pain (EQUUS-FAP). *Vet. J.* 220: 88–90.

Walsh, J., Eccleston, C., and Keogh, E. (2014). Pain communication through body posture: the development and validation of a stimulus set. *Pain* 155: 2282–2290.

Williams, A.C.D. (2002). Facial expression of pain: an evolutionary account. *Behav. Brain Sci.* 25: 439–435.

# 30

## Management of Pain

### The Pharmacologic Approach to Pain Management
*Rachel A. Reed*

## I Drug classes commonly utilized for management of pain in horses

### A Non-steroidal anti-inflammatory drugs (NSAIDs)

- ○ NSAIDs are the mainstay of acute and chronic pain management in equine patients.
- ○ NSAIDs inhibit cyclooxygenase enzymes in the arachidonic acid cascade resulting in decreased production of inflammatory mediators associated with tissue injury.
- ○ Adverse effects of NSAIDs in horses include gastric ulceration, right dorsal colitis, and renal toxicity.
- ○ Commonly used NSAIDs in horses include *phenylbutazone*, *flunixin meglumine*, and *firocoxib*.
- ○ For a more complete review of NSAIDs and their use in horses see Chapter 16.

### B Opioids

- ○ Opioid receptors are present throughout the body, within the central nervous system (CNS), and throughout the periphery. This receptor system represents an endogenous anti-nociceptive system within the body. Relevant opioid receptors include *mu*, *kappa*, and *delta*. Mu and kappa receptors are targeted by opioid agents administered for pain management in equine patients. (see Table 30.1)

#### Mu opioid receptors
- ○ Have been identified in the equine synovial membrane and are upregulated in the presence of inflammation. This upregulation can be prevented by administering NSAIDs at the time of insult to the joint. Taking advantage of this receptor upregulation, pure mu agonist opioids, especially *morphine*, are commonly administered intra-articularly for the management of joint pain.

*Manual of Equine Anesthesia and Analgesia*, Second Edition. Edited by Tom Doherty,
Alex Valverde, and Rachel A. Reed.

**Table 30.1**   Dosages of opioid agents in equine patients.

| Drug | Dose (mg/kg); route | Frequency | Comments |
|------|---------------------|-----------|----------|
| Morphine | 0.1; IV, IM, SQ, epidural | q4 hr | Histamine release, especially with IV administration. |
| Hydromorphone | 0.04; IV, IM, SQ | q12 hr | |
| Methadone | 0.2; IV, IM, SQ | q4 hr | |
| Meperidine | 0.5–1; IV, IM, SQ | q2 hr | Histamine release, especially with IV administration. Thus, not recommended for IV administration. |
| Fentanyl | 0.005–0.01; IV, Transdermal; two 10 mg patches for horses 115–585 kg | | Requires a CRI, 0.005–0.01 mg/kg/hr. Concentrations >1 ng/ml are achieved 1–14 hr after patch placement and maintained for 35 ± 15 hr. |
| Butorphanol | 0.02–0.05; IV, IM SQ | q2 hr | Minimal analgesic effect. |

IV, intravenous; IM, intramuscular; SQ, subcutaneous.

- Opioids can and do cause excitation when administered to non-painful, non-sedated horses. For reasons that are not understood, this effect is not commonly observed when opioids are administered to horses that are currently experiencing pain.
- Opioids decrease gastrointestinal (GI) motility via the effect of mu receptor agonism in the myenteric plexus of the GI. However, *this adverse effect of opioids is not a reason to withhold opioids in the management of patient pain*. Both prospective and retrospective studies of pure mu agonist opioids have shown that the effect of opioids on the GI tract does not commonly result in colic, and there is no clinically relevant difference in GI motility in horses that receive opioids vs. those that do not receive opioids for the management of existing pain.
- Transdermal application of fentanyl can be used in horses. The absorption of fentanyl is rapid and complete within 1–14 hours, and plasma concentrations consistent with analgesia in other species are maintained for up to 32 hours.
- These drugs are reversible with the opioid receptor antagonists *naloxone* and *naltrexone*.
- For a more complete review of opioids and their use in horses (see Chapter 12).

## C   α₂-adrenergic agonists

- $\alpha_2$-adrenergic agonists provide analgesic effects via inhibition of nociceptive impulses within the dorsal horn of the spinal cord.
- *Xylazine* is currently considered the drug of choice in the management of acute colic.
- Analgesic effects are accompanied by sedative effects and therefore, these drugs do not represent a viable option for management of pain in the long term.
- Available $\alpha_2$ agonists include *xylazine, detomidine, romifidine, medetomidine*, and *dexmedetomidine*. These drugs are commonly used for procedural sedation and sedation prior to induction of general anesthesia.
- $\alpha_2$ agonists can also be used as an *additive* in local blocks in order to prolong the duration of the blockade. The mechanism responsible for this effect is inhibition of hyperpolarization-activated cation current ($I_h$ current) and is unrelated to the activity of the drug at $\alpha_2$ receptors.

    ○ These agents are reversible with any $\alpha_2$ adrenergic antagonist (e.g. *tolazoline, yohimbine, atipamezole*). (see Table 30.2)

### D   N-methyl-D-aspartate receptor antagonists

    ○ *Ketamine* is commonly used for induction of general anesthesia in horses but can also be used at sub-anesthetic doses for provision of analgesia in anesthetized and awake horses. (see Chapter 12)

    ○ The opioid, *methadone*, is also an N-methyl-D-aspartate (NMDA) receptor antagonist. It is unknown how relevant this mechanism of action is in the clinical effect of methadone.

    ○ *Amantadine*, originally used as an anti-viral agent, has gained popularity in the management of chronic and neuropathic pain. Although this drug has some potential as an adjunct in the management of chronic pain in horses, there is currently no literature investigating its efficacy as an analgesic in horses.

### E   Local anesthetics

    ○ Regional anesthetic techniques should be used whenever possible.

    ○ Local blockade prevents transmission of the nociceptive impulse to the spinal cord and subsequently to the brain. This not only prevents pain as a conscious perception of nociceptive stimulation but also prevents centrally mediated chronic pain states as glutamate receptors within the spinal cord are not activated.

    ○ For more information about the indications and technique for specific blocks (see Chapters 22, 24, 25, 26, 27).

    ○ Systemic administration of lidocaine as an infusion provides many beneficial effects to the patient including analgesic effects, anti-inflammatory effects, free-radical scavenging, and antiarrhythmogenic effects. Lidocaine infusions are commonly used in the perioperative period with the additional effect of reducing the minimum alveolar concentration (MAC) of inhalant anesthetics. Lidocaine infusions can also be used in standing horses as an analgesic adjunct in a multimodal pain management plan. Care should be taken to avoid administering an inadvertent bolus or accidental overdose of the drug as central nervous system and subsequent cardiovascular toxicity can occur.

Table 30.2   Dosages and route of administration for alpha₂ adrenergic agonists.

| Drug | Dose (mg/kg) | Comments |
| --- | --- | --- |
| *Agonists* | | |
| Xylazine | 0.3–1.0; IV, IM | Fastest onset, shortest duration. |
| Detomidine | 0.005–0.02; IV, IM, | Oral transmucosal gel (dose 0.04 mg/kg). |
| Romifidine | 0.03–0.1; IV, IM | |
| Dexmedetomidine | 0.001–0.005; IV, IM | Slowest onset, longest duration. |

IV, intravenous; IM, intramuscular; SQ, subcutaneous.

F  **Gabapentin**

- ○ Gabapentin is a calcium-receptor antagonist, binding specifically at the $\alpha_2\delta$ subunit of the *voltage-gated calcium channel*. In binding, the drug disrupts cellular trafficking involved in pain processes.
- ○ The $\alpha_2\delta$ subunit of the voltage-gated calcium channel is upregulated over time in chronic pain states. With a higher density of these receptors in chronic pain patients, gabapentin is more effective in the management of chronic pain than acute pain.
- ○ Gabapentin is used extensively in human medicine for management of neuropathic pain.
- ○ There is some anecdotal evidence, including published case reports, that gabapentin may be effective in some cases of equine chronic pain. However, no controlled, prospective, blinded studies have shown a significant effect of gabapentin in the management of chronic pain in an equine model.

## II  Pain management

- Globally, improved recognition and the clinical management of pain in horses is a work in progress. In the last several years, an increased recognition of the importance of pain management in the well-being and performance of the equine patient has aided in the development of improved pain management techniques and recommendations.
- In 2019, the British Equine Veterinary Association published robust clinical guidelines for use by the practitioner in the management of common clinical scenarios of painful horses. The guidelines were completed in an effort to create evidence-based recommendations in light of the most recent literature. As such, they are a great resource for practitioners to implement multi-modal pain management plans within their practice(s).
- Similarly, in 2019, the Equine Veterinary Education Journal published an issue with a focus on pain management. Within the articles included in that issue, multimodal pain management was a primary focus. This emphasis on the use of multiple drugs to target multiple steps in the pain pathway is an example of "*balanced analgesia*."
- *Balanced analgesia* is a term used to describe any analgesic protocol utilizing more than one drug with the aim of targeting different steps in the pathway in an effort to provide optimum pain relief.
- Use of a balanced analgesia protocol often allows for a reduction in the required dose of some or all of the specific agents used. Consequently, there is a decreased incidence of adverse effects associated with those drugs.
- Selection of drugs to be used in the balanced analgesia plan should be aimed at choosing drugs with different targets. For example, an NSAID and an opioid.
  - ○ It does *not* enhance an analgesic plan to include two opioids.
  - ○ Additional consideration should be given in regard to the duration of action of each drug to aid in determining the frequency of administration, and whether a constant rate infusion (CRI) will be necessary.
  - ○ Lastly, it is necessary to identify the dose at which one would expect to see significant adverse effects associated with each specific drug included in the plan.
- In providing balanced analgesia, it is critical to consider the patient as an individual with very specific pain to be managed. The success of an analgesic plan in one horse does not mean that it will be successful in all horses. Therefore, the plan should be catered to the patient, the source of pain, and the severity of the pain *at the time*, recognizing that pain is a *dynamic* process that changes over the course of time. In order to successfully provide balanced analgesia, it is critical to assess the patient's level of pain regularly and titrate the dosages of different drugs to effect.

- At the outset of getting the patient's pain to a tolerable level, this may require high doses of each drug that is employed. Over time, with healing and resolution of the insult, the required doses to manage the pain will decrease and analgesic agents can be discontinued, one at a time. Each step down in the pain management plan should be followed with pain scoring to ensure that the patient's comfort level has not suffered.
- In general, it is a bad idea to discontinue or decrease the dose of multiple agents at one time. This could result in severe relapse of painful stimulation which may be more difficult to get under control the second time.

## III   Examples of case management using balanced analgesia

**Case 1**: A 12-year-old mare (550 kg) presenting for acute intractable colic, will undergo exploratory laparotomy. The tentative diagnosis is an acute large colon torsion. Pre-anesthetic bloodwork reveals a mild degree of hemoconcentration (packed cell volume [PCV] 50%) and a lactate of 4 mmol/l.

- *Xylazine* (200 mg, IV) is administered initially to control the mare for examination and to facilitate jugular catheter placement.
- *Flunixin meglumine* (600 mg) is administered IV.
- 2 l of 7.2% NaCl, is administered for cardiovascular support.

*Premedication:*

- An $\alpha_2$ agonist and an opioid is administered to provide presurgical sedation and analgesia:
  - *Xylazine* 1.1 mg/kg, IV.
  - *Hydromorphone* 0.04 mg/kg, IV.

*Induction:*

- *Ketamine*, an NMDA antagonist, for induction to induce hypnosis and analgesia, in combination with *midazolam*, a benzodiazepine, for muscle relaxation:
  - *Ketamine* 2.2 mg/kg, IV.
  - *Midazolam* 0.05 mg/kg, IV.
- Anesthesia will be maintained using a PIVA protocol to include a CRI *of lidocaine*, *xylazine*, and *ketamine* to provide intra-operative analgesia and reduce the MAC of *isoflurane*. This significant reduction (~ 70%) in MAC will serve to limit the cardiovascular depression and hypotension caused by high concentrations of isoflurane.
- CRI doses:
  - *Lidocaine*, 2 mg/kg loading dose (LD), IV over five minutes, followed by a CRI 3 mg/kg/hr.
  - *Ketamine*, a CRI of 1 mg/kg/hr.
  - *Xylazine*, a CRI of 1 mg/kg/hr.
- *Flunixin meglumine* administration will be continued postoperatively.

**Case 2**: A two-year-old stallion (450 kg) is presented for castration. The stallion is considered to be healthy based on the physical examination and history.

- A pre-anesthetic NSAID, (*flunixin meglumine* 1 mg/kg, IV) will be administered.

*Premedication:*

- An $\alpha_2$ agonist and an *opioid* is indicated to provide presurgical sedation and analgesia:
  - *Xylazine* 1.1 mg/kg, IV.
  - *Butorphanol* 0.02 mg/kg, IV. (*Note*: butorphanol is not a potent analgesic and is short acting; hence, it must not be used in place of an NSAID. A more potent opioid such as

> *morphine* (0.1 mg/kg, IV) or *hydromorphone* (0.04 mg/kg, IV) may be used in place of butorphanol.

### Induction
- Ketamine (2.2 mg/kg, IV) an NMDA antagonist for induction to induce hypnosis and analgesia.
- Midazolam (0.05 mg/kg, IV), a benzodiazepine for muscle relaxation.

### Local anesthesia:
- A testicular block using 2% *mepivacaine*, injecting a volume (e.g. 10 ml) that causes the testicle to become turgid (see Chapter 25).
  *Note: Mepivacaine was chosen because it is fast acting and its effects last up to four hours. In comparison, lidocaine has a maximum duration of action of about two hours.*
- Post-surgical analgesia should include continued oral administration of an NSAID for three days postoperatively (e.g. *flunixin meglumine* or *phenylbutazone*).

**Case 3**: A five-year-old Thoroughbred mare (570 kg) is presented for evaluation of a severe soft-tissue injury to the lateral and caudal aspects of the thigh after being hit by a truck. The patient presents with a pre-renal azotemia, contraindicating the use of an NSAID until her circulating volume is restored.
- *Detomidine* (10 μg/kg, IV) is administered to provide sedation and analgesia for initial evaluation of the wound.
- An *opioid* is indicated to manage pain due to the severity of the wound.
  – *Hydromorphone* (0.04 mg/kg) will be administered IV.
- Isotonic crystalloid replacement fluids are initiated to resolve dehydration prior to administration of an NSAID.
- Due to the severity of the wound, the horse will be hospitalized in order to facilitate wound healing and pain management.
  – *Flunixin meglumine* (1 mg/kg, IV, q8–12 hr) after correction of the fluid deficit.
  – *Hydromorphone*: it will not be necessary to repeat the dose as epidural *morphine* will be having an effect by the time a repeat injection is due.
  – An *epidural catheter* will be placed at the sacrococcygeal space or Co1–Co2 and advanced approximately 10 cm cranial toward the lumbosacral space.
    ▪ *Morphine* (0.1 mg/kg) will be administered epidurally q12–24 hours. (see Chapter 27)
  – If the horse is still in pain despite an NSAID and opioid administration, a *lidocaine* CRI will be administered: 2 mg/kg LD, IV over five minutes, and a CRI of 3 mg/kg/hr.

**Case 4**: A 20-year-old Arabian gelding (410 kg) is presented for evaluation of severe acute laminitis. No abnormalities were detected on bloodwork.
- An NSAID is indicated for management of pain and inflammation:
  – *Phenylbutazone* (4 mg/kg, IV) on presentation, and every 12 hours thereafter with reduction of the dose based on the pain level.
- A pure mu agonist opioid (e.g. *hydromorphone*, 0.04 mg/kg, IV) is indicated initially to get the pain under control.
- *Local anesthesia* of the palmar digital nerves is indicated. *Bupivacaine* combined with *dexmedetomidine* will provide local anesthesia for up to 12 hours.
  – 2 ml of 0.5% bupivacaine and 250 μg of dexmedetomidine over each nerve.
- A *lidocaine CRI* will be administered for further analgesic and anti-inflammatory effects, 2 mg/kg LD, IV over five minutes, and a CRI of 3 mg/kg/hr.
- *Cryotherapy*: Ice boots will be placed to cause vasoconstriction and provide an anti-inflammatory effect and further analgesia.

**Case 5**: A 17-year-old Quarter Horse gelding (525 kg) is presented for extraction of molar 207 utilizing standing sedation. Physical examination and bloodwork are within normal limits.

- ○ An NSAID (e.g. *phenylbutazone* 2 mg/kg, IV) is administered pre-anesthetically for preemptive pain management.
- ○ Sedation with an alpha$_2$ agonist and in combination with an opioid is indicated to provide surgical sedation and analgesia:
  - – Detomidine (0.005–0.01 mg/kg, IV).
  - – Hydromorphone (0.04 mg/kg, IV).
- ○ Maintenance of sedation can be achieved via top-ups of detomidine or a detomidine CRI (see chapter 20).
- ○ A *maxillary nerve block* will be administered using 10 ml of 0.5% bupivacaine (see Chapter 22).
  - – Dexmedetomidine can be added to extend the duration of the block.

## Suggested Reading

Bowen, I.M., Redpath, A., Dugdale, A. et al. (2019). BEVA primary care clinical guidelines: Analgesia. *Equine Vet. J.* 52: 13–27.
Equine Veterinary Education (2019) 31, 338–391.

## Rehabilitation Modalities for Acute and Chronic Pain in Horses
*Tena L. Ursini*

## I Introduction

- For any biologic system to function normally, it must be free from the restriction of pain.
- Horses are unique animals in that we ask them to perform routinely as premier level athletes. Thus, they are subject to a unique subset of acute and chronic pain conditions.
- The goal of a successful rehabilitation program is to return the patient to normal function.
- In the clinical setting, it is extremely rare for any one rehabilitation modality to be used in isolation. Similar to other branches of medicine, oftentimes a multimodal approach is used. Practitioners must rely on current literature and experience to develop comprehensive rehabilitation plans on a patient-by-patient basis until more comprehensive scientific evidence suggests significant clinical efficacy in horses.
- Appropriate pain medications have been discussed elsewhere in this book, but in addition, rehabilitation modalities can provide a non-pharmaceutical option for pain relief.

## II Pain assessment

- The most important aspect of developing any rehabilitation plan requires an accurate assessment of the patient.
- Assessing pain in horses requires a multifaceted approach as no one method is appropriate as a stand-alone measurement tool. Recording accurate baseline measurements are vital to determine if the patient is responding positively, negatively or not at all to the medical interventions being applied.
- Pain recognition in horses is discussed in chapter 29, and this section focusses on pain resulting from musculoskeletal issues.

## A   Lameness assessment

- Musculoskeletal pain often manifests as lameness.
- All lameness should be presumed to be caused by pain until proven otherwise.
- Lameness is any deviation from the normal gait pattern or symmetry. Therefore, it is a clinical sign caused by either pain or a mechanical restriction.
    - Pain is manifested by the horse avoiding to proper weight bearing or advancing the limb.
    - Whereas mechanical issues occur when scar tissue or conformational abnormalities do not allow the horse to move properly.
- Lameness can be assessed in several ways including subjective assessment based on a pre-determined scale or a more objective approach using inertial based sensors.
- It is the author's opinion that objective use of an *inertial sensor system* allows for a greater degree of consistency during repeat examinations. However, each method has its pros and cons, and no one system has been proven superior to another.

## B   Articular pain

- Intra- or extra-capsular articular pain can manifest as a restriction in joint motion. Again, this is likely a consequence of pain rather than a primary disease, as pain guarding leads overtime to decreased use and decreased elasticity of joint-related soft tissues.
- Passive range of motion can be determined easily and accurately by measuring the maximum flexion and extension comfortably obtained by the horse using a *goniometer*. (see Figure 30.1)

## C   Pressure algometry

- Pressure algometry is a method described in horses to determine the mechanical nociceptive threshold. (see Figure 30.2)

Figure 30.1   Goniometer assessing the range of motion of the left carpus.

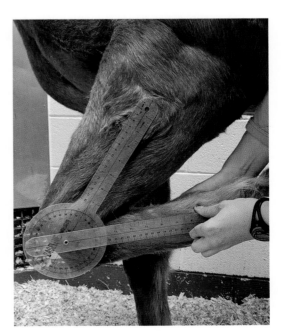

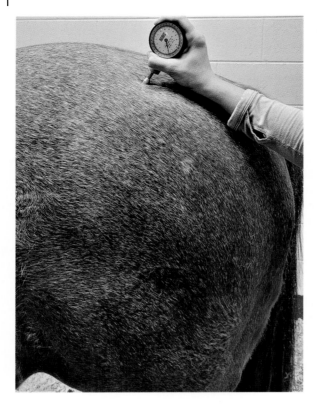

Figure 30.2   Pressure algometer assessing the mechanical nociceptive threshold of the middle gluteal muscle.

- It is defined as the minimum pressure required to induce an avoidance behavior (e.g. withdrawal or stomping of the stimulated limb). Pressure algometry has been validated and used in humans.
- Short-term intra-examiner reliability in horses has been shown to be fairly high; however, this figure fell when horses were re-examined three weeks later. Based on these findings, pressure algometry is *inappropriate* as a stand-alone assessment tool. However, in conjunction with other assessments previously described, it can allow practitioners to determine baseline and repeat pain levels.

## III   Rehabilitation modalities used to treat acute and chronic musculoskeletal pain

### A   Therapeutic laser *(Light amplification by stimulated emission of radiation.)* **(see Figure 30.3)**

- Laser energy is an artificial source of radiation emitted in the form of photons. Photons are then reflected, scattered, transmitted or absorbed by the body.
- When *chromophores* within the tissue absorb photons, a biologic effect is produced. Major chromophores in biologic systems include water, hemoglobin, and respiratory chain enzymes within the mitochondria.
- Direct effects of the photons induce a cascade of cellular interactions. Nitric oxide is disassociated from cytochrome C, allowing oxygen to bind and promote ATP production based on the electron gradient produced during aerobic respiration.

Figure 30.3   Class 4 therapeutic laser.

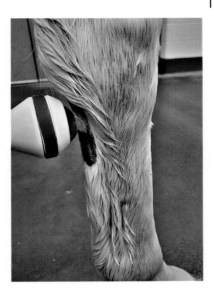

- ○ Laser photons also increase membrane permeability to calcium, increase cellular proliferation, and have anti-inflammatory effects.

*Analgesic effects of laser therapy*
- ○ The exact mechanism behind laser-induced analgesia is not completely understood.
- ○ Laser treatments result in decreases in prostaglandin E2 and cyclooxygenase 2.
- ○ Other less well supported theories for laser-induced pain modulation include decreased nociception of Aδ and C peripheral nerve fibers, suppressed central sensitization, and increased release of endorphins, enkephalins, and endogenous opioids.
- ○ Clinical trials in human beings have shown significant decreases in pain scores when laser therapy was incorporated into treatment plans for myofascial trigger point pain, diabetic neuropathic pain, and patellofemoral pain syndrome.
  - – Additionally, when laser therapy was included during palatal repair in children, there was a significant decrease in the need for analgesics postoperatively.
- ○ Clinical trials in animals regarding the use of laser in treating pain are lacking. However, in performance Quarter Horses, laser therapy has resulted in improved visual analog pain scores, epaxial muscle hypertonicity, and trunk stiffness when treating back pain.

## B   Acupuncture

- ○ Acupuncture has been employed for hundreds of years to treat musculoskeletal pain in many species. The mechanisms of acupuncture are explained in further detail later in this chapter.

## C   Cryotherapy

- ○ Ice treatment has been used for many years to mitigate musculoskeletal pain.
- ○ Studies have determined that the pain threshold increases immediately after a period of cooling.
- ○ The intensity of pain decreases as the skin temperature decreases, and intensifies as the skin temperature increases upon stopping the ice treatment.

- ○ Regional vasoconstriction occurs with ice treatment. Vasoconstriction post injury minimizes tissue edema which decreases the release of pro-inflammatory cytokines and other pain producing substances.
- ○ Additionally, a decrease in the peripheral temperature decreases nerve conduction, with the Aδ fibers being most affected. Unmyelinated C fibers are more resistant to this effect. Also, the application of cold stimulates cold sensory nerve fibers, and thus the use of a "*counterirritant*" could evoke the "gate-control theory," decreasing the degree of pain transmitted.
- ○ Superficial cold therapy can be reasonably applied to the horse using a variety of methods including but not limited to reusable ice packs, submersion in ice water, or circulating cold-water devices. It is of the author's opinion that cold therapy that includes moisture (i.e. water bath) is more effective at cooling tissues than "dry" cold techniques (i.e. ice packs). However, immersion in water is not appropriate for patients with postoperative incisions or lacerations.

### D  Thermotherapy

- ○ Superficial heat application has been proven to decrease pain in humans with chronic musculoskeletal conditions.
- ○ The mechanisms are the opposite of what happens with cold application. Increased local temperature induces vasodilation and thus increases blood flow. Vasodilation might also improve venous drainage and reduce tissue edema. Additionally, heat increases the conductance velocity and frequency of Aβ sensory nerve fibers. Sensory signals transmitted by Aβ nerves block transmission of impulses from Aδ and C fibers via the "gate control theory."
- ○ Heat is easily applied to the clinical patient in the form of UV radiation via a solarium, heating pad, or heat packs. Similar to cold therapy, heat is more effectively transferred via a moist interface. Horses sweat readily, and thus provide a moist interface for most heat application strategies.

### E  Electrical stimulation (Transcutaneous electrical nerve stimulation [TENS]) (see Figure 30.4)

- ○ TENS uses pulsed electrical currents delivered to the skin with the purpose of stimulating peripheral nerves.
- ○ Similar to other modalities presented in this chapter, the stimulation of non-nociceptive sensory nerves blocks transmission of nociceptive nerve impulses via the "gate-control theory."
- ○ A variety of protocols, from intermittent to pulsatile settings, have been used for pain relief. This wide variety of parameters has made it difficult to compare studies and prove efficacy. The limiting factor is the inability to blindly study participants to the TENS sensation. However, with limited contraindications, TENS is an easily applied modality as an adjunct treatment for pain relief.

### F  Extracorporeal shockwave therapy (see Figure 30.5)

- ○ Of all the modalities presented, extracorporeal shockwave therapy (ESWT) is the most widely investigated in horses.
- ○ Originally determined to have analgesic effects in human beings, several researchers have measured its effects in horses.

Figure 30.4 Electrical stimulation of the right gluteal.

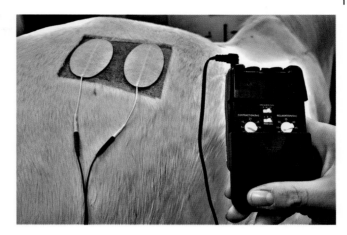

Figure 30.5 Extracorporeal shockwave therapy of the right proximal metacarpal region.

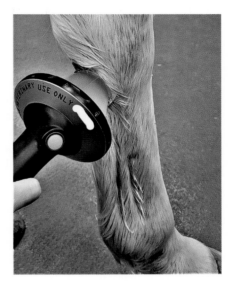

○ ESWT is a non-invasive high frequency pressure wave that can be applied to tissues in either radial or focused patterns. The mechanism causing analgesia after ESWT is poorly understood. Current theories include decreased substance P concentrations, conditioned pain modulation, unmyelinated nerve loss, and prolonged decreases in nerve conductance velocity.

○ In horses, ESWT has been reported to be effective at mitigating generalized back pain, proximal metacarpal and metatarsal sensitivity, distal forelimb lameness, and osteoarthritis. Cutaneous sensation is reported to be decreased for up to three days post treatment.

– The analgesic qualities of ESWT have led to many competition regulating bodies restricting its use before or during competitions.

## Suggested Reading

Keegan, K.G., Wilson, D.A., Kramer, J. et al. (2013). Comparison of a body-mounted inertial sensor system-based method with subjective evaluation for detection of lameness in horses. *Amer. J. Vet. Res.* 74: 17–24.

Millis, D.L. and Levine, D. (2014). *Canine Rehabilitation and Physical Therapy*, 2e. St. Louis: W.B. Saunders.

McGowan, C. and Goff, L. (2016). *Animal Physiotherapy*, 2e. Wiley: West Sussex, UK.

King, M. and Davidson, E. (2016). Innovations in equine physical therapy and rehabilitation. *Vet. Clin. North Am. Equine Pract.* 32: xiii–xiv.

Haussler, K.K., Manchon, P.T., Donnell, J.R., and Frisbie, D.D. (2020). Effects of low-level laser therapy and chiropractic care on back pain in quarter horses. *J. Equine Vet. Sci.* 86: 1–9.

Douglas, W.W. and Malcolm, J.L. (1955). The effect of localized cooling on conduction in cat nerves. *J. Physiol. Lon.* 130: 53–71.

McClure, S.R., Sonea, I.M., Evans, R.B., and Yaeger, M.J. (2005). Evaluation of analgesia resulting from extracorporeal shock wave therapy and radial pressure wave therapy in the limbs of horses and sheep. *Amer. J. Vet. Res.* 66: 1702–1708.

## Equine Acupuncture

*Neal Valk*

## I   Introduction

- Acupuncture is an ancient form of healing first described by the Chinese several thousand years ago. Early recognition that needle stimulation applied to various points on the body could relieve pain and dysfunction in local and distant anatomic structures lead to the development of medical acupuncture.
- Briefly, according to theory, twelve paired channels (or meridians) exist on either side of the body. Two additional meridians exist, the Governing vessel on the dorsal midline, and the Conception vessel on the ventral midline. The meridians serve to connect the surface of the body and the internal organs, and maintain harmony and equilibrium.
- Qi, the vital force or life energy of an organism, and blood circulate throughout the body via the meridians. Acupuncture points (acupoints) are located on the meridians, and can be stimulated to affect the body and its functions.
    - Pain occurs when the flow of Qi and/or blood is obstructed.
    - Stimulation of therapeutic acupoints restores the flow of Qi and/or blood and eliminates pain, hence its analgesic effect.
- While acupuncture is not a medical panacea, it can be a very effective treatment modality when performed by a trained practitioner. In addition, acupuncture appears to be relatively free of negative side effects when compared to allopathic medical and surgical therapy.

## II   Mechanism of acupuncture-induced analgesia

- It has generally been accepted that acupuncture-induced analgesia results from the central release of *opioid* peptides, and acupuncture has been associated with an increase in the cerebrospinal fluid concentration of *β-endorphin* in human beings.
- It has been postulated that needle penetration and manipulation at acupoints leads to deformation of collagen fibers which causes Transient receptor potential cation channel subfamily V member 2 proteins (TPRV2) to activate *mast* cells.
    - In support of this hypothesis, acupuncture-induced analgesia was inhibited in TRPV2 knockout mice, and this was accompanied by a decrease in the activation of mast cells at the stimulated acupoints.
- The increase in *histamine* concentrations locally leads to an increase in *adenosine* in the local tissues.

- Histamine and adenosine bind to $H_1$ and $A_1$ receptors, respectively, on nerve endings and generate excitatory signals that culminate in the central release of *opioid* peptides, and this is considered to generate the analgesic effect which persists after the needle is removed.
  - An injection of an adenosine $A_1$ receptor agonist or a histamine $H_1$ receptor agonist at an acupoint in an acute adjuvant induced arthritis model in rats was associated with an increase in β-endorphin concentration in the CSF.
- Nevertheless, it seems that mast cells may not be involved in mediating acupuncture-induced analgesia on all occasions. Mast cells were demonstrated to have a role in acupuncture-induced analgesia in a mechanically-induced model of nociception, but they did not appear to have a significant role in acupuncture-induced analgesia in thermally-induced nociception.

## III  Patient evaluation and treatment

- The goal of patient evaluation is to identify a pattern of disease based on traditional Chinese veterinary medicine (TCVM) theory so that a diagnostic plan can be established. The pattern is based on the concept that disease is caused by an imbalance in the body, and knowledge of the pattern allows the clinician to recognize the specific imbalance present in the patient.
- TCVM diagnostic evaluation of the horse is based on:
  - Patient history.
  - Palpation.
  - Examination of the tongue.
  - Assessment of the carotid pulses.
- A detailed description of the latter two is beyond the scope of this section, and the reader is referred to readily available resources to provide an overview of these techniques.
- Treatment entails the use of fine *needles* placed into acupoints to stimulate a desired response in the patient. (see Figure 30.6)
- This section will focus on the use of acupuncture to provide analgesia, but the technique can also be utilized to treat a myriad of other conditions.
- In TCVM, the Eight Principles are used as the initial step to determine a pattern, and consist of four opposing pairs:
  - Excess and deficiency.
  - Exterior and interior.
  - Hot and cold.
  - Yang and Yin.

### A  Acupuncture techniques

  - Acupuncture treatment can be delivered by using several different techniques.
  - All techniques result in the stimulation of the treated acupoints, which produces a response in the body.

#### *Acupressure*
  - Is the application of digital pressure to an acupoint, and the point is stimulated for the duration of pressure application.

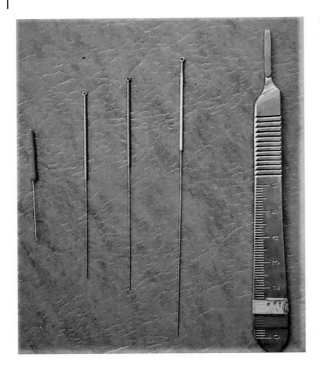

**Figure 30.6** A selection of acupuncture needles.

*Dry needle*
- This refers to the insertion of thin, solid needles into acupoints and leaving them in place for a period of time.

*Hemoacupuncture*
- This refers to bloodletting, whereby a small volume of blood is allowed to exit from an acupoint after puncture with a hypodermic needle.

*Aquapuncture*
- This involves the use of hypodermic needles and syringes to inject a liquid (usually vitamin B12, physiologic saline, a specific medication, or the patient's own blood) into an acupoint.
- Stimulation occurs until the injected substance is absorbed.

*Electroacupuncture* (EA)
- This method uses a device that passes an electrical current through needles placed into acupoints.
- EA provides stimulation of acupoints beyond that provided by other techniques, and is similar to TENS therapy, except that the stimulation is applied to the deeper tissues and not the skin surface alone.

*Moxibustion*
- This technique utilizes the burning of herbs near acupoints to provide a warming effect.

*Lasers and infrared light sources*
- The use of low power (5–30 mW) lasers and light sources effectively stimulates acupoints, and is performed by some practitioners.

*Implanted materials*

  o Various materials can be implanted into acupoints to provide chronic stimulation, and thus a much longer duration of therapeutic stimulation.

  o Short pieces of suture material, gold wire and gold beads are examples of materials used for acupuncture implantation.

## B Choice of technique

  o Choosing which technique to use depends on many factors including:
  - Practitioner preference.
  - Experience.
  - Patient tolerance.
  - Lesion location.
  - Equipment availability.
  - Severity of the condition being treated.

  o Some equine patients are averse to dry needle placement, but will tolerate aquapuncture.

  o Therapeutic points on the distal limbs are more sensitive to EA than those in heavily muscled regions.

  o The author prefers to use EA for analgesia when the patient is very reactive to palpation of diagnostic points, as this suggests a high level of pain in the affected area. As the condition improves and less sensitivity is noted, dry needle and/or aquapuncture may be used for subsequent treatments.

## C Number of treatments required

  o The number of treatments required to resolve a specific condition appears to be dependent upon the severity of pain, chronicity of the condition and response to therapy.

  o In general, a minimum of two to four treatments at intervals of one to two weeks for the treatment of moderate to marked musculoskeletal pain are recommended, though improvement is usually observed after one treatment.

  o However, equine athletes rarely have a single physical issue causing pain and/or poor performance, and subsequent examinations can reveal sensitivity in acupoints not previously recognized.

  o Furthermore, horses suffering from a musculoskeletal lesion often develop compensatory or secondary pain in other anatomic areas, and it is prudent to treat these problems as well, allowing for a more holistic approach to pain relief. If, after several treatments, there is no improvement, the patient is re-evaluated and the treatment strategy reassessed.

## IV Evaluation of the musculoskeletal system

- Assessment of the equine musculoskeletal system to identify sources of lameness and subclinical pain is performed by observing the horse while moving, and by "*scanning*" diagnostic acupoints.

- The *scanning* technique utilizes a blunt object or fingertip to apply pressure to the diagnostic acupoints in a consistent, predetermined sequence by tracing the path of the acupoints on both sides of the body.

- Acupoints that consistently elicit reactions are indicative of pain in the anatomic region with which the point is associated (joint, tendon/ligament, neck, etc.).

- Patient reaction varies from slight movement of the skin overlying the point to attempts to flee or bite and/or kick the examiner. As multiple points are diagnostic for each regional source of pain, reaction at more than one diagnostic point is needed to positively identify the region involved. Reactivity at only one single point is generally indicative of local pain.
- Acupuncture is commonly used to treat regional pain that is readily identified on physical examination without further ancillary diagnostics. For example, pain in the cervical, thoracolumbar or pelvic regions, without evidence of neurologic deficits, is often treated based solely on clinical findings. Lameness referable to the limbs and feet can be treated with acupuncture after ruling out serious underlying pathologies such as stress fractures and synovial infections.
- Acupuncture is especially helpful for diagnosing and treating subclinical conditions which contribute to overall "*poor performance*," but do not cause overt lameness in the equine athlete.

## V Environment

- The environment in which the horse will receive acupuncture treatment is of vital importance.
- Every attempt should be made to perform the treatment in an area that is clean, quiet and safe for both the patient and veterinarian.
- Distracted horses are more difficult to treat, and the procedure is best performed away from the daily activities of a busy barn or hospital. A place familiar to the patient, such as a stall, and in proximity to horses with which it is familiar, works well. A grooming or wash rack can also work, provided it is not located in the center of activity.
- Other environmental distractions, such as flies, can be minimized by using insect repellents. The patient should be reasonably well groomed, with obvious dirt and debris removed from the skin and hair coat prior to needle placement.

## VI Patient tolerance

- The vast majority of horses tolerate needle insertion surprisingly well, especially needles placed in the head, neck and body.
- Tolerant animals can be treated while restrained in cross ties. If the horse has not been treated before it is best to have an experienced handler restrain the patient, until its level of reactivity has been determined.
- Needles placed in the distal limbs can elicit a negative response, and extra care is taken when these regions are treated. If some type of additional restraint is necessary, it should be minimally offensive to the horse. Elevation of a forelimb, or temporary use of a lip chain or nose twitch can facilitate needle placement in a fractious horse.
- Chemical restraint may be indicated if the patient vigorously resists treatment, although the effect of sedatives on acupuncture treatment is debated. Some practitioners estimate that the use of sedatives reduces the effect of acupuncture in the horse by 30–50%, but, to the author's knowledge, this has not been documented.
- Rarely, one is presented with a patient who resists needle placement so vehemently that safety for the veterinarian and the handler becomes a concern, and acupuncture treatment should be reconsidered.

## VII  Needle placement

- The location of needle placement depends on the affected region and the diagnosis.
- Therapeutic *acupoints* can be local, regional and distant to the site of pain.
- A *combination* of acupoints in various locations is generally indicated, based on their therapeutic effect.
- Descriptions of specific therapeutic points and the indications for their use are readily available, and experience in acupuncture treatment lends familiarity to the treatment of most common problems.

## VIII  Treatment of musculoskeletal pain

- Equine acupuncture is most commonly used for the treatment of musculoskeletal pain caused by degenerative processes, trauma and repetitive use injury.
- These sources of pain tend to manifest as lameness, decreased or poor performance, abnormal behavior when working or pain on palpation/manipulation of a limb or anatomical region.
- Initial patient evaluation should include a thorough history, palpation and evaluation of the patient when moving, and use of ancillary diagnostics as indicated.
- Acupuncture treatment is often combined with *allopathic* therapy as part of a multi-modal approach. Most equine athletes experience multiple sources of musculoskeletal discomfort concurrently, some of which do not respond readily to systemically or locally administered medications (e.g. distal tarsitis combined with back pain). Acupuncture is useful in these cases by itself, and also as an adjunct therapy to Western medicine. This allows for a more holistic approach to treatment. Furthermore, TCVM techniques allow identification and treatment of subclinical conditions before they become clinically evident.
- Although it is common to see improvement following a single acupuncture treatment, many conditions require multiple (two to four or more) treatments before resolution or significant improvement is observed. This is especially true for chronic, long-standing conditions and those associated with severe pain. Good client communication is essential when planning an acupuncture treatment in order to prevent unrealistic expectations. No specific patient preparation is required prior to treatment, and many patients can return to light work immediately, unless contraindicated by the presenting medical condition.

### A  Foot pain

*Non-laminitic foot pain*
- Treatment of non-laminitic foot pain entails placement of acupuncture needles in the distal limb (local points) as well as the proximal limbs and body. (see Figure 30.7)
- The author rarely uses acupuncture as a stand-alone treatment for palmar foot pain. Most cases respond well to corrective farriery with or without intra-synovial medications unless significant boney changes are present radiographically. However, acupuncture can reduce or eliminate the need for analgesic medications in some patients. When severe degeneration exists, acupuncture can often improve lameness, but usually only for a very limited period of time, in the author's experience.

*Laminitic foot pain*
- Acupuncture can be an effective adjunct treatment for laminitis, but concurrent recognition and mitigation of the cause(s) is necessary to successfully treat the disease.

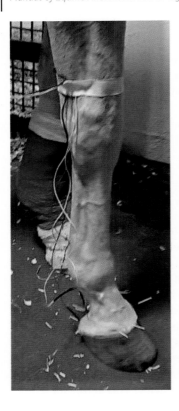

**Figure 30.7** Electroacupuncture and dry needle treatment for support limb laminitis.

- Hemoacupuncture is performed at the *ting points* (proximal to the coronary band).
- Dry needle, aquapuncture and/or electroacupuncture are performed at therapeutic acupoints located more proximally on the limbs and body.
- Results of a recent study indicate that acupuncture can be an effective treatment for chronic laminitis of varying or uncertain etiology. The author prefers to treat laminitis by identifying and eliminating the cause via dietary changes, pharmacologic management (as indicated) and corrective trimming and shoeing, where applicable.
- Acupuncture treatment of individuals with advanced inflammatory or supporting limb laminitis, including those with distal displacement of the third phalanx, have not been rewarding. Unfortunately, acupuncture treatment for these cases is often sought weeks or months after traditional therapy has been unsuccessful.
- However, the author has found acupuncture to be very effective for the treatment of compensatory pain in laminitic horses. These individuals generally exhibit significant pain in the muscles of the back, pelvic region and hind limbs due to the altered stance which is typically associated with severe bilateral forefoot pain. Acupuncture appears to significantly reduce muscle pain and spasms when performed on these horses.

B  Joint pain

- Rest, controlled exercise and anti-inflammatory medications are useful for traumatic synovitis, while more chronic conditions are often amendable to intra-articular medications for maintenance therapy.
- For horses normally maintained on intra-articular injections, the use of TCVM can allow for a decreased frequency of injections.

○ Acupuncture can be used as primary or adjunctive treatment of lameness caused by joint pathology. Acupuncture treatment has a regional effect and is not limited to the treatment of intra-articular pathology; periarticular structures that may be a source of pain, such as injured collateral ligaments, may also respond.

○ Response to treatment is generally better when only soft-tissue structures are affected, as in strain injuries.

### C   Tendon and ligament injuries

○ Pain caused by tendon and ligament injuries with minimal structural damage can be successfully treated with TCVM.

○ The author recently treated a horse with a two-year history of left-hind lameness attributed to proximal suspensory desmitis which failed to respond to intralesional platelet-rich plasma therapy, extracorporeal shock wave therapy and physical rehabilitation. Following three acupuncture treatments and eight weeks of Chinese herbal therapy the mare became sound, and has remained sound while in regular work.

### D   Cervical pain

○ Neck pain in the horse can cause a variety of clinical signs including obvious neck stiffness, abnormal head posture, unwillingness to work on the bit and forelimb lameness that cannot be localized to the limb.

○ Some relatively common sources of neck pain include:
  – Soft tissue injury.
  – Cervical vertebral fractures.
  – Osteoarthritis of the synovial facet joints.
  – Unstable fractures and severe osteoarthritis may result in compression of the spinal cord, which manifests as gait ataxia.

● Acupuncture is highly effective in treating neck pain, and clinical improvement is often observed after one treatment, but complete resolution usually requires three to six treatments, one to two weeks apart. (see Figure 30.8)

*Case report:*
A middle-aged gelding with a long history of severe neck pain was successfully treated by the author. Two and a half years prior, the gelding was found at pasture, unable to completely raise

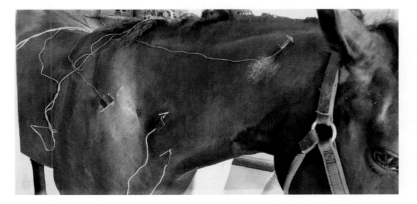

Figure 30.8   Electroacupuncture for cervical pain.

or lower his head. Lateral flexion of the neck to the left was limited, and the patient was unable to flex his neck to the right. Radiographs, ultrasound evaluation and nuclear scintigraphy were not diagnostic. Treatment with NSAIDs did not improve the condition. Clinical signs improved slightly following an extended period of rest. Acupuncture was performed, and significant improvement in neck mobility was observed after one treatment. The gelding was clinically normal following the third of three treatments performed two weeks apart. No recurrence of clinical signs has occurred in the 10 months following the last acupuncture treatment.

### E   Thoracolumbar pain

- ○ Acupuncture is highly effective for the treatment of back pain in the horse, and improvement is usually observed following a single treatment.
- ○ Severe or longstanding cases generally require several treatments one to two weeks apart to completely alleviate the clinical signs.
- ○ Acupuncture is also an excellent adjunct therapy in cases of back pain associated with lameness. Concurrent treatment of the back pain and the source of lameness allows for a more holistic approach to treating performance problems. This speeds recovery and shortens the convalescent period, allowing a quicker return to full function. (see Figure 30.9)

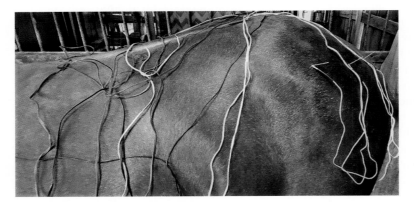

**Figure 30.9**   Electroacupuncture for thoracolumbar and pelvic area pain.

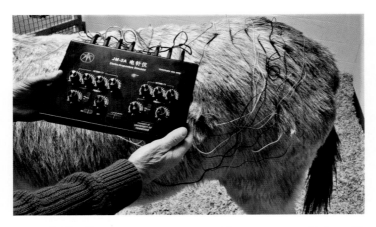

**Figure 30.10**   Electroacupuncture treatment for sacrococcygeal injury with urinary bladder paresis in a donkey.

F   Pelvic region pain **(see Figure 30.10)**

- ○ Acupuncture diagnostic scanning in the region of the pelvis often reveals areas of sensitivity indicative of regional pain.
- ○ Local diagnostic acupoints are useful for localizing pain to specific anatomic regions, and may not be associated with focal sources of pain.
- ○ Pain in the hips, sacroiliac joints, lumbosacral articulations and intertransverse joints are common findings, and response to treatment is usually very good. Improvement in the condition is verified by resolution of the presenting clinical problem and significantly reduced reactivity on palpation of the diagnostic acupoints on follow up evaluation.
- ○ The combination of thoracolumbar and pelvic pain is a common finding in the poor performing but otherwise sound horse, and the author has witnessed significant improvement following one-to-three treatment sessions. Increased flexion and extension of the back, greater hind limb impulsion and improved hind limb engagement are usually observed following acupuncture treatment.

G   Gastrointestinal pain

- ○ Acupuncture can be used to treat colic, but the author prefers a traditional allopathic approach, as most non-surgical ("simple") cases of colic respond readily and rapidly, and the treatment is very cost effective.
- ○ However, the author has successfully used acupuncture to treat post-operative ileus that was non-responsive to routine Western therapy.
  - – EA stimulation of points on the *bladder* meridian, which are associated with GI motility, can be quite successful, and gastric reflux often resolves following one or two daily treatments.

*Summary*

- ○ Acupuncture therapy is a useful primary or adjunctive method of treating pain in the equine patient. Though not a panacea, acupuncture affords the trained practitioner the ability to treat acute and chronic pain with minimal side effects. In many cases, it can allow for a reduction or cessation of the use of analgesic medications needed to control chronic pain, and improve performance and quality of life for the patient. Risk to the patient is minimal when performed by a trained veterinarian, and the worst-case scenario is that treatment is ineffective.

## Suggested Reading

Huang, M., Wang, X., Xing, B. et al. (2018). Critical roles of TRPV2 channels, histamine H1 and adenosine A1 receptors in the initiation of acupoint signals for acupuncture analgesia. *Sci. Rep.* 8: 6523.

Cui, X., Liu, K., Xu, D. et al. (2018). Mast cell deficiency attenuates acupuncture analgesia for mechanical pain using c-kit gene mutant rats. *J. Pain Res.* 11: 483–495.

Faramarzi, B., Lee, D. et al. (2017). Response to acupuncture treatment in horses with chronic laminitis. *Can. Vet. J.* 58: 823–827.

Schoen, A.M. (ed.) (2001). *Veterinary Acupuncture- Ancient Art to Modern Medicine*, 2e. St. Louis: Mosby.

Xie, H. and Preast, V. (eds.) (2007). *Xie's Veterinary Acupuncture*. Ames: Blackwell.

Xie, H. and Preast, V. (eds.) (2013). *Traditional Chinese Veterinary Medicine- Fundamental Principles*, 2e. Reddick, FL: Chi Institute Press.

Xie, H., Wedemeyer, M.A., Chrisman, M.A., and Kim, M.S. (eds.) (2015). *Practical Guide to Traditional Chinese Veterinary Medicine- Equine Practice*. Reddick, FL: Chi Institute Press.

31

# Anesthesia of Foals

*Tom Doherty and Alex Valverde*

- The normal full-term foal is well developed at birth but is in a transition phase to adult circulatory and pulmonary systems and, thus, is physiologically fragile.
- Pulmonary changes occur during the first few hours of life but the most important changes to the adult circulatory system take 48–72 hours.
  *Note: Foals lack fetal hemoglobin, and the left shift of the oxyhemoglobin dissociation curve is facilitated by having a low concentration of 2,3-diphosphoglycerate (2,3-DPG).*

## I Transition to adult life

### A Transition to adult circulation

- The equine fetal circulation has three major shunts present throughout gestation (*placental, foramen ovale, ductus arteriosus*), and blood is delivered from the dam via the umbilical vein.
  *Note: The ductus venosus closes early in gestation, and blood perfuses the hepatic capillaries throughout most of gestation.*
- The low fetal $PO_2$ and high concentrations of *prostaglandins* are responsible for the ductus arteriosus remaining patent.
  - Prostaglandins are secreted by the placenta and metabolized in the lungs.
- In addition, there is a high pulmonary vascular resistance (PVR) secondary to the relatively hypoxic environment in the pulmonary system, and the low systemic vascular resistance (SVR).
  - The high PVR causes blood to be shunted into the aorta from the pulmonary artery via the ductus arteriosus.
- Separation of the placenta from the circulation at birth results in an increase in SVR and blood pressure.
- Initial expansion of the lungs requires a high negative intrathoracic pressure, and results in a dramatic decrease in PVR as the pulmonary vascular bed dilates.
  - Endogenous *nitric oxide* plays a role in the transition of the fetal lung circulation by relaxing vascular smooth muscle.

*Manual of Equine Anesthesia and Analgesia*, Second Edition. Edited by Tom Doherty, Alex Valverde, and Rachel A. Reed.
© 2022 John Wiley & Sons, Inc. Published 2022 by John Wiley & Sons, Inc.

○ Right atrial pressure decreases as blood flow to the lungs increases, and blood flow into the left atrium from the pulmonary vein increases.
○ The left atrial pressure now exceeds right atrial pressure, and this results in closure of the *foramen ovale*.
○ Closure of the *ductus arteriosus* is primarily due to the increase in $PaO_2$ after birth.
   – The decrease in prostaglandin concentrations, consequent to removal of the placenta, also influences closure.

B   **Reopening of shunts**

○ Initial closing of fetal vascular shunts is not anatomically complete, and closure is a gradual process.
○ Permanent closure takes two to four weeks (longer if the foal is *premature*).
○ Shunts are more likely to remain open longer or re-open in systemically ill foals.
○ The *ductus arteriosus* is more likely to remain patent in *premature* foals due to the high concentration of *prostaglandins*.
○ Neonates have a reactive pulmonary vasculature and shunts can re-open under certain circumstances such as:
   – Hypoxia, acidemia, and increases in PVR are likely to result in right to left shunting.

## II   Respiratory system of the neonatal foal

- The metabolic cost of respiration is high in human neonates, and may be up to 15% of total oxygen consumption. Presumably, it follows a similar pattern in neonatal foals.
- There is increased overall oxygen consumption/kg (6–8 ml/kg/min) compared to the adult.

A   **Breathing pattern**

○ Increased respiratory rate.
○ Increased minute ventilation (L/kg).
○ Decreased tidal volume ($V_T$).
○ Increased chest-wall compliance.
○ Decreased lung elastance.
○ Decreased functional residual capacity (FRC).
   *Note*: Rapid shallow breathing decreases the elastic work of breathing, and thereby minimizes energy expenditure.

B   **Control of breathing**

○ There is a decreased sensitivity to changes in $PaO_2$ and $PaCO_2$.
○ Neural control of respiration is probably immature at birth.

C   **Arterial blood gas values in neonatal foals**

○ Foals can establish adequate pulmonary ventilation within a few minutes of birth and the major changes in ventilation occur in the first hour of life.
○ $PaO_2$ values are low (~40 mmHg) immediately following birth but increase (~60 mmHg) at one hour, and by four hours are up to 75 mmHg.

   – However, adult values are not achieved for about seven days.
   o Hypoxemia has been attributed to a right-to-left shunt which may be intrapulmonary or intracardiac in origin.
   o It is important to consider the effect of *lateral recumbency* when interpreting $PaO_2$ values.
      – $PaO_2$ values in the laterally recumbent foal may be 10–15 mmHg less than those in the standing foal.
   o $PaCO_2$ values are ~50 mmHg in the first hour of life and decrease thereafter.

## III   Cardiovascular system of the foal (see Table 31.1)

- The cardiac index (CO/kg; ml/kg/min) of the neonatal foal is greater than the adult, and this can be attributed to the relative higher metabolic rate in the neonate, which is fulfilled with a faster heart rate.
- The stroke volume index (ml/kg/heartbeat) is similar to the adult; but cardiac index is higher because of a higher heart rate.
- Mean arterial blood pressure (MAP) is lower in the neonate than in the adult horse, but increases as the sympathetic nervous system and baroreceptors mature (see Table 31.1)
- Systemic vascular resistance (SVR = MAP/CO) is higher in the foal than the adult horse, but when expressed as an index (SVRI = MAP/CI) it is actually lower in the foal than the adult horse, because the MAP is lower and the cardiac index is higher in foals. Foals do not tolerate increases in vascular resistance because it is already high and the contractile force

Table 31.1   Cardiovascular variables in foals of different ages and in the adult horse.

| Age | 2 h | 24 h | 6 d | 14 d | Adult |
|---|---|---|---|---|---|
| Heart rate (beats/min) | 83 | 84 | 104 | 95 | 36 |
| Mean arterial pressure (mmHg) | 95 | 84 | 97 | 100 | 123 |
| Cardiac index (ml/kg/min) | 155 | 197 | 214 | 222 | 70 |
| Cardiac output (l/min) | 7 | 8.9 | 12.4 | 15.8 | 32.9 |
| Stroke volume (ml/beat) | 86 | 106 | 126 | 161 | 900 |
| Stroke volume index (ml/beat/kg) | 1.9 | 2.4 | 2.2 | 2.3 | 1.9 |
| Systemic vascular resistance (dynes·s cm$^{-5}$) | 1086 | 755 | 626 | 506 | 299 |
| Systemic vascular resistance index (dynes·s cm$^{-5}$/kg) | 49 | 34 | 36 | 36 | 141 |
| Body weight (kg) | 45 | 45 | 57 | 71 | 470 |

Data in Table 31.1 were based on information in the following publications.
Hollis AR, Ousey JC, Palmer L et al. (2008) Effects of norepinephrine and combined norepinephrine and fenoldopam infusion on systemic hemodynamics and indices of renal function in normotensive neonatal foals. J Vet Intern Med 22, 1210–1215.
Lombard CW, Evans M, Martin L, Tehrani J (1984) Blood pressure, electrocardiogram and echocardiogram measurements in the growing pony foal. Equine Vet J 16, 342–347.
Solano AM, Valverde A, Desrochers A (2009) Behavioural and cardiorespiratory effects of a constant rate infusion of medetomidine and morphine for sedation during standing laparoscopy in horses. Equine Vet J 41, 153–159.
Tapio H, Raekallio MR, Mykkänen A et al. (2019) Effects of vatinoxan on cardiorespiratory function and gastrointestinal motility during constant-rate medetomidine infusion in standing horses. Equine Vet J 51, 646–652.
Thomas WP, Madigan JE, Backus KQ, Powell WE (1987) Systemic and pulmonary haemodynamics in normal neonatal foals. J Reprod Fertil Suppl 35, 623–628.

of the heart is still maturing, and the heart cannot cope with significant increases in vascular resistance. As a result, an increase in SVR decreases cardiac output significantly in foals.

## IV  Thermoregulation

- In utero, the fetus does not expend energy in maintaining its body temperature as the core temperature of the fetus is equal to or slightly above that of the mother.
- *Glucose* from the dam crosses the placenta and is normally adequate for fetal growth and glycogen storage.

### A  Heat production

- To maintain body temperature, the foal must be able to produce heat.
- Heat production requires *oxygen* and *glucose*. Hypothermia may result in:
  – Hypoglycemia.
  – Metabolic acidosis.
  – Decreased production of surfactant.
- Glycogen is mobilized after birth by *catecholamines*. However, glycogen reserves are depleted soon after birth in the foal, and hypoglycemia will develop if the foal does not ingest colostrum.
- Heat production can be achieved by:
  – Increased voluntary muscle activity (however, this will be inadequate in a sick foal or during anesthesia).
  – Increased involuntary muscle activity (generation of heat through increased muscle tone, shivering).
  – Non-shivering thermogenesis (*brown fat*) is vital to neonates of most species; however, foals have minimal or no *brown fat* deposits.

### B  Heat loss is exacerbated by:

- The foal's small body mass.
- High surface area to body mass ratio.
- Low body fat content.

### C  Neutral thermal environment

- It is the range of ambient temperatures within which body temperature can be maintained at minimum oxygen expenditure.
  – These temperatures are higher in the foal than in the adult, and the neutral thermal environment is narrow for neonates.
- Foals are especially prone to heat imbalances.

### D  Effects of anesthesia on heat balance

- Heat transfer from core to periphery is facilitated by:
  – Decreased vasomotor tone resulting in vasodilation.
  – Increased skin blood flow.
  – Impairment of central control mechanisms.
- Vasoconstriction is not triggered until core temperature is low.

E  Effects of hypothermia on anesthesia

      ○ Decreased minimum alveolar concentration (MAC).
        – Approximately 5% decrease in MAC per °C decrease in temperature.
      ○ Decreased tissue perfusion resulting in delayed drug elimination.
      ○ Decreased drug metabolism.
      ○ Increased bleeding (decreased clotting function).
      ○ Delayed recovery.
      ○ Increased oxygen consumption (e.g. from shivering in recovery).

# V  Drug metabolism and excretion

- Metabolic function develops in utero.
  - ○ Even though the placenta is primarily responsible for metabolic homeostasis, the fetal kidney has a role in regulating amniotic fluid volume.
- Metabolic pathways are not fully developed at birth in the foal, but they mature rapidly in the first few weeks of life.
- In comparison to other species, it appears that the mechanisms responsible for drug metabolism and excretion are well developed in the neonatal foal.
- However, differences in the pharmacokinetics of many drugs have been demonstrated as foals mature from the neonatal stage up to 1-month of age.
  - ○ For example, the ability of the liver to metabolize *diazepam* by oxidative pathways was low in foals at 4 days of age but was fully mature by 21 days.
- Dissimilarities in drug disposition can be attributed to differences in total body water (TBW), and hepatic and renal function. The TBW in foals is approximately 72–74% of body mass (kg), which is greater than the adult TBW of approximately 62%.
- Extracellular fluid (ECF) comprises 35–40% of body mass (kg) in foals up to one month of age, in comparison to a reported value of 25% in adult horses. This increase in ECF will result in differences in drug uptake and distribution, and changes in effect-site concentrations of drugs in comparison to the adult horse.
- Regardless of differences in hepatic function between the foal and adult, the clinical impression is that foals generally recovery quickly from anesthesia if attention is given to maintaining body temperature and avoiding the use of long-acting drugs.
- *Renal* function is relatively mature in the neonatal foal. However, the urine-specific gravity is low and the urine output per kg is higher than in the adult in the first few months of life.
  - ○ The foal kidney has adequate ability to manage sodium and water loads indicating a good ability to excrete drugs.

A  Injectable drugs

*Neonatal foals*

      ○ May require lower doses of injectable anesthetic agents than adults.
      ○ This may be due to:
        – A greater proportion of cardiac output going to the *vessel rich group* (heart and brain).
        – An immature central nervous system (CNS).
        – Increased sensitivity of receptors.
        – A more permeable blood-brain barrier.
        – Decreased plasma protein binding.

- However, the effects of the aforementioned factors may be offset by an increased in TBW and ECF.

*Older foals*

- ○ Older foals generally require higher doses per kg of injectable induction drugs than adults or neonates.
  - This may partly be a result of their excitable nature and an increased ECF volume compared to adults.

## B Inhalational anesthetics

- ○ Based on data from human beings and some other species, neonatal foals would be expected to have a lower MAC for inhalational anesthetics, but this has not been studied extensively. However, in one study, the MAC of isoflurane in foals was approximately 36% less in foals than in adult horses.
- ○ Proposed reasons for a reduced MAC in the neonate include:
  - Immature CNS.
  - Decreased pain sensitivity.
  - Increase in circulating *progesterone* concentrations.
  - Increased *endorphin* concentrations.

# VI  Sedation and general anesthesia

## A  Preoperative evaluation

- ○ It is especially important in the neonatal foal to determine if there are congenital cardiac defects which may increase the anesthetic risk.
- ○ Determination of *colostrum* intake is important, and a plasma transfusion should be considered if the IgG concentration is low (<800 mg/dl).
- ○ Blood *glucose* should be evaluated, as hypoglycemia can develop if the foal is not nursing or is bacteremic.

## B  Fasting

- ○ In general, the *neonatal foal* should be allowed to suck up to the time of anesthesia induction; however, if the foal is being tube fed, it may be necessary to withhold milk for a few hours as sick foals may have delayed gastric emptying.
- ○ *Older foals*, on solid food, may have food withheld from two to four hours.
  - However, it is uncertain if this is necessary.

## C  Sedation

*Neonates*

- ○ Neonatal foals usually become recumbent when sedated, and some may already be recumbent.
- ○ To prevent *hypothermia* and *hypoglycemia*, avoid keeping the neonatal foal sedated for long periods, and choose a technique that will allow a fast return to normal activity.
  - It is prudent to provide a heat source for neonates.
- ○ It is also advisable to provide $O_2$ via a mask or via nasal insufflation while the neonatal foal is sedated.

*Older foals*

- ○ Foals, one month or older, are generally treated as adults in regard to drug selection and dosage.
  - – In many cases, weanling foals may require higher doses than adults to achieve the same degree of sedation.

*Benzodiazepines*

> *Benzodiazepines are good choices for sedation of neonatal and sick foals*

- ○ In contrast to adult horses, benzodiazepines produce sedation in neonatal foals.
- ○ Sedation with a benzodiazepine is generally suitable for facilitating non-painful procedures such as imaging, a cast change, or arthrocentesis, or joint lavage in association with local anesthesia.
- ○ *Diazepam/midazolam* (0.05–0.1 mg/kg, IV) are the benzodiazepines most commonly used for sedation of *neonatal* foals.
  - – Because ataxia and sedation will develop after drug administration, the standing foal must be supported and helped into recumbency.
  - – Large doses or repeated dosing will produce prolonged ataxia.
- ○ A benzodiazepine may be combined with an opioid to cause more profound sedation and provide analgesia.

> e.g. Opioid/Benzodiazepine combinations for sedation of neonatal foal
> *Midazolam* (0.1 mg/kg, IV) + *Butorphanol* (0.1 mg/kg, IV).
> *Midazolam* (0.1 mg/kg, IV) + *Morphine* (0.05 mg/kg, IV).

- ○ The sedative effects of benzodiazepines can be reversed with *flumazenil.*
  - – However, this is rarely necessary.

*Opioids*

- ○ *Butorphanol* (0.05–0.1 mg/kg, IV, IM) is the most commonly used opioid in *neonatal* foals. However, *morphine* (0.05–0.1 mg/kg, IV), *methadone* (0.05 mg/kg, IV) or *hydromorphone* (0.02–0.04 mg/kg, IV) may also be used to provide sedation and provide analgesia, or can be used in conjunction with a *benzodiazepine* or an $\alpha_2$ *agonist* to provide a more profound effect.
- ○ *Neonates*, in contrast to adult horses, become sedated with *butorphanol* when it is administered alone, and do not exhibit the *behavioral* effects displayed by adults when administered butorphanol.
- ○ In one study, a *butorphanol* dose of 0.1 mg/kg, IV was necessary to provide analgesia in foals when using a thermal nociceptive model.

*$\alpha_2$ agonists*

- ○ Generally, it is not necessary to use $\alpha_2$ agonists in neonates as they sedate well with benzodiazepines ± an opioid.
- ○ However, a low dose of *xylazine* may be indicated to supplement sedation in a larger more vigorous younger foal.
  - – Nevertheless, $\alpha_2$ agonists should be used with caution (i.e. *low doses, administered to effect)* in the very young.
- ○ Avoid use of $\alpha_2$ agonists in the sick neonatal foal.

> *Benzodiazepines alone are **not** a good choice for sedation of an older robust healthy foal*

- *Older, healthy* foals may be sedated with an $\alpha_2$ agonist, as follows, with the higher end of the dose range being used for older and stronger foals.
  - *Xylazine*: (0.3–1.2 mg/kg, IV).
  - *Detomidine*: (0.005–0.01 mg/kg, IV).
  - *Medetomidine*: (0.0035–0.005 mg/kg, IV).
  - *Dexmedetomidine*: (0.002–0.005 mg/kg, IV).
  - *Romifidine*: (0.03–0.1 mg/kg, IV).
- $\alpha_2$ agonists may be combined with an opioid for more profound sedation and analgesia.

> e.g. $\alpha_2$/Opioid combinations for sedation of older, healthy foals
> *Xylazine* (0.5–1.0 mg/kg, IV) + *Butorphanol* (0.05–0.1 mg/kg, IV)
> *Xylazine* (0.5–1.0 mg/kg, IV) + *Morphine* (0.05–0.1 mg/kg, IV)

*$\alpha_2$ antagonists*
- $\alpha_2$ antagonists (yohimbine, tolazoline, atipamezole) can be used to reverse the sedative effects of $\alpha_2$ agonist.
- However, their use is rarely indicated.

*Caution: $\alpha_2$ antagonist administration has been associated with life-threatening hypotension, especially if administered intravenously as a bolus.*

D   Induction of anesthesia with intravenous drug(s)

- The choice of drug(s) is generally based on the experience and personal preference of the anesthetist.
- Induction occurs once the foal is appropriately sedated, as described above.

*Ketamine (2–3 mg/kg, IV)*
- Ketamine, usually with a co-induction drug (e.g., *midazolam, propofol*), is commonly used for induction of anesthesia.
- A co-induction drug may not be necessary if the foal was sedated with a benzodiazepine.

*Propofol* (2–4 mg/kg, IV) or *alfaxalone* (1–3 mg/kg, IV)
- May be used *alone* for induction, but they lack analgesic properties, and may be more likely than *ketamine* to induce apnea.
- The induction dose of these drugs will depend on the degree of sedation and the speed of administration.
- Regardless of drug choice, it is advisable to administer the drug *slowly*.
  - This will prevent overdosing (which may result in apnea).
  - Slow administration will allow the opportunity for $O_2$ to be provided, via a mask, during the induction process.

*Example induction protocols for neonatal foal*
- *Midazolam/diazepam* (0.05–0.1 mg/kg, IV) ± *Butorphanol* (0.05–0.1 mg/kg, IV) for sedation.
- *Ketamine* (1–2 mg/kg, IV) administered slowly to effect for induction.

Or

*Propofol* (1–3 mg/kg, IV) administered slowly to effect.
- Induction dose depends on the degree of sedation and speed of administration.
- Propofol is more likely to induce *apnea* than *ketamine*.

### Induction protocol for older, healthy foal

*Example 1*
- *Xylazine* (0.5–1.2 mg/kg, IV) ± *Butorphanol* (0.05–0.1 mg/kg, IV) for sedation.
  - The dose of *xylazine* will depend on the age and physical status of the foal.
- *Ketamine* (2.0–3.0 mg/kg, IV) + *Midazolam* (0.05–0.1 mg/kg, IV).
  - These drugs can be combined for administration.
  - The dose of *ketamine* will depend on physical status, temperament, and age of foal.

### Induction protocol for older foal

*Example 2 (Combining drugs)*
- *Xylazine* (1 mg/kg), *midazolam* (0.05 mg/kg), and *ketamine* (2 mg/kg) can be combined in the same syringe and administered slowly IV for induction.
- This protocol results in a smooth induction, and the authors have used this protocol in horses up to 300 kg.

E  **Induction of anesthesia with an inhalational anesthetic**

- This method has been recommended for foals, especially for *neonates*.

> *Sevoflurane* is less irritating to mucous membranes than is *isoflurane*

- Induction can be achieved following minimal or no sedation.
- The anesthetic can be delivered via a circle system using either a facemask or following nasotracheal intubation.
- While this method of induction is often advocated for sick foals, it must be understood that inhalational anesthetics have, in general, a lower therapeutic index than injectable agents.
- Inhalational anesthetic induction has been associated with an *increase in mortality*.
  - This higher mortality rate may be a consequence of the relatively rapid uptake of volatile agents in neonates.
- In *contrast*, not all studies support those findings, and the difference in outcome may be associated with the experience and skill of the personnel.
- Nevertheless, it is important to understand that volatile anesthetics have a rapid uptake in neonates; thus, they should be administered cautiously for induction.

### Reasons for rapid uptake of volatile anesthetics in neonate
- High alveolar ventilation (l/min) relative to FRC.
- Lower anesthetic solubility in blood.
  - Due to differences in plasma constituents (e.g. albumin, triglycerides).
- Lower anesthetic solubility in tissues.
  - Due to a higher water content and decreased protein and lipid concentration.
- The cardiac output is preferentially distributed to the *vessel rich group* (e.g., brain/heart).

**F Maintenance of anesthesia**

- As in the case of induction agents, the choice of maintenance drugs is often based on operator experience and personal preference.
- The merits of maintenance with inhalational anesthetics, total intravenous anesthesia (TIVA), and partial intravenous anesthesia (PIVA) are discussed in Chapter 21.

*Volatile anesthetics*

- Volatile anesthesia is the most common method of anesthesia maintenance in neonatal foals. The popularity of volatile anesthesia is probably due to the familiarity of clinicians and technicians with this method, but also because of the widely held belief that neonatal foals are going to have a delayed recovery due to inadequate metabolism and clearance of injectable anesthetics.
- The disadvantages of using a volatile anesthetic include:
  - No *antinociceptive* effect.
  - No blunting of the *stress response* to surgery except at very high doses.
  - More likely to be associated with *hypotension* than TIVA or PIVA.

*Partial intravenous anesthesia (PIVA)*

- This method in which injectable anesthetics are combined with volatile anesthetics has become more popular in equine anesthesia. It has advantages over volatile anesthesia in that it provides *antinociception*, *decreases the MAC* of the volatile agent and thereby lessens the incidence of *hypotension*, and may blunt the *stress response* to surgery, depending on the choice of drugs.

*Neonatal foal – Example PIVA protocol*

- *Lidocaine* combined with *ketamine,* in association with *isoflurane* or *sevoflurane,* for maintenance of anesthesia.
- *Lidocaine:*
  - A loading dose of 3 mg/kg/15 min. The loading dose is administered slowly because it is a relatively big dose.
  - A CRI of 100 µg/kg/min for the first hour, decreasing to 70 µg/kg/min thereafter.
- *Ketamine:*
  - A CRI of 20–30 µg/kg/min.
  - The induction dose serves as the loading dose.
- Both infusions are discontinued approximately 15 minutes prior to the end of the procedure.
- Based on the end-tidal concentration of isoflurane required, it appears that this regimen is associated with a 40–50% decrease in MAC.
- In the authors' experience, this regimen is not associated with a delayed recovery.

*Older foal - Example of PIVA protocol*

- *Lidocaine* combined with *xylazine*, and *ketamine* for infusion, in association with *isoflurane or sevoflurane.*
- *Lidocaine:*
  - A loading dose of 3 mg/kg/15 min.
  - A CRI of 100 µg/kg/min for the first hour, decreasing to 70 µg/kg/min thereafter.
  - The *lidocaine* infusion is discontinued approximately 15 minutes prior to the end of the procedure.

- ○ *Ketamine:*
  - – A CRI of 20–30 μg/kg/min.
  - – The induction dose serves as the loading dose.
- ○ *Xylazine:*
  - – A CRI of 0.5–1.0 mg/kg/h.
  - – The sedation dose serves as the loading dose.
- ○ It appears that this regimen is associated with at least a 70% decrease in MAC, based on the end-tidal concentrations of the volatile anesthetic (i.e., 0.5% isoflurane) required to prevent movement during anesthesia.

### Total intravenous anesthesia (TIVA)

- ○ TIVA is most likely to be used for relatively short procedures, and in *larger older foals* rather than in neonates.
- ○ The most commonly used regimen is a mixture of *xylazine* and *ketamine*, in *guaifenesin*. This drug mixture is colloquially referred to as *Triple Drip*.
- ○ Infusions of *propofol* or *alfaxalone* have been used for TIVA, but are less practical than *Triple Drip*, are more likely to cause hypoventilation, and they lack antinociceptive properties.

*Example 1*: 150 kg foal – *TIVA using Triple Drip* (see Box 31.1)
- ○ 60-minute procedure.

*Example 2*: 150 kg foal – *Intermittent injections*
- ○ For shorter procedures, up to 30 minutes, intermittent boluses of xylazine & ketamine can be administered approximately every 10–15 minutes after induction, at ⅓ to ½ of the initial dose of each drug.

## VII   Monitoring and patient care

### A   Positioning and padding

- ○ As with *all anesthetized patients, attention should be given to proper positioning and padding.* (see Figure 31.1)
- ○ The relatively long limbs of the foal need to be supported and bony prominences should be protected. (see Figure 31.2)

---

**Box 31.1   Example of TIVA: Foal 150 kg, Anesthesia for 60 Minutes**

- • **Sedation**: *Xylazine:* (1.3 mg/kg, IV)
- • **Induction**: *Midazolam:* (0.1 mg/kg, IV)
          *Ketamine:* (2.5 mg/kg) IV
- • **CRI** with "*Triple drip*"
- – *Xylazine:* 300 mg
- – *Ketamine:* 600 mg
- – Add to 200 ml 5% *guaifenesin*
- – Infuse at ~3 ml/minute

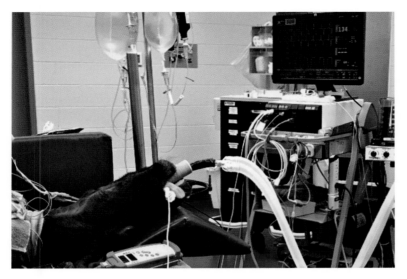

Figure 31.1   Foal anesthetized and breathing spontaneously immediately post induction. Notice that the ECG is counting double for heart rate.

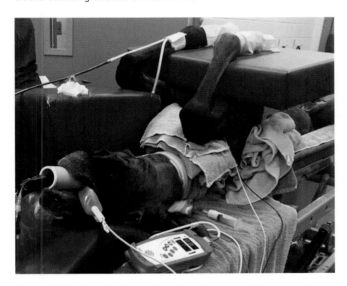

Figure 31.2   Positioning and padding to support limbs of a foal and protect bony prominences. A wedge-shaped pad is placed under the nasal bones to prevent over-extension of the neck.

B   Monitoring (see Chapter 19)

- Monitoring of vital functions during anesthesia is especially important in the neonate.
- Monitoring, ideally, should include the following:

*Depth of anesthesia*

- In addition to monitoring the various relevant reflexes, an *anesthetic agent monitor* is particularly useful as the end-tidal anesthetic concentration is an indication of the effect-site concentration of the volatile anesthetic.

*Cardiovascular system*

- o Basic cardiovascular monitoring consisting of *digital* evaluation of the arterial pulse quality and cardiac auscultation may suffice for healthy older foals undergoing short periods of sedation and light general anesthesia. However, more in-depth monitoring is warranted for longer procedures, for neonatal foals, and sick foals of all ages.
- o The *electrocardiogram* (ECG) should be displayed and *arterial blood pressure* should be measured in all but the shortest anesthetic events.
- o Blood pressure can be measured using *non-invasive* or *invasive methods*; however, the latter are more desirable and give a beat-to-beat display.
  - – Catheters are usually placed in either a *facial, transverse facial,* or *lateral metatarsal* artery, depending on the position of the foal on the surgery table and the surgical procedure.
- o It appears that the anesthetized neonatal foal can have a lower blood pressure than that which is acceptable in the adult horse and still have adequate tissue perfusion.
  - – A MAP of 50–60 mmHg appears to be acceptable in the anesthetized neonate.
  - – Cardiac output is heart rate dependent in foals; therefore, bradycardia (<50 beats/min) is generally unacceptable.
  - – However, cardiac output is rarely monitored in clinical cases.
- o *Hypotension* should be dealt with as described in Chapter 38.

*Respiratory system*

- o Basic monitoring of the respiratory system includes counting the respiratory rate and observing the respiratory rhythm.
- o Neonatal foals are prone to respiratory depression from anesthetic drugs, and there is a risk of *hypoxemia* and *hypercarbia*. In addition, respiratory depression is compounded by their *immature* lung, *decreased FRC*, and easily *fatigued* respiratory muscles.
  - – This is especially problematic if the foal is breathing room air.
- o Monitoring *hemoglobin oxygen saturation* (SpO$_2$) with a portable pulse oximeter is feasible nowadays. However, this method has its limitations, and *blood gas analysis* is a more accurate and informative method of determining the adequacy of gas exchange.
- o *Capnography*, the continuous recording of CO$_2$ in respiratory gases, is a useful, non-invasive method of monitoring alveolar ventilation. Modern units display a number (*capnometry*) depicting the partial pressure of CO$_2$ in expired gases and a waveform (*capnogram*).
- o Mechanical ventilation is commonly employed in anesthetized neonatal foals to maintain the PECO$_2$ in the normal range (35–45 mmHg).
  - – Tidal volumes are in the range 6–8 ml/kg.
  - – A respiratory rate of 12–25/minute is usually employed.
  - – The airway pressure should not exceed 12 cm H$_2$O.

*Body temperature*

- o Foals are likely to develop *hypothermia* for the reasons previously described. Thus, body temperature should be monitored.
- o Most multipurpose monitors have electronic temperature probes that give a continuous display of temperature.
  - – The probe is most commonly inserted into the esophagus via the ventral meatus.
- o Heat losses should be minimized, and *active warming* applied, as necessary.

*Blood glucose*

- o Hypoglycemia in neonatal foals at presentation is associated with sepsis, systemic inflammatory response syndrome (SIRS), and a poor prognosis.
- o *Glycogen* stores become depleted soon after birth in the foal.
- o Blood glucose should be recorded at baseline and regularly during long procedures, especially, if it is trending downwards.
- o Routine administration of *dextrose*, in the absence of monitoring, may cause hyperglycemia. This may result in hyperinsulinemia and re-bound hypoglycemia if the foal does not have an energy source (e.g. milk or further IV dextrose) soon after recovery.
- o Sick foals on total parenteral nutrition (TPN) should have their blood glucose closely monitored if the TPN is discontinued in the peri-operative period.

## VIII  Recoveries

- Foals should be placed on a pad of suitable thickness, and the pad should be covered with absorbent material to help keep the foal dry.
- Foals should be kept warm in recovery, and excess moisture on the foal's coat should be removed (e.g. with a hair dryer).
- A forced warm-air blanket will help to restore/maintain body heat.
- The foal should remain intubated, and have supplemental oxygen until it is ready to be extubated.
  - o A portable $SpO_2$ monitor applied to the tongue can be used to monitor hemoglobin saturation with oxygen.
- Hand assisted recovery is recommended for foals. (see Figure 31.3)

## IX  Managing the mare at induction and recovery

- Most mares will become distressed if separated from their foal, especially a neonatal foal. How the mare is managed will depend on her temperament and the age and health of the foal.
- In most cases, the mare is sedated if she is to be separated from the foal, and the choice of drugs will depend on the expected duration of separation and the temperament of the mare.

*Examples of sedation regimens for the mare*

- *Acepromazine* (0.02–0.03 mg/kg, IV) + *Detomidine* (0.005–0.01 mg/kg, IV).
  - o Acepromazine is especially indicated for longer procedures.
  - o *Acepromazine* and *detomidine* can be combined in the same syringe and administered IV.
- *Xylazine* (0.2–0.5 mg/kg, IV) alone may be sufficient for short procedures.

*Induction phase*

- o If a *neonatal* foal is in the same stall as the mare or within sight of the mare, and can be easily placed on a gurney, the mare can be sedated in the stall prior to placing the foal on the gurney, and she can be left in her stall for the duration of the procedure.

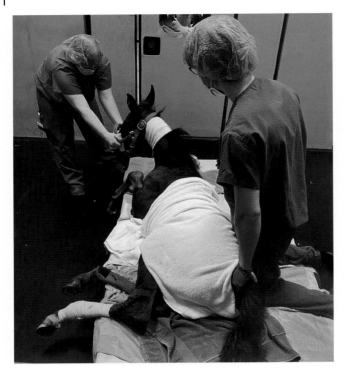

**Figure 31.3** Hand recovering a foal. One person supports the head and another holds the tail to prevent the foal lunging forward and to support the foal when standing.

- For *older* and stronger foals that are difficult to control, it is generally best to lead the mare to the induction area with the foal following along. Once the foal is induced, the mare should be sedated and lead back to the stall. (see Figure 31.4)
- The administration of the sedating drugs needs to be timed properly so that the mare does not become over sedated and has difficulty ambulating.

*Recovery phase*
- If foals are ambulatory after recovery, especially in the case of older, stronger foals, it is best to bring the mare back to the recovery area to bond with the foal.
- This must be handled carefully, as the mare will generally dash into the recovery area to meet the foal and this can pose a threat to personnel, especially if the mare is aggressive by nature.
- At this stage, most foals will want to suck the dam briefly, and the mare can then be led back to the stall with the foal following.

## X Analgesia for the neonatal foal

- Foals are neurologically mature at birth; thus, the provision of analgesia is an important component of patient care. However, identification of behaviors known to be associated with pain in adults are not well documented. Thus, procedures considered to be painful in adults should also be considered to be painful in foals, and analgesics should be administered accordingly.

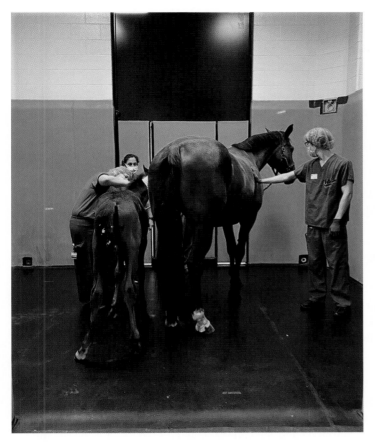

Figure 31.4   Mare and foal in induction area. The foal will be induced with the mare present and the mare will be sedated and led back to its stall once the foal is induced.

- For foals undergoing surgical procedures under general anesthesia, *balanced anesthesia* techniques should be employed, where applicable, to decrease the *stress* response to surgery and provide *analgesia* in the post-operative period.

*Examples of balanced anesthesia*
- ○ Administration of infusions or boluses of *ketamine, lidocaine,* $\alpha_2$ *agonists*, and/or *opioids* as adjuncts to inhalational anesthesia, as deemed appropriate.
- ○ Use of *local/regional* anesthesia where feasible.
- ○ Administration of an non-steroidal anti-inflammatory drugs (NSAIDs).
   - – However, NSAIDs should not be the sole agents for analgesia.
- The pharmacokinetics of some analgesic drugs, particularly NSAIDs, change as the neonatal foal gets older. Changes in kinetics arise because of differences in the volume of distribution and drug clearance.

*NSAIDs*
- ○ Doses of commonly used NSAIDs are generally higher in foals than in adults, but the dosing interval may be longer.

    ○ As in adults, the risks of toxicity (renal and gastrointestinal especially) must be considered, and the duration of treatment should be limited. Toxicity may be more likely to occur in sick foals.

*Flunixin meglumine*

    – Despite a decreased elimination of *flunixin* in neonatal foals, dosages of 1.1 mg/kg, IV q 24–36 hours seem to be safe.

    – Although licensed for IM use, its administration in this manner has been associated with *Clostridial myositis.*

*Phenylbutazone*

    – Neonates under 24 hours of age have a decreased ability to eliminate phenylbutazone.

    – A dose of 2.2 mg/kg IV or orally q12–24 hours. seems appropriate.

*Meloxicam*

    – A dose of 0.6 mg/kg, IV or orally q12–24 hours. has been recommended.

*Opioids*

    ○ *Butorphanol* is the most commonly used opioid analgesic in horses.

    ○ Foals, unlike adult horses, do *not* exhibit behavior effects when administered *butorphanol*, and neonatal foals become sedate.

    ○ For the purpose of analgesia, foals seem to need higher doses of *butorphanol* than do adults.

        – In foals aged from 1 to 8 weeks, a *butorphanol* dose of 0.1 mg/kg, IV provided 150 minutes of analgesia in a thermal model of nociception. A dose of 0.05 mg/kg, IV was *not* associated with analgesia.

    ○ The pure mu agonists, *morphine* and *methadone*, may be used at adult doses; thus, it would seem reasonable to assume that *hydromorphone* can also be used in foals at adult doses. However, PK/PD data on these drugs are limited in foals.

        – *Morphine* (0.05–0.1 mg/kg, IV, IM).

            ■ Intraarticularly administered *morphine* (0.05 mg/kg) has been recommended for treating foals with septic arthritis undergoing joint lavage.

        – *Methadone* (0.05–0.1 mg/kg, IV, IM).

        – *Hydromorphone* (0.02–0.04 mg/kg, IV, IM).

    ○ *Buprenorphine* (0.01 mg/kg, IM) significantly increased the nociceptive withdrawal reflex in 2-day old foals, but not in 11-day old foals.

        – It is of interest that these foals displayed typical opioid-induced *behavioral* changes, including increased locomotor activity.

## XI   Anesthesia for foals with uroabdomen

● Rupture of the urinary bladder is a condition that requires prompt surgical attention, and affected foals often have significant cardiovascular and metabolic derangements.

● This condition was originally thought to occur mainly in colt foals, and was considered to be due to the increase intraabdominal pressure when the foal was passing through the pelvic canal. However, recent studies indicate that this assumption may not be entirely true.

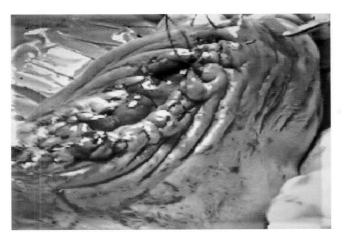

Figure 31.5   Repair of a tear in urinary bladder.

- Many foals that develop uroperitoneum have comorbidities, and urinary tract infections and sepsis is associated with uroabdomen in foals of both sexes.
- It is postulated that urinary tract infections and sepsis result in ischemia of the urinary bladder and ultimately to urinary leakage into the abdomen (see Figure 31.5).

## A   Clinical presentation

- There is a large range of ages at diagnosis. A recent study reported that the age at presentation ranged from 0 to 42 days, with a mean age of 6.2 days.
- Many foals with uroabdomen will already be hospitalized for treatment of infection and sepsis; hence the speculation that a focal infection and ischemia may be the cause of the uroabdomen.

### Clinical signs

- Clinical signs will depend on whether comorbidities are present and include:
  - Depression and loss of interest in sucking.
  - Dehydration.
  - Straining to pass urine.
    - The volume of urine passed will depend on the size of the defect in the bladder and its anatomical location.
  - Abdominal distension.
    - Occurs over time and causes pain and compromise of lung function.
  - The severities of clinical and metabolic changes are dependent on the age of the foal and whether any urine can be voided.

## B   Metabolic changes

- Electrolyte abnormalities are the most common abnormality.
- The main changes are a decrease in plasma $[Na^+]$ and $[Cl^-]$ and an increase in $[K^+]$.
- However, foals hospitalized and receiving IV fluids are less likely to have electrolyte abnormalities than foals presented specifically for uroabdomen.

*Hyponatremia ([Na$^+$] < 125 mEq/l)*

- Is the result of an increase in ECF volume due to abdominal distention with urine.
- Results in depression, muscle weakness and anorexia.
- Central nervous system changes are uncommon, probably because the change in plasma [Na$^+$] occurs slowly.

*Hyperkalemia ([K$^+$] > 5.5 mEq/l)*

- The accumulation of urine with a high [K$^+$] in the abdominal cavity results in the re-absorption of potassium into the systemic circulation resulting in *hyperkalemia*.
- The myocardial resting membrane potential is increased (less negative) which results in an increase in cell membrane excitability.
- Signs of hyperkalemia are [K$^+$] dependent, and mainly involve the cardiovascular and neuromuscular (muscle weakness) systems.
- ECG changes include:
  - Arrhythmias (e.g. heart block).
  - Tall T waves (occur at plasma [K$^+$] ≥ 5.5 mEq/l).
  - Widened QRS (usually indicates that plasma [K$^+$] ≥ 6.5 mEq/l).
  - Atrial asystole (no P wave indicates that plasma [K$^+$] ≥ 6.5 mEq/l).
  - Prolonged P-R interval (indicates that plasma [K$^+$] ≥ 6.5 mEq/l).

## C  Preoperative treatment

- Although it is important to decrease the plasma [K$^+$] it must be remembered that many foals with uroabdomen have co-morbidities that must also be managed.
- The plasma [K$^+$] should be decreased to less than <6 mEq/l and cardiovascular function should be optimized before proceeding with anesthesia.
- Although it is technically possible to drain the abdomen of urine, it is very time consuming and is poorly tolerated by the foal.
- Administration of large volumes of isotonic IV fluids will further dilute the plasma Na$^+$ and distend the abdomen.
- IV *potassium penicillin* may increase [K$^+$] and should be used with caution.

*Plasma volume expansion*

- 7.2% hypertonic saline (5 ml/kg) will increase intravascular volume and increase plasma [Na$^+$] by approximately 8 mEq/l.
  - The aim is to increase the [Na$^+$] to the value at which neurological signs are allayed rather than return the [Na$^+$] to normal.
  - Also, increasing plasma [Na$^+$] may counteract the effects on hyperkalemia on cardiac arrhythmias as has been demonstrated experimentally in dogs.
- Potassium-free replacement fluids (e.g. 0.9% NaCl) are recommended during anesthesia.

*Reduce plasma [K$^+$]*

- Expand intravascular volume (e.g. with hypertonic saline, isotonic saline solution).
- Transfer potassium into cells:
- *Dextrose*
  - A dextrose infusion will increase endogenous insulin release; however, the onset of its effect is slow, and it is *not reliable* in reducing plasma [K$^+$].

○ *Insulin*
  – Regular insulin (0.1–0.2 IU/kg, IV) in 5% *dextrose* (3–5 ml/kg).
  – Should reduce the plasma $[K^+]$ to <5.5 mEq/l by the end of the 30-minute infusion.

○ *$\beta_2$ agonists* (e.g. albuterol)
  – Administration results in *adenylate cyclase* activation which stimulates the production of cyclic adenosine monophosphate, and this is used by the $Na^+$-$K^+$ ATPase pump to transfer $K^+$ intracellularly.
  – It can be administered (10–20 mg) IV over 15 minutes.
  – The maximum effect on plasma $[K^+]$ occurs between 30 and 60 minutes.
  – Not commonly administered due to slow onset of effect compared with insulin/dextrose.

○ *Correct metabolic acidosis*
  – A decrease in pH causes an increase in plasma $[K^+]$.
  – However, significant metabolic acidosis is not a common finding.

○ *Sodium bicarbonate*
  – $NaHCO_3$ may *not* be effective in lowering plasma $[K^+]$ in foals that are not acidemic.
  – Administration of $NaHCO_3$ does *not* appear to protect against hyperkalemia-induced arrhythmias. There appears to be minimal benefit to alkaline therapy for emergency cases of hyperkalemia. Any benefit to $NaHCO_3$ treatment in hyperkalemia may be due to *sodium loading*.
  – $NaHCO_3$ administration may also result in a reduction in plasma *ionized calcium* which would be especially detrimental in this situation.
  – Thus, $NaHCO_3$ therapy in hyperkalemic patients should be reserved for the treatment of those with severe metabolic acidosis.

*Reverse membrane effects of hyperkalemia*
  ○ To reduce the arrhythmogenic effects of hyperkalemia, the following are recommended:
    – *Beta$_1$ agonists* (e.g. *dobutamine*) may be efficacious in heart block. In the authors' experience, dobutamine administration acts relatively rapid in restoring sinus rhythm in hyperkalemia foals. However, the effect is short lived, and a CRI may be necessary; thus, its use is intended for emergency situations.
    – *Calcium chloride* (1 ml/10 kg of a 10% solution) or *calcium borogluconate* (0.25–0.5 ml/kg) can be infused slowly (15–30 minutes).
    – *Hypertonic saline* – Increasing plasma $[Na^+]$ with hypertonic saline is reported to have a protective effect against hyperkalemia-induced arrhythmias, as mentioned above.

D **Anesthesia** (see sections E and F)

  ○ Electrolyte imbalances and fluid deficits should be corrected to *safe* values prior to anesthesia.
  ○ Drugs likely to cause *bradycardia* (e.g. $\alpha_2$ agonists) are best avoided, unless the foal is older and healthy and has no electrolyte imbalances.

*Sedation*
  ○ If considered necessary for the neonatal foal, a *benzodiazepine* $\pm$ *butorphanol* can be administered.
    – For example, *Midazolam* (0.05–0.1 mg/kg, IV) $\pm$ *Butorphanol* (0.05–0.1 mg/kg, IV)

*Induction*

- ○ The dose of all injectable induction drugs will depend on the foal's physical status and whether it is sedated.
  - – Induction drugs should be administered *slowly* to effect.

  e.g., *Ketamine* (1.0–2.0 mg/kg) + *Midazolam* (0.05–0.1 mg/kg – *if not already sedated*).

  e.g., *Propofol* (2–3 mg/kg) or *Alfaxalone* (1–2 mg/kg, IV), alone or in combination with *ketamine*, are injectable options for induction.

  e.g., *Mask induction*
  - – Some clinicians prefer to induce neonatal foals with a volatile anesthetic.
  - – *Sevoflurane* is less irritating than *isoflurane* to mucous membranes.
  - – The process is less stressful for the foal if it is sedated.

*Maintenance*

- ○ Anesthesia may be maintained with inhalational anesthetics.
  - – e.g. *isoflurane* or *sevoflurane*.
- ○ To reduce the chances of arrhythmias occurring, a lower concentration of inhalational anesthetics can be delivered.
  - – An infusion of *ketamine* (3 mg/kg/h) should reduce MAC by at least 20% and supply analgesia.
- ○ Ventilation should be controlled, as hypoventilation is likely to occur due to the effects of anesthetic drugs and the increased intra-abdominal pressure.
  - – Additionally, decreasing the $PaCO_2$ by 10 mmHg decreases the plasma $[K^+]$ by 0.5 mEq/l.

E   Monitoring

- ○ In addition to routine monitoring, plasma *glucose* and electrolytes should be checked periodically.

  *Note: It is important that the abdomen be slowly drained of urine to avoid inducing hypotension.* (see Figure 31.6)

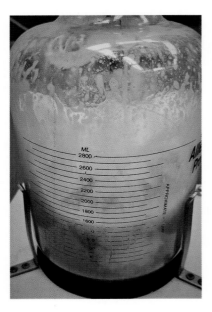

**Figure 31.6**   Urine in suction jar after removal from abdomen. It is important to drain the urine slowly from the abdomen to decrease the likelihood of inducing arterial hypotension.

## F   Analgesia

○ Analgesics should be administered as previously described.

## Suggested Reading

Arguedas, M.G., Hines, M.T., Papich, M.G. et al. (2008). Pharmacokinetics of butorphanol and evaluation of physiologic and behavioral effects after intravenous and intramuscular administration to neonatal foals. *J. Vet. Intern. Med.* 22: 1417–1426.

Baggot, J.D. and Short, C.R. (1984). Drug disposition in the neonatal animal, with particular reference to the foal. *Equine. Vet. J.* 16: 364–367.e

Carrick, J.B., Papich, M.G., Middleton, D.M. et al. (1989). Clinical and pathological effects of flunixin meglumine administration to neonatal foals. *Can. J. Vet. Res.* 53: 195–201.

Crisman, M.V., Wilcke, J.R., and Sams, R.A. (1996). Pharmacokinetics of flunixin meglumine in healthy foals less than twenty-four hours old. *Am. J. Vet. Res.* 57: 1759–1761.

Driessen, B. (2019). Anesthesia and analgesia for foals. In: *Equine Surgery*, 5e (eds. J.A. Auer, J.A. Stick, J.M. Kümmerlee and T. Prange), 313–330. Elsevier.

Dunkel, B., Palmer, J.E., Olson, K.N. et al. (2005). Uroperitoneum in 32 foals: influence of intravenous fluid therapy, infection, and sepsis. *J. Vet. Intern. Med.* 9: 889–893.

Goodwin, W., Keates, H., Pasloske, K. et al. (2012). Plasma pharmacokinetics and pharmacodynamics of alfaxalone in neonatal foals after an intravenous bolus of alfaxalone following premedication with butorphanol tartrate. *Vet. Anaesth. Analg.* 39: 503–510.

Kaplan, J.I., Eynon, A., Dalsey, W.C. et al. (2000). Hypertonic saline treatment of severe hyperkalemia in nonnephrectomized dogs. *Acad. Emerg. Med.* 7: 965–973.

Lombard, C.W., Evans, M., Martin, L. et al. (1984). Blood pressure, electrocardiogram and echocardiogram measurements in the growing pony foal. *Equine. Vet. J.* 16: 342–347.

McGowan, K.T., Elfenbein, J.R., Robertson, S.A. et al. (2013). Effect of butorphanol on thermal nociceptive threshold in healthy pony foals. *Equine. Vet. J.* 45: 503–506.

Ragno, V., Driessen, B., Bertolotti, L. et al. (2013). Perianesthetic morbidity and mortality in the equine: a retrospective study. *Vet. Surg.* 42: E68.

Robertson, S.A., Carter, S.W., Donovan, M. et al. (1990). Effects of intravenous xylazine hydrochloride on blood glucose, plasma insulin and rectal temperature in neonatal foals. *Equine. Vet. J.* 22: 43–47.

Spensley, M.S., Carlson, G.P., and Harrold, D. (1987). Plasma, red blood cell, total blood, and extracellular fluid volumes in healthy horse foals during growth. *Am. J. Vet. Res.* 48: 1703–1707.

Steffey, E.P., Willits, N., Wong, P. et al. (1991). Clinical investigations of halothane and isoflurane for induction and maintenance of foal anesthesia. *J. Vet. Pharmacol. Ther.* 14: 300–309.

Wilcke, J.R., Crisman, M.V., Sams, R.A., and Gerken, D.F. (1993). Pharmacokinetics of phenylbutazone in neonatal foals. *Am. J. Vet. Res.* 54: 2064–2067.

## 32

# Anesthesia of Horses with Intestinal Emergencies (Colic)
*Tom Doherty*

- The overall risk of mortality in anesthesia of intestinal colic cases is about 10 times that of elective cases.
  - The increased risk is due to a number of factors. Cardiovascular compromise, endotoxemia, and accidents during recovery are important contributors.
  - Factors for the owner to consider when deciding on abdominal surgery include the horse's health status, its prognosis for an athletic career, and the cost of surgery and postoperative care.
- Horses anesthetized for abdominal problems vary greatly in physiological status.
  - Those with chronic intermittent colic are usually physiologically stable, as are horses in the early stages of a large colon displacement.
  - Horses with advanced small intestinal obstruction and those with large colon torsion can be in extremis at presentation.

## I  Preoperative evaluation

- Horses may be in a state of cardiovascular compromise due to a shift of fluids and electrolytes into the distended intestine, which over time causes a decrease in fluid content in all body compartments (i.e. intracellular and extracellular) and dehydration.
  - This results in a decrease in intravascular volume resulting in reduced preload and cardiac output.
  - Hemoconcentration increases blood viscosity, which increases the resistance to blood flow and the work of the heart, and impairs organ perfusion.
- Change in cardiovascular function is reflected in high heart rates, weak peripheral pulses, increased capillary refill times, and pale or cyanotic mucous membranes.
- Pain, resulting from intestinal distension and stretching of mesentery, may make the horse uncontrollable without sedation and analgesia.
- Abdominal distension (e.g. from large bowel torsion) can also compromise respiratory and cardiovascular function.

*Manual of Equine Anesthesia and Analgesia*, Second Edition. Edited by Tom Doherty, Alex Valverde, and Rachel A. Reed.
© 2022 John Wiley & Sons, Inc. Published 2022 by John Wiley & Sons, Inc.

- Gastric distension, if unrelieved may result in:
  - Aspiration of gastric contents subsequent to reflux into the pharynx.
  - Gastric rupture.
- Passage of a *nasogastric tube* is part of the initial evaluation process, and the tube is usually kept in place during anesthesia.


## II   Preparation for anesthesia

- Once the decision to perform surgery is reached, the horse usually needs to be treated rapidly, and this generally includes:


### A   Fluid therapy

- In most cases the intravascular volume will be reduced significantly.
- To facilitate rapid administration of fluids it may be necessary to place two large bore jugular catheters.

*Isotonic fluids (e.g. lactated Ringer's)*
- Large volumes (40–60 ml/kg) are needed (i.e. 20–30 l for a dehydrated 500 kg horse).
  - This takes a relatively long time to administer.
  - Large volumes contribute to interstitial edema.
- Isotonic fluids do not remain in the circulation long, especially in shock states.

*Hypertonic saline*
- Is an effective alternative to isotonic fluids.
- Solutions of ~5–7% NaCl appear to be most efficacious and practical.
- Small volumes are effective (e.g. 4–6 ml/kg of 7.2% NaCl).
- It can be administered rapidly (10–15 minutes).
- The "*efficiency ratio*" is about 2, meaning that if 2 l are administered the blood volume should expand by about 4 l, and this effect should last for about 30 minutes.
- It has a positive *inotropic* action.
- It has an *anti-inflammatory* effect (e.g. via decreased prostaglandin formation).

*Synthetic colloids*
- Are solutions containing large molecules (e.g. Hetastarch) which exert an oncotic effect and thereby expand the intravascular volume.
- Relatively small volumes (5–10 ml/kg) are efficacious.
- Hetastarch has the ability to "plug" leaks in endothelium.
- Decrease formation of adhesion molecules by LPS-stimulated endothelium.
- Longer dwell time in vascular space.
- Decrease volume of isotonic crystalloid needed for resuscitation.
  *Comment:* In an adult horse (500 kg), hypertonic saline (~7%) is the most practical treatment. A volume of 2–3 l (4–6 ml/kg) is sufficient and causes significant improvement in cardiac output. For a more prolonged effect, hypertonic saline can be combined with a colloid (5–10 ml/kg), colloquially referred to as "*turbostarch*."

*Acid-base correction*
- ○ Is generally unnecessary, as few of these cases have significant metabolic acidosis.

## B Sedation and analgesia

- ○ May be necessary in order to control a painful horse during the evaluation process.

*α₂ agonists*
- ○ Provide sedation and analgesia.
- ○ Low doses (e.g. *xylazine*, 0.3 mg/kg, IV) may be given as needed.

*Non-steroidal anti-inflammatory drugs (NSAIDs)*
- ○ Examples include *flunixin, phenylbutazone*, and *ketoprofen*.
- ○ Used for analgesia, and anti-inflammatory effects in endotoxemic horses.

*Opioids*
- ○ May be given IV with an α₂ agonist or given alone IM.
- ○ The onset of action is not as rapid as α₂ agonists, and large doses can cause excitement; however, this is less likely to happen if the horse is painful.
  - – *Morphine* (0.1 mg/kg IV).
  - – *Hydromorphone* (0.04 mg/kg, IV).
  - – *Butorphanol* (0.02–0.05 mg/kg, IV) is less efficacious than *morphine* but seems to be associated with a favorable outcome when given as a constant rate infusion in the postoperative period.
  - – *Methadone* (0.05–0.1 mg/kg, IV).

*Phenothiazines*
- ○ Generally contraindicated in colic patients due to their vasodilating actions, which have a negative effect on preload in the volume-depleted horse. But can be used safely in a physiologically stable horse undergoing colic surgery.

## C Anti-endotoxin therapy

- ○ A high percentage of horses are either endotoxemic at presentation or become so as surgery progresses.

*Polymyxin B*
- ○ Has a high affinity for the lipid A component of LPS.
- ○ Dose: 1000–6000 IU/kg, IV.
  - – The dose is generally added to 1 l of isotonic fluid and administered slowly (~30 minutes).

*NSAIDs*
- ○ Efficacious at decreasing prostaglandin formation in response to LPS administration (e.g. flunixin meglumine 1.1 mg/kg, IV).

## D Antimicrobial therapy

- ○ Usually consists of a β lactam (e.g. *K penicillin*) and an aminoglycoside (e.g. *gentamicin*).
- ○ Since dramatic decreases in blood pressure can follow the administration of *K penicillin* to the anesthetized horse, it should ideally be given (slowly) prior to induction.
  - – Otherwise, administer slowly (~15 minutes) during anesthesia.

○ It may be beneficial to administer anti-endotoxin therapy prior to antimicrobials.
  – Administration of β-lactam antimicrobials cause an increase in the plasma concentration of LPS due to their actions on the bacterial cell wall.

## III  Sedation and induction

- In horses with poor circulatory status, the onset of drug effect may be prolonged.
- Examples of sedation/induction regimens include:
  ○ α$_2$ agonist (e.g. *xylazine* [0.5–1.1 mg/kg, IV]) for sedation followed by *ketamine* (2.2 mg/kg, IV) + *midazolam* (0.05 mg/kg, IV) to induce anesthesia.
    – The *xylazine* dose should be based on the horse's physiological status, and whether the effects of xylazine administered during the examination process are still present.
  ○ *Xylazine + butorphanol* (0.02 mg/kg, IV) for sedation followed by *ketamine/ midazolam*.
  ○ *Xylazine* for sedation followed by *guaifenesin* (~50–100 mg/kg) + *ketamine* (2 mg/kg) for induction.

## IV  Intubation and oxygenation

- To decrease the risk of aspiration of gastric contents, intubation in sternal recumbency is recommended if reflux of gastric contents is occurring (see Figure 4.8).
- Oxygen supplementation and positive pressure ventilation (IPPV) are particularly important if the abdomen is distended (e.g. large colon torsion).
  ○ A *demand valve* is an effective way to deliver O$_2$ immediately following induction (see Figure 32.2).
- IPPV is generally performed throughout the anesthetic period.
  ○ With severe abdominal distention due to dilation of the gastrointestinal tract (see Figure 32.1), relatively high airway pressures will be required to ventilate the lungs.
  ○ In these circumstances, the goal of ventilation is to improve O$_2$ delivery rather than to reduce end-tidal CO$_2$ to normal.

**Figure 32.1**  Distended and fluid-filled small intestine with compromised blood flow.

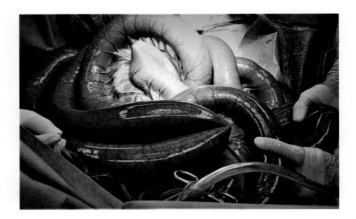

– It may not be possible to achieve an end-tidal $CO_2$ in the normal range until the abdomen is opened and the distended viscera is removed from the abdominal cavity, without the use of excessive airway pressures.

## V Maintenance of anesthesia

- Endotoxemic horses anesthetized for colic surgery often appear to need lower doses of maintenance anesthetics.
  - This may be a direct result of endotoxemia as LPS administration to laboratory rodents causes a significant decrease in MAC.
- The potential advantages of PIVA are worth considering (see Chapter 21).

## VI Intraoperative support

### A Fluid therapy

*Isotonic fluids*
  - Are a suitable choice (e.g. lactated Ringer's).
  - Infusion rates of ≥20 ml/kg/h may be required.

*Colloids*
  - Not commonly indicated.
  - Indicated if hypoproteinemia is present (see Chapter 10).
    – A volume of 5–10 ml/kg (e.g. Hetastarch) may be necessary, and this can be infused slowly in association with isotonic fluids.
    – Colloids will also decrease the volume of isotonic fluid needed.

### B Cardiovascular support (see Chapter 38)

  - Hypotension is a common complication.
  - Treatment of hypotension consists of improving *preload* and providing *inotropic* support.

*Preload*
  - Is improved by fluid replacement as previously described.

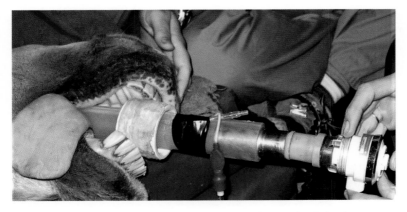

Figure 32.2 Use of a demand valve to ventilate a horse after induction.

*Inotropic support*

- ○ Is best achieved with a cardioselective $\beta_1$ adrenergic agonist.
- ○ Endotoxemic horses seem to require higher doses of a $\beta_1$ agonist to maintain an acceptable blood pressure.
- ○ $\beta_1$ agonists.
  - – *Dobutamine* and *ephedrine* are "first-line" inotropic agents.
  - – *Dobutamine* (~0.5–5 µg/kg/min) is a cardioselective $\beta_1$ agonist.
  - – *Ephedrine* (0.05–0.1 mg/kg, as a slow bolus) is not as effective as *dobutamine,* but can be given as a bolus.
- ○ Vasopressors (e.g. *norepinephrine, phenylephrine*) are not commonly used, and are reserved for patients in circulatory shock.
- ○ Horses in vasodilatory shock may not respond to $\beta_1$ agonists and remain hypotensive, despite increases in cardiac output. These horses benefit from vasoconstriction from α-adrenergic drugs (e.g. *phenylephrine*; 1–4 µg/kg, IV).

*Calcium infusions*

- ○ Many colic cases develop low plasma concentrations of ionized calcium.
- ○ Calcium can be infused *slowly* over the course of the surgery.
  - – A 23% *calcium borogluconate* solution is the most commonly used preparation.
  - – 0.5 l can be administered to an adult horse (400–500 kg) over the course of the surgery.
  - – The effect of supplementation can be monitored via serial determination of plasma electrolyte concentrations throughout anesthesia and surgery.
- ○ Commercial preparations for large animals generally contain ~10 g of calcium and variable amounts of dextrose and magnesium (<3 g).
- ○ Calcium will provide some *inotropic* support.

**C   Respiratory support** (see Chapter 38)

- ○ Hypoxemia is a common complication due to overdistension of the abdomen and V/Q mismatch.
- ○ Management of hypoxemia should consider all steps depicted in Chapter 38 (i.e. IPPV, positive end-expiratory pressure, alveolar recruitment maneuvers, aerosolized albuterol).
  - – Hypoxemia may persist despite treatment, but oxygen delivery may be adequate if the cardiac output and (Hb) are sufficient.

## VII   Recovery

- • The airway needs to be protected from aspiration of gastric contents.
  - ○ Leaving the orotracheal in place until the horse is standing will reduce the risk of aspiration.
    - – The head can be tilted downwards to facilitate pharyngeal drainage.
- • If it is planned to remove the endotracheal tube in recovery nasal instillation of *phenylephrine* is recommended to maintain airway patency.
  - ○ 5 ml of 0.15% phenylephrine (adult, full-sized horse) squirted into each nostril in the ventral meatus by elevating the nose and allowing contact with the nasal mucosa, about 30 minutes before extubation, will reduce nasal edema.
- • In most cases, horses recover slowly and quietly following colic surgery.
- • Many horses undergoing colic surgery have relatively long recoveries, and seem content to rest.

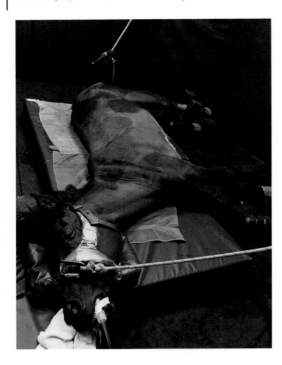

Figure 32.3 Horse on pads in recovery. An orotracheal tube is in place.

- o It is best to allow the horse time to recover, and myopathy does not seem to be a concern in long recoveries if the horse is recovered on a *padded* surface (see Figure 32.3).
- o Recovery may be assisted as deemed appropriate.
- It is common to remove the *nasogastric tube* as the end of surgery approaches. Generally, gastric reflux will have ceased by then.
  - o It should be removed slowly and carefully to prevent nasal bleeding.
  - o However, some clinicians prefer to leave the nasogastric tube in place for recovery. Whether this is more likely to promote regurgitation of stomach contents is undetermined.

## VIII   Intraoperative use of phenylephrine

- When *nephrosplenic entrapment* of intestine is present, *phenylephrine* may be used intraoperatively to contract the spleen and facilitate surgical correction of the problem.
- Low doses of *phenylephrine* (e.g. 1–2 µg/kg, IV, over 5 minutes) may be effective.
  - o It is prudent to start with low doses to avoid causing extreme hypertension.
  - o Phenylephrine will *not* be effective if the splenic blood vessels are occluded.

## Suggested Reading

Adami, C., Westwood-Hearn, H., and Bolt, D.M. (2020). Prevalence of electrolyte disturbances and perianesthetic death risk factors in 120 horses undergoing colic surgery. *J. Equine. Sci.* 84: 102843.

Boesch, J.M. (2013). Anesthesia for the horse with colic. *Vet. Clin. North Am. Equine Pract.* 29: 193–214.

33

# Anesthesia of the Geriatric Horse
*Reza M. Seddighi*

- Although age is not a disease per se, aging is associated with a myriad of disorders that increase morbidity and mortality.
- Older horses are more likely to be presented for management of conditions including gastrointestinal emergencies, dental disease, sinus infections, musculoskeletal problems, neoplasia, esophageal choke, and ocular diseases.
- The number of older horses that require veterinary care has increased, and this may be an indication of their importance as companion animals. However, horses differ from small companion animals in that they have to remain active and must be able to ambulate.

## I  Definition of geriatric

- A variety of criteria have been used to classify aging including:

*Chronological age*
  - This simply refers to how long an animal has been alive.
  - Many factors may affect the aging process, and therefore evaluating an animal based solely on its chronological age may not accurately reflect its physiological capabilities.
  - Older horses vary greatly in their physiologic and physical status and, like their human counterparts, chronological age does not always reflect physiologic age.
  - Therefore, when evaluating the animal for anesthetic purposes, chronological age is not the only factor to be considered.

*Physiologic age*
  - This describes how the animal functions when compared to a younger animal.
  - In physiologically aged animals, the compensatory mechanisms to cope with stress and the increased demand at times of crisis, including perianesthetic periods, are reduced.

*Demographic age*
  - Describes how an animal compares in age with others of the same species.
  - According to common definitions, animals at the last 25% of their average life expectancy for the species are considered geriatric or aged.
  - The average life expectancy for horses and ponies is 25 and 30 years, respectively.
    - Thus, horses may be considered geriatric after the age of 20, and ponies may be considered geriatric after age 25.

*Manual of Equine Anesthesia and Analgesia*, Second Edition. Edited by Tom Doherty, Alex Valverde, and Rachel A. Reed.
© 2022 John Wiley & Sons, Inc. Published 2022 by John Wiley & Sons, Inc.

## II Mechanisms of aging

- Much of what is known relative to the mechanisms of aging has come from the study of geriatric human beings.
- Aging is associated with a gradual loss of functional reserve in most organ systems.
- Multiple mechanisms are presumed to be responsible for aging and the associated physiologic changes.
- Mitochondrial dysfunction and oxidative stress are considered to be the two main mechanisms responsible for the aging process. Oxidative stress damages the cell membrane phospholipid layer, proteins, and DNA, and negatively modulates cell signaling pathways and gene expression, and cumulatively results in aging.

## III The impact of aging on body systems

- Aging may affect the function of most of the body systems, and therefore, the knowledge of the changes in organ function is an important step in counteracting their potential negative impact on the anesthetic outcome.
- The main physiologic changes in the function of body systems are summarized below.

### A Nervous system

- o Multiple structural changes in the central and peripheral nervous systems are reported in aged horses, which may result in a variety of functional changes.
- o In addition to the reported gross progressive reduction in brain mass in horses aged 7–23 years, microscopic changes including neuronal damage and depletion, and arterial wall degeneration are reported. These changes resemble changes occurring in elderly human beings, and are suspected to be associated with cognitive dysfunction.
- o A reduction in brain mass is associated with a decrease in cerebral metabolic rate and depletion of neurotransmitters including catecholamines, serotonin, and acetylcholine, and cumulatively may affect memory and motor function.
- o Differences in the anesthetic requirement in geriatric horses have not been compared with non-geriatric animals; however, the minimum alveolar concentration of volatile anesthetics (MAC) decreases with age in humans and dogs.
  - – Nevertheless, any decrease in MAC is not likely to be of clinical significance, and it is of interest that the bispectral index (BIS) value does not change in geriatric human beings despite a decrease in MAC.
- o An example of biochemical alterations potentially affecting anesthesia is the lower plasma *albumin* concentration in geriatric animals that may affect pharmacokinetics and pharmacodynamics of anesthetics. Alterations in N-methyl-D-aspartate (NMDA) binding capacity in geriatric dogs have been reported as an element that may result in a lower anesthetic requirement in geriatric dogs compared with younger ones.
- o Potential age-associated alterations in the peripheral nervous systems have not been evaluated in horses, but changes such as loss of motor, sensory and autonomic fibers, a decrease in afferent and efferent conduction velocities, and a decrease in the efficiency of nerve to muscle coupling, are reported in humans.

- ○ The presence and clinical importance of these changes in geriatric horses are unclear.
- ○ There is no specific anesthetic regimen to prevent anesthetic-related insults to the nervous system, but considering potential age-associated changes in the nervous system in geriatric horses, maintaining perioperative homeostasis as close to normal as possible may minimize the risk of central nervous imbalances resulting from general anesthesia.

## B Cardiovascular system

- ○ An increased age-associated fatality rate has been reported in horses with cardiovascular disease.
- ○ A fatality rate of 5.1% was reported in horses aged 15–23 years compared with 8.5% for older horses (≥24 years old). Among a variety of cardiovascular changes that may occur with increased age, *valvular heart* diseases are more prevalent in older horses compared with myocardial disease or pericarditis.
- ○ It is also important to consider that some of the cardiovascular-related increased mortality in aged horses may be associated with congenital lesions, such as *ventricular septal defect* or *patent ductus arteriosus*, as clinical signs of heart failure in the affected animals may not develop until later years.
- ○ A decrease in the ability of the cardiovascular system in older patients to cope with stress is expected and, at least in humans, it has been reported that aging results in a decline in the responsiveness of β-adrenergic receptors, and replacement of compliant cardiac and vascular tissue by a stiff, fibrotic tissue. These changes blunt chronotropic and inotropic responses of the heart and impair diastolic filling.
- ○ Although such age-related changes are not thoroughly evidenced in horses, fibrous scarring of the left ventricular apex is reported to occur in 60% of hearts from horses older than 20 years of age, which may result in decreased ventricular compliance and diastolic filling, and ultimately reduce the cardiac output.
- ○ A decrease in the maximal heart rate and myocardial aerobic capacity has been reported in aged horses.

*Valvular heart diseases in geriatric horses*

- ○ Valvular heart disease has a prevalence of >23% in horses 16 years of age or older.
- ○ Advancing age is a significant risk factor for mortality associated with aortic and mitral insufficiency in horses.
  - – Aortic valve pathology accounts for 82% of valvular abnormalities, and the greatest incidence of aortic regurgitation is in horses aged 15–20 years.

*Age-associated arrhythmias*

- ○ A variety of arrhythmias may appear in horses with cardiac diseases; however, these arrhythmias are rarely recognized on physical examination, and require ambulatory and exercising electrocardiographic studies to document their presence.
- ○ General anesthesia may predispose older animals to develop arrhythmias, and in one report, 30% of horses >20 years experienced an arrhythmia during inhalational anesthesia compared to 16% in younger horses.
- ○ Horses with *aortic valve insufficiency* appear to be at risk of developing supraventricular and ventricular arrhythmias, while other arrhythmias, such as premature ventricular beats or ventricular tachycardia, may reflect myocarditis.
- ○ An increase in left atrial pressure secondary to mitral regurgitation may increase left atrial diameter, and predispose the animal to the development of atrial fibrillation.

*Vascular changes in aged horses*

- ○ Vascular changes result in arterial and venous rigidity, an increase in systemic vascular resistance, and a decrease in venous compliance.
- ○ In older horses, mineralization of the intimal layer of the cerebral arteries, capillaries, and veins is a common finding, although its clinical importance is not clear. In one study, there was no difference in arterial blood pressures in horses less than 15 years compared with those over 20 years.

*Hypotension*

- ○ In a study of anesthetized horses, age did not affect the response to *dobutamine* therapy, indicating that there was no decrease in the responsiveness of β-receptors. Nevertheless, there is some evidence that geriatric horses are more prone to the cardiovascular depressant effects of inhalational anesthetics.
- ○ Other factors predisposing to hypotension, particularly in aging, may include diminished sensitivity of baroreceptors and a decrease in the response of the renin/aldosterone/angiotensin system.

## C Aging and the pulmonary system

- ○ The main age-associated anatomical and physiologic changes in the pulmonary system include increased compliance and decreased elastic recoil of the lungs, respiratory muscle function, and chest wall compliance.
- ○ The latter changes increase residual and closing volumes, and dead-space ventilation. In elderly human beings, the dynamic lung compliance becomes frequency-dependent and, as breathing rate increases, lung expansion becomes less effective and ventilation to perfusion (V/Q) mismatch increases.
- ○ Similar pathophysiology may be responsible, at least in part, for the development of V/Q mismatch in geriatric horses. These changes, along with a decrease in alveolar surface area, result in decreased gas exchange efficiency, manifested by lower arterial oxygen partial pressures ($PaO_2$), and greater alveolar-arterial difference in oxygen pressure (A–a difference).
- ○ Lower $PaO_2$ (90 mmHg in geriatric versus 101 mmHg in young horses) and greater A–a differences are reported for awake horses older than 20 years of age when compared to a group of younger horses.
- ○ In addition, a decrease in $PaCO_2$ and a subsequent increase in pH values are described in aged horses, compared to the younger animals, indicating compensatory hyperventilation.
- ○ In recumbent horses under inhalational anesthesia, functional residual capacity and residual volume are reduced, and $PaO_2$ values are often decreased, despite the use of a high fraction of inspired oxygen.

*Pulmonary diseases*

- ○ In addition to the age-associated anatomic and physiologic changes in the pulmonary system, disease conditions may exaggerate the effect of aging on the pulmonary function.
- ○ *Recurrent airway obstruction* (RAO) (heaves) is the most common respiratory disorder in older horses, and this can cause permanent pulmonary remodeling and fibrosis.
- ○ Exercise intolerance, respiratory distress, chronic coughing, mucopurulent nasal discharge, abnormal pulmonary sounds, and an enlarged field of percussion are usually noted during physical examination of horses suffering from RAO.
- ○ Pulmonary arterial pressure is increased, gas exchange is compromised, and end-expired lung volume is increased.

○ Airway smooth muscle and pulmonary epithelial hypertrophy may result in a net loss of intra-alveolar septae and pulmonary capillaries, with an increased number of intra-alveolar pores and deposition of collagen.

○ These changes will result in an overall decrease in respiratory functional reserve, greater (A-a) oxygen difference, V/Q mismatch, and lower $PaO_2$ and $PaCO_2$ values in geriatric horses.

○ Therefore, providing mechanical ventilation during general anesthesia to correct blood gas abnormalities is imperative. In addition, as these horses usually suffer from increased pulmonary resistance, bronchodilators such as aerosolized *albuterol*, are efficacious in relieving smooth-muscle contraction in the lower airways and may improve oxygenation and ventilatory parameters.

## D   Aging and the musculoskeletal system

○ *Sarcopenia* is defined as age associated loss of skeletal muscle strength and function.

○ Sarcopenia is recognized in veterinary patients, and several factors may have a role in its development including changes in central and peripheral nervous system innervation, hormonal status, inflammation, and altered caloric and protein intake.

○ Mechanisms involving dysfunction of highly energetic cell types in skeletal muscle are the cause of many age-related disorders such as sarcopenia. Skeletal muscle is dependent on mitochondria for energy production and functioning of contractile elements.

○ In addition to the loss of muscle mass, age-associated functional changes in muscles may include changes in spatial organization and physiological properties of motor units, regulation of contractile speed and force generation capacity of muscle fibers, and functional properties of myosin.

○ There is also disorganization of coordinated expression of contractile, sarcoplasmic reticular and mitochondrial protein isoforms in aging skeletal muscle. Therefore, a reduction in contractile strength, proprioception, and coordination are among the other effects of aging on neuromuscular function, and may have a clinical impact on geriatric horses, particularly those recovering from general anesthesia.

○ Sarcopenia may also contribute to increased heat loss under general anesthesia as lean animals with less fat insulation and a higher ratio of body surface area to body mass lose core temperature faster than animals with sufficient muscle mass and fat tissue.

○ Musculoskeletal diseases in aged horses are very common and periarticular and osteoarthritic degenerative changes affect the overall function of the musculoskeletal system and may compromise the quality of recovery from general anesthesia.

  – In morbidity/mortality studies, fractures are more commonly reported in older horses, associated with comorbidities like osteoporosis, arthritis, and fatigue.

○ There is a decrease in bone density with age which may lead to bone fractures during recovery from anesthesia.

## E   Aging and the endocrine system

○ A variety of endocrine diseases may be manifested in geriatric animals; however, only Cushing's disease and hypothyroidism, the two most common conditions in horses, are discussed here.

*Cushing's disease (pituitary pars intermedia dysfunction – PPID)*

○ Cushing's disease is one of the most common endocrine abnormalities of older horses. (see Figure 33.1)

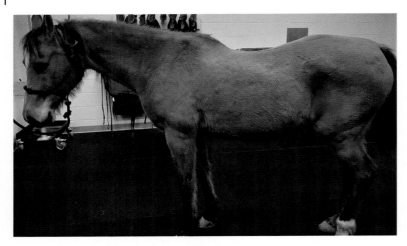

Figure 33.1    22-year-old horse with Cushing's disease (*pituitary pars intermedia dysfunction* – PPID).

- ○ Cushing's disease is the result of excessive production of *glucocorticoids* and is primarily observed in horses 18–21 years old.
- ○ Muscle wasting, fat redistribution, corticosteroid-induced changes such as hepatopathy, immunosuppression, and osteoporosis may be seen in horses with Cushing's disease.
- ○ These changes may cumulatively affect drug metabolism, pulmonary function (development of pulmonary infections, i.e. pneumonia), and ultimately may result in an increase in sensitivity to sedative and anesthetic drugs and affect the quality of recovery.
- ○ Cardiopulmonary changes associated with Cushing's disease including tachypnea, tachycardia, and hypertension, are not uncommon. Interestingly, these cardiovascular changes may counteract some of the cardiovascular instabilities expected in geriatric horses undergoing general anesthesia (e.g. bradycardia and hypotension). Nevertheless, vasoconstriction and hypovolemia may result in reduced tissue perfusion, and therefore, *volume loading* of these animals before anesthesia is recommended.
- ○ Other coexisting conditions with Cushing's, such as secondary diabetes mellitus or insipidus, and hyperhidrosis may result in blood glucose, fluid, hypovolemia, and electrolyte abnormalities.
- ○ Sarcopenia may also be present in horses with Cushing's as the result of the catabolic effect of corticosteroids, and this may increase the need for supporting ventilation and assisting recovery.
- ○ Horses receiving medications such as *dopamine* agonists or *serotonin* antagonists for treatment of Cushing's may be prone to some adverse effects including hypotension, agitation, cardiac arrhythmias, and sedation.

*Hypothyroidism*
- ○ Hypothyroidism may be seen in aging horses in either primary (autoimmune) or secondary hypothyroidism.
- ○ Secondary hypothyroidism is the more prevalent form and may occur due to hyperadrenocorticism or following surgical thyroidectomy.
- ○ Physiologic changes of hypothyroidism that may affect general anesthesia include *bradycardia* and *decreases in cardiac output*, which may result in *hypotension*, decreases in respiratory rate, and body temperature.

– Therefore, evaluation of thyroid abnormalities and correcting the imbalances should be performed before anesthesia, and particularly in horses with secondary hypothyroidism, the underlying cause should be identified and treated.

## IV Pharmacologic considerations in geriatric horses

- Alterations in pharmacokinetics and pharmacodynamics of many drugs, including anesthetics, may be observed in geriatric animals.
- Changes in the pharmacokinetics of anesthetic drugs may be due to the changes in physiologic variables such as a decreased metabolic rate and cardiac output, increased ratio of fat-to-muscle tissue, and a decrease in the concentration of plasma protein, and volume of distribution of particular drugs.
- The decreased lean body mass in geriatric animals, results in a smaller fraction of the drug being distributed into the muscles, and therefore, a greater fraction will be distributed to the brain. It is reported that geriatric horses experience more intense and longer-lasting analgesia with *butorphanol* and *morphine* for standing sedation, and the above mechanisms may be responsible for such differences.
- The pharmacodynamics of anesthetic drugs in geriatric animals may also be altered due to several factors including changes in receptor sensitivity and hepatic and renal clearance of drugs.
  ○ Alterations in receptor activity of opioids and benzodiazepines and a decrease in the MAC of isoflurane have been reported in geriatric human beings and dogs, respectively.
- Clearance of the anesthetic drugs with a high extraction ratio (e.g. *ketamine* and *morphine*) may be affected by a decrease in liver blood flow during anesthesia. In contrast, anesthetic drugs with a low extraction ratio (e.g. *diazepam* and *thiopental*), clearance is limited by the metabolizing capacity of the liver.
- Renal clearance of drugs may also be affected by the aging process; however, in a study of healthy horses older than 20 years, no abnormality in serum urea nitrogen, creatinine, albumin, liver enzyme activities, or electrolytes was found.
- In addition to the above-mentioned changes, a greater proportion of adipose tissue in geriatric animals may act as a "sink" for lipid-soluble drugs (e.g. many anesthetic agents) and prolong the clearance of the drugs, and therefore, the recovery from anesthesia.

## V Anesthetic considerations in geriatric horses

- Anesthetic-associated morbidity and mortality in horses increase with aging. In a study on more than 41 000 horses, older animals (≥14 years) were at greater risk of mortality (odds ratio of 1.42).
- In the latter study, the two main reasons for increased mortality in older horses were an increased likelihood of co-existing diseases affecting the outcome and an increased risk of long-bone fracture during recovery.
  ○ Older mares are reported to be at an increased risk of long-bone fracture, and bone density studies have reported decreased metacarpal breaking strength in some older mares up to 40 weeks post-parturition.

A   Preanesthetic evaluation

- A thorough physical examination of a geriatric horse including evaluation of the cardio-pulmonary system (such as heart and lung auscultation, evaluating mucous membrane color, capillary refill time, and pulse quality), exercise tolerance, and the ability to rise from recumbency should be performed prior to anesthesia.
- Exercise may unmask diseases such as RAO and cardiac diseases that are not apparent at rest.
- Routine laboratory analysis in healthy geriatric horses may be limited to basic laboratory tests (hematocrit and total protein determination); however, in sick horses, a complete and differential blood count and biochemical analysis may be indicated.
- If significant cardiac murmurs or arrhythmias are present, a complete cardiac evaluation, including echocardiography, is recommended.
- Age-associated physiologic changes in geriatric horses make them more prone to anesthetic complications. However, by administering a balanced anesthesia regimen, closely monitoring during anesthesia, and assisting with recovery, as well as controlling pain, the anesthetic outcome can be optimized.

B   Anesthetic protocols for geriatric horses

- Surgical and diagnostic procedures in horses may be performed either using standing sedation or general anesthesia. Drug regimens used and the duration of anesthesia for each of these methods depend on several factors including the health status of the animal, the available facility, and the purpose of sedation or anesthesia.
- In general, protocols for sedation (see Chapter 20) and general anesthesia (see Chapter 21) are similar to those reported for younger horses. However, it is generally advisable to administer the lower end of the drug dose range initially in geriatric horses and observe the effects.
  - In the case of *acepromazine,* a normal dose (0.05 mg/kg, IM) may be associated with clinically important hypotension, but a smaller dose (e.g. 0.02 mg/kg, IM) may have beneficial effects in protecting against cardiac arrhythmias and may improve cardiac output by decreasing afterload.

C   Anesthetic monitoring

- Monitoring during anesthesia is important because geriatric horses may have limited physiologic reserve.

*Body temperature*
  - Geriatrics are predisposed to hypothermia thus measures to preserve body heat, and apply active heating when feasible, should be employed.

*Blood pressure*
  - Arterial blood pressure measurement, preferably a direct measurement, is recommended.
  - A minimum mean blood pressure of 70 mmHg should be maintained, using an inotrope (e.g. *dobutamine*), if necessary.

*Electrocardiography (ECG)*
  - The ECG should be monitored closely due to the increased incidence of arrhythmias in older horses.

*Blood gas analysis*
- Arterial blood gas analysis monitoring is advisable due to the increased incidence of hypoxemia in this age group.

*Positioning*
- Due to their reduced muscle mass proper positioning and padding is important to prevent muscle and nerve damage.

## D Recovery

- Assisted recoveries may be recommended in many cases due to the aforementioned muscle and joint problems.
- It is recommended that the horse be placed on a pad of suitable thickness, and sedated in the hope of having a slower more deliberate recovery.

## Suggested Reading

Betros, C.L., McKeever, K.H., Kearns, C.F., and Malinowski, K. (2002). Effects of aging and training on maximal heart rate and $VO_{2max}$. *Equine Vet. J. Suppl.* 34: 100–105.

Bidwell, L.A., Bramlage, L.R., and Rood, W.A. (2007). Equine perioperative fatalities associated with general anesthesia at a private practice – a retrospective case series. *Vet. Anaesth. Analg.* 34: 23–30.

Davis, E. and Rush, B.R. (2006). Respiratory disease in the geriatric equine patient. In: *Equine Geriatric Medicine and Surgery* (ed. J.J. Bertone), 179–192. St Louis, MO: Saunders Elsevier.

Derksen, F.J., Olszewski, M.A., Robinson, N.E. et al. (1996). Aerosolized albuterol sulfate used as a bronchodilator in horses with recurrent airway obstruction. *Am. J. Vet. Res.* 60: 689–693.

Doherty, T.J. (2003). Invited review: aging and sarcopenia. *J. Appl. Physiol.* 95: 1717–1727.

Doherty, T.J. and Brown, W.F. (1993). The estimated numbers and relative sizes of thenar motor units as selected by multiple point stimulation in young and older adults. *Muscle Nerve* 116: 355–366.

Donaldson, L.L. (2006). Anesthetic Considerations for the Geriatric Equine. In: *Equine Geriatric Medicine and Surgery* (ed. J.J. Bertone), 25–37. Saunders Elsevier: St Louis, MO.

Donaldson, L.L. (1988). Retrospective assessment of dobutamine therapy for hypotension in anesthetized horses. *Vet. Surg.* 17: 53–57.

Else, R.W. and Holmes, J.R. (1972). Cardiac pathology in the horse. 1. Gross pathology. *Equine Vet. J.* 4: 1–8.

Glade, M.J. (1993). Effects of gestation, lactation, and maternal calcium intake on mechanical strength of equine bone. *J. Am. Coll. Nutr.* 12: 372–377.

Johnston, G.M., Eastment, J.K., Wood, J.L.N., and Taylor, P.M. (2002). The confidential enquiry into perioperative equine fatalities (CEPEF): mortality results of Phases 1 and 2. *Vet. Anaesth. Analg.* 29: 159–170.

Love, S. (1993). Equine Cushing's disease. *Br. Vet. J.*: 149139–149153.

Magnusson, K.R., Scanga, C., Wagner, A.E., and Dunlop, C. (2002). Changes in anesthetic sensitivity and glutamate receptors in the aging canine brain. *J. Gerontol. A Biol. Sci. Med. Sci.* 55: B448–B454.

Marr, C.M. and Bowen, M. (2006). Cardiac Disease in the Geriatric Horse. In: *Equine Geriatric Medicine and Surgery* (ed. J.J. Bertone), 39–49. Saunders Elsevier: St Louis, MO.

Messer, N.T.T. and Johnson, P.J. (2007). Evidence-based literature pertaining to thyroid dysfunction and Cushing's syndrome in the horse. *Vet. Clin. North Am. Equine Pract.* 23: 329–364.

Nyman, G., Lindberg, R., Weckner, D. et al. (1991). Pulmonary gas exchange correlated to clinical signs and lung pathology in horses with chronic bronchiolitis. *Equine Vet. J.* 23: 253–260.

Robinson, N.E., Derksen, F.J., Olszewski, M.A., and Buechner-Maxwell, V.A. (1996). The pathogenesis of chronic obstructive pulmonary disease of horses. *Br. Vet. J.* 152: 283–306.

Sage, A.M. (2002). Cardiac disease in the geriatric horse. *Vet. Clin. North Am. Equine Pract.* 18: 575–589.

Seddighi, R. and Doherty, T. (2012). Anesthesia of the geriatric equine. *Vet. Med. (Auckl)* 3: 53–64.

Sojka, J.E. (1995). Hypothyroidism in horses. *Compend. Contin. Educ. Prac. Vet.* 17: 845–852.

Stevens, K.B., Marr, C.M., Horn, J.N. et al. (2009). Effect of left-sided valvular regurgitation on mortality and causes of death among a population of middle-aged and older horses. *Vet. Rec.* 164: 6–10.

Traub-Dargatz, J.L., Long, R.E., and Bertone, J.J. (2006). What is an "old horse" and its recent impact. In: *Equine Geriatric Medicine and Surgery* (ed. J.J. Bertone), 1–4. Saunders Elsevier: St Louis, MO.

Vischer, C.M., Foreman, J.H., Constable, P.D. et al. (1999). Hemodynamic effects of thyroidectomy in sedentary horses. *Am. J. Vet. Res.* 60: 14–21.

# 34

## Anesthesia and Pregnancy

*Lydia Donaldson*

- The need for anesthesia during pregnancy occurs under two general conditions:
  - Surgical procedures unrelated to the pregnancy.
  - Obstetric procedures.
- Although the overall concerns are similar, obstetric procedures must also focus on the delivery of a *viable foal*.
- Maintaining maternal blood pressure and oxygenation are critical under both circumstances, but minimizing fetal exposure to longer acting, compromising anesthetic agents is also important for success.

## I Physiology of pregnancy (see Table 34.1)

- The following observations are from studies of pregnant women. Information regarding pregnant mares will be included where available.

### A Cardiovascular

- Hematocrit, hemoglobin concentration, and total protein (albumin more so than globulin) are decreased due to dilution.
  - This is secondary to the relatively greater increase in plasma volume than red cell mass or protein.
- Blood pressure may be normal or slightly below normal.
- Cardiac output is increased.
- Procoagulant activity is increased.
  - In pregnant mares, increases occur in fibrinogen, Factor VIII: C, and von Willebrand factor.

### B Respiratory

- There is a greater potential for hypoxemia due to increased $O_2$ consumption, decreased functional residual capacity, and increased closing volume.
  - Total $O_2$ transport is greater due to:

*Manual of Equine Anesthesia and Analgesia*, Second Edition. Edited by Tom Doherty, Alex Valverde, and Rachel A. Reed.

Table 34.1  Physiologic changes identified during pregnancy in women.

| | |
|---|---|
| Cardiovascular | Increase plasma volume (~40%) |
| | Increase RBC mass (~20%) |
| | Increase ventricular end-diastolic volume and wall thickness |
| | Increase fractional shortening and stroke volume (~20–50%) |
| | Increase resting heart rate (20–30%) |
| | Increase cardiac output (30–50%) |
| | Increase systemic & pulmonary vascular resistance (20–30%) |
| | Increase procoagulant activity |
| Respiratory | Increase metabolic rate |
| | Increase minute ventilation (~70%) |
| | Decrease functional residual capacity (~20%) |
| | Increase closing volume |
| | Decrease $PaCO_2$, increase pH and normal $PaO_2$ |
| Renal | Increase blood flow |
| | Increase glomerular filtration rate |
| Uterus | Increased blood flow |
| | Altered vascular response to catecholamines |
| Brain | Increased progesterone and endogenous opioids |

- Respiratory alkalosis increasing $O_2$ uptake at the lung.
- Greater total hemoglobin.
- Increased cardiac output.
 ○ Fetal $O_2$ uptake is facilitated by:
    - Increased $O_2$ delivery.
    - Higher maternal 2,3-DPG facilitating $O_2$ unloading at the placenta.
    - A lower P50 for fetal hemoglobin (although not structurally different from adult hemoglobin).

**C   Renal**

 ○ Increased renal blood flow, glomerular filtration rate, and plasma result in decreased serum blood urea nitrogen and creatinine.

**D   Uterus**

 ○ Uterine blood flow is increased.
 ○ Uterine vascular control is altered.
    - $\alpha_1$-adrenoceptor mediated vasoconstriction is increased.
    - $\alpha_2$-adrenoceptor mediated vasodilation (nitric oxide mediated) is enhanced.
    - $\beta_2$-adrenoceptor mediated vasodilation is reduced.

## II  Factors affecting drug disposition during pregnancy

### A  Maternal

- Increased plasma volume dilutes the anesthetic agent.
- Decreased serum albumin increases the *free* fraction of protein bound drugs.
- Increased body fat provides a larger redistribution compartment.
- Increased pulmonary blood flow, minute ventilation, and decreased functional residual capacity hasten the uptake and elimination of less soluble inhalants.
- Increased circulating progesterone and endogenous opioids are partially responsible for the observed minimum alveolar concentration (MAC) decrease for inhalants, and dose decreases for local anesthetics, as well as some sedatives and analgesics.
- Greater cranial spread of epidurally administered local anesthetics or analgesics.
  - The epidural space is reduced in volume due to blood volume increases causing vertebral venous engorgement.
  - This increases sensitivity to local anesthetics.

### B  Placental

- The equine placenta is relatively primitive.
  - Horse placenta is classified as diffuse and epitheliochorial, where the fetus is in contact with the allantoamnion inside the chorioallantois, which creates a complete set of layers that include the endometrial epithelium, maternal connective tissue, and maternal endothelial cells, all attached to the endometrium.
  - The capillary-to-capillary distance is very small (~12 µm) within the microcotyledons.
  - Capillary bed flow of the two circulations is countercurrent.
- In the pregnant mare, uterine blood flow is approximately twice that of umbilical blood flow.
  - *Uterine blood flow* is affected by factors that influence cardiac output and blood pressure (e.g. inotropes, vasopressors, vascular volume, anesthetic drugs, autonomic nervous system activity).
  - *Uterine vascular resistance* is affected by a number of factors (e.g. hypoxemia, hypercarbia, and extreme hypocarbia, stress, pain, anesthetic drugs).
- Maternal-to-fetal drug exchange across the lipoprotein barrier occurs by *diffusion*.
  - It is dependent on the concentration gradient, protein binding, lipid solubility, ionization, and size of the molecule.
- The placenta has metabolic activity (e.g. cytochrome P450, several transferases, sulfating enzymes).

### C  Fetal

- The equine fetal circulation does not include a *ductus venosus*, as it is lost early in gestation.
  - Thus, all umbilical venous blood flows through the liver sinusoids before reaching the right ventricle.
  - Drugs can be metabolized or sequestrated in the fetal liver.

○ Fetal albumin concentration is ≥ than that of the mare (2.3–4.2 mg/dl).

○ Anesthetics reaching the fetal brain are diluted by the 50–60% of cardiac output that does not flow through the placenta, some hepatic metabolism, and mixing with left ventricular blood through the ductus arteriosus.

○ The fetal blood–brain barrier is immature allowing more direct access.

○ Fetal heart rate (FHR) is *increased* by factors such as adrenosympathetic response, acidosis, slow-onset hypoxia, activity, atropine, and acepromazine.

○ FHR is *decreased* by factors such as acute hypoxia, acidosis, sleep, $\alpha_2$ agonists, and opioids.

## III  Anesthesia concerns in the pregnant mare

### A  Compression of the vena cava

○ It is sometimes recommended that mares undergoing cesarean section *not* be placed squarely on their backs as this may result in life-threatening hypotension from compression of the caudal vena cava.

  – However, there is no evidence that this is beneficial in horses, and tilting the mare to one side is going to increase the likelihood of myopathy.

○ Some obstetric procedures (e.g. assisted vaginal delivery under general anesthesia) are performed using the Trendelenburg position (head down), which can exacerbate negative cardiovascular and respiratory changes.

### B  Hypoventilation, hypoxemia, and impaired gas exchange

○ Hypoventilation resulting from the effects of anesthesia and recumbency is compounded by the gravid uterus impinging on the diaphragm, further reducing thoracic volume and compliance.

○ Reduced cardiac output, atelectasis, and decreased thoracic compliance contribute to ventilation/perfusion mismatch and shunt.

### C  Myopathy

○ The risk is greater due to the increased body mass and increased likelihood of hypotension and hypoxemia.

### D  Recovery

○ Brood mares are often older, overweight, or heavy with their pregnancy, arthritic, unfit, and less dependent on man than the average horse in training.

○ These factors contribute to difficulty getting to their feet and being uncooperative during recovery.

## IV  Anesthetic management in pregnancy

○ Drugs given to the mare can affect the fetus either *directly*, by crossing the placenta to alter neurologic or cardiovascular function, or *indirectly* by altering uterine blood flow.

○ In general, molecules that cross the blood–brain barrier also cross the placenta.

○ Equine fetal stress is indicated by persistent bradycardia and an increase followed by a decrease in activity.

## A   Sedation and premedication

*Acepromazine*
○ Fetal and maternal heart rates increase for ~25 minutes after *acepromazine* (0.1 mg/kg, IV) administration to the mare.
○ Fetal aortic blood flow does not change at this dose.

*α₂ agonists*
○ Have proven to be clinically safe, although fetal bradycardia is as profound as and of longer duration than maternal bradycardia.
○ Fetal aortic blood flow decreases 66% after *detomidine* (10 μg/kg, IV) is administered to the mare.
○ *Detomidine* decreases spontaneous uterine contractility in late pregnancy.
○ These drugs increase uterine contraction for up to 30 minutes post administration, but do not interfere with pregnancy.

*Opioids*
○ Readily cross the placental barrier.
  – Increased fetal activity was reported in pony fetuses after *pentazocine* administration to the mares.
  – Morphine has a lower lipid solubility and higher molecular weight than other opioids, which delays and restricts transfer across the placenta.

*Flunixin meglumine*
○ Blocks prostaglandin-$F_2\alpha$ release and protects against fetal loss after uterine manipulation.
○ Near term, non-steroidal anti-inflammatory drugs (NSAIDs) can mediate premature ductus arteriosus closure resulting in pulmonary hypertension.

## B   Induction

*Ketamine*
○ Has *no* cardiovascular effects on the fetus.
○ Decreased responsiveness and muscle rigidity has been seen in human neonates at birth.

*Diazepam*
○ Benzodiazepines, including diazepam and midazolam, cross the placenta readily due to their high lipid solubility and unionized form.
○ In humans, diazepam administration pre-partum can cause profound muscle relaxation (hypotonia), depression, and hypothermia in the neonate, which result in low Apgar scores.

*Midazolam*
○ Does not accumulate in the fetus but may cause respiratory depression in the neonate.
○ Has lower fetal-to-maternal plasma concentrations than diazepam; therefore it can be considered preferable to diazepam.

*Guaifenesin*
- Can cause a decrease in systemic vascular resistance and hypotension.
- Readily crosses the placenta.
  - Nevertheless, it has been successfully used in total intravenous anesthesia (TIVA) for controlled vaginal delivery, as well as induction and maintenance for cesarean delivery of viable foals.

## C   Maintenance

- Positive pressure ventilation and supplemental $O_2$ should be used to prevent hypoventilation and hypercarbia and to optimize oxygenation, regardless of the anesthetic technique.

*Inhalational anesthetic MAC*
- Pregnancy reduces MAC 25–40% in other species, so a significant reduction would be expected in the late-term mare.
  - Nevertheless, the bispectral index (BIS) value does not change in pregnant women despite a decrease in MAC and the decrease in MAC is not clinically relevant.
- Inhalational agents dose-dependently decrease maternal blood pressure, cardiac output, uterine blood flow, uterine tone and contractile activity.
- Umbilical blood flow and fetal blood pressure is also decreased, but pH is maintained in procedures lasting less than an hour.

*TIVA*
- *Guaifenesin/ketamine/detomidine* maintains maternal blood pressure and uterine blood flow better than *halothane*, but fetal bradycardia is comparable.

*Partial intravenous anesthesia (*PIVA*)*
- Has not been studied in pregnant mares.
- A constant rate infusion of *lidocaine* appears to be safe. In women undergoing a cesarean delivery, a lidocaine infusion perioperatively was associated with a decreased stress response in the mother, and Apgar scores did not differ from the control group.
- Lidocaine does not affect uterine blood flow.
  *Note*: The non-ionized form of lidocaine crosses into the placenta more readily than the ionized form, and this could result in "ion trapping" when $H^+$ ions bind to the non-ionized form of lidocaine. The fetal pH is generally less than the maternal pH and this favors ion trapping which would increase the concentration of lidocaine in the fetal circulation, especially in fetal acidosis. However, this is not likely to be of clinical significance under normal circumstances.
- *A dexmedetomidine* infusion has been associated with good fetal and maternal outcomes in human beings.

## D   Specific monitoring

*Direct blood pressure*
- Measurement of blood pressure is critical to ensure sufficient pressure for uterine perfusion.

*Arterial blood gas analysis*
- Helps to optimize uteroplacental $O_2$ delivery.

- Hypoxemia and hypercarbia activate the sympathetic nervous system causing uterine artery constriction.
- Hypocarbia decreases cardiac output and increases uterine vascular resistance.

*Electrocardiography*
- Allows detection of arrhythmias which could compromise cardiac output and uterine blood flow.

*FHR*
- Is an indicator of fetal well-being and can be detected as early as the 120th day of pregnancy.
- Positioning or surgical manipulations prohibit electrocardiogram (ECG) lead placement for FHR monitoring, but pre- and post-anesthetic readings may be informative of fetal status.
- Heart rate is decreased by:
  - Acute onset hypoxemia.
  - Acidemia.
  - Sleep or the direct effect of sedatives, anesthetics, or analgesics.
- Heart rate is increased by:
  - Slow-onset hypoxemia or recovery after acute hypoxemia. This activates the fetal adreno-sympathetic system causing increased FHR and blood pressure.

E   Cardiovascular supportive measures

- *Ephedrine* improves cardiac output and causes no decrease in uterine blood flow.
- *Dobutamine* is also satisfactory.
- *Atropine* crosses the placenta whereas *glycopyrrolate* does not.
- For uterine surgery, intensive fluid therapy may be necessary to compensate for blood loss, particularly with inhalational anesthesia where decreased uterine tone hinders hemostasis.

F   Recovery

- Oxygen should be administered by demand valve and/or insufflation.
- The heavily pregnant, unfit, older mares may need assistance.
- Those that have been in labor for a long time will also be exhausted.
- Following a cesarean or controlled vaginal delivery, care should be taken to dry the recovery stall floor of amniotic fluids and obstetrical lubricant.
- Multiparous mares may emerge from general anesthesia anxiously searching for the foal.

G   Pain management

- The long-term administration of analgesics during the first trimester of pregnancy may alter normal fetal development, and during later pregnancy may induce tolerance in the fetus with withdrawal after delivery.
- Epidural opioids have minimal maternal or fetal cardiovascular effects during late pregnancy.

## V   Managing anesthesia in the pregnant mare

- *Elective surgery* should be avoided. If this is not possible, the mare and fetus are at the least risk during the middle trimester, i.e. after differentiation and development of the fetus but before rapid growth burdens the mare.

### A   Non-obstetric procedures

*Abdominal surgery for intestinal emergency*
- Short-term survival rate of pregnant mares with surgical colic (61%) is reported to be no different from that of non-pregnant horses (65%).
- Fetal loss (12%) is comparable regardless of the stage of pregnancy.
  - It is linked to maternal endotoxemia and to hypoxemia and/or hypotension in mares <60 days to term.
- Uterine manipulation in early equine pregnancy frequently results in fetal loss.
- Attentive volume support, pre-oxygenation, mechanical ventilation and maintenance of blood pressure and oxygenation are important as with any colic case.
  - Hypovolemia may be less easily identified in the pregnant mare due to expanded blood volume and dilutional anemia and hypoproteinemia.

*Trauma*
- Many wounds, fractures, ocular injuries, etc. require induction of anesthesia regardless of the stage of pregnancy.
- The stress of these injuries, as with abdominal surgery, may be as detrimental to pregnancy as are anesthesia and surgery.

### B   Obstetric procedures

*Uterine torsion*
- A 70% survival rate has been reported for the mare and fetus.
- Rotation of the uterus on its long axis compromises perfusion.
- Correction of the torsion may be done with the mare standing, through a flank incision, or may require general anesthesia with rolling or celiotomy.
- Anesthetic concerns are those of non-obstetric late-term procedures plus any hemodynamic instability caused by uterine manipulation during surgery or additional cardiopulmonary compromise created by lifting and rolling the heavily pregnant mare.

*Dystocia/Cesarean section* (see Table 34.2)
- Mare survival-to-discharge rates for dystocia, whether resolved by vaginal or cesarean delivery, are 70–94%.
- Foal survival varies from 11 to 30% with time from onset of labor to delivery being a significant factor in foal outcome.
  - From 30 minutes of the onset of stage 2 labor (chorioallantoic rupture), there is a 10% increased risk of delivering a dead foal or a 16% increased risk of the fetus not surviving discharge for each 10 minutes of delay.
- Elective cesarean section has considerably better survival rates: 100% of mares and 90% of foals.

**Table 34.2** Suggested general anesthetic management of a mare with a live foal dystocia for controled delivery or cesarean section.

- All members of the team must be prepared and understand the need for efficiency
- In general, mares presented for dystocia are in good hemodynamic status
- Premedicate with an $\alpha_2$ agonist (e.g. *xylazine* 0.3–0.5 mg/kg, IV) to effect $\pm$ *butorphanol* (0.01 mg/kg, IV)
- Insufflate $O_2$ as soon as the mare will tolerate it
- It is generally best to induce with a protocol that the anesthesia team is familiar with
  - e.g. Guaifenesin (40–100 mg/kg) and ketamine (2 mg/kg, IV), alternatively,
  - Substitute a GABA$_A$ agonist (e.g. midazolam or propofol) for guaifenesin
- Anesthesia is primarily maintained with an inhalational agent; however, PIVA using $\alpha_2$ agonists have been used successfully in women, and result in favorable maternal and fetal outcome
  - $\alpha_2$ agonists (e.g. *xylazine* or *dexmedetomidine*) decrease MAC, decrease the stress response, and provide analgesia
- Positive pressure ventilation is generally recommended, but avoid hyperventilation as a PaCO$_2$ < 30 mmHg decreases cardiac output and uterine blood flow
- Measure arterial blood pressure directly and support if necessary
- Measure blood gases
- If a cesarean is necessary, anticipate increased blood loss and administer crystalloid as needed and adjust ventilation as needed
- *Oxytocin* will help control uterine bleeding but it should be administered over 30 minutes to prevent hypotension developing. Hypotension may result from a decrease in systemic vascular resistance and a subsequent decrease in venous return and cardiac output
- In recovery, supplement oxygen and assist ventilation with a demand valve, as needed
- Prevent the mare attempting to stand too soon with the use of sedatives and mild physical restraint
- Consider using assisted recovery, if available
- Provide a dry footing by removing any uterine fluids and obstetric lubricant

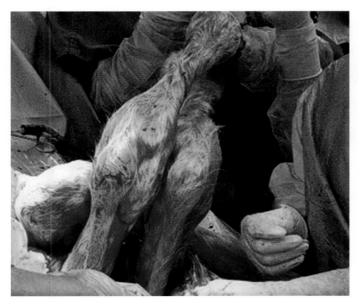

**Figure 34.1** Delivery of live foal, lifting by hindlimbs out of uterus. *Source:* Image courtesy of Dr. Blake Everett, DVM, Dip ACVS-LA.

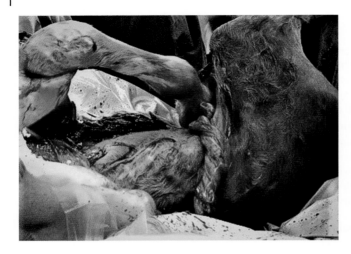

Figure 34.2   Delivery of live foal; hindlimbs, abdomen, and thorax exiting uterus. *Source:* Image courtesy of Dr. Blake Everett, DVM, Dip ACVS-LA.

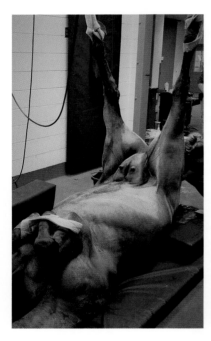

Figure 34.3   Positioning of mare for attempted vaginal delivery of the fetus. A wedge-shaped pad can be placed under the lumbar area to give support.

*Live foal at presentation* (see Figures 34.1 and 34.2)

- ○ Efforts at delivery should proceed rapidly from a quick assessment of the standing mare to assisted delivery to general anesthesia with controlled vaginal delivery or cesarean section.
- ○ Efforts should be made to minimize fetal exposure to anesthetics by choosing agents that do not accumulate in the fetus, limiting the time between induction and delivery, and dosing to effect.
- ○ A plan must be in place for resuscitation of the foal if deemed necessary.

*Dead foal at presentation*
  - Stabilizing the mare becomes as important as removing the fetus.
  - Once the mare is rehydrated, with electrolytes and acid–base status corrected, the above steps should proceed in an orderly fashion.
  - Controlled vaginal delivery often involves *raising the mare's hindquarters* to shift the fetus back into the abdomen for repositioning. This places an additional load on the diaphragm and lungs and encourages abdominal venous return if the gravid uterus is not occluding the caudal vena cava. (*see* Figure 34.3)

Oxytocin administration intraoperatively
  - *Oxytocin* should be administered *slowly* to avoid vasodilation and hypotension.

## Suggested Reading

Li, A., Jinlin Shi, J., Bai, Y. et al. (2019). Effectiveness and safety of intravenous application of dexmedetomidine for cesarean section under general anesthesia: a meta-analysis of randomized trials. *Drug Des. Devel. Ther.* 13: 965–974.

Byron, C.R., Embertson, R.M., Bernard, W.V. et al. (2002). Dystocia in a referral hospital setting: approach and results. *Equine Vet. J.* 35: 82–85.

El-Tahan, M.R., Warda, O.M., Diab, D.G. et al. (2009). A randomized study of the effects of perioperative i.v. lidocaine on hemodynamic and hormonal responses for cesarean section. *J. Anesth.* 23: 215–221.

Freeman, D.E., Hungerford, L.L., Schaeffer, D. et al. (1999). Caesarean section and other methods for assisted delivery: comparison of effects on mare mortality and complications. *Equine Vet. J.* 31: 203–207.

Maaskant, A., De Bruijn, C.M., Schutrups, A.H., and Stout, T.A.E. (2010). Dystocia in Friesian mares: prevalence, causes and outcome following caesarean section. *Equine Vet. Educ.* 22: 190–195.

Norton, J.L., Dallap, B.L., Johnston, J.K. et al. (2007). Retrospective study of dystocia in mares at a referral hospital. *Equine Vet. J.* 39: 37–41.

Rioja, E., Cernicchiaro, N., Costa, M.C., and Valverde, A. (2012). Perioperative risk factors for mortality and length of hospitalization in mares with dystocia undergoing general anesthesia: a retrospective study. *Can. Vet. J.* 53: 502–510.

Sanghavi, M. and Rutherford, J.D. (2014). Cardiovascular physiology of pregnancy. *Circulation* 130: 1003–1008.

Wilson, D.V. (1994). Anesthesia and sedation for late-term mares. *Vet. Clin. North Am. Equine Pract.* 10: 219–236.

## 35

## Anesthesia for Equine Imaging
*Carrie A. Davis*

## Magnetic resonance imaging

## I   Introduction

- Magnetic resonance imaging (MRI) of horses has become relatively common, and while most imaging involves the distal limbs, imaging of more proximal portions of the limbs and head is also performed.
- The type or strength of the MRI system, high-field (typically 1.5–3.0 Tesla, utilized in anesthetized recumbent horses), or low-field MRI (usually 0.27 Tesla, utilized in standing sedated horses), dictates the management of the case and the issues confronting anesthesia personnel.
- Although no significant difference has been reported in the incidence of postanesthetic myopathy/neuropathy or anesthetic-related mortality in horses undergoing anesthesia for MRI in comparison with non-MRI procedures, anesthetizing horses for MRI presents unique challenges.

### A   Specific challenges

- ○ The presence of a continuous magnetic field.
  - – This can cause safety issues such as the magnetic field turning ferrous objects (e.g. oxygen cylinders) into projectiles.
  - – In addition, the magnetic field can damage sensitive equipment such as anesthetic monitors that are not MRI compatible.
- ○ There may be limited access to the patient which may hinder patient monitoring.
- ○ There is limited ability to pad the horse's extremities within the bore of the magnet.
- ○ There are positioning challenges in acquiring diagnostic images, in addition to the physical effort required to position the horse.
- ○ Motion artifact affects the quality of the images. Thus, movement of the horse, or rapid breathing, or movement of the MRI patient table must be minimized.

*Manual of Equine Anesthesia and Analgesia*, Second Edition. Edited by Tom Doherty,
Alex Valverde, and Rachel A. Reed.
© 2022 John Wiley & Sons, Inc. Published 2022 by John Wiley & Sons, Inc.

   ○ There is a requirement for MRI compatible anesthetic machines, patient table, fluid poles, and monitoring equipment.

     *Note*: Non-MRI compatible monitors may be used but they must be located remotely from the magnet.

   ○ MRI equipment must be protected.

     – This includes preventing the horse flailing its legs while in the bore of the MRI.

     – There is a risk of *urine* getting into the magnet when a horse's penis or vulva are positioned close to the gantry (see *urinary catheter* below).

## II  MRI safety

- There are potential hazards to human beings with MRI given that the magnetic field and the radiofrequency (RF) field are capable of producing detrimental biologic effects if they are of sufficient intensity. However, human MRI-related data are limited, and there are no quantitative data in relation to safe exposure. Nevertheless, guidelines on patient and operator exposure have been published in some countries. In the USA, the FDA has issued guidelines for evaluating the risk. For equine hospitals, these guidelines would apply to the MRI operator rather than the patient. Although the MRI operator in an equine hospital is unlikely to be exposed for long periods to electromagnetic radiation, the liability issues related to MRI exposure should not be ignored. Due to potential health hazards and liability concerns, it is prudent to exclude individuals with cardiac pacemakers, those with metallic clips (e.g. aneurysm clips), and pregnant women from the MRI suite at all times. In human medicine, MRI safety is a major liability concern, and the most common type of injury in patients results from burns.
  - Some veterinary institutions and private practices require that the anesthesia personnel do not remain in the MRI suite with the patient, and that patients be monitored from the control room.
- Personnel training is paramount for ensuring safe working conditions.
  - Warning signs should be posted outside the MRI room (see Figure 35.1), and access to the room should be limited.

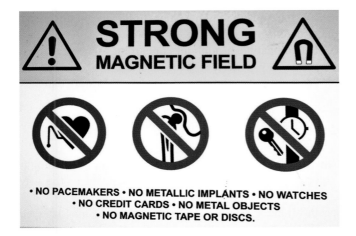

Figure 35.1   Warning signage posted outside of the MRI room.

- Ferromagnetic projectiles are the most likely injury risks to the patient and staff (see Gauss lines below). Strict procedures should be in place to prevent ferromagnetic objects (e.g. gas cylinders, non-MRI safe anesthetic equipment, fluid poles, halters with metal buckles, clippers, hobbles, or personal effects) from entering the MRI room.
  - Personal items that could be damaged by the magnetic field include credit cards and cellular phones).
- Ferromagnetic items are not only safety concerns, but when close to the imaging portion of the magnet they can cause image artifacts from magnetic field disruption.
- Implanted magnetic material (e.g. embolic coil implants, aneurysm clips, cardiac pacemakers) pose a danger to the individual secondary to motion in the case of implants or aneurysm clips), or the magnetic field may change the pacemaker settings.
- RF pulses required to generate the MRI signal may cause burns when conducting material (e.g. electrocardiogram [ECG] cables) capable of creating electric currents and heat are attached.
- To prevent burns at ECG electrode attachments and from associated cables, avoid looping or crossing of cables. Cables should be insulated from the patient by padding.
  - MRI-compatible ECG leads and electrodes are essential to avoid such hazards.
- *Fentanyl patches*
  - Although it is unlikely that an adult horse has a *fentanyl* patch in place prior to an MRI, there is a slight chance that a foal may have. Not all brands of fentanyl patches contain metal (e.g. aluminum foil) in the backing layer, but those that do have the potential to create the following problems for a patient undergoing an MRI, if the patch is located on a body part that is located within the bore of the magnet.
    - *Skin burns*: Metal in the patch acts as a conductor and induces electrical currents. These eddy currents result in intense local heat production and potentially to skin burns which may not become evident for a number of hours.
    - *Increased drug absorption*: The local increase in temperature may result in an increase in drug absorption, potentially causing an increase in plasma fentanyl concentrations. This is most likely to occur in the case of a patient (e.g. foal) with its body in the bore of the magnet for a prolonged period; however, it is unlikely to cause a clinically important problem as the temperature of the patch will decrease when the patient is removed from the magnet.
    *Note*: Generally, there is *no* reason to remove a fentanyl patch, unless it contains metal and is located within the bore of the magnet.
- Due to the noise level (~110 dB), MRI-compatible headphones or earplugs should be worn by staff remaining in the MRI room.
  - Placing cotton in patient ears reduces noise stimulation and the risk of auditory damage.

## III   MRI scanning room equipment

- To avoid accidental damage when moving the horse into the MRI room and positioning it in the scanner, all anesthetic equipment should be strategically placed out of the way beforehand.
- Depending on manufacturer specifications and limitations, the equipment may later be moved into position for use; however, non-MRI compatible equipment should remain as far away as possible from the scanner.

A   MRI-*safe* equipment

- Implies there is no *safety* hazard; however, there is no guarantee of correct function or lack of interference with the scanner.

B   MRI-*compatible* equipment

- Implies that the equipment is MRI safe, functions normally, and does not interfere with imaging, if instructions are adhered to.
- Thus, MRI compatible monitoring equipment is recommended, as this allows the anesthetist to remain in the MRI room with the monitoring equipment and directly assess the horse at all times. *Whether or not the latter is allowed will depend on guidelines in use by the practice.*

C   Use of non-ferrous anesthetic equipment

- Specialized non-ferrous anesthetic machines and pneumatic ventilators, and aluminum oxygen cylinders should be used.
- Alternatively, oxygen may be piped from a central source.
- The patient table and attachments must be constructed of non-ferrous material.
  - Table padding must be of appropriate dimensions (see Chapter 18) while allowing the correct height for matching up to the magnet when moving the area of interest into the bore, in the case that the height of the table is not adjustable.

D   Use of ferromagnetic equipment

- Because the magnetic field decreases in strength with distance from the bore, in general, ferromagnetic equipment may be safely placed outside the 5 G line; however, this boundary will differ based on the magnet strength and shielding.
  - Regardless of Gauss-line boundaries, equipment outside this line should be secured to a wall to prevent accidental crossing into the magnetic field.
  - Because the risk of interference with imaging equipment remains, the effect of ferromagnetic equipment should be considered when troubleshooting image degradation.
  - If ferromagnetic equipment is being considered for use in the MRI scanning room, the manufacturer of both the MRI unit and equipment should be consulted before use.
- Ferromagnetic or non-MRI compatible monitoring equipment and fluid pumps may be used if located outside the scanning room (e.g. in the control room) using extensions adapted for that purpose.
  *Note*: If the anesthetist has located in the control room, he/she should have visual access to the patient and monitors at all times, and make intermittent hands-on evaluation of the patient between scans.

## IV   Patient preparation

- Planning is key to success when anesthetizing a horse for an MRI. Designation of staff roles during preparation, movement into the MRI room, and patient positioning is necessary to produce high-quality images in a safe and timely manner.

- An anesthetic duration greater than 90 minutes has been associated with a ninefold increase in the incidence of myopathy, and most MRIs are reported to last 110 minutes. Therefore, detailed attention to positioning, padding, and preventing motion that result in repeat scans is paramount.
- Due to size limitations within the imaging portion of the closed-bore magnet, MRI is limited to the head and limbs of most adult horses.
  - Limbs up to and including the carpus and tarsus are commonly imaged, and possibly the stifle and cranial neck in select horses.
  - Individual limitations that should be considered prior to imaging include limb length, thoracic width and depth, hindquarters width, and neck length.
- Enquire with the owner to confirm the absence of *ferromagnetic devices* or *implants*.
- *Shoes* must be removed from *all* feet of horses entering the MRI room.
  - Radiographs should be performed to ensure that there are no nail fragments in the hoof wall that may induce an artifact when imaging the foot.
  - Debris on the hoof wall that may lead to artifact must be removed.
- A preanesthetic physical examination should be performed, and further diagnostic tests performed as deemed necessary.
- A catheter should be placed in the jugular vein that will be uppermost when the patient is positioned for the scan. If the head is to be imaged, fluid line extensions should be attached to the jugular catheter, or a hindlimb catheter can be placed for easy access once the patient is anesthetized.
- After anesthetic induction, an endotracheal tube with a bell-type silicone connector should be placed, or a tube with a non-ferromagnetic metal adapter.
- The patient should be positioned on the padded table while outside the MRI room using a hoist and hobbles.
- Ensure that ferromagnetic objects are removed from the patient or table (e.g. halter, hobbles).
- A lubricant may be applied to the table (e.g. *diluted dish soap or a silicone-based shine product*) immediately prior to induction to facilitate movement of the patient during positioning once in the MRI room.
- A sterile urinary catheter is placed. A closed system for collection of urine is essential in the MRI suite to avoid hazards to personnel resulting from urine spillage onto the floor, and especially to avoid urine leakage into the MRI unit.
- Ensure that the patient's anesthetic depth is appropriate prior to moving the table into the MRI suite and during positioning.

## V  Patient positioning

- The area of interest is manually moved into the magnet, potentially using ropes to pull the legs.
  *Note: It is important that the dependent eye is protected as the horse is moved.*
- Placing the horse in lateral recumbency, with the limb to be imaged on the dependent aspect to minimize movement during image acquisition is routine at some facilities.
  - However, depending on the imaging system, and when imaging the proximal portion of the limb, the upper limb may be more easily positioned into isocenter.

- o A plan should be rehearsed to ensure rapid positioning and image acquisition.
- Depending on the area of interest, and size limitations of the individual horse, the limb may be pulled tightly with a rope and tied to the wall. This may allow the area of interest to reach isocenter.
  - o However, too much traction may induce artifact secondary to respiratory or cardiac motion, particularly when applied to the upper limb (see Box 35.1).
- Limb movement may be minimized with padding and sandbags; however, this needs to be done properly to avoid injury.
- The nondependent limb, which is also in the core of the magnet, must be padded and supported in a parallel placement.
  - o Postanesthetic neuropathy and myopathy has been reported in the nondependent limb.
- The table in the magnet core has limited room for padding, but, if possible, padding should be used for any part of the patient in contact with the scanner/gantry.
- If the proximal *hindlimbs* are the areas of interest, ensure that the tail is tucked into the gantry.
- The limbs remaining outside the gantry should be appropriately placed, padded, and supported.
  - o Postanesthetic neuropathy and myopathy has been reported following MRI in limbs not being scanned, outside the gantry (see Chapter 18).
- When the *thoracic limbs* are the area of interest, particularly the carpus, the patient is pulled maximally into the magnet. Attention should be directed at the periphery of the bore to ensure that the jugular veins and trachea are not compressed.
  *Note*: A custom cutout of the gantry will minimize such complications. In addition, this cutout permits the horse to be positioned further into isocenter to ensure successful carpal studies in shorter limbed horses. A narrow bore (60 cm) MRI is too small to allow an adult horse to be pulled deep into the magnet. (see Figure 35.2)
- When the pelvic limbs are in the magnet, ensure that the hindquarters are not pressed against the gantry resulting in muscle compression.
  *Note*: This is only going to be an issue if the gantry is modified to allow the horse to be pulled in deep into the magnet as described above.
  - o This is more likely to be a problem when imaging the proximal portion of the limbs of short-legged horses with heavily muscled hindquarters.

---

**Box 35.1   Avoid Excessive Traction on Limbs**

Excessive traction on the limb must be avoided. In the author's opinion, which is based on clinical experience, excessive stretching of the limb seems to be associated with clinically important nociception, presumably from stretching of peripheral nerves. This conclusion is based on the observed increase in arterial blood pressure which is directly associated with the application of traction, and the blood pressure returns to pre-stretching values once traction is removed.

In addition, traction on the limb may be associated with the development of neuropathy or myopathy. Pelvic limb neuropathy has been reported following an MRI in horses, and traction on the limb was suggested as a risk factor. The author has also witnessed *femoral* neuropathy in a limb that was stretched.

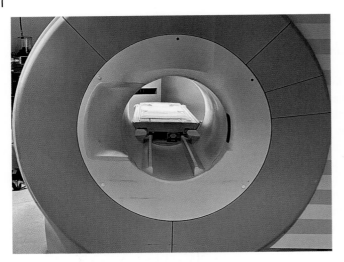

Figure 35.2   Custom cutout of the gantry of a 3.0 Tesla MRI allows for the horse to be positioned further into isocenter for imaging of proximal portions of the limbs.

## VI   Anesthesia and monitoring

### A   Anesthesia (see Chapter 21)

- The anesthetic plan is based on the personal preference of the anesthetist. ET intubation is advised to provide the ability for intermittent positive pressure ventilation (IPPV) to control respiratory motion and to guarantee airway patency.
- Partial intravenous anesthesia (PIVA) is an appropriate option as this will minimize the likelihood of sudden awakening in comparison to inhalant-only anesthesia. TIVA (e.g. *Triple drip*) may be considered for shorter scans.

### B   Monitoring

- Monitoring should be employed to the same standard as used in the surgical suite. (see Chapter 19)
- Monitoring the horse remotely from the control room is *not* ideal, and the author recommends that the patient be monitored directly in the MRI suite, but this may not be an option depending on the guidelines of the institution/practice. The patient should be evaluated *constantly* for the following reasons:
  - To avoid motion that may alter image quality if the horse were to move, as this necessitates repeating the imaging which adds to the duration of anesthesia.
  - To avoid catastrophic damage to the MRI equipment if the horse thrashes with its limbs in the bore.
  
  *Note*: If a horse falls from the table in the MRI suite there is no hoist access to reposition the horse on the table, so it would have to be manually dragged out of the room to be hoisted.
- Be prepared to stop IPPV briefly for specific scans (T2-weighted) to minimize respiratory motion artifact.

*Blood pressure*
- A catheter should be placed in an accessible artery once the horse is positioned.
- Ensure that the transducer is non-ferrous.

*Urine collection*
- A closed collection urinary catheter system should be placed, and patency ensured frequently by visual confirmation that there is no leakage around the urinary catheter that might cause urine to flow into the magnet.
  - The author places a towel around the penis or vulva to ensure that urine does not leak into the gantry.
  - It is also important to check that the penis is not trapped between the patient table and MRI unit during positioning.

*Assessing anesthetic depth*
- When the head is the area of primary interest, access is limited for assessing eye reflexes. A padded stick may be used to evaluate the palpebral reflex, in addition to assessing depth through other avenues such as anal tone.
- End-tidal anesthetic gas analysis is advised as a guide to estimating anesthetic depth.

*ECG*
- ECG electrodes are placed close together to avoid artifacts, but RF pulses can interfere with the signal making ECG evaluation difficult and nondiagnostic during some scans.
- As mentioned under MRI safety, MRI-compatible ECG electrodes and cables must be used, avoid coiling of cables within the magnet and avoid having cables in direct contact with the patient by using padding.

*Pulse oximetry*
- Non-ferromagnetic cables should be used.
- Sequence interference and equine tongue dimensions limits the use of pulse oximetry.
- When scanning the head, avoid coiling of the cable within the bore.

*Temperature*
- As the body temperature is likely to decrease, the horse should be covered with a blanket to minimize heat loss.

## VII  MRI contrast media

- Gadolinium-based contrast enhanced MRI is rarely performed in horses but has been reported in brain, laryngeal, and septic arthritis studies.
- Gadolinium contrast agents are considered safe with lower reaction rates than *iodinated* CT (computed tomography) and radiography contrast agents.
- Several gadolinium agents have higher than normal physiologic osmolality, but the small volume administered IV (~50 ml/horse, 0.02–0.04 mmol/kg) creates only a small, transient increase in plasma osmolality.
- In horses, transient decreases in blood pressure immediately following IV administration have been reported, but no other adverse effects have been documented.

- MRI contrast agents are considered non-nephrotoxic.
  - Nevertheless, nephrogenic systemic fibrosis (NSF) is an adverse effect reported to occur on rare occasions in human beings with preexisting renal disease.
  - Although NSF has not been reported in veterinary species, preanesthetic renal value screening is advised prior to gadolinium contrast.

## Low-field standing MRI

### I Introduction

- Standing, low-field MRI (0.27-T) has become more available for use in horses.
- This open unit is mounted vertically at floor level; therefore, imaging is limited to the distal limbs (from foot to carpal or tarsocrural joints). It features a "U" or "C" shape design which can be raised or lowered, and the horse is standing as the magnet coil is placed around the area to be imaged. (see Figure 35.3)
- The unit should ideally be located in a quiet area to avoid stimulating the sedated horse.

#### A Advantages of low-field MRI

  - It eliminates the need and risk of general anesthesia.
  - It is less ferromagnetic, thus permitting the use of standard monitoring equipment.
  - It is easy to position and access the patient.
  - Less manpower is required.

#### B Disadvantages of low-field MRI

  - The areas imaged are limited to the distal limbs.
  - The risk of motion artifact increases as sites imaged move proximally from the foot; however, anti-motion software may assist with this problem.

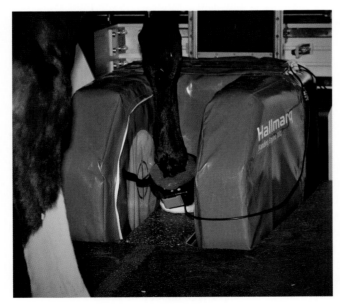

Figure 35.3   Low-field MRI used for imaging of standing horses.

○ There may be difficulty in maintaining appropriate patient restraint and getting the horse to stand still for motionless imaging. However, excessive sedation may induce tremors, knuckling, swaying, ataxia, or even recumbency, and pose a danger to staff. On the other hand, light sedation may result in the horse being hypersensitive to stimulation and cause too much movement.
  – Thus, acquisition of the images with a standing MRI unit may potentially be more time consuming, depending on the sites imaged and patient cooperation.
○ Success depends to a great extent on the experience of the anesthetist and appropriate patient selection.

## II   MRI safety

- Despite the low-field strength (e.g. 0.27 Tesla) the same safety precautions are adhered to as with high-field MRI.

## III   Patient preparation

- A pre-sedation physical examination should be performed.
- *Tip*: *It is recommended to place the patient in a freshly bedded stall prior to scanning to encourage urination before entering the MRI room.*
- The patient is prepared in much the same way as for a high-field MRI; however, shoes need only be removed from the foot that is being imaged, and the halter may remain in place.

*Patient limitations*
  ○ Patient selection is important in achieving successful sedation and image quality with a standing MRI. It may be difficult to maintain an appropriate level of sedation in a fractious or stressed horse.
  ○ Safety must be a priority because imaging is often performed in a confined space.
  ○ Consider the horse's level of lameness and pain, as this may alter its ability to stand motionless on the affected limb long enough to acquire images.
    *Note:* Do not perform local blocks to the affected area in an effort to assist analgesia and weight bearing cooperation for the scan. Seek input from the radiologist prior to such decisions due to the induced image artifact from the injection.

## IV   Standing sedation for image acquisition

- Management of standing sedation is based on personal preference and experience. (see Chapter 20)
  ○ However, a good sedation protocol and well-trained staff are mandatory to obtain diagnostic images.
- $\alpha_2$–adrenergic agonists are the mainstay of sedation protocols.
  ○ Increased urine production is an adverse effect which can induce not only hazardous floor conditions but risk damaging expensive equipment.
    *Tip: It may be best to take breaks during the imaging process to allow the horse to rest in a freshly bedded stall to encourage it to urinate.*

- In order to protect the equipment, the horse should be sedated appropriately prior to moving the area of interest into position.
- The goal is to provide reliable sedation with minimal ataxia, and adequate analgesia, if required.
  - A horse undergoing a standing MRI may require minimal or no analgesia. But if the horse is in pain, it will likely require analgesia to enable it to stand on the affected limb for imaging.
  - However, the addition of an analgesic (e.g. *morphine*, *hydromorphone* IM) with or without *acepromazine* will augment sedation and decrease the need for $\alpha_2$ agonists, potentially decreasing the degree of ataxia.
  - These drugs (e.g. *acepromazine + morphine*) can be administered IM 30–45 minutes prior to removing the horse from its stall (see Chapter 20).
- A dedicated handler should remain at the head of the horse. A second person is necessary to run the MRI and maintain communication throughout the procedure (they are in the same MRI scanning room as the horse).
- Blinders and ear plugs are options to reduce stimulation once the horse is sedated.

### A Concerns in standing sedation

  - Personnel safety is a priority, and the anesthetist should assume responsibility for this.
  - A good rule of thumb is to plan for the worst.
  - Have escape routes planned, and a skilled handler to manage the horse in a stressful situation.
  - Consider the footing in the facility. If the horse falls it must be able to get up safely.

## V Monitoring

- Monitoring should be employed at the same standard as used in any standing procedure (see Chapter 20). At the minimum, manual evaluation of heart rate and rhythm and respirations is advised.
- Documentation of drugs and recorded timeline of scan durations, notation of changing sites and breaks should be included.
- A steady plane of sedation is ensured through an attentive handler/anesthetist and communication with the technologist running the scanner to permit timely repeat of drug boluses if a CRI is not being used.
- Abnormal events should be documented and addressed accordingly.
- If the scan is an outpatient procedure, the patient should be recovered appropriately from sedation prior to release for trailering.
- Administration of an alpha$_2$ antagonist (e.g. *tolazoline HCl*) may be indicated. (see Chapter 20)

## Computed tomography

- CT is an imaging technique that is becoming more commonly performed with the availability of conventional recumbent anesthetized systems and modifications being made to standard CT units to obtain standing scans of the horse's head.

- Units designed specifically for imaging the distal aspects of the limbs, the head, and potentially the neck, of the *standing* horse are also becoming available.
- Equipment limitations dictate areas that can be imaged, but the head, cranial cervical spine and distal limbs can be imaged in the adult horse.

## I  Introduction

- Equine CT is often limited by the need for general anesthesia, which may put horses at a greater risk during recovery, especially those with *neurologic* disease.
  - The benefits of performing a CT should outweigh the associated risks.
  - The advantages of having the horse anesthetized for the CT are that it eliminates motion artifact, avoids risk of injury to handlers maneuvering a sedated ataxic horse into position, and decreases risk of radiation exposure to anesthesia staff.
- Custom or specialized CT scanners for obtaining images in the *standing* sedated horse may avoid risks associated with general anesthesia and recovery, and in addition, permit a follow-up CT without assuming these risks.

## II  Radiation safety

- CT imaging produces a large amount of ionizing radiation and the potential for scatter.
- During image acquisition, the anesthetist monitoring the horse under general anesthesia should temporarily move to a shielded area, returning to the horse's side for monitoring between scans.
- During a standing CT, the horse handler should remain as far as possible from the radiation source, use a mobile shield, and wear appropriate protection.
- Monitoring radiation exposure of staff, particularly those restraining horses for standing CT, is essential.
- The radiation safety principle, ALARA (as low as reasonably achievable) should be followed.

## III  Equipment and facilities

### A  Conventional recumbent CT under general anesthesia

- The closed construct bore diameter (common ranges 30–90 cm) limits imaging regions in adult horses to the head, neck (up to C4 or C6 depending on the size of the horse), and limbs up to the elbow and stifle joints.
- A commercially available horse CT table or one that is custom-made is required. (see Figure 35.4)
  - The equine CT table may be coupled to integrate with the standard table drive and advance automatically. Alternatively, the CT gantry may advance onto a stationary table.
  - The equine CT table should ideally be adjustable and padded with the ability for limb support as with any recumbent horse. (see Chapter 18)

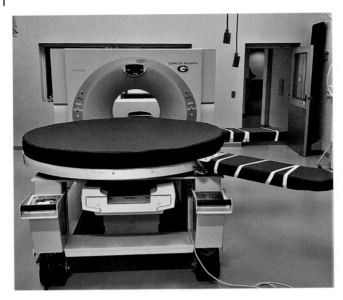

Figure 35.4   Table used for equine CT under general anesthesia.

- Ropes and positioning pads should be available.
- Physical efforts to move the table and the horse, in addition to positioning alterations once on the table are to be expected.

### B   Standing CT

- Although the risk of complications associated with general anesthesia is eliminated, a heavily sedated horse, or more likely a sedated neurologic horse, may fall and injure itself, personnel, or equipment.
- The flooring in the preparation area, CT room and on the platform should be constructed of non-slip material, which will allow the horse to gain sufficient traction in order to stand back up if it were to fall.
- The main challenge to the anesthetist is the need to limit motion by maintaining an adequate plane of sedation, and at the same time, avoiding heavy sedation which may result in ataxia, hindering image quality or causing recumbency. It could be catastrophic if a horse were to become recumbent in a confined space!
- The stocks should be designed with one open side or have the ability to quickly swing open the side bar. (see Figure 35.5)
  - The horse handler/anesthetist should have an escape route planned.
- Blindfolds or hoods with blinders should be available for use in select horses to aid positioning and to limit distraction-induced motion.
- Sandbags should be available for placement on the neck to limit motion during image acquisition. (see Figure 35.6)

*Performing a head CT in a modified, adapted standard CT scanner:*
- The horse stands in a pit in front of the gantry (reversed presentation) on a platform that is coupled to the standard CT table to drive the horse into the MRI bore. (see Figure 35.7)

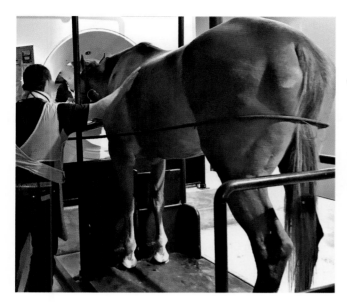

Figure 35.5   Stocks used for CT in the standing horse with open side.

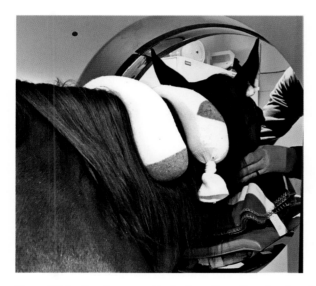

Figure 35.6   Sandbags used to limit motion of head and neck during image acquisition.

- ○ The platform is mounted on air skates to allow smooth frictionless movement when the table moves the area to be scanned into the bore.
- ○ A removable riser platform should be available to accommodate shorter horses being positioned into the bore for imaging.
- ○ An air compressor for driving the platform is required. The compressor is loud and may stimulate the horse, so it needs to be activated slowly, and ear plugs may be helpful to limit stimulating the horse. Distracting the horse during this maneuver with whistling or other technique may be helpful.

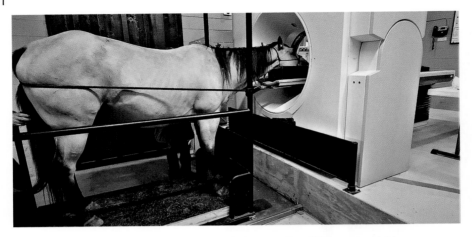

Figure 35.7   Platform for horse to stand on during standing CT image acquisition.

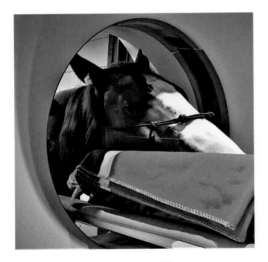

Figure 35.8   Horse's head in CT gantry.

- A V-shaped trough should be available to cradle the head in a motionless position. (see Figure 35.8)
- A rope halter is recommended to avoid artifact, and to assist in positioning the head throughout imaging.

## IV   Patient preparation for CT

- Horseshoes and nails need to be removed only if they will be in the field of view.
- An IV catheter should be placed in anticipation of repeat injections in the case of standing sedation, and potentially IV fluid or contrast administration during any CT.
  - For lateral recumbency, catheter placement in the non-dependent jugular vein is advised.

- The mouth should be rinsed thoroughly prior to imaging the head to avoid artifact from debris in the oral cavity.
- Preanesthetic examination should include neurologic status, and additional testing should be performed based on the horse's health.
  - Consider evaluating hydration and renal status if contrast is expected to be used.

### A Conventional recumbent CT

- Patient preparation is as for any general anesthetic event. (see Chapter 21).

### B Standing head CT in a modified scanner

- Patient selection is the key to success.
- Limitations of height and neck length should be considered.
- Horses with a severe head tilt and ataxia or of excitable behavior may not be amendable to safe sedation for a successful standing CT.
- Sedate the patient as close as possible to the stocks of the CT to limit walking distance, especially if the horse is ataxic.
- Changing to a rope halter prior to entering the CT area is advised.

## V Anesthesia, sedation, and image acquisition

### A Conventional recumbent CT under general anesthesia

- Because of the relatively short duration of anesthesia for a CT (usually less than 60 minutes) and the inconvenience of attaching the horse to an anesthetic machine, TIVA is commonly employed for maintenance using "*Triple drip*". (see Chapter 21)
  - However, inhalational anesthesia or PIVA may also be used.
- It is prudent to perform ET intubation if the horse is anesthetized using TIVA to ensure a patent airway, and oxygen can be supplied.

### B Standing CT of the head

- Management of standing sedation is based on clinician preference and experience. (see Chapter 20).
- However, a good sedation protocol and well-trained staff is mandatory to obtain quality images safely for patient and personnel.
- Acquisition of images should be rapid, depending on sites imaged, equipment and patient cooperation.
- Several people are needed to position the sedated horse completely forward in the stocks to ensure successful placement of the head in the bore to capture the area of interest.
- The rear gate of the stocks is closed once the horse is settled.
- With smaller horses, the stocks may be too large relatively and allow a patient to back up, away from the scanner. In such situations, a rope may be placed around the rump and held taut by the handler to keep the horse forward in the stocks to maintain the appropriate position during image capture.

- ○ After appropriate sedation, the horse's head is placed in the extended position into a V-shaped trough on the CT table. A weight, such as a sandbag, may be placed on the neck to minimize motion during image acquisition. (see Figure 35.6)
- ○ A handler remains present in the trench, adjacent to the horse's shoulder, throughout the procedure to monitor depth and patient reaction. The handler maintains an appropriate level of sedation, calms the horse during platform motion and the noise of air compressor release, and assists in emergency release if a horse thrashes in the confined space.

## VI  Monitoring

- Monitoring should be employed tot the same standard as used in the surgical suite for anesthetized horses or as for any standing sedated procedure. (see Chapters 19 and 20)
- A dedicated anesthetist should be present to ensure the depth of anesthesia or sedation is kept as stable as possible to avoid any motion that may alter image quality or result in repeat scans. Catastrophic damage to the CT equipment or the patient could result if a horse becomes light and thrashes. Furthermore, avoiding the patient falling from the table or collapsing from the standing platform is paramount, particularly if the flooring is not optimal for recovering and there is no hoist available.
- The head of the patient should be accessible for monitoring eye reflexes.

## VII  CT contrast media

- *Iodinated* contrast media are commonly administered during CT imaging.
  - ○ Low osmolar iodinated contrast media are two to three times higher in osmolarity than normal plasma.
- Intraarterial injection may be indicated for limb studies. In that case, catheter size is important to avoid high flow rates that might induce vascular trauma or rupture.
  - ○ An 18-gauge catheter using a flow rate of 2 ml/s is recommended.

### A  Adverse effects

- ○ Adverse effects are uncommon in horses, and are generally mild and do not require treatment. The incidence is comparable to what is reported for human beings.
- ○ More severe adverse events include anaphylactoid reactions, seizures, hypo- and hypertension, and bronchospasm. (see Chapter 38)
- ○ Reported delayed adverse effects in horses include hyperthermia and urticaria or facial edema, which usually resolve without treatment; however, anti-inflammatories or antihistamines may be indicated on occasion.
- ○ Organ-specific adverse events have not been reported in horses.
- ○ Intravascular volume status should be evaluated to avoid the horse becoming dehydrated.
- ○ Extravasation of contrast medium may not cause a problem, or may result in swelling, erythema, and pain that peak up to 48 hours following injection. Rarely, skin ulceration and necrosis develop.

# Radiographic myelography

- Radiographic myelography is the technique of administering a water soluble, nonionic iodinated contrast agent into the subarachnoid space prior to radiography. It is the most accurate test in horses to diagnose cervical vertebral stenotic myelopathy.
  - There is a continued need for equine radiographic myelography because currently available CT and MRI equipment are not capable of imaging the caudal neck of most adult horses or of obtaining flexed views.

## I Introduction

- The myelographic study should be performed quickly, not only to reduce recumbency time, but because radiographic contrast visibility may decrease with time through dilution and reabsorption, ultimately limiting study quality and diagnostic value.
- Anesthesia of equids for radiographic myelography presents challenges for the anesthetist, including:
  - Horses presenting for myelography have mild to severe neurologic disease with correlating proprioceptive deficits and ataxia that present an additional danger/risk to the animal and staff throughout the induction and recovery phases.
  - The reported incidence of adverse events during myelography and including recovery is 12.9%.
    - Larger volumes of contrast and longer anesthetic duration increase the risk of adverse events.
    - The limited padding under the patient, particularly when the horse is placed on the floor or when a myelogram table is used, may increase the risk of developing myopathy and peripheral neuropathy.
  - Multiple position changes result in the need for:
    - Constant vigilance to protect the eye, IV catheter, and fluid line.
    - Ensuring ET tube safety and patency (if used).
    - Protection of anesthetic equipment.

## II Radiation safety

- Radiography is associated with the production of ionizing radiation and the potential for scatter.
- The same safety procedures as described for CT should be implemented.

## III Patient and procedure preparation

- Planning with all personnel involved to ensure safety and efficiency is advised.
  - To expedite the procedure, designated roles should be assigned for anesthetic preparation, induction, movement into the imaging area, patient padding and positioning, and image acquisition.

- Supplemental oxygen, intubation supplies and the ability to ventilate (e.g. demand valve) should be available.
- Preparation for potential complications, such as management of seizures, and having the ability to re-anesthetize during recovery in the event of an emergency are recommended.
- Preanesthetic evaluation should include age, temperament, and the degree of ataxia.
  - Further diagnostic tests may be performed as deemed necessary.
  - Survey radiographs may be requested on the standing horse, and particular care must be taken with ataxic patients.
- A catheter should be placed in the non-dependent jugular vein.
- The horse should be brought to the induction area prior to premedication, if possible, because of the worsening of ataxia once sedated.
  - Horses that are severely ataxic or recumbent may have to be anesthetized in a stall equipped with a hoist, and returned to the stall for recovery.
  - Select cases may benefit from sling support to assist recovery.
- Adverse reactions associated with general anesthesia or myelographic technique (e.g. inadvertent needle puncture of the spinal cord during removal of cerebrospinal fluid (CSF), reactions associated with the administration of iodinated contrast material, or secondary to manipulation of the head and neck) may occur during the procedure or during recovery.

## IV   Anesthesia, monitoring, and procedure

### A   Anesthesia

- General anesthesia is necessary for cervical myelography. Clinician preference, patient factors, facility design and variability in procedure duration are some factors that may drive the decision for inhalant vs. TIVA protocols.
  - Due to positioning changes, frequent disconnection of the breathing circuit is required. This increases personnel exposure to the anesthetic if inhalation anesthesia is used.
- If the patient is intubated, overinflation of the endotracheal (ET) tube cuff and manipulation of the neck for positioning to obtain flexed views are risk factors for damage to the tracheal mucosa. Furthermore, such manipulation may result in occlusion of the ET tube. Therefore, the neck should be returned to the neutral position after image capture. *Author's preference: For the aforementioned reasons the author does not routinely intubate horses during myelograms and prefers to use a TIVA protocol, but has the necessary supplies available to maintain an airway if needed in an emergency. Additionally, many radiologists prefer to have the ET tube removed for ventrodorsal views.*
- With the possible exception of cisternal puncture, the patient receives minimal noxious stimulation; therefore, maintaining a light plane of anesthesia is acceptable.

### B   Monitoring

- Monitoring is routine as for any anesthetized procedure (see Chapter 19).
- At minimum, the depth of anesthesia, heart rate, pulse quality and rhythm, respiratory rate, pulse oximetry, arterial blood pressure should be monitored.

○ Adverse events reported during myelography and recovery may include generalized and focal seizures, muscle fasciculations, hyper- or hypotension, cardiac arrhythmias, decreased cardiac contractility, bronchospasm, and pulmonary edema.
  – Corneal ulceration may occur if the horse thrashes around during a seizure.
○ Larger volumes of contrast and longer anesthetic duration increased the risk of adverse events.

## C Procedure

○ Although the anesthetist is dedicated to monitoring the patient, assistance with maneuvering, may be involved.
○ After aseptic preparation, anesthetic depth is ensured, and CSF collection is followed by contrast administration.
  – The *head should then be elevated* to prevent cranial migration of contrast material.
  – A table that can position the horse in reverse Trendelenburg position can be used to assist with head elevation and spread of the contrast material caudally.
○ Lateral images of the neck in a neutral position are often obtained initially to diagnose an obvious lesion which may negate the need to further manipulate the neck and exacerbate a lesion.
○ The physical effort required for myelography will vary based on the facility and available equipment, but manual assistance for flexed and extended "stressed" views is necessary while ensuring careful manipulation to avoid exacerbation of any dynamic component to the compression.
  – Positioning changes may be necessary to acquire ventrodorsal views.
○ A specialized table, standard table, or the floor may be used with the horse in lateral recumbency for the myelogram. Regardless, the best efforts for padding, eye lubrication and protection must be practiced, along with attention to limb positioning and support during the procedure. (see Chapter 18)
  – Radiolucent cushions should be available to aid positioning in true lateral for the duration of myelogram image acquisitions.
  – Efficient myelogram studies are encouraged with quick movement of the horse from the floor or myelogram table to an appropriate pad for recovery.

## V Myelographic contrast media

• Iodinated contrast media (e.g. Iohexol) 240–350 mg iodine/ml is administered intrathecally in equine myelography (volume 50 ml).
  *Note*: Contrast outside the range of 140–350 mg iodine/ml is contraindicated for intrathecal administration.
• Larger volumes of contrast medium increase the risk of adverse events.
• Only *non-ionic* iodinated products are appropriate for subarachnoid spaces to avoid minor alterations in blood pressure and heart rate.
• Adverse reactions to contrast material are infrequently reported in horses, but adverse renal events are reported in dogs, cats, and human beings (see CT contrast media adverse events section of this chapter).

- Additionally, adverse reactions to intrathecal injection of contrast may occur secondary to volume-induced changes in craniospinal pressure after removal of CSF, or CSF leakage secondary to dural and arachnoid puncture, or from direct injury to spinal cord from misplacement of spinal needle or neurotoxicity of iohexol.

## VI   Recovery

- Recovery in a dark quiet stall is recommended with the horse on a pad of appropriate dimensions and attention to limb placement and support. Assisted recovery is recommended if the facilities are available. A padded *helmet* may be used to decrease the risk of head injury.
    - ○ The patient should remain in the recovery stall until it is able to ambulate safely.
- Preparation for complications in recovery including generalized and focal seizures, muscle fasciculations, peripheral neuropathy or myopathy, blindness, hyperesthesia, dull mentation, stargazing, temporary worsened ataxia/neurologic signs and a prolonged recovery is recommended.

## Suggested Reading

Franci, P., Leece, E.A., and Brearley, J.C. (2006). Post anesthetic myopathy/neuropathy in horses undergoing magnetic resonance imaging compared to horses undergoing surgery. *Equine Vet. J.* 38: 497–501.

Moreno, K.L., Scallan, E.M., Friedeck, W.O., and Simon, B.T. (2020). Transient pelvic limb neuropathy following proximal metatarsal and tarsal magnetic resonance imaging in seven horses. *Equine Vet. J.* 52: 359–363.

Mullen, K.R., Furness, M.C., Johnson, A.L. et al. (2015). Adverse reactions in horses that underwent general anesthesia and cervical myelography. *J. Vet. Intern. Med.* 29: 954–960.

Nelson, B.B., Goodrich, L.R., Barrett, M.F. et al. (2017). Use of contrast media in computed tomography and magnetic resonance imaging in horses: techniques, adverse events and opportunities. *Equine Vet. J.* 49: 410–424.

## 36

# Anesthesia of Donkeys and Mules

### Anatomic, Physiologic, and Behavioral Differences
*Suzanne L. Burnham*

> *When I hear somebody talk about an animal being stupid, I figure it's a sure sign that the animal has outfoxed them.*
>
> –Tom Dorrance, (1910–2003) horse trainer

- The domestic horse, *Equus caballus*, and the domestic donkey, *Equus asinus*, share a common ancestor but are now morphologically distinct species. Although donkeys differ, but not greatly, from horses as regards the management of anesthesia, they have some anatomic, physiologic, and behavioral differences worth considering.

## I   Anatomical differences

- Besides the obvious anatomic differences of longer ears, smaller feet and a switch for a tail, donkeys have numerous other physical differences from horses, only some of which may be relevant to medical management and anesthesia for surgical interventions.

### A   Upper airway

- The anatomy and physiology of the horse airway have been studied extensively to better understand respiratory diseases of horses.
- The airways of donkeys have been typically investigated to better understand their vocalization, the *bray*, as a mere curiosity.
- Anatomic differences in the upper airways of donkeys (including the nasal passages, pharynx, and larynx) create challenges for passing endotracheal or nasogastric tubes.

### B   Endotracheal intubation (see Airway management Chapter 4)

- A slightly smaller tube relative to a horse of similar body mass is usually necessary.
- Intubation can be difficult in donkeys due to the relatively large pharyngeal diverticulum. (see Figure 36.1)

*Manual of Equine Anesthesia and Analgesia*, Second Edition. Edited by Tom Doherty, Alex Valverde, and Rachel A. Reed.

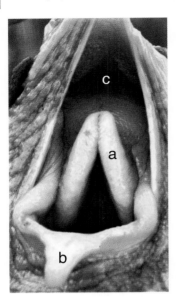

**Figure 36.1** Pharyngeal/laryngeal anatomy of the donkey; (a) arytenoid cartilages; (b) pointed epiglottis; (c) caudal pharyngeal mucosal diverticulum.

### C   Nasogastric intubation

- The *ventral meatus* of donkeys and mules is much narrower than that of a horse of similar size.
- After the nasogastric tube passes through the tight ventral nasal passage the neck will need to be flexed more intentionally than when tubing a horse. Otherwise, the tube is likely to become trapped in a dead-end pouch extending 4–6 cm in the caudal pharynx.
- This *pharyngeal diverticulum* extends caudally from the dorsal part of the pharyngeal recess that is proportionally larger in donkeys than in horses. (see Figure 36.1)
- Besides having a deeper pharyngeal recess compared with horses, the recess is situated at a different angle than the horse pharyngeal recess and has multiple additional saccules and ventricles in the vocal fold area.
- The *epiglottis* is shorter and more pointed on a donkey.
- The difference in the angle of the nasopharynx may cause difficulty in visualizing the trachea or guttural pouches with an endoscope.
- Excessive bleeding during passage of a nasogastric tube in donkeys has been reported as a common occurrence, probably due to the use of a too large diameter tube, excessive manipulation in the larynx/pharynx or to tube entrapment in the diverticulum. The tissue in this area is highly vascular and fragile.

### D   Jugular catheterization

- The jugular furrow is partially concealed in the donkey; the middle third is overlaid by a well-developed *cutaneous colli* muscle. The jugular vein is best approached in the lower third or upper third of the jugular furrow. (see Figure 36.2)
- Larger donkeys and draft mules have *thick skin* even in the jugular area.
- Slapping and jabbing is not recommended in donkeys or mules.
- Donkeys tend to lean into pressure. Quietly and slowly massage the skin with swab or hand. Place the needle against the skin and let the donkey lean into the needle stick.
  *Note: If you miss the vein in an untrained, highly agitated mule, you may not get a second chance.*

**Figure 36.2**  Jugular vein traveling deep to the *cutaneous colli* muscle.

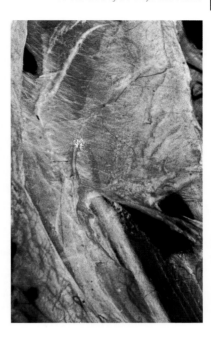

E   **Epidural anesthesia**

- The donkey's *sacrum*, like the horse, has five segments, but often the first coccygeal vertebra is fused to the sacrum with occlusion of the sacrococcygeal space.
- The donkey sacrum is curved dorso-ventrally, directing the spinal canal ventrally in the caudal segments. The sacral spines point backwards and rapidly decrease in length caudally.
- The first intercoccygeal space in the donkey is narrower than the second space. For the epidural approach, it is best to aim for the wider second intercoccygeal space directing the needle at an angle of 30° from the horizontal. The anesthetic can be injected cranially under the second coccygeal spine.
- In the horse, the anesthetic drug is injected in the first intercoccygeal or sacrococcygeal space at an angle of 30–90° from the horizontal.

F   **Miscellaneous anatomic differences**

*Distal colon*
- The haustrations in the distal colon differ from those of the horse.
- Haustrations are less defined in the donkey, and fecal material is already formed and dry there.

*Nasolacrimal duct*
- Location of the distal opening of the nasolacrimal duct is out on the lateral flare of the nostril rather than on the floor of the nostril.

*Dentition*
- Donkey teeth erupt on a slower schedule than horses making aging donkeys problematic.

*Vertebral formula*
- The vertebral formula for the *donkey*: C7, T18, L5, C15–17.
- The vertebral formula for the *horse*: C7, T18, L6, C15–21.

## II   Physiologic differences

- It can be difficult to assess the body condition of donkeys. A thin appearing donkey with prominent ribs and backbone can easily have a deposit of 5–8 in. of belly fat along the entire midline. Obese donkeys have very large fat deposits around the tail head, along the back, and on the crest of the neck.
- Obese donkeys may be prone to life-threatening *hyperlipemia* when stressed.
- Donkeys digest feed more efficiently than do horses.
- Transit time for feedstuffs is longer.
    - This may be clinically relevant when assessing fecal output after fasting for surgery.
- Differences in metabolism of glucose and glycogen in response to work and stress have been documented between donkeys and horses.

### A   Evolution in a desert environment

- Similar to camels, donkeys are physiologically desert-adapted animals. They can graze long distances from water and can digest coarse vegetation even after 24 hours without water.
- Donkeys have specialized their thermal and water regulatory mechanisms to make them more efficient for desert survival by conserving blood volume.
- Donkeys are similar to ruminants in that their hind gut acts to store water.
- During periods of water deprivation fecal water loss is reduced.
- Urine output is less than in the horses under normal conditions.
- Water balance, particularly plasma volume, is maintained during dehydration by reducing urine output, reducing evaporative water loss, and regulating body temperature. Thus, rather than concentrating their urine, donkeys simply produce less urine which will only be mildly concentrated compared to other species, even the *camel*.

    *Note*: Because of the aforementioned adaptations to water deprivation, changes in total protein are not a reliable indicator of dehydration in donkeys.

## III   General behavioral characteristics

- Donkeys and mules have a strong sense of self-preservation, tending to be suspicious of new things and people. When approaching a donkey or mule, it is advisable to take your time, move slowly and purposefully, give the donkey or mule some time to study you.
- Donkeys have a cautious, but curious nature. Given time, they will approach you.
- Donkeys will tend to avoid drinking water from unknown sources.
- Similar to cattle, a group of donkeys can be herded more easily than led.
- Donkeys roll in the sand and stand without shaking the sand and dirt off. This dirt turns to mud on the surface of the skin when it gets wet.

    *Tip: As you approach and stand near the shoulder or head, casually breathe in deeply and exhale long, slowly, and loudly, demonstrating that you are totally relaxed. Most of the time, it will relax your patient.*

## IV   Preoperative evaluation

- Emphasis should be placed on physical examination and recent history, and further testing should be based on the results of these findings.
- Clinical signs for colic, pneumonia, or severe pain are subtle when compared to a horse with the same condition.
- Donkeys tend to be stoic.
- Donkeys do not demonstrate pain the way horses do. For example, rather than display all the typical signs associated with visceral pain that a horse does, a donkey may lie down or stand with its head lowered. A donkey with respiratory distress or laminitis will do the same thing.
- Interpreting donkey clinical signs depends on understanding the following key differences.
  - A bright, alert, and responsive donkey will bring its ears forward and appear relaxed unless frightened by noise or threat.
  - A depressed donkey does not come for feed or attention, may have drooping head and ears, tense upper eyelids, and/or be lying down.
  - An agitated or painful donkey will give his tail a quick twitch.
  - Donkeys with severe colic typically do not thrash, roll, and bite at their sides.
  - Donkeys breathe shallowly when their lungs are congested and no rales are detectable until the donkey has been trotted for a few minutes.
  - A donkey's normal temperature is diurnally variable and will rise with an increase in ambient temperature.
  - *Normal* temperature range can be as low as 98.6 °F (37 °C) in the morning to 104 °F (40 °C) during a very hot day.
  - Because donkeys can tolerate dehydration by preserving plasma volume, total serum protein is not a reliable indicator of hydration status.

### A   Blood and chemistry differences

- Differences exist in some laboratory values between donkeys and horses. (see Chapter 2)
- Gamma glutamyl transferase activity is approximately two to three times higher in donkeys than horses.
- The donkey red blood cells (RBC) is larger than the horse RBC, resulting in the inaccurate interpretation of anemia.
- The coagulation parameters most commonly determined in equine practice are different in donkeys compared with horses. Thus, the use of normal reference ranges reported previously for healthy horses in donkeys might lead to a misdiagnosis of coagulopathy in healthy donkeys, and unnecessary treatments in sick donkeys.

## Suggested Reading

Burnham S (2002) Anatomical differences of the donkey and mule. Proceedings of the AAEP 102–109.

Jamdar, M.N. and Ema, A.N. (1982). A note on the vertebral formula of the donkey. *Brit. Vet. J.* 138: 209–211.

Kasirer-Izraely, H., Choshniak, I., and Shkolnik, A. (1994). Dehydration and rehydration in donkeys: the role of the hind gut as a water reservoir. *J. Basic Clin. Physiol. Pharmacol.* 5: 89–100.

Lindsay, F.E. and Clayton, H.M. (1986). An anatomical and endoscopic study of the nasopharynx and larynx of the donkey (Equus asinus). *J. Anat.* 144: 123–132.

Maloiy, G.M. (1970). Water economy of the Somali donkey. *Am. J. Physiol.* 219: 1522–1527.

Mendoza, F.J., Perez-Ecija, R.A., Monreal, L., and Estepa, J.C. (2011). Coagulation profiles of healthy Andalusian donkeys are different than those of healthy horses. *J. Vet. Intern. Med.* 25: 967–970.

Shoukry, M., Saleh, M., and Fouad, K. (1975). Epidural anesthesia in donkeys. *Vet. Rec.* 97 (23): 450–452.

Yousef, M.K., Dill, D.B., and Mayes, M.G. (1970). Shifts in body fluids during dehydration in the burro, *Equus asinus. J. Appl. Physiol.* 29: 345–349.

# Sedation and Anesthesia of Donkeys and Mules

*Tom Doherty*

## I Differences in drug dosages compared to horses

- Differences in metabolism and responses to anesthetics and analgesics have been documented between donkeys and horses, and among breeds of donkeys.
- In general, donkeys eliminate anesthetic drugs faster than do horses, and this would indicate more frequent dosing for a specific blood concentration to be maintained.
- Generally, for anesthetic drugs, donkeys, and mules require the dose of injectable drug to be ~30% higher than that used for the horse.
- In comparison with horses, mules administered *xylazine* (0.6 mg/kg, IV) exhibited less intense sedation and sedation was of shorter duration than in horses. Pharmacokinetic analysis indicated that the xylazine elimination half-life was shorter in mules (32 minutes) than in the horse (47 minutes), which may account for the shorter duration of sedation.
- *Acepromazine* (0.05 or 0.1 mg/kg, IV) was not associated with clinically important sedation or analgesia in donkeys.
- *Acepromazine* (0.05 mg/kg, IV) did not augment the sedating effects of *xylazine*.

## II Sedation of donkeys and mules

- The drugs used for sedation in horses can be used in donkeys and mules, but the dose usually has to be *higher* to achieve the same effect.
  *Note: it is of interest that donkeys commonly sneeze and/or rub their faces against a forelimb after IV administration of an $\alpha_2$ agonist.*

- Common IV doses of sedatives include:
  - *Xylazine* (1.0–1.5 mg/kg).
  - *Detomidine* (0.02–0.04 mg/kg).
  - *Dexmedetomidine* (0.002–0.005 mg/kg).
  - *Romifidine* (0.1–0.15 mg/kg).
  - *Morphine* (0.1 mg/kg, IV, 0.3 mg/kg, IM) in conjunction with an $\alpha_2$ agonist for more profound sedation.
  - *Butorphanol* (0.02–0.05 mg/kg, IV, IM) in conjunction with an $\alpha_2$ agonist for more profound sedation.

- Unruly donkeys and mules may have to be sedated with an IM injection to allow safe handling and jugular catheter placement.
    - For this purpose, IM doses of *xylazine* (3 mg/kg), *detomidine* (0.04 mg/kg) or *romifidine* (0.2 mg/kg) plus or minus *morphine* (0.3 mg/kg) will provide effective sedation in about 20–30 minutes.
    - Once approachable, IV sedation (e.g. $\alpha_2$ agonist) may be given, as needed.
    - *Detomidine gel:* A dose of 40 μg/kg has been recommended for producing mild to moderate sedation in donkeys when administered by the oral transmucosal route. However, this dose was *not* associated with mechanical hypoalgesia.

      Based on findings in horses, it is to be expected that *intravaginal* administrations of detomidine in the gel formulation would also be efficacious.

## III Induction of anesthesia

- As in the horse, a variety of drugs and drug combinations may be used.
- Induction drugs are to be administered following *heavy sedation with an $\alpha_2$ agonist.*
- The drug regimens outlined below are only intended for *short-duration* procedures.
- Doses are for IV administration.

*Ketamine* (2.5–3 mg/kg)
- Muscle relaxation is poor.
- Duration of surgical anesthesia is short (5–10 minutes).
- Premedication with *detomidine* or *romifidine* may give a slightly longer duration of surgical anesthesia than *xylazine* premedication.

*Ketamine* (2.5–3 mg/kg) + *benzodiazepine* (e.g. *diazepam/midazolam* 0.05–0.1 mg/kg)
- Improved muscle relaxation.
- Does not increase the duration of surgical anesthesia.

*Ketamine* (2.5 mg/kg) + *Propofol* (0.5–1.0 mg/kg)
- Propofol is used instead of a benzodiazepine.
- Provides a deeper plane of anesthesia.
- Improves muscles relaxation over ketamine alone.
- Duration of anesthesia (10–15 minutes).

*Propofol* (2.0 mg/kg)
- Provides 10–15 minutes of anesthesia.
- No analgesia with propofol.

*Alfaxalone* (2.0 mg/kg)
- Provides 10–15 minutes of anesthesia.
- No analgesia with *alfaxalone.*

*Thiopental* (5–8 mg/kg)
- Provides 10–20 minutes of anesthesia.
- Use lower end of dose range if animal is heavily sedated.
- No analgesia with *thiopental.*

*Tiletamine* + *zolazepam* (1–2 mg/kg)
- Use high end of dose range in smaller donkeys.
- Longer period of surgical anesthesia (up to 15 minutes) than with *ketamine* or ketamine and a benzodiazepine.

- ○ Good inductions.
- ○ Recoveries not as good as with *ketamine* but are acceptable.
  - – Reversal of *zolazepam* seems to improve recovery speed and quality (author's observations).

## IV  Maintenance of anesthesia

### A  Inhalational anesthetics

- ○ May be used in the same manner as in the horse.
- ○ There is no reason to believe that minimum alveolar concentration (MAC) values differ significantly from those of horses.

### B  Total intravenous anesthesia (TIVA)

- ○ *Xylazine* and *ketamine* in a solution of *guaifenesin* is the most commonly used combination (*Triple drip*).
- ○ *Guaifenesin* is used primarily for muscle relaxation.
- ○ Care must be taken to avoid overdosing with *guaifenesin*, especially when anesthetizing small donkeys.
  - – It is probably never necessary to use more than a 5% solution even in the largest mules, and the solution should be further diluted before use in small donkeys.

*Example of TIVA*: donkey (150–200 kg)
- ○ Induce anesthesia with *ketamine* (2.5 mg/kg)/*midazolam* (0.1 mg/kg) after sedation with *xylazine* (1.5 mg/kg).
- ○ Administer the triple combination, at a constant rate, for maintenance of anesthesia.
  - – A rough guide for a 45-minute procedure, is to put *xylazine* (2 mg/kg) and *ketamine* (3 mg/kg) in 0.5 l of Lactated Ringer's Solution (LRS) or 0.9% normal saline solution.
  - – Add 10–15 g of *guaifenesin*.
  - – If a longer duration of anesthesia is desired, the doses of *xylazine* and *ketamine* should be increased accordingly.

### C  Partial intravenous anesthetic (PIVA)

- ○ As described for the horse. (see Chapter 21)

## V  Recovery from anesthesia

- Donkeys and mules take longer to stand, preferring to wait until fully recovered.
- Recovery from anesthesia is usually smooth.
- The same care should be taken to protect the airway as in the horse.

## VI  Analgesia

- Evaluation of pain can be difficult in donkeys.
- Nevertheless, analgesics should be provided in the postoperative period for procedures that would be considered to cause pain in horses.

## A  Non-steroidal anti-inflammatory drugs (NSAIDs)

- May be used for the treatment of acute or chronic pain.
- May be combined with opioids for the treatment of acute pain.
- Generally, NSAIDs have a shorter elimination half-life than in the horse.
  - However, *carprofen* is metabolized more slowly in donkeys.
  - Miniature donkeys may metabolize some NSAIDs faster than do standard sized donkeys.

*Phenylbutazone*
- A dose of 2.2–4.4 mg/kg, IV q12 hrs, is typically used for donkeys.
- More frequent dosing may be necessary in miniature donkeys because clearance is more rapid.

*Flunixin meglumine*
- 1.1 mg/kg, IV, q12–24 hrs.

*Meloxicam*
- The mean residence time after an IV dose of 0.6 mg/kg in donkeys was extremely short (0.6 hrs vs. 9.6 hrs in the horse).
- Thus, the use of meloxicam in donkeys may not be plausible.

*Carprofen*
- 0.7–1.3 mg/kg, q24 hrs.

## B  Opioids

- Are safe to use at the horse doses for post-operative analgesia; however, there is little information on their efficacy in donkeys.
- The risk of ileus in equids administered opioids seems to be less than was previously though.

*Butorphanol*
- 0.02–0.05 mg/kg; IV, IM.
- Duration 30–60 minutes.

*Morphine*
- 0.1 mg/kg, IV; 0.3 mg/kg, IM.
- Duration two to four hours.

*Hydromorphone*
- 0.04 mg/kg, IV, IM.

*Buprenorphine*
- 0.006 mg/kg, IV, IM
- Duration four to six hours.

## Suggested Reading

Bidwell LA (2010) How to anesthetize donkeys for surgical procedures in the field. AAEP Proceedings 38–40.

Lizarraga, I., Sumano, H., and Brumbaugh, G.W. (2004). Pharmacological and pharmacokinetic differences between donkeys and horses. *Equine Vet. Educ.* 16: 102–112.

Lizarraga, I., Castillo-Alcala, F., Varner, K.M., and Robinson, L.S. (2016). Sedation and mechanical hypoalgesia after sublingual administration of detomidine hydrochloride gel to donkeys. *J. Am. Vet. Med. Ass.* 249: 83–89.

Lucas Castillo, J.A., Gozalo-Marcilla, M., Werneck Fonseca, M. et al. (2018). Sedative and cardiorespiratory effects of low doses of xylazine with and without acepromazine in Nordestino donkeys. *Equine Vet. J.* 50: 831–835.

Maney, J.K. and Dzikiti, B.T. (2019). Evaluation of xylazine-alfaxalone anesthesia for field castration in donkey foals. *Vet. Anaesth. Analg.* 46: 547–551.

Sinclair, M.D., Mealey, K.L., Matthews, N.S. et al. (2006). Comparative pharmacokinetics of meloxicam in clinically normal horses and donkeys. *Am. J. Vet. Res.* 67: 1082–1085.

## Donkey Pain Assessment Scales

*Machteld van Dierendonck and Thijs van Loon*

## I  Natural pain responses in donkeys

- Donkeys are not small horses with large ears.
  - Not anatomically, not physiologically and also not behaviourally.
  - Donkeys are by considered to be "stubborn" by people who are not familiar with them, but veterinarians and equine ethologists describe donkeys more as "*stoic.*"
- Donkeys are extremely social, even when ill, so they should always have a social companion with them, for instance when they are transported to a clinic, and also as far as possible, while in the clinic.
- A donkey's first response to a potential threat to its individual integrity is opposite to the response of a horse.
  - Donkeys normally *freeze* initially, then *fight*, then *flight*.
  - Donkeys are known to mask and hide their signs of stress, pain and/or unrest.
- The combination of these two different responses makes pain assessment in donkeys more difficult than in horses, even qualitatively.
- *Rule of thumb*: when you think a donkey is in pain *act*, because it might be an emergency.

## II  Pain assessment scales for acute pain in equids

### A  Current types of pain assessment scales

- There are several pain assessments methods for horses in a box, in hand, or ridden. (see Chapter 29)
- The current most valid, reliable, and objective assessment methods for acute pain in equids can be divided into two types:

*Composite Pain Scales (CPS)* consisting of:
  - Behavioral parameters (sometimes including locomotion scores).
  - Physiologic parameters.
  - Interactive parameters.

*Facial expression-based Pain Scales (FAP)* consisting of:
  - Head-related behavioral parameters.
  - Interactive parameters.

B   **Basic set-up of pain assessment scales**

- All elements are as quantitative as possible and divided into distinct simple descriptive scales (SDS), i.e. 0-1-2 or 0-1-2-3.
- They should be recorded within a certain fixed time frame.
- The SUM of ALL scores presents the final score for that moment.
    - In some methods an individual weighting factor can be appointed by multiplying a particular score.
- There are research-based *cut-off values* to differentiate between painful animals and non-painful animals.
    - The higher the score, the more likely the donkey is to be experiencing acute pain.

C   **Primary use and advantages of using pain scales**

- To determine a starting (pain) level for baseline reference.
- To allow "quantitative" evaluation of a treatment effect of an analgesic protocol.
- Pain scales can be used reliably in a clinical environment with multiple staff members over time due to high inter-observer reliability.
- Pain scales can be used to compare results over longer time periods (weeks to months).

## III   Donkey pain assessment scales for acute pain

- For donkeys with acute pain two objective acute pain assessment scales were developed.
    - The DCPS.
    - The Donkey Facial Expression-based Pain Scale.
- Both scales are validated for:
    - Acute orthopedic pain.
    - Acute colic.
    - Postoperative pain.
    - Acute head-related (dental, eye, head trauma) pain.
- The higher the score, the more likely the donkey is to be experiencing acute pain (maximum score cannot be reached since some parameters prevent others from being expressed).

*Note:* Due to the differences in behavior between horses and donkeys, pain scales developed for horses will most likely underestimate the intensity of pain that donkeys are experiencing.

A   **Donkey composite pain scale** (Donkey CPS)

- The *Equine Utrecht University Scale for Donkeys Composite Pain Assessment* the (*EQUUS-Donkey-COMPASS*).
    - The Equine version is the EQUUS-COMPASS.
- This scale includes:
    - Locomotion scores.
    - Physiologic parameters.
    - Behavioral parameters.
    - Interactive parameters.
- Scores for individual parameters range from 0 (no pain) to 3 (severe pain).

B   **Donkey facial expression-based pain scale**

   ○ The *Equine Utrecht University Scale of Donkey Facial Assessment of Pain* the (*EQUUS-Donkey-FAP*)
      – The Equine version is the EQUUS-FAP.
   ○ Scores for individual parameters range from 0 (no pain) to 2 (associated with severe pain).

C   **Which scale to use**

   ○ The EQUUS-DONKEY-COMPASS is most useful to assess:
      – Acute orthopedic pain.
      – Postoperative pain.
   ○ The EQUUS-DONKEY-FAP is most useful to assess:
      – Acute colic.
      – Head-related pain.

D   **How to carry out a COMPASS and/or FAP for acute pain manually**

   *Preparation (See Table 36.1)*
   ○ Preferably stay at a comfortable distance (3–5 m when possible) from where the donkey can be observed with as few distractions as possible.
   ○ If necessary, the donkey can be kept on the leading rein on a headcollar by a familiar handler.
   ○ Be aware that the donkey might *freeze*, as a coping mechanism, when an unfamiliar person is close by.
   ○ Check that the donkey is not resting upright/sleeping.
      – This can be done by making the donkey aware of your presence when starting.
   ○ Make sure that the donkey is not distracted (or as little as possible).
   ○ If necessary, wait a few minutes before the assessment starts, to allow the donkey to behave naturally and not to go into the *freeze* mode.
   ○ Keep doors and (field) gates closed.
   ○ Be aware of the weather conditions: in very warm and/or humid weather conditions, some behaviors (for instance flaring of nostrils) can be influenced.
   ○ Make sure all involved, including the donkey, are safe.
   ○ Do *not* use these pain scales in sedated or premedicated animals.

E   **How to carry out a COMPASS and/or FAP for acute pain by means of EPWA (the Equine Pain and Welfare App)**

   ○ The presented pain scales are incorporated in EPWA.
   ○ The app can be downloaded: www.epwa.nl
   ○ It is available free for Android and iOS phones.
      – Minimal requirements: Android v4.1 or higher; iPhone iOS v8.0 or higher.
   ○ For CPS and Facial expression-based Pain Scale assessments.
   ○ For "Veterinary personnel" and non-vet owners.
   ○ "Veterinary personnel": people which are reliable able to determine:
      – Heart Rate.
      – Respiratory rate.

**Table 36.1** Preparation details – EQUUS donkey composite pain assessment scale for acute pain.

- Preferably stay at a comfortable distance (3–5 m when possible) from where the donkey can be observed with as few distractions as possible.
  - If necessary, the donkey can be kept on the leading rein on a headcollar by a familiar handler.
  - Be aware of the chance that the donkey might *freeze* as a coping mechanism when an unfamiliar person is close by.
- Be sure the donkey is not "resting upright"/sleeping.
  - This can be done by making the donkey aware of your presence when starting.
- Make sure that the donkey is not distracted (or as little as possible).
- If needed, wait a few minutes before the assessment starts, to allow the donkey to behave naturally and not to go into the *freeze* mode.
- Keep doors and (field) gates closed.
- Be aware of the weather conditions: in very warm and/or humid weather conditions, some behaviors (for instance flaring of nostrils) can be influenced.
- Make sure all involved, including the donkey, are safe.

**Table 36.2** EQUUS donkey composite pain assessment scale for acute pain.

**PREPARATION** for scoring manually. (For detailed Instructions, see Table 36.1)

**During 5 minutes:**

**1. COUNT (for instance by tallying) or indicate directly (**Dark Gray 6 parameters)

**2. Observe from a distance** (Middle Gray 8 parameters)

**After 5 minutes: mark the most appropriate score for these two parts**

| | Pain Sounds | Score | Place to tally | Episodes of Tail Flicking (Excluding flicking to insects) | Score |
|---|---|---|---|---|---|
| | No audible signs of pain | 0 | | No tail flicking, tail in normal position | 0 |
| | Occasional teeth grinding or moaning (1 or 2 times/5 min) | 1 | | Occasional tail flicking (1 or 2 times/5 min) | 1 |
| | Frequent teeth grinding or moaning (3 or 4 times/5 min) | 2 | | Frequent tail flicking (3 or 4 times/5 min) | 2 |
| | Excessive teeth grinding or moaning (>4 times/5 min) | 3 | | Excessive tail flicking (>4 times/5 min) and/ or lifted or tucked in tail | 3 |
| | **(Attempts to) Lie down, rolling** (Excluding auto grooming) | **Score** | | **Looking or kicking at Abdomen** | **Score** |
| | Does not lie down or rests lying down | 0 | | Quietly standing, no kicking | 0 |
| | Attempts to lie down or is lying down <50% of the time | 1 | | Looking at abdomen | 1 |

*(Continued)*

Table 36.2   (Continued)

| | Score | | Score |
|---|---|---|---|
| Lying down >50% of the time | 2 | Lifting up hind legs, may kick 1x or 2x at abdomen | 2 |
| Lies down in abnormal position: on its side with stretched limbs or on its back and/or is repeatedly rolling | 3 | Extensive kicking at abdomen (>2 times/5 min) | 3 |

| **Pointing or pawing at floor** (with one or both front feet) | Score | **Respiratory Rate** | Score |
|---|---|---|---|
| Quietly standing, does not paw at floor | 0 | 12–28 breaths/min | 0 |
| Points limb | 1 | 29–32 breaths/min | 1 |
| Occasional pawing at floor (1 or 2 times/5 min) | 2 | 33–36 breaths/min | 2 |
| Extensive pawing at floor (>2 times/5 min) | 3 | > 36 breaths/min | 3 |

### OBSERVE FROM DISTANCE

| **Overall Appearance** | Score | **Posture** | Score |
|---|---|---|---|
| Alert and/or is interacting with companion/group | 0 | Quietly standing and/or one hind leg resting | 0 |
| Mildly "depressed" and/or restless and/or decreased interaction with group companion/group | 1 | Slightly tucked up abdomen and/or mild weight shifting | 1 |
| Moderately "depressed" and/or aggressive or no reaction to companion/group | 2 | Extremely tucked up abdomen and/or hunched back and/or stretching limbs/body and/or mild muscle tremors | 2 |
| Severely "depressed" | 3 | Sits on hind quarters and/or extreme muscle tremors | 3 |

| **Head Carriage** | Score | **Sweating** | Score |
|---|---|---|---|
| Ear base above withers or eats/drinks (from the ground) | 0 | No signs of sweating | 0 |
| Ear base at the level of the withers | 2 | Signs of sweating (wet spots visible, no droplets or streams) | 2 |
| Ear base below the withers | 3 | Excessive sweating (streams or droplets) | 3 |

| **Position of the Ears** (>75% of the time) | Score | **Changes in Behavior of Companion/Group** | Score |
|---|---|---|---|
| Normal position | 0 | Patient is in the group | 0 |
| Abnormal position (backwards/sideways/flat) | 3 | Companion/group leaves / has left patient (excluding normal herd behavior) | 3 |

| **Weight Distribution** | Score | **Eating** (present some food – NB only if the animal is allowed to eat) | Score |
|---|---|---|---|
| Normal weight distribution | 0 | Eats normally or fasts | 0 |
| | | Eats less and/or slowly | 2 |

Table 36.2    (Continued)

| Abnormal weight distribution | 3 | Not interested in food | 3 |
|---|---|---|---|

**INTERACT GENTLY** After the 5 minutes approach the donkey at a slow pace and in a quiet manner; some stimulation to move the donkey is allowed.

| **Reaction to Observer(s)** | **Score** | **Movement** (0 = no lameness – 5 = severe lameness ["on three legs"]) | **Score** |
|---|---|---|---|
| Reaction to observer(s) | 0 | No reluctance to move and normal gait | 0 |
|  |  | Mildly abnormal gait (1 or 2 out of 5) and/or stiff walk | 1 |
| Mild reaction to observer(s) | 2 | Reluctance to move when motivated and/or severely abnormal gait (3–5 / 5) | 2 |
| No reaction to observer(s) | 3 | No movement or is lying down | 3 |

| **Heart Rate** | **Score** | **Digestive Sounds** | **Score** |
|---|---|---|---|
| 32–52 beats/min | 0 | Normal motility | 0 |
| 53–60 beats/min | 1 | Decreased motility | 1 |
| 61–68 beats/min | 2 | No motility | 2 |
| >68 beats/min | 3 | Hypermotility or steel band | 3 |

| **Rectal Temperature** | **Score** | **Reaction to Palpation of the Painful Area** (only when safe) | **Score** |
|---|---|---|---|
| 35.7–38.0 °C | 0 | No reaction to palpation | 0 |
| 35.3–35.6 °C or 38.1–38.5 °C | 1 |  |  |
| 34.7–35.2 °C or 38.6–39.0 °C | 2 | Mild reaction to palpation | 2 |
| <34.6 °C or > 39.1 °C | 3 | Severe reaction to palpation | 3 |

**To calculate FINAL ACUTE CMPASS PAIN SCORE:** Determine per element what score (0 1 2 3) fits the best Sum the total score

| *If the total COMPASS score is ≥ 5 the donkey might be in acute pain* | **Total composite pain score (max score = 60)** |
|---|---|

Table 36.3    EQUUS donkey facial assessment of pain scale for acute pain.

**PREPARATION** for scoring manually. (For detailed instructions see Table 36.1)

Observe from a comfortable distance or helper holds donkey on a leading rein. **OBSERVE BOTH SIDES OF THE HEAD**

**During 2 minutes:**
**1. "COUNT" and mark the most applicable score** (Dark Gray 3 parameters)
**2. Observe from a distance and mark the most applicable score** (Middle Gray 8 parameters)
**After 1 minute make an attractive sound** (Light gray 1 parameter)

| | **Teeth Grinding and/ or Moaning** | **Score** | | **Flehmen/Yawning/ Smacking** | **Score** |
|---|---|---|---|---|---|
| | Not been heard | 0 | | Not seen | 0 |
|  | Heard | 2 |  | Seen | 2 |

**Table 36.3** (Continued)

| | Startle/Headshaking | Score | | Ear Response | Score |
|---|---|---|---|---|---|
| | No startle/headshaking | 0 | | Clear response with both ears or ear closest to source | 0 |
| | | | | Delayed/reduced response to sounds | 1 |
| | At least one startle (a sudden abrupt movement with the head as if suddenly aware of danger)/period of head shaking | 2 | | No response to sounds | 2 |

| OBSERVE FROM DISTANCE | | | | | |
|---|---|---|---|---|---|
| | **Focus** | **Score** | | **Muscle Tone Head** | **Score** |
| | Focused on environment | 0 | | No fasciculations or increased tension | 0 |
| | Less focused on environment | 1 | | Mild fasciculations or increased tension | 1 |
| | Not focused on environment | 2 | | Obvious fasciculations or increased tension | 2 |

| | **Eyelids** | **Score** | | **Nostrils** | **Score** |
|---|---|---|---|---|---|
| | Opened | 0 | | Relaxed | 0 |
| | More opened eyes or tightening of eyelids | 1 | | A bit more opened, nostrils lifted, wrinkles seen | 1 |
| | Obviously more opened eyes (sclera visible) or obvious orbital tightening of eyelids | 2 | | Obviously more opened, nostril flaring, possibly audible breathing | 2 |

Table 36.3 (Continued)

| Head | | Score | Corners Mouth/Lips | | Score |
|---|---|---|---|---|---|
| | Normal movement | 0 | | Relaxed | 0 |
| | Less/no or more/exaggerated movement | 2 | | Lifted | 2 |
| **Ear Position** | | Score | Sweating Behind the Ears | | Score |
| | Normal position | 0 | | No signs of sweating | 0 |
| | Abnormal position (hang down/backwards) | 2 | | Signs of sweating | 2 |

**To calculate FINAL ACUTE Facial Assessment of Pain SCORE:** Determine per element what score (0, 1, 2) fits the best. Sum the total score.

*If the total COMPASS score is ≥2 the donkey might be in acute pain*

**Total Facial Assessment of Pain score** (max. score = 24)

- Rectal temperature.
- Borborygmi (abdominal sounds).

*Preparation*

- Preferably stay at a comfortable distance (3–5 m when possible) from where the donkey can be observed with as few as distractions as possible.
- If needed, the donkey can be kept on the leading rein on a headcollar by a familiar handler.
- Be aware that the donkey might *freeze*, as a coping mechanism, when an unfamiliar person is close by.
- Check that the donkey is not resting upright/sleeping.
  - This can be done by making the donkey aware of your presence when starting.
- Make sure that the donkey is not distracted (or as little as possible).
- If necessary, wait a few minutes before the assessment starts, to allow the donkey to behave naturally and not to go into the *freeze* mode.
- Keep doors and gates closed.
- Be aware of the weather conditions: in very warm and/or humid weather. Conditions, some behaviors (for instance flaring of nostrils) can be influenced.

- ○ Make sure all involved, including the donkey(s), are safe.
- ○ Do *not* use these pain scales in sedated or premedicated animals.
- ○ *THE EQUUS-donkey COMPASS and FAP for acute pain assessment* via *the APP*
  - − Open the app and fill in the required fields the same as with the manually performed assessment.
  - − The counting and calculating of the total pain scores are performed within the app.

## IV Donkey pain assessment scales for chronic pain

### A The Donkey Chronic pain scale (See Table 36.4)

- ○ For donkeys with chronic pain the Donkey Chronic Pain Scale (DCPS**)** is used.
- ○ The DCPS is a combination of:
  - − The objective Donkey Chronic Pain – Composite Pain Scale (DCP CPS)
  - − Scores range from 0 (no pain) to 3 (associated with severe pain) for individual parameters.
  - − And the aforementioned EQUUS-Donkey-FAP scale to be referred to now as DCP-FAP.
  - − Scores range from 0 (no pain) to 2 (associated with severe pain).
- ○ The DCPS has been used in animals with:
  - − Osteoarthritis.
  - − Chronic laminitis.
  - − Dental disease.
- ○ The higher the score, the more likely the donkey is to be experiencing chronic pain (maximum score cannot be reached since some parameters prevent others from being expressed).

### B THE DCP CPS for chronic pain assessment to perform manually

#### Preparation

- ○ Preferably stay at a comfortable distance (3–5 m when possible) from where the donkey can be observed with as few as distractions as possible.
  - − If needed, the donkey can be kept on the leading rein on a headcollar by a familiar handler.
- ○ Be aware that the donkey might *freeze*, as a coping mechanism, when an unfamiliar person is close by.
- ○ Check that the donkey is not resting upright/sleeping.
  - − This can be done by making the donkey aware of your presence when starting.
- ○ Make sure that the donkey is not distracted (or as little as possible).
- ○ If necessary, wait a few minutes before the assessment starts, to allow the donkey to behave naturally and not to go into the *freeze* mode.
- ○ Keep doors and (field) gates closed.
- ○ Be aware of the weather conditions: in very warm and/or humid weather conditions, some behaviors (for instance flaring of nostrils) can be influenced.
- ○ Make sure all involved, including the donkey, are safe.

Table 36.4    Donkey chronic pain – composite pain scale for chronic pain.

**PREPARATION** for scoring manually. (For detailed instructions, see Table 36.1)

**During 5 minutes: 1. Observe from a distance and mark the most applicable score** (Middle Gray 10 parameters)

### OBSERVE FROM A DISTANCE

| General Appearance | Score | Body Posture | Score |
|---|---|---|---|
| Alert and/or is interacting with mate/group | 0 | Quietly standing and/or one hind leg resting | 0 |
| Mildly depressed and/or restless and/or decreased interaction with mate/group | 1 | Slightly tucked up abdomen | 1 |
| Moderately depressed and/or aggressive or no reaction mate/group | 2 | Extremely tucked up abdomen and/or hunched back and/or stretching limbs/body and/or mild muscle tremors | 2 |
| Severely depressed | 3 | Sits on hind quarters and/or extreme muscle tremors | 3 |
| **Weight Distribution** | **Score** | **Weight shifting of front limbs** | **Score** |
| Normal weight distribution | 0 | Not seen | 0 |
| Less weight on one leg and/or body displaced slightly backwards | 1 | Mild weight shifting, 25% of time | 1 |
| Less weight on one leg, with only the tip on the ground | 2 | Moderate weight shifting, 50% of time | 2 |
| One leg obviously lifted and/or body obviously displaced backwards | 3 | Severe weight shifting, >75% of time | 3 |
| **Body Condition Score (BCS)** | **Score** | **Muscles loss** (epaxial, gluteal, hamstring and cervical muscles) | **Score** |
| Normal BSC (3/5) | 0 | Symmetric muscles, no muscle loss | 0 |
| Increased or decreased BCS (2/5 or 4/5) | 1 | Mild muscle loss | 1 |
|  |  | Moderate muscle loss | 2 |
| Severely increased or decreased BCS (1/5 or 5/5) | 3 | Obvious (a)symmetric muscle loss | 3 |

*(Continued)*

Table 36.4   (Continued)

| Pressure sores on skin | Score | Changes in behavior to mate/group | Score |
|---|---|---|---|
| No pressure sores on skin | 0 | Donkey is in the group | 0 |
| Mild pressure sores on skin | 1 | Donkey is not in the group, but with his/her mate | 1 |
| Moderate pressure sores on skin | 2 | | |
| Severe pressure sores on skin | 3 | Mate/group leaves or has left Donkey (excluding herd behavior) | 3 |
| **Head carriage** | **Score** | **Eating** (present some food – NB only if the animal is allowed to eat) | **Score** |
| Ear base above withers or eats/drinks (from the ground) | 0 | Interested and eats normally or fast | 0 |
| Ear base at the level of the withers | 1 | Reluctant to take food, but eats normally | 1 |
| Ear base below the withers | 2 | Reluctant to take food and drops the food | 2 |
| Nose to ground (not eating) | 3 | Not interested in food | 3 |

**INTERACT GENTLY** After the 5 minutes approach the donkey at a slow pace and in a quiet manner; some stimulation to move the donkey is allowed.

| Reaction to observer(s) | Score | Movement (0 = no lameness – 5 = severe lameness ["on three legs"]) | Score |
|---|---|---|---|
| Reaction to observer(s) and ear movements toward observer | 0 | No reluctance to move and normal gait | |
| Mild decreased reaction or ear movements to observer(s) | 1 | Mildly abnormal gait (1 or 2 out of 5) and/or stiff walk, not reluctant | |
| Moderate decreased reaction or ear movements to observer(s) | 2 | Reluctance to walk when motivated and/or severely abnormal gait (3–5 / 5) | |
| No reaction or ear movements to observer(s) | 3 | Does not want to walk or is lying down | |
| **Pain reaction to palpation of the back** | **Score** | **Pain reaction to standardized flexion of both distal limb and carpus/tarsus** | |
| No reaction to palpation | 0 | No reaction to standardized flexion of limbs | |
| Mild reaction to palpation | 1 | Mild reaction to standardized flexion of limbs | |

Table 36.4    (Continued)

| | | |
|---|---|---|
| Moderate reaction to palpation | 2 | Moderate reaction to standardized flexion of limbs |
| Severe reaction to palpation (ears backward, tends to bite) | 3 | Severe reaction to standardized flexion of limbs |
| **Carrot/apple test** (only in chronic dental cases) | **Score** | |
| Normal biting and eating of carrot/apple | 0 | |
| Reluctant to or difficulties with eating carrot/apple | 2 | |
| Does not want to eat the carrot/apple | 3 | |

To calculate FINAL COMPOSITE PAIN SCALE for CHRONIC PAIN: Determine per element what score (0, 1, 2, 3) fits the best. Sum the total score.

Total chronic composite pain score (max. score = 45)

PERFORM THE EQUUS DONKEY FACIAL ASSESSMENT OF PAIN scale – SEE Table 36.2

Total Facial Assessment of Pain score (max. score= 24)

SUMMARIZE BOTH SCORES (maximum score cannot be reached since some parameters prevent others from being expressed)

If the total DCPS score is ≥6 the donkey might be in acute pain

Total Donkey Chronic Pain Scale score (max. score = 69)

## V    Donkey grimace scale (DGS)

- Recently, the first steps in the development of the Donkey Grimace Scale were described for recognizing pain in donkeys after castration.
- Nine donkeys were castrated, and they were observed by 12 observers before and after castration (see Orth, Suggested reading).

## VI    Pain assessment in mules and hinnies

- Mules are a hybrid between a jack (male donkey) and a mare (female horse).
- Hinnies are a hybrid between a stallion (male horse) and a jenny (female donkey).
  - Often the term mule is used for both mules and hinnies since mules are more common.
- On almost every aspect (anatomy, physiology, ethology, pain assessment) they are also a hybrid of the characteristics of horses and donkeys, independent whether the dam is a mare of a Jenny or the father is a stallion or a Jack.

 o Due to epigenetic influences, there can be differences between mules and hinnies, especially in temperament.
- No specific studies on the use of pain scales in mules/hinnies have been published to date.

## Suggested Reading

de Grauw, J.C. and van Loon, J.P.A.M. (2016). Systematic pain assessment in horses. *Vet. J.* 209: 14–22.

Matthews, N. and Loon, J.P.A.M. (2013). Anaesthesia and analgesia of the donkey and the mule. *Equine Vet. Educ.* 25: 47–51.

Matthews, N. and van Loon, J.P.A.M. (2019). Anesthesia, sedation, and pain management of donkeys and mules. *Vet. Clin. North Am. Equine Pract.* 35: 515–527.

Orth, E.K., Navas González, F.J., Iglesias Pastrana, C. et al. (2020). Development of a donkey grimace scale to recognize pain in donkeys (Equus asinus) post castration. *Animals* 10: 1–22.

van Dierendonck, M.C., Burden, A.F., Rickards, K. et al. (2020). Monitoring acute pain in donkeys with the equine Utrecht university scale for donkeys composite pain assessment (EQUUS-DONKEY-COMPASS) and the Equine Utrecht University Scale for donkey facial assessment of pain (EQUUS-DONKEY-FAP). *Animals* 10: 354.

VanDierendonck, M.C. and van Loon, J.P.A.M. (2016). Monitoring acute equine visceral pain with the Equine Utrecht University Scale for Composite Pain Assessment (EQUUS-COMPASS) and the equine Utrecht University scale for facial assessment of pain (EQUUS-FAP): a validation study. *Vet. J.* 216: 175–177.

van Loon, J.P.A.M. and van Dierendonck, M.C. (2018). Objective pain assessment in horses (2014–2018). *Vet. J.* 242: 1–7.

van Loon, J.P.A.M. and Van Dierendonck, M.C. (2017). Monitoring equine head-related pain with the Equine Utrecht University scale for facial assessment of pain (EQUUS-FAP). *Vet. J.* 220: 88–90.

van Loon, J.P.A.M., de Grauw, J.C., Burden, F. et al. (2021). Objective assessment of chronic pain in donkeys using the donkey chronic pain scale (DCPS): a scale-construction study. *Vet. J.* 267: 105580.

# 37

# Remote Capture of Equids
*Nigel Caulkett*

- Remote drug delivery can facilitate sedation or immobilization of wild or feral equids.

## I General considerations

### A The decision to use remote delivery

- ○ Remote delivery can be used at distances of 1–40 m.
- ○ Remote delivery will facilitate drug delivery in situations where:
  - – An animal *cannot be closely approached* for safety reasons.
  - – When the *flight distance* is such that the drug cannot be delivered via hand injection.
- ○ The decision to use remote delivery must be weighed against the risk, and the least traumatic technique should be used.

### B Trauma reduction

- ○ Trauma from remote delivery equipment is related:
  - – To the energy of the dart impact.
  - – The speed of drug injection.
  - – The injection site.
- ○ Impact energy is described by the following equation:

$$KE = M / 2 \times V^2$$

where KE = Kinetic energy
M = Mass of the dart
V = Velocity

- ○ From the above equation it is apparent that *high velocity* is the major factor that will result in trauma.
  - – A good general rule is to use the lowest velocity that will result in an accurate trajectory at a given distance.
- ○ Drugs should be delivered into a *large muscle mass* to facilitate uptake and decrease the risk of trauma to underlying structures.

*Manual of Equine Anesthesia and Analgesia*, Second Edition. Edited by Tom Doherty,
Alex Valverde, and Rachel A. Reed.
© 2022 John Wiley & Sons, Inc. Published 2022 by John Wiley & Sons, Inc.

- The muscles of the thigh, neck, or shoulder are generally considered to be good locations for dart placement.
  ○ High-velocity injection can induce trauma, especially when using large volumes.
  ○ Ideally, low volumes (< 5 ml) should be delivered via slow injection darts, to reduce the risk of trauma.

## C Environment

○ Anesthesia can be hazardous in field situations; therefore, appropriate supportive care, personnel and emergency drugs and equipment should be readily available.
○ With client-owned animals the client must be informed of the increased risk of morbidity and mortality when remote capture is used.

## II Equipment

### A Choice of delivery equipment

*Distance*
○ *Pole syringes* can be used to extend the reach by up to 4 m.
○ *Blow pipes* can be used up to 10 m.
  - Traditional blow pipes should *not* be used with potent immobilizing drugs.
○ *Pistols* are generally effective up to 20 m.
○ A *rifle* (pneumatic or cartridge powered) is required for > 20 m.

*Trauma*
○ The least traumatic technique should always be chosen.
○ Gas-powered dart rifles with pressure gauges such as the Dan-injectR or Pneu-DartR EX-Caliber are very adjustable for close or long-range dart delivery.

*Familiarity*
○ Practice with equipment is vital to ensure accurate dart placement and to reduce the risk of trauma.

### B Equipment options

*Pole syringe*
○ Is most useful for ranges of 1–3 m.
○ Is typically used to deliver drugs to confined animals or to top up anesthesia in recumbent, but lightly anesthetized animals.
○ Generally, *short*, 14–16-gauge needles should be used, as this will decrease the risk of a bent or broken needle, and of hitting bone. Care should be taken to avoid lacerations.

*Blow pipe*
○ Is useful as a short-range (5–10 m), limited-volume (3–5 ml) system.
○ Mouth-operated blowpipes should not be used with potent drugs. Systems are available that use a $CO_2$ or air-powered pistol grip to project darts.
○ The discharge mechanism in most blowpipe darts is compressed air or *butane*.
  - This results in low-velocity injection and minimal tissue trauma.
○ Practice is vital to ensure accurate dart delivery.

*Pistol*
- Pistols are generally useful up to ranges of 20 m.
- They are compact and easy to transport.
- Projection of the dart is powered by compressed air or carbon dioxide.
- Dart volume is generally limited to a maximum of 5 ml.

*Rifles (see Figure 37.1)*
- Are useful up to ranges of 20–40 m.
- Compressed air, $CO_2$, or a .22 caliber cartridge powers projection of the dart.
- Dart volumes of up to 10 ml may be delivered.
- Velocity adjustment is via *pressure selection* in pneumatic rifles, and via *charge selection* or a velocity dial in cartridge powered rifles.

## III  Pharmacology

### A  Choice of drugs

- Drug(s) must be *potent* enough to be delivered in small volumes.
- Must be stable in solution with other capture drugs.
- Ideally, a drug(s) should confer a rapid, smooth induction and have minimal cardiovascular and respiratory side effects.
- The ability to antagonize immobilization drugs is also desirable.

### B  $\alpha_2$ agonists and antagonists

- $\alpha_2$ agonists may be used to induce sedation of fractious horses, or to facilitate capture of feral domestic horses or wild horses.

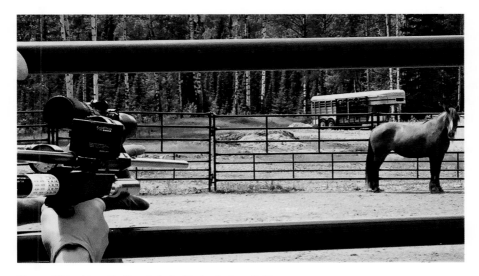

**Figure 37.1**  Use of a Dan-inject rifle to dart a wild horse.

*Xylazine*
   o Is useful for sedation or to improve muscle relaxation when combined with potent narcotics or dissociative agents.
   o The major limitation to its use is the concentration of the commercial drug, as volume requirements are high with commercial preparations.
   o Compounded xylazine may be sourced at a concentration of 300 mg/ml.

*Detomidine*
   o Is better suited to remote delivery as it is more potent, and volume requirements are decreased compared to xylazine.

*Romifidine*
   o Has been used in combination with Telazol®, for immobilization.

*Medetomidine*
   o It is the most useful $\alpha_2$ agonist for remote delivery due to its potency.
   o Concentrations of 20–30 mg/ml are ideal for remote delivery.

*Yohimbine* (0.1–0.2 mg/kg, IM) or *tolazoline* (2–4 mg/kg, IM).
   o May be used to antagonize xylazine, romifidine and detomidine.

*Atipamezole*
   o (3–5 times the medetomidine dose) is required to antagonize medetomidine.

## C  Phenothiazines and butyrophenones

   o *Acepromazine* (0.05 mg/kg, IM) can be used as an adjunct to sedation, in combination with alpha$_2$ agonists.
   o *Azaperone* (0.2 mg/kg, IM) Used in combination with potent opioids or alpha$_2$ agonists to provide tranquilization.

## D  Opioids and opiates

*Morphine*
   o Can be used in combination with *detomidine* ± *acepromazine* to facilitate sedation of fractious horses.
   o Dose: 0.1–0.2 mg/kg, IM.

*Butorphanol*
   o May be substituted for morphine at a dose of 0.025–0.05 mg/kg, IM.

*Thiafentanil*
   o Can be delivered at a small volume and is readily reversible with naltrexone.
   o It is being investigated for wild horse capture; further studies are required to determine its efficacy when compared to etorphine.

*Etorphine*
   o Has proven useful for immobilization of wild and domestic horses.
   o It should be combined with acepromazine, azaperone, or an alpha$_2$ agonist to decrease muscle rigidity.

## E  Dissociative anesthetics

*Ketamine*
   o Is useful in combination with medetomidine.
   o High volumes of ketamine are required when it is combined with xylazine.
   o Compounded ketamine may be sourced at a concentration of 200 mg/ml.

*Telazol* (Zoletil®)
- ○ Is a combination of tiletamine and zolazepam.
- ○ The powered drug form can be reconstituted with an α2 agonist to produce a satisfactory combination for capture of feral horses.

## IV    Monitoring and supportive care

### A    Field anesthesia

- ○ Field anesthesia increases the risk.
- ○ Down time should be minimized and supportive care should be provided.

### B    Monitoring

- ○ Monitoring of pulse and respiration should be performed every five minutes.
- ○ Pulse oximetry assesses hemoglobin saturation and guides $O_2$ therapy.
- ○ Non-invasive blood pressure monitoring can be useful to monitor trends.

### C    Oxygenation

- ○ The simplest way to provide supplemental inspired $O_2$ is via nasal insufflation.
- ○ An ambulance-type regulator is sturdy and simple to use in the field. E (660 L) or D (350 L) cylinders can be transported to most field situations (*see* Figure 37.2)
- ○ Flows of 8–15 l/minute are generally required to maintain oxygenation in mature horses. Flow can be adjusted to provide a minimum flow that will maintain a percent hemoglobin saturation of 95–97%.
    - – Consider the duration of a full cylinder at these flow rates (44–83 minutes for an E cylinder; 23–44 minutes for a D cylinder).

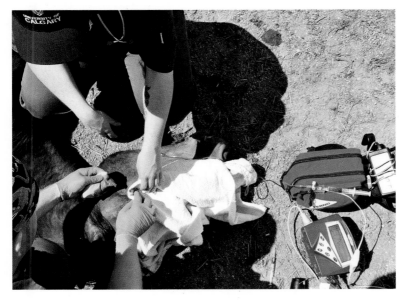

Figure 37.2    Delivery of supplemental inspired oxygen in the field. An E-cylinder with an ambulance type regulator will facilitate delivery of intranasal oxygen.

**D   Position and padding**

- ○ Generally, dorsal recumbency should be avoided as V/Q mismatching is most pronounced in this position. This will contribute to hypoxemia.
- ○ If intubation is not performed, ensure head and neck extension, to maintain a patent airway.
- ○ The horse should be maintained on a soft, level surface.
- ○ The legs should be hobbled or tied to prevent injuries to handlers (from kicks), during light anesthesia.
  - – Control of the limbs is particularly important if narcotic-based anesthesia has been used.

## V   Sedation of fractious horses

**A   The decision to use IM sedation**

- ○ Generally, IM sedation is considered when IV drug administration will put handlers at significant risk of injury.
- ○ Drugs may be delivered via a *pole syringe* or *blow dart* to penned animals.
  - – Longer-range delivery equipment may be required in the field.
- ○ IM sedation can be used to facilitate IV delivery of additional sedatives or to facilitate delivery of IV anesthetics.

**B   Sedative protocol**

- ○ A mixture of *detomidine* (20–40 µg/kg), plus *morphine* (0.1–0.2 mg/kg) is administered by IM injection.
  - – Ideally, *morphine* should be used at a concentration of 50 mg/ml to facilitate low-volume delivery.
- ○ *Acepromazine* (0.05 mg/kg) can also be combined with this mixture.
  - – If it is used in breeding stallions the risk of *priapism* should be discussed with the owner.
- ○ The animal should be left alone to facilitate drug uptake and sedation.
- ○ After 15–20 minutes approached cautiously, and handle the horse, if possible.
  - – Additional *detomidine* (5 µg/kg, IV) will provide further sedation, if necessary.
- ○ The horse should be watched for at least two hours after drug administration, as there is a risk of CNS stimulation if the detomidine is metabolized prior to the morphine.
  - – Additional *detomidine* or *acepromazine* can be used to treat excitement.
- ○ Alternatively, *butorphanol* (0.05 mg/kg) may be substituted for *morphine*, but sedation may be less profound.

## VI   Sedation and anesthesia of captive feral horses

**A   Technique**

Physical capture of feral horses may be possible with well-trained wranglers.

Once in captivity a well-designed chute system should be used to restrain the horse prior to sedation and anesthesia (*see* Figure 37.3).

- ○ *Medetomidine* 0.02–0.04 mg/kg, *acepromazine* (0.05 mg), and butorphanol (0.02 mg/kg) are administered IM by hand injection.
  - – Total injectate volume is typically 2.5 ml in the 400 kg horse.

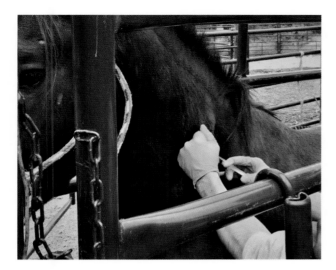

**Figure 37.3**   Wild horse restrained in a chute system to facilitate intramuscular administration of sedatives.

- The horse is held in the chute until first signs of sedation.
- The horse is released into a pen and allowed to develop deep sedation. Horses are often very ataxic.
- Once deep sedation is apparent anesthesia can be induced with diazepam (0.02–0.04 mg/kg, IV) combined with ketamine (2.0–2.5 mg/kg, IV).
- The horse must be approached with caution as they may snap out of sedation or ataxic horses may fall on the operator.
- This technique is typically sufficient for minor surgical procedures such as castration.
- If recovery time is prolonged, *atipamezole* can be considered at a dose of 3–5 times the medetomidine dose administered IM.

## VII   Remote capture of free-ranging feral horses

### A   Techniques

- A variety of techniques have been used for capture.
- Physical capture may be possible with well-trained wranglers.
- *Telazol*-based protocols are probably the most readily available and user friendly.

### B   Telazol - $\alpha_2$ mixtures

- *Telazol* can be reconstituted with an $\alpha_2$ agonist to decrease volume.
- *Telazol* (3.5 mg/kg) + *butorphanol* (0.07 mg/kg) + *xylazine* (3 mg/kg) has been used, successfully, to capture feral horses.
  - Volume is large.
  - It is possible to reduce the volume considerably if concentrated xylazine (300 mg/ml) can be sourced.
- The combination is more readily available to the general practitioner than potent narcotics.
- *Alternatively,* Telazol (3.5 mg/kg) + *medetomidine* (0.15 mg/kg) has been advocated.
  - Medetomidine may be antagonized with *atipamezole* at 2–5 times the medetomidine dose.

- ○ Induction and recovery can be rough when high doses of Telazol are used.
- ○ The addition of *acepromazine* 0.05 mg/kg ± *butorphanol* 0.02 mg/kg to the Telazol – medetomidine mixture can be considered to reduce Telazol and medetomidine dose requirements by approximately 20–30%.

## VIII   Wild equids

### A   Techniques

- ○ In general, remote delivery is required for capture of wild equids.
- ○ Drug choice will depend on availability of drugs and supportive care.
- ○ It is important to note that drug requirements are generally greater in free-ranging animals compared to captive animals.

### B   Zebra

- ○ A variety of combinations have been advocated; most are narcotic based.

*Adult Grevy's zebra*

- ○ *Etorphine* (0.02 mg/kg) + *azaperone* (0.2 mg/kg), induces anesthesia that can be antagonized with 2 mg *diprenorphine*/mg of *etorphine*.
- ○ *Diazepam* or *xylazine* can be administered IV to improve muscle relaxation once the animal is immobilized.

*Common zebra*

- ○ *Etorphine* has also been recommended.
- ○ *Etorphine* (0.02 mg/kg) + *azaperone* (0.2 mg/kg), induces anesthesia that can be antagonized with 2 mg *diprenorphine*/mg of *etorphine*.
  - – *Diazepam* or *xylazine* can be administered IV once the animal is immobilized to improve muscle relaxation.
- ○ If a *non-narcotic* based protocol is desired, captive zebra can be immobilized with 1.8 mg/kg of Telazol combined with 0.35 mg/kg of *romifidine*.
- ○ Supplemental $O_2$ should be provided as hypoxemia is common with all combinations.

### C   Przewalski's horse

- ○ The combination of choice for capture of free ranging animals is:
  - – *Etorphine* 0.008 mg/kg + *detomidine* 0.033 mg/kg + *butorphanol* 0.033 mg/kg.
  - – This combination can be antagonized with 0.16 mg/kg of *naltrexone* and 0.04 mg/kg of *atipamezole* administered IV.
- ○ If a *non-narcotic* based protocol is desired, captive Przewalski's horses can be immobilized with *medetomidine* (0.1 mg/kg) + *ketamine* (2 mg/kg).
  - – *Atipamezole* is recommended for antagonism of immobilization, at a dose of 0.3 mg/kg, split IV (25%) and subcutaneously (75%).
- ○ Transient hypoxemia and bradycardia were noted with the above protocol.
- ○ *Telazol* (3.3 mg/kg) + *romifidine* (0.6 mg/kg) has also been used.

## Suggested Reading

West G, Heard D, Caulkett N. (2014) Zoo Animal and Wildlife Immobilization and Anesthesia 2, Wiley-Blackwell. Ames, Iowa.

# 38

# Complications

## Intraoperative Hypotension

*Christopher K. Smith and Tom Doherty*

$$\text{MAP} = \text{CO}\left(\text{stroke volume} \times \text{heart rate}\right) \times \text{SVR}$$

- A decrease in cardiac output (CO) or systemic vascular resistance (SVR) or both will result in a decrease in the mean arterial pressure (MAP).
  - Causes for reduced CO include anesthetic drugs, bradycardia, hypovolemia, endotoxemia, and cardiac disease, including arrhythmias.
  - Causes for reduced SVR include anesthetic drugs, endotoxemia, systemic inflammatory response syndrome (SIRS), anaphylaxis.
- Intraoperative hypotension is a common occurrence in the anesthetized horse, especially when inhalational anesthetics are used for the maintenance of anesthesia.
  - Vasodilation in these instances results in a *relative* hypovolemia.
- The incidence of hypotension decreases, as does the degree of hypotension, when anesthesia is maintained with injectable anesthetics (TIVA) or a combination of injectable and inhalational anesthetics (PIVA).
- Hypotension, if not corrected, may impair organ perfusion causing irreversible ischemic damage.
  - In human beings, uncorrected hypotension is associated with neurologic deficits, cardiomyopathy, and renal dysfunction.
  - In *adult* horses, there is a strong correlation between intraoperative hypotension and post-operative myopathy.
  - Maintaining the MAP > 70 mmHg reduces the incidence of myopathy.
- *Neonatal foals* have lower blood pressure than do adults due to lower vascular tone and responsiveness.
  - A MAP of 50–60 mmHg during general anesthesia is generally acceptable in the neonate.

## I Common causes of hypotension

### A Inhalational anesthetics

  - Hypotension is particularly likely to occur during the early phase of general anesthesia if the horse is exposed to a high-inspired concentration of a volatile anesthetic following induction.

*Manual of Equine Anesthesia and Analgesia*, Second Edition. Edited by Tom Doherty, Alex Valverde, and Rachel A. Reed.
© 2022 John Wiley & Sons, Inc. Published 2022 by John Wiley & Sons, Inc.

- ○ The halogenated inhalational anesthetics (*desflurane, sevoflurane, isoflurane*, and *halothane*) decrease the MAP in a dose-dependent manner.
- ○ This decrease in MAP with inhalational anesthetics (with the exception of *halothane*) is mainly due to a decrease in SVR.
- ○ Halothane decreases the MAP by directly affecting myocardial contractility, resulting in a decrease in CO.
- ○ Sevoflurane has a less negative inotropic effect than isoflurane. In one study, sevoflurane anesthetized horses (1.5 MAC) had higher CO than isoflurane and halothane-anesthetized horses, but MAP did not differ among treatments.
- ○ Comorbidities, such as *endotoxemia* (e.g. gastrointestinal emergencies, neonatal bacteremia), contribute to cardiovascular depression.
  - – Hypotension may result from a direct effect of *lipopolysaccharide* (LPS) on the myocardium and/or result from a decrease in *ionized calcium* secondary to endotoxemia.
  - – A decrease in *ionized calcium* may also occur in healthy horses administered volatile anesthetics, and result in reductions in both *inotropy* and *vascular tone*.

## B  Hypovolemia

- ○ Hypotension is more likely to occur if the patient is hypovolemic because hypovolemia results in a decrease in preload, stroke volume, and systemic filling pressures.
  - – Ideally, hypovolemia is corrected prior to surgery, but this may not always be possible in emergency cases.
  - – In emergencies, such as in the case of a horse with severe GI colic, rapid, small volume fluid replacement with 7.2% NaCl (4–6 ml/kg) may be the only feasible option.
- ○ Routine parameters evaluated on physical examination may indicate that a horse is hypovolemic (e.g. *tachycardia, poor pulse quality, decrease vessel wall turgor*) but none is specific for this clinical state.

*Static measures of preload*
- ○ Previously utilized techniques, such as central venous pressure (CVP) measurement, are unreliable methods for evaluating volume status, or the need for fluids.
- ○ This is largely because CVP is affected by many factors (e.g. *venous return, myocardial compliance, pleural pressure*), including recumbency in the horse. Therefore, while the animal's volume status may be reflected in its CVP, so are many other variables, thus making interpretation of this parameter difficult.

*Dynamic measures of preload*
- ○ There is no practical way of determining "*intravascular volume status*" or "*fluid responsiveness*" in the horse; thus, clinicians rely on arterial blood pressure measurement changes to judge responses to fluid administration.
  - – However, MAP is affected by several variables, making interpretation difficult at times.
  - – For example, a horse presenting acutely ill may have a normal, or even increased MAP despite being significantly dehydrated or hypovolemic.
- ○ The dynamic measurement of *preload indices*, or *volume responsiveness*, are techniques that rely on physiologic changes to venous return and CO that occur when positive pressure ventilation is instituted.
- ○ The increase in intrathoracic pressure that occurs during the inspiratory phase of positive pressure ventilation affects normal cardiovascular physiology.
  - – Right atrial pressure increases.

- Venous return decreases.
- Right ventricular afterload increases.
- Right and left ventricular COs decrease.
- Transmural aortic pressure decreases.
- LV afterload decreases.

○ Ultimately, these changes lead to a reduction in CO and possibly MAP.
○ The *dynamic indices* include:
  - Pulse pressure variation (PPV).
  - Systolic pressure variation.
  - Stroke volume variation.
  - Plethysmographic variability index.

*Note: Literature on the use of these dynamic indices in horses is lacking.*

*PPV*

○ PPV has been validated in humans, and has been shown to reasonably predict fluid responsiveness in veterinary patients.
○ PPV represents the changes observed in pulse pressure (PP) over the course of the respiratory cycle during positive pressure ventilation.
  - An increased variability in PP suggests that there is "*cycling*" occurring due to changes in CO.
○ PPV = (PPmax – PPmin)/(PPmax + PPmin/2) x 100.
  - Modern multiparameter monitors will generate this parameter automatically (see Figure 38.1).
  - However, one can easily calculate PPV manually with variables obtained from invasive blood pressure measurement.
○ Studies in human beings and animals report that for a patient to be "*fluid responsive*" the PPV should not be less than 14%.
  - This would likely place the patient on the so-called ascending limb of the Frank-Starling curve and thus, administration of a fluid bolus would lead to an appreciable increase in CO and MAP.
  - Typical fluid boluses administered to animals are between 5 and 20 ml/kg of isotonic crystalloids.
○ Arrhythmias, low tidal volumes, spontaneous ventilation, and vasoactive agents can alter the reliability of PPV. Thus, caution should be used when interpreting PPV under these scenarios.

**Figure 38.1** Multiparameter anesthetic monitor indicating pulse pressure variation.

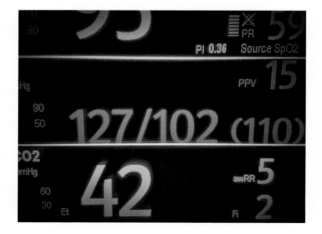

### C Bradycardia

- Bradycardia is an uncommon cause of hypotension in horses.
- Bradycardia in horses is arbitrarily defined by some clinicians as a heart rate of <25 beats/min in an adult horse. However, the resting heart rate depends on the breed and the level of fitness.
- Occasionally, the heart rate may decrease to <20 beats/min following induction of anesthesia, and is most commonly associated with $\alpha_2$ agonist administration. In these instances, it is more common to see bradycardia accompanied by hypertension.
  - Increasing the heart rate in this instance is contraindicated.
- Bradycardia associated with $\alpha_2$ agonist sedating drugs is usually transient, and generally only needs to be addressed if the blood pressure is also low.

*Treatment*

- Anticholinergics, (e.g. *atropine, glycopyrrolate, butylscopolammonium bromide [Buscopan]*) may be used to increase the heart rate, if deemed appropriate.
  - *Atropine* has been associated with the development of *ileus* in horses, but this is not likely to occur after a single dose.
- If bradycardia is accompanied by hypotension, a sympathomimetic drug (e.g. *ephedrine*) may be administered to increase heart rate and MAP.

## II Treatment of hypotension

- Although it is important to consider *decreasing anesthetic depth*, if appropriate to do so, there is no rapid response in blood pressure using this strategy alone.
  - If the inspired concentration of the volatile anesthetic is decreased, it is usually necessary to administer injectable drugs to maintain an adequate depth of anesthesia.
- *Fluid deficits* are not generally a cause of hypotension in healthy horses undergoing general anesthesia for elective procedures.
  - A rapid increase in MAP is not going to happen due to the time required to administer a fluid bolus, and other measures (e.g. an inotrope) to improve blood pressure should be instituted concurrently.
  - Additionally, crystalloids only remain in the vascular system for a short time.

### A Positive inotropic agents

- Positive inotropic agents such as *dobutamine* or *ephedrine* are generally the *first-line* treatments for hypotension in the anesthetized horse, and the following are the most commonly used inotropes.

*Dobutamine*

- Dobutamine is primarily a $\beta_1$-adrenergic selective drug that increases myocardial contractility.
- Dobutamine, when administered as an infusion (0.5–3 µg/kg/min), generally results in a relatively rapid increase in the MAP.
  - The increase in MAP is due to an increase in CO, because SVR does not increase, and usually decreases.
  - The increase in CO is due to an increase in SV because HR does not change significantly at clinically relevant doses.

- In healthy isoflurane-anesthetized horses, *dobutamine* (3 μg/kg/min) increased CO, MAP, and heart rate, and blood flow to the jejunum and colon.
- Horses in vasodilatory shock may remain hypotensive, despite increases in CO. These horses benefit from vasoconstriction from α-adrenergic drugs (e.g. *phenylephrine*; 1–4 μg/kg, IV) in combination with dobutamine.
- Dobutamine has a relatively short half-life (two to three minutes) in plasma, hence the need to administer an infusion.
- The onset of effect is fairly rapid (one to two minutes), but the peak effect may take 10 minutes.
- The lower end of the dose range is usually sufficient to maintain the desired MAP in otherwise healthy patients.

    *Adverse Effects*:
    - In one study, dobutamine administration to *halothane*-anesthetized horses resulted in atrioventricular block, premature atrial contractions and atrioventricular dissociation. This effect is likely to be dose-related.
    - The incidence of arrhythmias appears to be lower in isoflurane-anesthetized horses than in halothane-anesthetized horses.
    - *Tachycardia* may occur with high infusion rates. Tachycardia will increase myocardial oxygen demand and reduce filling times, which may compromise CO.

*Ephedrine*

- Dose (0.05–0.1 mg/kg, IV).
- *Ephedrine* predominantly acts indirectly on adrenergic receptors.
    - It causes presynaptic release of *norepinephrine*.
- It is an agonist at $\alpha_1$, $\beta_1$, and $\beta_2$ receptors.
- It increases myocardial contractility, heart rate, and CO, resulting in an increase in systolic, diastolic, and MAP.
- Repeated dosing may cause *tachyphylaxis*, and this is probably due to depletion of *norepinephrine* stores.
- It has the advantage that it can be given as a bolus IV or IM.
    - However, the onset of action after IM administration is longer than with IV making it a less practical route of administration.
- Ephedrine crosses the *blood-brain-barrier,* and may cause CNS stimulation. However, this is unlikely to be a concern at clinically relevant doses.

*Dopamine*

- It has agonist activity at $\alpha_1$ and $\beta_1$ receptors and causes the release of endogenous *norepinephrine*.
- Dopamine (4 μg/kg/min) in healthy isoflurane-anesthetized horses increased CO but *decreased* MAP. It caused a small increase in heart rate.
- Dopamine (5 μg/kg/min) in healthy isoflurane-anesthetized horses increased CO, but *decreased* SVR, MAP, and colonic blood flow.
- Its *inability* to increase MAP limits the usefulness of dopamine as an inotrope in equine anesthesia.

    *Adverse Effects*:
    - Dopamine administration has been associated with cardiac arrhythmias in anesthetized horses.

*Epinephrine*

- ○ Epinephrine is *not a first-line* drug to treat intraoperative hypotension.
  - – Its use is generally reserved for the treatment of *cardiac arrest* or *anaphylaxis*.
- ○ Epinephrine has agonist activity at α- and ß-adrenergic receptors, particularly $α_1$ and $ß_1$ receptors.
- ○ Due to its effect on both types of receptors, the administration of epinephrine can result in *hypertension* (due to $α_1$-receptor mediated vasoconstriction) or *hypotension* (due to $ß_2$-receptor mediated arterial dilation), depending on the dose administered.
  - – *Low doses* of epinephrine (0.01–0.03 µg/kg/min) have primarily $ß_2$ effects and may decrease the MAP due to arterial vasodilation.
  - – *Intermediate doses* (0.02–0.1 µg/kg/min) have $ß_1$ and $ß_2$ effects resulting in increases in MAP and heart rate.
  - – *High doses* (0.1–1 µg/kg/min), have primarily $α_1$ effects resulting in hypertension due to vasoconstriction.
- ○ High doses of epinephrine are associated with the occurrence of *premature ventricular beats*, and this may be more likely to occur if the horse is *hypercarbic*.
- ○ A bolus dose of 1–2 µg/kg can be used to treat horses with severe hypotension.

*Calcium salts*

- ○ Administration of *calcium gluconate* increased CO and MAP in anesthetized horses and ponies. Heart rate decreased with calcium gluconate infusion.
  - – *Too rapid administration can cause vasodilation, decreased blood pressure, cardiac arrhythmias and cardiac arrest.*
- ○ The effects of a calcium infusion on cardiovascular function are more likely to be beneficial in patients that are hypocalcemic.
- ○ In the authors' practice, *calcium gluconate* is commonly administered as a slow infusion in intestinal surgeries, as these patients are more likely to develop a decrease in ionized calcium. Approximately 1 ml/kg of a 23% solution is administered over the course of the surgery.

# B    Vasopressors

*Norepinephrine* (NE)

- ○ NE is *not* used routinely in healthy anesthetized horses to treat hypotension; rather it is reserved for the patient in *circulatory shock*.
- ○ NE is an endogenous catecholamine with *potent* α-adrenergic activity and *modest* β-receptor activity.
  - – Hence its potent *vasoconstrictor* effect and mild *inotropic* and *chronotropic* effects.
- ○ In healthy, isoflurane-anesthetized adult *horses*, NE (0.1–0.5 µg/kg/min) increased MAP and SVR, but did *not* improve CO or intestinal perfusion.
- ○ In *foals* with isoflurane-induced hypotension, NE increased cardiac index and MAP.
- ○ In septic patients, NE's effect on renal and splanchnic blood flow may be improved by co-administering *dobutamine*.

*Phenylephrine*

- ○ Phenylephrine is an $α_1$-adrenergic receptor agonist. It has *no* ß receptor activity.
  - – Thus, phenylephrine is suitable for increasing blood pressure that is primarily due to anesthetic-induced vasodilation.

- Its administration is commonly associated with a baroreceptor reflex-mediated decrease in heart rate.
- CO decreases due to decreased stroke volume resulting from increased afterload.
- In healthy horses anesthetized with either isoflurane or sevoflurane, *phenylephrine* administration (1–3 µg/kg/min) was associated with increases in MAP and SVR, and decreases in CO and heart rate.
- Phenylephrine may be administered either as bolus doses (1–2 µg/kg, IV) or as a continuous infusion (0.5–3 µg/kg/min).
  - The effect of the bolus is short lasting.

*Vasopressin*
- Vasopressin is *not a first-line* treatment for healthy horses with volatile anesthetic-induced hypotension.
  - Rather, its use should be reserved for patients in *septic* shock.
- Endogenous plasma concentrations of vasopressin are likely to be increased in the early phase of septic shock, but decreased thereafter.
- In one study, horses admitted for colic surgery had higher arginine vasopressin plasma concentrations than did normal horses.
- Vasopressin acts on V1, V2, V3, and oxytocin-type receptors (OTR).
- V1 vascular receptors are located on vascular smooth muscle, and are responsible for causing vasopressin-induced vasoconstriction, and the subsequent increases in blood pressure.
- In hypotensive isoflurane-anesthetized *foals*, administration of vasopressin (0.3 and 1.0 IU/kg/min) was associated with an increase in arterial blood pressure.
  *Caution – the administration of vasopressin to isoflurane-anesthetized horses that were made hypotensive by increasing the anesthetic depth, resulted in the immediate death of four of five horses administered a bolus dose of vasopressin (0.2 IU/kg, IV) and four or five horses administered vasopressin as an infusion (0.08 IU/kg/min).*
  *These doses of vasopressin are within the recommended range for horses.*

## Suggested Reading

Araos, J., Kenny, J.S., Rousseau-Blass, F., and Pang, D.S. (2020). Dynamic prediction of fluid responsiveness during positive pressure ventilation: a review of the physiology underlying heart–lung interactions and a critical interpretation. *Vet. Anesth. Analg.* 47: 3–14.

Dancker, C., Hopster, K., Rohn, K., and Kästner, S.B. (2018). Effects of dobutamine, dopamine, phenylephrine and noradrenaline on systemic haemodynamics and intestinal perfusion in isoflurane anaesthetised horses. *Equine. Vet. J.* 50: 104–110.

Donaldson, L.L. (1988). Retrospective assessment of dobutamine therapy for hypotension in anesthetized horses. *Vet. Surg.* 17: 53–57.

Grosenbaugh, D.A. and Muir, W.W. (1998). Cardiorespiratory effects of sevoflurane, isoflurane, and halothane anesthesia in horses. *Am. J. Vet. Res.* 59: 101–106.

Ludders, J.W., Palos, H.M., Erb, H.N. et al. (2009). Plasma arginine vasopressin concentration in horses undergoing surgery for colic. *J. Vet. Emerg. Crit. Care* 19: 528–535.

Ohta, M., Kurimoto, S., Ishikawa, Y. et al. (2013). Cardiovascular effects of dobutamine and phenylephrine infusion in sevoflurane-anesthetized thoroughbred horses. *J. Vet. Med. Sci.* 75: 1443–1448.

Trim, C.M., Moore, J.N., and White, N.A. (1985). Cardiopulmonary effects of dopamine hydrochloride in anaesthetised horses. *Equine. Vet. J.* 17: 41–44.

Valverde, A., Giguère, S., Sanchez, L.C. et al. (2006). Effects of dobutamine, norepinephrine, and vasopressin on cardiovascular function in anesthetized neonatal foals with induced hypotension. *Am. J. Vet. Res.* 7: 1730–1737.

Wollanke, B., Reimold, R., and Gerhards, H. (2015). Vasopressin is life threatening for horses under isoflurane anaesthesia. *Pferdeheilkunde* 31: 341–345.

Young, L.E., Blissitt, K.J., Clutton, R.E., and Molony, V. (1998). Haemodynamic effects of a sixty minute infusion of dopamine hydrochloride in horses anaesthetised with halothane. *Equine. Vet. J.* 30: 310–316.

## Intraoperative Hypertension

*Tom Doherty*

## I  Characterization

- In human beings, a diagnosis of hypertension is based on a systolic pressure > 140 mmHg and/or a diastolic pressure > 90 mmHg.
- Pre-existing hypertension such as *primary* (i.e. idiopathic or "essential") hypertension or *secondary* (e.g. renal, endocrine, or pregnancy-induced) hypertension are conditions which are rarely diagnosed in horses. However, there is some evidence that hypertension may occur in horses with equine metabolic syndrome.

## II  Causes of hypertension in anesthetized horses

### A  Inadequate plane of anesthesia

- This is the most common cause of hypertension.
- A sudden increase in arterial pressure may occur with surgical stimulation.
  - This is less likely to occur when administering multimodal anesthesia vs. inhalation anesthesia only.
  - Check that the horse has not become disconnected from the machine or from an anesthetic drug infusion, or that the vaporizer is empty.
- Signs indicating a light anesthetic plane may accompany hypertension.
  - *Purposeful* movement.
  - Ocular signs (active palpebral reflex, nystagmus).

  *Note*: A heart rate increase usually does *not* accompany hypertension in this case.
- Hypertension should resolve upon deepening the anesthetic plane.

### B  Medications

*α₂ agonists*

- Administration of an $\alpha_2$ agonist causes a temporary increase in arterial pressure.
- This increase in pressure is usually short-lived after a bolus of the $\alpha_2$ agonist, and a slight decrease in heart rate may occur concurrently.

    ○ Arterial pressures usually remain relatively high when $\alpha_2$ agonists are administered as an infusion.

*Sympathomimetic drugs*

    ○ Hypertension may result from overzealous administration of sympathomimetic (e.g. *dobutamine*) drugs for cardiovascular support.

    ○ The magnitude of hypertension can be dramatic if a $\beta_1$ agonist (e.g. *dobutamine*) is administered following a parasympatholytic drug (e.g. *atropine*).

      – Tachycardia will accompany hypertension in these cases.

    ○ *Phenylephrine*, when used intraoperatively as a vasopressor or in cases of nephrosplenic entrapment, will cause hypertension due to vasoconstriction.

      – This is usually accompanied by bradycardia.

## C   Nociception

    ○ Nociceptive stimuli can result in hypertension.

*Somatic*

    ○ e.g. Surgical incision and manipulation.

*Visceral*

    ○ e.g. Distended viscus, distended urinary bladder, traction on mesentery.

*Sympathetic*

    ○ e.g. *Tourniquet-induced pain* has been implicated as a cause of hypertension in anesthetized horses.

      – Tachycardia may be present concurrently.

      – Hypertension develops soon after tourniquet placement, and may increase in magnitude over time.

      – Hypertension resolves once the tourniquet is removed.

## D   Miscellaneous causes

    ○ Severe *hypercarbia*.

      – May be accompanied by excessive oozing from surgical site (see hypercarbia).

    ○ Severe *hypoxemia*.

      – The horse may be tachypneic, trying to "*buck*" the ventilator, or gasping (see hypoxemia).

    ○ *Hyperthermia*

      – (see hyperkalemic periodic paralysis [HYPP] and malignant hyperthermia [MH]).

## Suggested Reading

Copland, V.S., Hildebrand, S.V., Hill, T. 3rd et al. (1989). Blood pressure response to tourniquet use in anesthetized horses. *J. Am. Vet. Med. Assoc.* 195: 1097–1103.

Abrahamsen, E., Hellyer, P.W., Bednarski, R.M. et al. (1989). Tourniquet-induced hypertension in a horse. *J. Am. Vet. Med. Assoc.* 194: 386–388.

## Hypoxia and Hypoxemia
*Rachel A. Reed*

### I  Introduction

- Inadequate oxygen delivery to the tissues leads to ischemic injury to vital organs and skeletal muscle.
- Ischemic injury to vital organs can lead to life-threatening organ failure, whereas ischemic injury to skeletal muscle can lead to *myopathy* in the recovery period.

### II  Hypoxia

- Is a state of inadequate *tissue* oxygenation.
- Regardless of the cause, insufficient $O_2$ eventually results in the cessation of aerobic metabolism and oxidative phosphorylation leading to *cell death*.
- The presence of hypoxemia does *not* necessarily imply that tissues are hypoxic.
  - *Oxygen delivery* (DO$_2$) to the tissues and tissue *oxygen demand* must be considered when determining whether tissues are likely to be hypoxic (see Box 38.1).

#### A  Causes of hypoxia

- *Stagnant hypoxia*: decreased perfusion.
  - Decreased CO.
  - Vascular occlusion.
  - Vascular injury.
  - Edema.
- *Hypoxic hypoxia:* hypoxemia leading to decreased Hb saturation.
- *Anemic hypoxia:* decreased oxygen carrying capacity of blood.
  - Anemia.
  - Hemoglobinopathy (*rare* in horses).

---

**Box 38.1  Calculation of Oxygen Delivery to Tissues**

$DO_2(mL/min) = CaO_2 \times CO$

$$DO_2 = \left( 1.36 \times Hb \times \frac{Hb\%Sat}{100} \right) + \left( 0.003 \times PaO_2 \right) \times CO$$

- 1.36 (*Hufner's* constant) = ml of $O_2$ at 1 atm bound by 1gr Hb. Varies from 1.34 to 1.39 based on how determined and presence of non-functional Hgb (i.e. methemoglobin, carboxyhemoglobin, sulfhemoglobin)
- $CaO_2$ = Arterial $O_2$ content
- CO = Cardiac output (l/min)
- Hb = Hemoglobin (g/dl)
- 0.003 (ml) is the constant representing the volume of oxygen dissolved in plasma. Approximately 0.003 ml of $O_2$ will dissolve in 100 ml of blood for every 1 mm Hg of $PO_2$, at normal body temperature.

○ *Histotoxic hypoxia:* inability of the cell to utilize the oxygen delivered.
  – e.g. *cyanide* toxicity.

## III  Hypoxemia

- *Hypoxemia* refers to subnormal oxygen partial pressure in arterial blood.
- An arterial partial pressure of oxygen ($PaO_2$) < 60 mmHg at sea level is considered the cutoff point for hypoxemia.
- However, this rigid definition may be misleading in some cases.
- This definition would not apply to animals breathing room air at higher altitude.
  ○ e.g. the expected $PaO_2$ at 6000 ft (1829 m) is ~60 mmHg.
- A $PaO_2$ of 50 mmHg may be normal, for a 12-hour old foal in lateral recumbency.
- A $PaO_2$ > 60 mmHg can also be subnormal (e.g. if the horse is breathing a higher fraction of oxygen).
- Hypoxemia may also been defined as a resting $PaO_2$ which is >2 standard deviations below the normal $PaO_2$ for that animal's age at the particular inspired $O_2$ fraction.

### A  Causes of hypoxemia

○ There are five basic causes of hypoxemia:

*Ventilation-Perfusion (V/Q) mismatch*
  – Dead space ventilation.
  – Lung regions with a low V/Q have a relative increase in perfusion.
    ▪ Examples include pneumonia, recurrent airway obstruction.
  – V/Q mismatch is characterized by:
    ▪ An increased $P(A\text{-}a)O_2$ gradient.
    ▪ It usually responds well to oxygen supplementation.

*Shunt (Low V/Q mismatch)*
  – Shunt is the extreme of V/Q mismatch.
  – Blood enters the left side of the heart without taking part in gas exchange in the lungs.
  – It is normal to have a small shunt fraction (<3% of CO) due to blood from *bronchial* and coronary veins emptying into the left side of the heart.
  – Shunt is characterized by:
    ▪ Increased $P(A\text{-}a)O_2$ gradient.
    ▪ A minimal response to oxygen supplementation.
  – Examples: intracardiac shunts (VSD, atrial septal defect [ASD])

*Hypoventilation*
  – Hypoventilation contributes to hypoxemia by virtue of the fact that an increase in alveolar partial pressure of $CO_2$ ($PACO_2$) reduces the $PAO_2$, and thus the $PaO_2$, according to the alveolar gas equation.
    ▪ $PaCO_2 \propto 1/VA$ (alveolar ventilation)
  – $PaCO_2$ is greater than normal in hypoventilation.
  – Hypoventilation ultimately leads to low $PAO_2$ followed by a low $PaO_2$.
  – The $P(A\text{-}a)O_2$ gradient is usually normal. However, prolonged hypoventilation, may result in atelectasis and an increasing $P(A\text{-}a)O_2$ gradient.

    – Hypoxemia due to hypoventilation can usually be corrected by supplying *supplemental oxygen*, even in the face of hypoventilation and hypercarbia.

### Diffusion impairment

    – A decrease in oxygen transport across the alveolar-capillary membrane due to impaired diffusion is a relatively uncommon cause for hypoxemia in horses.
    – Diffusion impairment is characterized by:
       ■ Increased $P(A-a)O_2$ gradient.
       ■ It usually responds well to oxygen supplementation.
       ■ $PaCO_2$ is usually normal because of its good diffusability relative to oxygen.

### Low-inspired oxygen

    – The $PaO_2$ is directly proportional to the inspired oxygen fraction ($FIO_2$); thus, a decrease in the $FIO_2$ will result in a decrease in the $PaO_2$.

$$PAO_2 = FiO_2\left(PB - PH_2O\right) - \frac{PaCO_2}{R}$$

$FIO_2$ = Inspired oxygen fraction (~0.21)
PB = Atmospheric pressure (mmHg)
$PH_2O$ = Water vapor pressure (~50 mmHg at body temperature of horse)
R = Respiratory gas exchange ratio (~0.8)

## B   Other factors likely to exacerbate hypoxemia

    ○ Factors decreasing mixed venous $O_2$ (e.g. ↓ CO, ↑ $O_2$ consumption) exacerbate the effects of V/Q mismatch and shunt on hypoxemia.
    ○ Distension of abdominal contents causing atelectasis (e.g. large colon impaction).
    ○ Pre-existing respiratory pathology (e.g. recurrent airway obstruction).

## C   Clinical signs of hypoxemia

    ○ May be difficult to appreciate in an anesthetized horse.
    ○ The horse may be tachypneic, "*bucking*" the ventilator, or gasping.
    ○ Cyanosis may be present.
    ○ Tachycardia and hypertension due to hypoxia-induced catecholamine release are less commonly observed.

## IV   Problems with oxygen delivery

    ● Problems with oxygen delivery can occur at various points between the oxygen source and the patient.
    ● An in-line *oxygen analyzer* will decrease the likelihood of this problem going unnoticed.

## A   Central supply

    ○ The liquid oxygen tank may have been inadvertently filled with the incorrect gas (e.g. nitrogen).

- A gas leak may be present.
- Cylinders may be empty.
- Cylinders may not be adequately opened.
- An incorrect cylinder may be attached.

### B Anesthetic machine

- Check the oxygen pressure gauge to determine if there is a problem with oxygen supply to the machine.
- Check the flowmeter setting.
  - The $O_2$ *flow* should be adequate to match the patient's $O_2$ *consumption* (~2.5 ml/kg/min in adult horse), and allow for loss due to leaks, and the volume of $O_2$ aspirated (150–250 ml/min) from the system by the gas analyzer.
  - Small leaks in the system will be more likely to noticeably affect the $FIO_2$ if the fresh gas flow is low.
- Check the flowmeter for cracks.
- Engage the $O_2$ flush valve to see if the rebreathing bag or ventilator bellows fills.
  - If the rebreathing bag/bellows does *not* fill, check visible (accessible) $O_2$ hoses on the anesthetic machine.
  - If a disconnected $O_2$ hose is not visible, the leak may be inside the machine.

### C Anesthesia circuit

- Check that the circuit is connected to the machine and endotracheal (ET) tube.
- Check the circuit for leaks.

### D Endotracheal tube

- Check for esophageal intubation.
- Check for accidental extubation.
- Check that the cuff is adequately inflated.
- Check for *endobronchial* intubation if the patient is a small/minature foal.
  - However, this is very unlikely to occur due to the horse's relatively long neck.
- Check that the endotracheal tube is tightly attached to the Y- piece.

### E Ventilator

- Check that the circuit is properly connected to the anesthetic machine.
- If *compressed air* is being used to drive a ventilator bellows, a decrease in $FIO_2$ can result if a leak develops in the bellows allowing air to enter the bellows.
- Check settings (tidal volume, respiratory rate, minute volume).

## V  Improving arterial oxygen partial pressure (PaO₂)

### A Correct mechanical failures

- Check anesthetic machine and ventilator as described above.

**B  Institute intermittent positive pressure ventilation**

- Instituting positive pressure ventilation from the beginning of anesthesia is more effective in maintaining arterial oxygenation than trying to recruit collapsed alveoli.
  - However, the resulting increase in intrathoracic pressure decreases venous return and, hence, CO.
- Optimize tidal volume (10–15 ml/kg).
- Respiratory rate ranges are 6–8 breaths/min for adults and 8–12 for foals (up to 25 for neonates).
- If the horse is bucking the ventilator, check that the depth of anesthesia is adequate.
  - Neuromuscular blockade is rarely indicated to correct this problem.

**C  Optimize the inspiratory: expiratory ratio**

- An increase in inspiratory time may optimize alveolar ventilation.
- This may be especially important in cases of recurrent airway obstruction.

**D  Increase the FIO$_2$**

- Increasing the FIO$_2$ should increase the PaO$_2$.
  - This will not be true in the presence of a shunt.

**E  Positive end-expiratory pressure (PEEP)**

- In some cases, application of PEEP (5–10 cm H$_2$O) may decrease atelectasis.
- However, the increase in alveolar pressure may interfere with capillary circulation.
- When PEEP approaches central venous pressure, venous return is reduced.

**F  Alveolar recruitment maneuvers (ARMs)**

- In one study in which PEEP was maintained at 10 cm H$_2$O, imposing ARM improved PaO$_2$ values in horses in dorsal recumbency but *not* in horses in lateral recumbency.
  - The improvement in PaO$_2$ values lasted into the recovery period.
  - The ARM consisted of three consecutive breaths up to a peak inspiratory pressure of 80 cm H$_2$O.

**G  Aerosolized albuterol**

- *Albuterol* ($\beta_1$ and $\beta_2$ agonist), administered as an aerosol, is reported to be beneficial in the treatment of hypoxemia in the anesthetized horse.
  - *Albuterol* is more selective for $\beta_2$ receptors, thus its principle effect is *bronchodilation*.
- A dose of 2 µg/kg into the airways is recommended for adult horses. It is generally administered at the Y-piece of the breathing circuit during the inspiratory phase of the ventilator cycle.
- *Albuterol* treatment prior to anesthesia may benefit horses with recurrent airway obstruction.
  *Caution: Aerosolized albuterol in anesthetized horses has been associated with adverse effects including ventricular tachycardia and hypotension. Sweating is a common occurrence.*

## VI  Postoperative hypoxemia

### A  Causes

- ○ Hypoventilation following the cessation of intermittent positive-pressure ventilation (IPPV), a decrease in $FIO_2$, and an increase in $O_2$ demand may all contribute to hypoxemia during the recovery period.
- ○ Pulmonary issues contributing to *shunting* are the main reason for postoperative hypoxemia in otherwise healthy horses; however, n*on-shunting* reasons, such as airway obstruction, need to be addressed quickly.

*Pulmonary shunting may result from*:

- ○ A decrease in the functional residual capacity (FRC) of the lung occurs in the anesthetized horse; this results in atelectasis and shunting which persist into the recovery period.
- ○ Accumulation of secretions in the small airway compounds the effects of a decrease in FRC on atelectasis.
- ○ Increased $O_2$ consumption during attempts to stand in recovery, or as a result of shivering, will decrease mixed venous $O_2$ thus exacerbating the effects of shunting and V/Q mismatch.
- ○ Inhalational anesthetics inhibit *hypoxic pulmonary vasoconstriction* which may contribute to shunting and V/Q mismatch.
- ○ Aspiration pneumonia contributes to atelectasis; however, it is an uncommon occurrence in the horse post-anesthesia.
    - – It is most likely to occur in a horse with GI colic subsequent to inhalation of refluxed gastric contents.

*Airway obstruction*

- ○ Decreased airway patency will contribute to hypoxemia.
- ○ A patent airway must be established upon extubation.
- ○ Nasal or naso-tracheal tube placement, and/or intra-nasal *phenylephrine* administration will improve airway patency (see Chapter 4 – Airway Management).

### B  Supplemental oxygen

- ○ Increasing the $FIO_2$, especially if $O_2$ is delivered intratracheally (10–15 l/min), may increase $PaO_2$.

## Suggested Reading

Hopster, K., Duffee, L.R., Hopster-Iversen, C.C.S. et al. (2018). Efficacy of an alveolar recruitment maneuver for improving gas exchange and pulmonary mechanics in anesthetized horses ventilated with oxygen or a helium-oxygen mixture. *Am. J. Vet. Res.* 79: 1021–1027.

Hopster, K., Rohn, K., Ohnesorge, B., and Kästner, S.B.R. (2017). Controlled mechanical ventilation with constant positive end-expiratory pressure and alveolar recruitment manoeuvres during anaesthesia in laterally or dorsally recumbent horses. *Vet. Anaesth. Analg.* 44: 121–126.

## Hypercarbia

*Tom Doherty*

- Defined as a $PaCO_2$ above normal.
  - A $PaCO_2 > 45\,mmHg$.
- Hypercarbia is common during general anesthesia due to the depressant effects of anesthetic drugs on the respiratory center.
- Hypercarbia reflects inadequate ventilation (*hypoventilation*) relative to carbon dioxide production.
  - On occasions, hypercarbia results from problems with the anesthetic machine or ventilator.
  - On rare occasions, hypercarbia results from increased production of $CO_2$.
    - e.g. HYPP.

## I  Causes of hypercarbia

### A  Decreased $CO_2$ elimination

$$PaCO_2 = VCO_2/VA \ (VCO_2 = CO_2 \text{ production}; VA = \text{Alveolar ventilation})$$

*Inadequate ventilation*
  - This is the most likely cause of hypercarbia under anesthesia.
    - Check ventilator settings.
    - The minute ventilation may be too low.
  - Central depression (due to anesthetic drugs) in spontaneously ventilating horse.
    - Institute IPPV.
  - Residual neuromuscular block.
    - Reversal of block is indicated.

*Decreased lung compliance*
  - Distended abdomen (e.g. due to colonic displacement/impaction).
  - Capnoperitoneum during laparoscopy.
  - Diaphragmatic hernia (uncommon, most likely in mares *post-partum*, but may be a chronic condition).
  - Head-down position.
  - Partial obstruction of airway.
    - COPD.
    - Bronchospasm (uncommon in the horse).
    - Kinking of endotracheal tube.

### B  Increased $CO_2$ production

  - Due to an increase in body temperature.
    - HYPP.
    - MH (extremely unlikely cause).
    - Sepsis.
    - $NaHCO_3^-$ administration.
    - $CO_2$ administration (e.g. during laparoscopy).

C   Increased $CO_2$ delivery to lungs

- $CO_2$ rebreathing. This will be easy to detect if an end-tidal monitor is in use.
  - Check that expiratory *valve* on anesthetic machine is not *stuck open*.
  - Check $CO_2$ absorbent.

## II   Effects of hypercarbia on the cardiovascular system

- In a study in isoflurane anesthetized horses, the effects of hypercarbia on cardiovascular function were considered to be *biphasic*. In that study, horses were ventilated, and $CO_2$ was added to the inspired gases to manipulate the $PaCO_2$.
- The cardiovascular effects of three levels of hypercarbia were investigated.

A   Mild increase in $PaCO_2$ (55–65 mmHg) was associated with:

- Bradycardia (small decrease in heart rate).
- Decrease in CI and $DO_2$.
- Increase in SBP, MAP, SVR.
- Increase in venous admixture.

B   Moderate increase in $PaCO_2$ (75–85 mmHg) was associated with:

- Increases in CI, SI, SBP, MAP, peak airway pressure (PAP).
- Increases in $CaO_2$, $CvO_2$, $DO_2$.

C   Severe increase in $PaCO_2$ (>90 mmHg) was associated with:

- Increases in HR, CI, SI, SBP, PAP.
- Decrease in SVR.
- No change in MAP – probably due to the decrease in SVR.

- The hypercarbia-induced cardiovascular stimulation is considered to result from *catecholamine* release, and plasma *norepinephrine* concentrations increase with increasing $PaCO_2$ values.

## III   Other effects of hypercarbia

- Hypercarbia can contribute to *hypoxemia*, especially if a horse is breathing a low-inspired oxygen fraction.
  - See alveolar gas equation.
- Increased cardiac irritability resulting in *arrhythmia*s has *not* been associated with hypercarbia in anesthetized horses.
- Decrease in pH.
  - The pH decreases by ~0.1 pH unit for every 20 mmHg acute increase in $PaCO_2$.
  - Thus, a $PaCO_2$ of 70 mmHg would decrease the pH by ~0.15 units.
- Effect on plasma $[K^+]$.
  - Decreasing the $PaCO_2$ by 10 mmHg decreases the plasma $[K^+]$ by ~0.5 mEq/l.
    - This is likely to be of clinical significance in patients with *uroperitoneum*.

## IV   Management of hypercarbia

- As mentioned, hypercarbia in the anesthetized horse is usually due to hypoventilation.
  - However, other causes of hypercarbia that would require prompt attention (e.g. HYPP) should be considered.
- If hypercarbia is due to a distended colon, it is best to tolerate a high $PaCO_2$ until the pressure on the diaphragm can be relieved, in order to avoid excessive airway pressures.
- Ensure that oxygenation and ventilation are adequate.
- Check that the *one-way valves* on the anesthetic machine are functioning.
- Institute-controlled ventilation if the horse is breathing spontaneously.
- If the horse is already being ventilated check:
  - That the *tidal volume* is adequate (10–15 ml/kg, in an adult).
  - That the *ventilation rate* is adequate (6–8/min, in an adult).
  - That the *bellows* is intact and filling adequately to deliver an adequate tidal volume. Improper filling of the bellows may be a result of leaks in the system.

## Suggested Reading

Khanna, A.K., McDonell, W.N., Dyson, D.H., and Taylor, P.M. (1995). Cardiopulmonary effects of hypercarbia during controlled intermittent positive pressure ventilation in the horse. *Can. J. Vet. Res.* 59: 213–221.

## Pulmonary Edema as a Consequence of Airway Obstruction
*Tom Doherty*

- Pulmonary edema has been reported in horses during recovery.
- It can be fatal if not treated promptly. However, every effort must be directed at preventing it occurring.
- In addition to airway obstruction, pulmonary edema has been reported in 17% of horses recovering in the Hydro-Pool system.

## I   Clinical signs

- Exaggerated inspiratory effort.
- Tachypnea and tachycardia.
- Cyanosis of mucous membranes.
- Presence of blood-tinged frothy fluid in the endotracheal tube or from the nostrils in the post-obstruction period.

## II   Proposed pathogenesis

- Pulmonary edema subsequent to obstruction of the upper airway has been described as negative pressure pulmonary edema.

- In attempting to inhale forcibly against an obstruction, the horse generates an exceedingly high negative intrathoracic pressure with a resultant increase in venous return to the heart.
- However, CO decreases due to a decrease in pulmonary venous drainage into the left atrium.
- There is an increase in pulmonary vascular resistance, and this may be a result of the increased pulmonary interstitial pressure and vasoconstriction due to sympathetic discharge.
  - This may result in an increase in right ventricular pressure and, in severe cases, ventricular septal displacement may cause a decrease in left ventricular compliance.
- There is an increase in *pulmonary capillary pressures, intraalveolar* pressures decrease, and there is a disruption of *alveolar cell junctions.*
  - This results in fluid movement into *interstitial* and *alveolar spaces.*
  - Pulmonary edema persists even after relieving the airway obstruction.
- The process is exacerbated by hypoxia and the resulting *hyperadrener*gic state.

## III   Treatment

- Relieving the obstruction is the primary step. However, this may be difficult if the horse is awake and anxious.
  - Be prepared to perform an *emergency tracheostomy.* It may be necessary, in some cases, to wait until the horse collapses to perform a tracheostomy (see Chapter 4).
- Correct the hypoxemia by providing $O_2$.
  - If possible, pass an orotracheal or nasotracheal tube, otherwise an emergency tracheostomy is required.
  - A *demand valve* is a practical method to supply oxygen and ventilate the horse.
- It may be necessary to sedate the horse *post-obstruction* to decrease anxiety and stress. This will also decrease oxygen consumption.
  - In human beings, *morphine* has been shown to be efficacious in treating patients with pulmonary edema, and it decreases the tone of airway smooth muscle.
- Although diuretics *(e.g. furosemide)* and corticosteroids *(e.g. dexamethasone)* are generally recommended, their efficacy is debated.
- *β₂ agonists*, although primarily used to relieve bronchospasm which is not likely to be a factor in post-obstruction pulmonary edema, may be beneficial in relieving edema by *increasing alveolar fluid clearance.*

## Suggested Reading

Abrahamsen, E.J., Bohanon, T.C., Bednarski, R.M. et al. (1990). Bilateral arytenoid cartilage paralysis after inhalation anesthesia in a horse. *J. Am. Vet. Med. Assoc.* 197: 1363–1365.

Senior, M. (2005). Post-anaesthetic pulmonary oedema in horses: a review. *Vet. Anaesth. Analg.* 32: 193–200.

## Endotoxemia

*Tom Doherty*

- LPS, also known as *endotoxin*, is a major component of the outer membrane of the cell wall of Gram-negative bacteria.
- High concentrations of LPS are found in the large intestine of horses; however, LPS is mostly restricted from entering the circulation by the intact intestinal mucosal barrier. The small amount of LPS that enters the circulation under normal conditions is effectively removed by the Kupffer cells in the liver.
- If the intestinal barrier is damaged, LPS molecules enter the circulation and evoke a sequence of biologic responses that result in the clinical condition described as *endotoxemia*.
- Endotoxemia is present in up to 35% of horses undergoing emergency abdominal surgery for GI problems. In addition, endotoxemia occurs in up to 50% of foals suspected to be suffering from bacteremia.
- The horse is among the most sensitive of species to the toxic effects of LPS.
  - Only man and the chimpanzee are more sensitive than the horse to LPS.

## I    Treatment of endotoxemic horses

- Treatment is aimed at:
  - Cardiovascular support (fluids, inotropes).
    - *Hypertonic saline* has been shown to improve cardiac contractility and *has anti-inflammatory* effects in sepsis.
  - Reducing the release and effects of inflammatory mediators.

## II    Drugs used in the treatment of endotoxemic horses

### A    Non-steroidal anti-inflammatory drugs (NSAIDs)

- NSAIDs are effective in blocking the clinical effects of LPS in experimental models in horses.
- NSAIDs inhibit COX enzymes associated with early hemodynamic responses to LPS.
- They decrease the production of prostaglandins by inhibiting LPS-induced COX enzyme induction in a variety of tissues.
- NSAIDs, except *phenylbutazone*, inhibit the production of nuclear factor κB (NFκB), which is important in cytokine gene transcription.

### B    Polymyxin B (PB)

- *PB*, a polypeptide antibiotic, is not generally administered systemically as an antimicrobial due to its potential for inducing *nephrotoxicity* at anti-bacterial doses.
  - The anti-bacterial dose is 15 000–25 000 units/kg/day divided q12 hour., IV.
- At sub-therapeutic doses, *PB* has a high affinity for lipid A, the common component of LPS molecules. *PB* forms a stable complex with lipid A, thus preventing it from interacting with inflammatory cells.

- ○ *PB* reduces the adverse effects of LPS in horses and reduces cytokine production.
- ○ The effects of *PB* are dose-related.
    - – Doses of 1000–6000 units/kg can be administered pre-surgery or intraoperatively.
    - – *PB* is usually diluted (e.g. in 1 l 0.9% NaCl), and infused slowly (15–30 minutes).

## C  Lidocaine

- ○ Lidocaine has a number of properties that may be beneficial to horses suffering from endotoxemia.
    - – It decreases the expression of inducible *nitric oxide synthase*.
    - – It inhibits NFkB.
    - – It decreases chemotactic factors and cytokines.
    - – It decreases albumin extravasation and microvascular permeability.
    - – It inhibits the sequestration, migration, and activation of polymorphonuclear cells.
    - – It inhibits the adherence of polymorphonuclear cells to endothelial cells.

## D  Dimethyl sulfoxide (DMSO)

- ○ DMSO has anti-inflammatory actions and was efficacious in experimental models of endotoxic shock in rodents.
    - – DMSO decreased cytokine production (e.g. ↓ TNFα production).
- ○ Doses up to 1 g/kg, IV q24 hours, have been used clinically in horses.
- *Note: There is no study indicating that DMSO is efficacious for treating horses suffering from endotoxemia. In one experimental study in horses, DMSO administration did not alleviate the clinical signs associated with LPS administration, but it ameliorated LPS-induced fever.*
- ○ DMSO should be diluted in a large volume (3–5 l) of balanced electrolyte solution for infusion.
- ○ Overdosing of DMSO can result in *pulmonary edema*.
- ○ High concentrations can cause *hemolysis*.
- ○ DMSO has human health hazards.
    - – Hospital personnel must take precautions when using DMSO (e.g. wear gloves).
    - – DMSO is excreted mainly (~70%) via the lungs, so good ventilation is important to avoid inhalation by hospital personnel.

## Suggested Reading

Barton, M.H., Parviainen, A., and Norton, N. (2004). Polymyxin B protects horses against induced endotoxaemia *in vivo. Equine. Vet. J.* 36: 397–401.

Semrad, S.D., Hardee, G.E., Hardee, M.M. et al. (1987). Low dose flunixin meglumine effects on eicosanoid production and clinical signs induced by experimental endotoxaemia in horses. *Equine. Vet. J.* 19: 201–206.

Kelmer, G., Doherty, T.J., Elliott, S. et al. (2008). Evaluation of dimethyl sulphoxide effects on initial response to endotoxin in the horse. *Equine. Vet. J.* 40: 358–363.

## Postanesthetic Myopathy

*Krista B. Mitchell*

- Defined as postanesthetic muscle swelling, weakness, and pain resulting from ischemic muscle damage due to hypoperfusion.
- Historically a common complication of equine anesthesia.
- In halothane-anesthetized horses, postanesthetic myopathy has been directly related to a long duration of recumbency and intraoperative hypotension.
- The most severe form of the condition, *rhabdomyolysis*, is potentially fatal in cases in which the horse is unable to stand in recovery or suffers renal damage due to *myoglobinuria*.
- Myopathy appears to be less common nowadays, and this may be due to more emphasis on maintaining an adequate arterial blood pressure and providing better padding and limb support for the anesthetized horse.
- Myopathy can occur in two forms:
  - Localized.
  - Generalized.

## I  Localized myopathy

- Refers to ischemic muscle damage, usually occurring in dependent muscles; however, non-dependent muscles may be affected.
- Particularly susceptible muscle groups include:
  - *Triceps*, *gluteals*, *quadriceps,* and *masseter* in lateral recumbency.
  - *Longissimus dorsi, gluteals,* and *adductor*s in dorsal recumbency.
- The condition has been compared to *compartment syndrome* in human beings.
  - Compartment syndrome is a term used to describe local muscle ischemia, and subsequent muscle contracture, resulting from edema and increased pressure within osteofascial compartments.

### A  Contributing factors

- Hypotension.
- Inadequate padding of body and support of limbs.
- Improper positioning.
  - e.g. Horse tilted to one side while in dorsal recumbency.
- Large body mass of horse.
  - More likely to occur in drafts and large warmbloods.
- Hypoxemia.
- Horse's nutritional/health status.

### B  Pathogenesis

*Decreased perfusion*
  - Muscles are divided functionally into compartments separated by fascial sheaths, which prevent fluid movement between compartments.

○ Muscle perfusion pressure = MAP – Intracompartmental muscle pressure or venous pressure.
  – Thus, increases in intracompartmental pressure will decrease the muscle perfusion pressure.
○ Intracompartmental muscle pressure is a function of:
  – Duration of the intracompartmental pressure increase.
  – Metabolic rate of tissues.
  – Vascular tone.
  – Local arterial blood pressure.
  – Venous drainage.
  – Surface pressure on the muscle compartment (affected by padding and mass of horse).
○ Intracompartmental pressure has been determined to be 30–60 mmHg in dependent muscle groups.
○ If venous drainage from a muscle group is occluded, compartmental pressure increases, or if the MAP falls below compartmental pressure/venous pressure, muscle perfusion is diminished leading to ischemia.

*Ischemic injury*
  ○ Ischemia of muscle capillaries leads to increased permeability of the capillary walls and *edema* formation.
  ○ Edema perpetuates the increase in compartmental pressure.
  ○ Unless the arterial flow can be restored (e.g. by repositioning the horse) in a timely manner and before a "*critical*" pressure develops, serious consequences for the muscle may result.

*Reperfusion of ischemic muscle*
  ○ May be partially responsible for muscle damage due to excess production of *oxygen free radicals* initiating membrane lipid peroxidation and membrane protein alterations.

## C   Clinical signs

  ○ Signs depend on the severity of the condition and the location of muscle damage.
  ○ Usually, clinical signs do not become evident until the horse attempts to stand or up to one hour after recovery.
  ○ Signs include:
    – Difficulty in recovery due to inability to bear full weight on affected limb(s) (e.g. a dropped elbow stance with triceps myopathy, unwillingness to bear weight on hind limbs with gluteal myopathy).
    – Lameness (mild to severe).
    – Localized swelling and varying degrees of hardness of muscle(s).
    – Sweating (due to pain) may be severe.
    – Muscle fasciculations may be present.
    – Myoglobinuria.
    *Comment*: It may sometimes be difficult to differentiate *triceps myopathy* from *radial nerve* damage. Usually with *radial nerve* injury there is no muscle swelling or pain; however, it is possible that both conditions may co-exist.

*Laboratory data*
  ○ Serum creatine kinase (CK) activity *increase quickly* following myocyte damage.

○ In contrast to CK, aspartate aminotransferase (AST) activity increase more slowly and persist longer in plasma following muscle damage.

○ The urine may be "*coffee colored*" depending on the myoglobin concentration, and will test positive for blood with urine test strips (see Chapter 2).

*Non-dependent limb myopathy*

○ The development of a myopathy in the *non-dependent* limb has been documented.

○ The cause has been hypothesized to be due to decreased hydrostatic pressure if the limb is elevated above heart level.

## II  Generalized myopathy

- Postanesthetic generalized myopathy is an uncommon condition in horses, and has a guarded prognosis.
- Pathologic changes occur in multiple muscle groups resulting in generalized muscle swelling, weakness and pain.
- The condition has been compared to MH.

### A  Clinical signs

○ Tachycardia.

○ Tachypnea.

○ Sweating.

○ Myoglobinuria.

○ May progress to cardiovascular shock leading to metabolic acidosis and hyperkalemia.

### B  Pathogenesis

○ The pathogeny is unknown, but theories include:
  – Local ischemic lesions caused by systemic hypotension and hypoxemia may become generalized due to the stress of anesthesia or release of free radicals when the muscle is reperfused.
  – Inherited muscle disorders may be exacerbated by the stress of surgery and anesthesia (e.g. polysaccharide storage myopathy, recurrent exertional myopathy).

## III  Reducing the incidence of postanesthetic myopathy

- Decrease the duration of recumbency.
- Provide adequate padding.
- Position the horse properly (see Chapter 18).
  ○ Place horse squarely on its back when in dorsal recumbency.
  ○ Avoid extreme flexion or extension of limbs.
  ○ Position upper limbs parallel to table when horse is in lateral.
  ○ Do not place support padding on top of the lower limb in an effort to support the upper limb, as this may affect venous drainage of the lower limb.
- Avoid intraoperative hypotension.
  ○ MAP > 70 mmHg.

- Muscle perfusion is also a function of CO and SVR; therefore, mucous membrane color, capillary refill time, heart rate, serum lactate, and fluid status should be assessed as well as blood pressure.

*Dantrolene*
- *Dantrolene* decreases calcium release from the sarcoplasmic reticulum by inhibiting *ryanodine* receptors in skeletal muscle cells.
- There is some evidence that *dantrolene* is effective in preventing postanesthetic myopathy.
  - In a crossover study, oral administration of dantrolene (6 mg/kg) in hypotensive horses subjected to 90 minutes of anesthesia with isoflurane was not associated with an increase in serum CK activity over baseline values at any time point, indicating that muscle damage did not occur. However, dantrolene administration was associated with an increase in serum [K$^+$] and a decrease in CO in comparison to the placebo treatment. In addition, one horse developed bradycardia (15 beats/min), and another developed an AV block that necessitated treatment.
- There is evidence that dantrolene may be effective in preventing *exertional rhabdomyolysis* (ER) in horses.
  - In a crossover study, oral administration of 800 mg of dantrolene sodium to Thoroughbred horses, one hour before exercise, caused a small but significant decrease in the difference between the pre- and post-exercise plasma CK activity relative to the control treatment. In addition, no horse in the dantrolene treatment developed ER, and 3 of 77 horses in the control treatment developed ER.
  - In horses with *recurrent ER*, dantrolene administered orally at 4 mg/kg, decreased the plasma CK activity after exercise in four of five horses.
- Reported complications associated with pre-operative dantrolene administration include hyperkalemia, muscle weakness, and prolonged post-anesthetic recovery in clinical cases.

## IV  Sequelae

- Injury (e.g. long-bone fracture) in the recovery period due to incoordination and weakness.
- Renal damage from myoglobinuria.
- Muscle wasting (may be chronic).

## V  Treatment

- Some horses may need assistance to stand during and following recovery.
- If the horse is recumbent, provide adequate padding and nursing care.
- Mild cases should benefit from light exercise (i.e. walking), starting on the day following recovery from anesthesia.
- Maintain hydration.
  - However, infusions of large volumes of isotonic fluid may be detrimental as this may increase intracompartmental pressure.
- *Mannitol* has been shown, in experimental models of ischemic myopathy, to reduce intracompartmental pressure and improve tissue oxygenation.

- It may also provide protection against myoglobin-induced renal tubular damage.
  - A bolus of *mannitol* (0.25 g/kg, IV) may be repeated two to three in the first 24 hours.
- Provide analgesia.
  - NSAIDs should suffice in mild cases.
  - More severe cases require more intensive analgesia.
- *Methocarbamol*, a centrally acting muscle relaxant, is sometimes used to treat tying-up in horses. The injectable form is Food and Drug Administration (FDA) approved for treatment of muscle spasm in horses resulting from inflammatory conditions.
  - A dose of 15–25 mg/kg, IV (administered slowly) has been recommended for acute rhabdomyolysis. This dose may be repeated up to 4 times daily.
  - However, the efficacy of methocarbamol for treating horses with rhabdomyolysis is unproven.
- Provide *vitamin E* and *selenium*, if deemed to be deficient.
- Local treatment of affected muscle (e.g. various massage modalities, ultrasound therapy).
- *Dantrolene* has been recommended for the treatment of horses with post-anesthetic myopathy, but there is no evidence that it is beneficial once the muscle damage occurs.
  - Doses of 2–4 mg/kg, IV (administered slowly) have been recommended during an acute MH crisis in human patients and this may have to be repeated at four-to-six hour intervals.
  - Oral doses of 2–8 mg/kg have been used in horses.
  - *Note: The administration of dantrolene IV to horses may not always be feasible due to cost and logistical issues associated with its preparation. (see malignant hyperthermia)*
  - The adverse effects of dantrolene should be considered prior to its administration.
- Other treatments that have been recommended include DMSO.

## Suggested Reading

Edwards, J.G.T., Newton, J.R., Ramzan, P.H.L. et al. (2003). The efficacy of dantrolene sodium in controlling exertional rhabdomyolysis in the Thoroughbred racehorse. *Equine. Vet. J.* 35: 707–711.

Grandy, J.L., Steffey, E.P., Hodgson, D.S. et al. (1987). Arterial hypotension and the development of postanesthetic myopathy in halothane-anesthetized horses. *Am. J. Vet. Res.* 48: 192–197.

Klein, L., Ailes, N., Fackelman, G.E. et al. (1990). Postanesthetic equine myopathy suggestive of malignant hyperthermia: A Case Report. *Vet. Surg.* 18: 479–482.

McKenzie, E.C., Valberg, S.J., Godden, S.M. et al. (2004). Effect of oral administration of dantrolene sodium on serum creatine kinase activity after exercise in horses with recurrent exertional rhabdomyolysis. *Am. J. Vet. Res.* 65: 74–79.

McKenzie EC, Mosley C (2009) Dantrolene sodium prevents myopathy in horses undergoing hypotensive anesthesia (abstr), in *Proceedings*. 15th Int Vet Emerg Crit Care Symp 717.

McKenzie, E.C., Di Concetto, S., Payton, M.E. et al. (2015). Effect of dantrolene premedication on various cardiovascular and biochemical variables and the recovery in healthy isoflurane-anesthetized horses. *Am. J. Vet. Res.* 76: 293–301.

Oosterlinck, M., Schauvliege, S., Martens, A. et al. (2013). Postanesthetic neuropathy/myopathy in the nondependent forelimb in 4 horses. *J. Equine. Vet. Sci.* 33: 996–999.

Parish, S.M. and Valberg, S.J. (2009). Nonexertional rhabdomyolysis. In: *Large Animal Internal Medicine*, 4e (ed. B.P. Smith), 1400–1411. St. Louis, Mo: Mosby/Elsevier.

Richey, M.T., Holland, M.S., McGrath, C.J. et al. (1990). Equine postanesthetic lameness. A retrospective study. *Vet. Surg.* 19: 392–397.

Serteyn, D., Mottart, E., Deby, C. et al. (1990). Equine postanaesthetic myositis: a possible role for free radical generation and membrane lipoperoxidation. *Res. Vet. Sci.* 48: 42–46.

Valverde, A., Boyd, C.J., Dyson, D.H. et al. (1990). Prophylactic use of dantrolene associated with prolonged postanesthetic recumbency in a horse. *J. Am. Vet. Med. Assoc.* 197: 1051–1053.

White, N.A. and Suarex, M. (1986). Change in triceps intracompartmental pressure with repositioning and padding of the lowermost thoracic limb of the horse. *Am. J. Vet. Res.* 47: 2257–2260.

Young, S.S. (2005). Post anaesthetic myopathy. *Equine. Vet. Educ.* 15: 60–63.

## Neuropathy

*Rachel A. Reed*

- Anesthesia-related nervous system injuries occur in the horse.
- Most commonly, the insult involves *peripheral nerves* (e.g. radial, facial).
    - On rare occasions it may involve the *spinal cord.*
- Many of the factors involved in the development of postanesthetic myopathy are also important in the development of neuropathy.
- Clinical signs:
    - Are dependent on the severity of the condition and the location of the nerve damage.
    - Signs are generally noticed when the horse attempts to stand.
    - Mild cases may not be noticed until the horse attempts to walk.
    - Peripheral nerve damage usually occurs in *dependent* nerves; however, *non-dependent* nerves may be affected.

## I  Factors contributing to peripheral nerve damage

- Large body mass of horse.
- Long duration of recumbency.
- Inadequate padding of body and support of limbs.
    - Direct pressure from hard surface or object (e.g. a halter buckle causing *facial nerve* damage).
- Improper positioning.
    - The lower thoracic limb should be pulled forward to release the triceps muscle and radial nerve from under the thoracic cage.
    - If *radial nerve* damage has occurred in the *non-dependent* limb, it may be that the brachial plexus has been damaged by malposition of the limb.
- Overextension of limbs.
    - e.g. *Femoral nerve* paralysis may result from overextension of the pelvic limbs when the horse is in dorsal or lateral recumbency.

## II  Radial nerve injury

### A  Clinical signs

- Vary with the severity of the injury.
- Signs may be evident when the horse attempts to stand or may not develop for some hours after recovery.

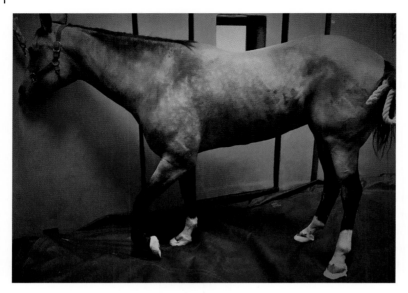

Figure 38.2    Horse with radial nerve injury following recovery from anesthesia.

- – It is not always easy to differentiate radial nerve damage from triceps myopathy.
- ○ Inability to bear weight on affected forelimb.
- ○ Elbow is "dropped" due to lack of triceps tone (see Figure 38.2).
- ○ Inability to extend the thoracic limb.
- ○ Generally, no pain in affected area unless triceps myopathy co-exists.
- ○ In cases where the onset of clinical signs of radial nerve damage is delayed, it is likely that the nerve damage occurred from swelling of the triceps as a result of myopathy.

B    Sequelae

- ○ Difficult recovery from anesthesia.
  - – Assisted recovery may be necessary.

C    Outcome

- ○ Most cases regain neurologic function in a few days.
- ○ Permanent nerve damage results in some cases.

## III    Femoral nerve injury

- • Probably results from overextension of the pelvic limbs with the horse in dorsal recumbency.
- • May also result from overextension of the pelvic limbs in lateral recumbency, such as may occur when a horse is undergoing an MRI and the limbs are pulled tightly into the gantry.

### A   Clinical signs

- May involve one or both pelvic limbs.
- Inability to stand if both pelvic limbs are involved.
- Inability to *extend* the stifle (see Figure 38.3).
- *Flexion* of hock is evident.
- The condition appears to the painful, and affected horses may sweat profusely and have tachycardia initially.
- Usually no swelling of muscles in pelvic limb unless myopathy coexists.

### B   Sequelae

- Difficult recovery or unable to stand.
- Further injury (e.g. long-bone fracture) likely to result if horse makes repeated attempts to stand.
- Mild cases should resolve in a few days.

## IV   Peroneal nerve injury

- Uncommon occurrence.
- Usually occurs in *dependent* limb with the horse in lateral recumbency.

### A   Clinical signs

- Horse is usually able to stand.
- Inability to *flex* the hock and *extend* the foot.

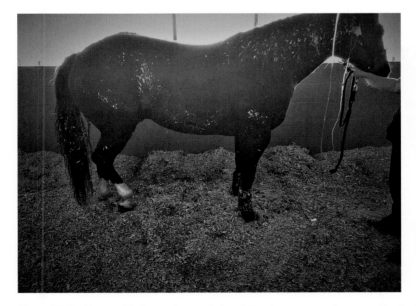

Figure 38.3   Horse with femoral nerve injury following recovery from anesthesia. *Source:* Dr. Carrie A. Davis.

**B Sequelae**

  ○ Mild cases should resolve in a few days.

## V Facial nerve injury (see Figure 38.4)

  • Usually results from the *halter buckle* applying pressure over the nerve with the horse in lateral.

### A Clinical signs

  ○ Motor paralysis of facial muscles.
  ○ Drooping of lip is most common sign.

### B Sequelae

  ○ Mild cases resolve in a few days.
  ○ Condition may be permanent in some cases.

## VI Spinal cord myelomalacia

  • Myelomalacia or hemorrhagic myelopathy has been described following anesthesia in horses.
  • Horses are usually young (6–24 months), rapidly growing, and of the heavier breeds.

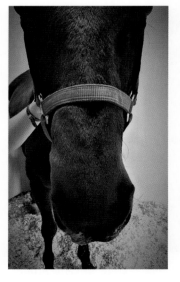

**Figure 38.4**  Horse with facial nerve injury following recovery from anesthesia.

- Most reported cases were horses that had been positioned in dorsal recovery. Many were anesthetized for short periods.
- Hemorrhagic poliomyelomalacic lesions of the spinal cord have been described in some cases.
- The condition is thought to be ischemic in origin and may be associated with low arterial pressure or fibrocartilagenous emboli.

## A   Clinical signs

- The horse may initially have pelvic limb weakness or be unable to stand.
- The condition progresses caudally resulting in the loss of deep pain and movement in the pelvic limbs and loss of anal tone.
- The horse may "*dog-sit*" or adopt *Schiff-Sherrington* posture.
- Horse does not seem to be in pain.

## B   Sequelae

- Little chance of recovery.

## VII   Myelogram associated neuropathy

- Myelograms generally cause deterioration in neurologic function in the post anesthetic period.
- It is common for horses to show an increased neurological deficit (usually a one-grade change) for a few days after a myelogram.
- Prior administration of NSAIDs may lessen the adverse effects of the myelogram.
- On rare occasion, horses may have temporary *blindness*.

## VIII   Cerebral cortical necrosis

- Signs of cerebral cortical injury have been reported to develop within a few hours of recovery from anesthesia or up to seven days later.
- May be linked to cerebral ischemia during the anesthesia period.

## A   Clinical signs

- Blindness.
- Behavioral disturbances such as:
  - Compulsive pacing.
  - Head pressing.
  - Lethargy.
  - Seizures.

## B   Sequelae

- Recovery is unlikely.

## IX   Treatment of peripheral neuropathies

- Treatment of peripheral neuropathies is very similar to treatment of myopathies and is mainly supportive.
- Some horses may need assistance to stand during and following recovery.
  - ○ Consider using a *sling* if the horse has difficulty in standing (see Chapter 39).
- If recumbent, provide adequate padding and nursing care.
- Maintain hydration.
- Anti-inflammatories (e.g. NSAIDs).
  - ○ NSAIDs will also provide analgesia if there is associated myopathy.
- Other recommended treatments include DMSO, but its efficacy is unproven.
- Local treatment of affected area, including various massage modalities and ultrasound therapy, have been recommended.

## Suggested Reading

Ragle, C., Baetge, C., Yiannikouris, S. et al. (2011). Development of equine post anaesthetic myelopathy: Thirty cases (1979–2010). *Equine. Vet. Ed.* 23: 630–635.

Spadavecchia, C., Jaggy, A., Fatzer, R., and Schatzmann, U. (2001). Postanaesthetic cerebral necrosis in a horse. *Equine. Vet. J.* 33: 621–624.

## Hyperkalemic Periodic Paralysis (HYPP)

*Alanna N. Johnson and Rachel A. Reed*

## I   Introduction

- HYPP is a genetic condition that causes altered conduction in the muscle membrane.
- HYPP affects about 4% of Quarter Horses, and also affects Quarter horse-crossbred horses, and Paints.
- Affected horses are usually heavily muscled.

### A   Triggers for HYPP

- ○ The condition can be triggered by a number of factors including:
  - – Stress.
  - – Exposure to cold.
  - – Transportation.
  - – Changes in diet or fasting.
  - – High potassium diets (e.g. alfalfa, soybean meal).
  - – Pregnancy.
  - – Sedation or general anesthesia.

## II   Pathogenesis

- HYPP is an autosomal dominant trait.
- The disorder results in a point mutation in the SCN4A gene.
- An increase in the resting membrane potential occurs due to the failure of this subpopulation of $Na^+$ channels to inactivate after depolarization. This results in an influx of $Na^+$ and an efflux of $K^+$ and culminates in a persistent depolarization of the muscle cell, and results in the clinical signs of muscle fasciculations and weakness.

## III   Clinical signs

### A   Awake horses

- Some HYPP affected horses may not exhibit clinical signs.
- Others may exhibit signs on a daily basis.
- Signs may include:
  - Sweating.
  - Focal muscle fasciculations.
  - Prolapse of the nictitating membrane.
  - Generalized muscle fasciculations may occur and these will be aggravated by movement.
  - Weakness is a common sign, and horses may stagger or dog-sit and may become recumbent.
  - Respiratory signs subsequent to pharyngeal and laryngeal collapse can result in stridor and respiratory distress.
- Horses are normal between episodes.
- Death associated with an HYPP episode is awake horses is uncommon.

### B   Anesthetized horses

- Focal muscle fasciculations may be evident.
- Hyperthermia.
- The heart rate decreases as hyperkalemia progresses but may increase initially.
- Hypercarbia due to increased muscle activity. An increase in $ETCO_2$ occurs despite the horse been ventilated. The horse will likely be bucking the ventilator at this stage.
  - The soda lime cannister will turn color more rapidly than expected and the temperature of the cannister will increase noticeably.
- Electrocardiogram (ECG) changes will develop as hyperkalemia progresses.
  - T wave becomes taller.
  - QRS complex widens.
  - P wave becomes smaller and disappears as the serum $[K^+]$ increases.
  - Bradycardia.
- Prolonged recovery is common and assistance to standing is indicated in most cases.

## IV  Laboratory findings

- During an HYPP episode the most significant change is hyperkalemia.
- $[K^+]$ may increase to 9 mEq/l.
- $[Na^+]$ may be mildly increased.
- Serum *creatine* activity may increase slightly for a few hours.
- Mild hemoconcentration may occur.

*Diagnosis*

- A definitive diagnosis of HYPP is based on genetic testing.
- Hair samples with the roots attached can be submitted to the Veterinary Genetics Laboratory, at the University of California, Davis, CA for testing.

## V  Perioperative preparation and anesthesia

### A  Owner education

- The owner should be advised regarding the risk of anesthesia and related risk factors (e.g. transportation, hospitalization), and how to decrease the associated stress.

### B  Diuretic therapy prior to anesthesia

- Potassium excretion can be promoted using the diuretics *acetazolamide* or *hydrochlorothiazide*. They should be administered for at least two days prior to anesthesia.
  - *Acetazolamide*: 2 mg/kg, orally; q12 hours.
  - *Hydrochlorothiazide*: 0.5–1.0 mg/kg, orally; q12 hours.

### C  Patient evaluation

- A detailed history of the horse should be obtained especially in relation to whether it is heterozygous or homozygous for the mutation.
  - Although both types are susceptible to an HYPP episode, homozygous horses are generally more severely affected.
  - Determine if the horse has had episodes of HYPP and inquire about its diet or recent dietary changes.
- In addition to a physical examination, an ECG and serum chemistry should be performed. It is especially important to have a baseline value for serum $[K^+]$.
- Determine if the horse is being administered drugs with the potential to increase serum $[K^+]$ such as potassium sparing diuretics (e.g. *spironolactone*).

### D  Pre-anesthetic sedation

- It is important to reduce stress, and the horse should be appropriately sedated if placement of an IV catheter is likely to induce stress.
  - Drugs may be administered IV or IM depending on the horse's disposition.
  - For example, *Xylazine* ± an opioid administered IV or IM initially to induce sedation prior to catheter placement.
  - Allow sufficient time for sedation to develop after IM drug administration.

E    Anesthesia

- ○ Anesthesia can be induced, based on the preference of the clinician, once the horse is adequately sedated.
- ○ It is important that stress be reduced to a minimum by employing a noise-free setting.
- ○ It may be beneficial to maintain anesthesia with a PIVA protocol to reduce *stress* and to provide *analgesia* into the recovery period.

## VI    Intraoperative monitoring

- • *Blood pressure* – ideally measured directly.
  - ○ A decrease in blood pressure is to be expected with hyperkalemia.
- • *ECG* – important to detect changes occurring subsequent to hyperkalemia.
- • *Electrolytes* – especially to monitor [$K^+$], and repeat every 30 minutes.
- • *Capnography* is ideal to continuously measure the end-tidal $CO_2$, otherwise, blood gases should be checked frequently to monitor $PaCO_2$ in particular.
- • *Body temperature* should be monitored continuously. The temperature will increase dramatically during an HYPP episode and may reach 42 °C (108 °F).
- • *Blood glucose* should be monitored if *dextrose* and *insulin* are administered (see below).

## VII    Managing an episode of HYPP during anesthesia

- • If monitoring is adequate, the signs (e.g. muscle fasciculations, increase in body temperature, increase in $ETCO_2$, decrease in blood pressure) will predict the impending HYPP episode and will allow time to initiate treatment.

A    Hyperkalemia (for a more complete description see Chapter 31)

- ○ Treatment is initially aimed at counteracting the cardiac effects of *hyperkalemia*. Depending on the severity of the condition the following treatments should be started.

*Calcium borogluconate*
- ○ An infusion should be started to counteract the cardiac effects of hyperkalemia.
- ○ A dose of 0.25–0.5 ml/kg of a 23% solution can be administered over 15–30 minutes. The ECG should be monitored closely during the infusion.

*Dextrose*
- ○ A bolus of *dextrose* (0.25–0.5 ml/kg of a 50% solution) can be administered to promote the release of *insulin* and facilitate a shift in $K^+$ into the cells.
- ○ However, the response is not rapid, and it may be necessary to administer exogenous *insulin* concurrently to facilitate this process.

*Insulin*
- ○ Insulin administration in association with dextrose is a more rapid and reliable method of decreasing the serum [$K^+$].
- ○ A dose of 0.1–0.2 IU/kg, IV is usually effective.

*Dobutamine*

- An infusion of dobutamine, administered to effect, may be efficacious in temporarily restoring sinus rhythm if heart block is present.

*Hypertonic saline*

- Hypertonic saline, by increasing plasma $[Na^+]$ has a protective effect against hyperkalemia-induced arrhythmias.
  - A dose of 4–6 ml/kg can be infused over 10 minutes.

*$\beta_2$ agonists*

- For example, *Albuterol*, transfer $K^+$ intracellularly, but the onset of action is slow, and thus is not a *first-line* treatment.

*Sodium bicarbonate*

- There appears to be no benefit in administering $NaHCO_3$ to hyperkalemic patients that are not acidemic. Although horses experiencing an HYPP episode under anesthesia are likely to experience severe respiratory acidosis, the pH in this instance should be controlled by decreasing the $PaCO_2$.
- Additionally, administration of $NaHCO_3$ is likely to decrease the ionized calcium concentration which would be contraindicated in hyperkalemia.

## B   Hyperthermia

- Measures should be put in place to decrease the horse's body temperature.
- Surgical drapes should be removed where possible, and *ice packs*, *cold enemas*, and room temperature IV fluids administered.
- Changing the soda lime and/or the anesthetic machine will decrease the temperature of the inspired gases.

## C   Decrease $PaCO_2$

- Controlled ventilation should be initiated, if not already in place, to decrease the $PaCO_2$.
  - The decrease in pH secondary to respiratory acidosis will further increase the serum $[K^+]$.
- Changing the *soda lime* may help to decrease the $PaCO_2$.

# VIII   Recovery

- Electrolyte abnormalities should be corrected prior to the recovery period and the horse should be recovered on a pad of suitable thickness in a noise-free environment.
- The horse should be sedated to promote a slow controlled recovery.
- A prolonged recovery is to be expected and plans should be in place to assist recovery.
- A patent airway should be assured by leaving the endotracheal tube in place or by replacing it with a nasotracheal tube.

## Suggested Reading

Pang, D.S., Panizzi, L., and Paterson, J.M. (2011). Successful treatment of hyperkalaemic periodic paralysis in a horse during isoflurane anesthesia. *Vet. Anaesth. Analg.* 38: 113–120.

# Malignant Hyperthermia
*Alanna N. Johnson and Rachel A. Reed*

## I  Introduction

- MH is an autosomal-dominant inherited mutation of the gene encoding the skeletal muscle *ryanodine 1 receptor (RyR1)* (C7360G) responsible for the efflux of calcium out of the sarcoplasmic reticulum.
- The mutated receptor is associated with a lower threshold of activation and an increased threshold for deactivation.
- Excessive release of calcium from the sarcoplasmic reticulum results in a hypermetabolic state.
- MH has been described in several breeds including the Quarter Horse, Paint horse, Thoroughbred, Appaloosa, and Arabian. The estimated prevalence is <1%.
- MH episodes can be incited by inhalant anesthetics (especially halothane), depolarizing neuromuscular blocking agents (i.e. succinylcholine), and stress.
  - Prognosis is poor for horses experiencing an MH episode under anesthesia.

## II  Clinical signs and immediate diagnostic findings

- Clinical signs are associated with the hypermetabolic state:
  - Muscle rigidity/tremors.
  - Increased body temperature.
  - Tachycardia.
  - Sweating.
- Diagnostic findings include the following:
  - Hypercarbia.
    - If the patient is anesthetized, the carbon dioxide absorbent will rapidly change color and heat up as the absorbent capacity is depleted.
  - Mixed respiratory and metabolic acidosis.
  - Electrolyte derangements including hyperkalemia, hypochloremia, and hyperphosphatemia. Plasma calcium and sodium concentrations may be increased or decreased.
  - Elevated CK activity.

## III  Diagnosis

- If MH is suspected based on history, clinical signs, and diagnostics, genotyping should be performed to confirm the *RyR1* mutation.
  - Hair samples (20–30 hairs, with roots) can be submitted to the University of California-Davis Veterinary Genetics Laboratory.

## IV  Treatment

- Identify the inciting cause and eliminate it.

- *Non-anesthetized patients:* reduce stress, sedation (e.g. acepromazine, alpha$_2$ adrenergic agonists).
  - *Anesthetized patients:* discontinue inhalant anesthetics immediately, flush anesthetic circuit of the inhalant anesthetic, shift to total intravenous (IV) anesthesia, recover as soon as possible.
- Efforts should be made to cool the patient using the following where appropriate:
  - Ice packs.
  - Soak with cold water or alcohol.
  - Cool IV fluids.
  - Cold saline enemas.
- Dantrolene
  - Dantrolene is an *RyR1* receptor antagonist available as an IV (2 mg/kg) or oral formulation (4 mg/kg).
  - The IV formulation is often difficult to obtain and is very expensive, and is not likely to be at hand in a veterinary hospital as it has no other use. The cost of dantrolene, at the time of writing, is between $30 and $70 per vial. The product is supplied in powder form (20 mg per vial) which needs to be reconstituted in normal saline solution. For a horse of 500 kg, receiving the minimum dose of 2 mg/kg, IV, it would be necessary to reconstitute 50 vials, a time-consuming process considering that treatment must be administered promptly once MH is suspected.
  - Adverse effects of dantrolene reported in horses include hyperkalemia, muscle weakness, and prolonged recovery.
- Oxygen supplementation
  - Non-anesthetized patients may tolerate supplemental oxygen via nasal cannula.
  - Anesthetized horses should receive 100% oxygen via endotracheal tube.
- Ventilation
  - Anesthetized patients should be ventilated intensively in pursuit of normocapnia.
- Address acid-base and electrolyte abnormalities:
  - Patients suffering from severe metabolic acidosis (pH < 7.2) should receive sodium bicarbonate (0.5–1 mEq/kg, IV).
- Patients with severe hyperkalemia should receive standard therapy to reduce potassium (see HYPP and Chapter 31). Patients suspected of having MH *should not* receive calcium containing solutions.

## V   Prevention

- For horses with confirmed *RyR1* mutation and those where a strong suspicion exists, avoid stressful environments and inhalant anesthetics and depolarizing neuromuscular blocking agents.
- If anesthesia is unavoidable, consider the following:
  - Acclimating the horse to the hospital environment prior to anesthesia.
  - Pre-treating with oral *dantrolene* (4 mg/kg, PO, 30–60 minutes prior to anesthesia).
  - Using a total intravenous anesthesia protocol (see TIVA Chapter 21).
  - Monitoring arterial blood gases and electrolytes throughout the anesthetic.
  - Monitoring body temperature continuously.
  - Assisting recovery.

## Suggested Reading

Aleman, M., Nieto, J.E., and Magdesian, K.G. (2009). Malignant hyperthermia associated with ryanodine receptor 1 (C7360G) mutation in Quarter Horses. *J. Vet. Intern. Med.* 23: 329–334.

Michelson, J.R. and Valberg, S.J. (2015). The genetics of skeletal muscle disorders in horses. Ann Rev. *Anim. Biosc.* 3: 197–217.

Nieto, J.E. and Aleman, M. (2009). A rapid detection method for the ryanodine receptor 1 (C7360G) mutation in Quarter Horses. *J. Vet. Intern. Med.* 23: 619–622.

Valberg, S.J. (2018). Muscle conditions affecting sport horses. *Vet. Clin. of North Am. Equine.* 34: 253–276.

## Delayed Awakening and Recovery

*Tom Doherty*

- Delayed awakening from anesthesia is unusual in healthy adult horses.
  - On the contrary, *early and sudden* awakening and attempts to stand post-surgery are more likely, and should be prevented in order to improve the quality of recovery.
- An *unexpected, delayed awakening* after general anesthesia is a *cause for concern*, as this may be due to an intraoperative event such as *cerebral hypoxia*, *hemorrhage*, or *embolism*.
- *Prolonged recoveries* (two hours or more), or more specifically *prolonged periods before attempting to stand*, are not uncommon following a lengthy surgery (e.g. intestinal surgery).
  - These horses are *awakening* normally, but appear to be content to lie in lateral recumbency, especially if placed on a thick pad.
  - The prolonged recovery in these cases may be a result of becoming fatigued from the colic episode prior to undergoing general anesthesia.
  - In general, these horses make an uneventful recovery.

## I  Delayed awakening

- A number of factors affect *awakening* from anesthesia, including:
  - Patient factors.
  - Drugs.
  - Surgery and anesthesia.
  - Metabolic derangements.
  - Surgery-induced changes.
- Most cases of delayed awakening in the horse are due to the *residual effects of anesthetic drugs*, and should resolve with time.
- *Non drug-related* causes of delayed awakening are likely to have a much more serious outcome.

### A  Patient factors

*Age*
  - Extremes of *age* are associated with delayed emergence from anesthesia in human beings; however, this issue has not been investigated in horses.

○ Plasma drug concentrations may be higher in *geriatric* patients due to a decrease in the volume of distribution, clearance rate, and plasma protein binding.

○ Neonatal foals are more prone to *hypoglycemia* which may delay recovery.

### Hypothermia

○ *Hypothermi*a is likely to be greater in *neonatal foals* due to their relatively larger body surface area, and *hypothermia* may slow drug metabolism and awakening.

○ However, hypothermia may also be a significant problem in adults and has been shown to delay recovery time in adult horses (see Chapter 11).

### Genetic factors

○ Genetic factors affecting drug metabolism are not well documented in the horse.

○ Prolonged recovery is likely in horses with HYPP, although this is not related to delayed drug metabolism.

### Body condition score

○ Horses with an increase in body fat mass are more likely to have a delayed awakening if anesthetized for a prolonged period with a more soluble volatile anesthetic (e.g. *halothane*).

○ Some underweight horses may have difficulty regaining the standing position, due to muscle weakness, especially geriatric horses with advanced *sarcopenia*.

### Comorbidities

○ In an apparently healthy horse that is capable of exercise, the existence of an underlying condition, such as cardiovascular of respiratory disease, likely to affect recovery from anesthesia would be extremely *rare*.

○ In contrast, metabolic derangements occurring during surgery may affect recovery.

## B Drugs

○ Pre- or postoperative administration of sedatives or tranquilizers (e.g. *acepromazine*) may delay the horse attempting to stand; however, their administration is usually not associated with prolonged *somnolence*.

○ Recovery, after longer procedures, may be slightly longer with the more lipid soluble inhalation anesthetics (e.g. *halothane*) than the less lipid soluble anesthetics (e.g. *sevoflurane*). However, this is also influenced by the duration of the procedure.

○ *Hypoventilation* resulting from drug-induced respiratory depression increases the time required to exhale *volatile* anesthetics, and thus delays recovery. Prolonged periods of anesthesia increase tissue uptake of the drug, and this depends on the drug concentration administered (end-tidal concentration), and the solubility of the drug.

○ In the case of *intravenous* anesthetics, drug accumulation may occur with drugs that have a long context-sensitive half-life or in the case of drugs that have *active metabolites*. But this was more relevant when barbiturates were used for anesthesia.

– Nevertheless, it may be prudent to decrease the infusion rate of certain injectable anesthetics over time during prolonged anesthetic events.

○ Long-acting sedative/tranquilizers (e.g. *acepromazine*) are generally not administered to neonatal *foals* either as premedication or in recovery, as a speedy recovery is desirable to get the foal back with the dam.

○ *Drug interactions* affecting awakening and recovery are not well described for the horse.

– Administration of *midazolam* as a co-induction drug with *ketamine,* was associated with prolonged recoveries in horses being treated with *fluconazole*.

– This was thought to be due to inhibition of the enzyme CYP3A4 by *fluconazole*, as this enzyme is responsible for the metabolism of *midazolam* in other species.

## C   Anesthesia-associated pathological changes

The following may contribute to prolonged recoveries:
- Hypoxia.
- Hypoventilation.
  - A $PaCO_2 > 90\,mmHg$ results in CNS depression.
  - Delays elimination of volatile anesthetics if the horse is breathing spontaneously.
- Hypotension.
- Acid-base abnormalities.
- Electrolyte abnormalities such as:
  *Hyperkalemia*
  - e.g. HYPP, urinary blockage, uroabdomen.
  *Hypokalemia*
  - e.g. diuretic use, insulin/glucose administration.
  *Hyponatremia*
  - Most commonly seen with *uroabdomen*, in which case *hyperkalemia* is also present.
  *Hypocalcemia*
  - May cause muscle weakness.
- Hypoglycemia
  - Is more likely to occur in neonates.
- Hypothermia
  - Is more likely to occur in foals and miniature horses, but can occur in all ages and sizes.
  - It decreases the MAC of volatile anesthetics.
  - It may decrease metabolism of anesthetic drugs.

## II   Surgically-induced pathological changes

- The following may cause prolonged awakening:
  - Embolus lodging in the central nervous system (CNS).
  - Bleeding from the surgical site leading to hypotension and shock.

## III   Management of delayed awakening

- Diagnosis of the underlying cause is important for appropriate management; however, regardless of the cause, it is imperative that the initial management is to maintain an *airway*, and to support *breathing* and *circulation*.

## Suggested Reading

Krein, S.R., Lindsey, J.C., Blaze, C.A., and Wetmore, L.A. (2014). Evaluation of risk factors, including fluconazole administration, for prolonged anesthetic recovery times in horses undergoing general anesthesia for ocular surgery: 81 cases (2006–2013). *J. Am. Vet. Med. Assoc.* 244: 577–581.

Voulgaris, D.A. and Hofmeister, E.H. (2009). Multivariate analysis of factors associated with post-anesthetic times to standing in isoflurane-anesthetized horses: 381 cases. *Vet. Anaesth. Analg.* 36: 414–420.

## Paraphimosis and Priaprism
*Meggan Graves and Jim Schumacher*

- Paraphimosis and priapism, although uncommon, are potentially serious complications of sedation, tranquilization, and anesthesia.

## I  Definitions

### A  Paraphimosis

- ○ Inability to retract the protruded penis into the internal and external preputial cavities.
- ○ *Note:* The internal lamina, the non-haired portion of the prepuce, doubles on itself to form the preputial fold when the penis of a horse is retracted, thus dividing the preputial cavity into an internal cavity and an external cavity. The opening of the internal preputial cavity is termed the preputial ring, and it appears as a thick band on the protruded penis. The opening to the external preputial cavity is the preputial orifice.
- ○ Paraphimosis is commonly the result of prolonged penile protrusion, of which there are many causes, such as priapism.

### B  Priapism

- ○ Persistent erection without sexual stimulation (see Figure 38.5).
- ○ The persistently erect penis cannot be retracted, and therefore, priapism is a cause of paraphimosis.

## II  Causes of Paraphimosis and Priapism

- The causes of paraphimosis, accompanied, or unaccompanied by priapism, associated with general anesthesia are similar.

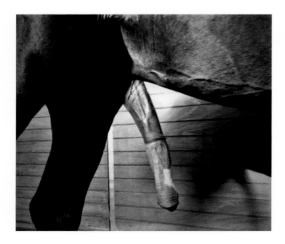

Figure 38.5  Priapism in standing horse following recovery from general anesthesia. *Source:* Courtesy of Dr. Anne Josson-Schramme.

- Paraphimosis occur most commonly from administering a *phenothiazine-derivative* tranquilizer, such as *acepromazine*, or the rauwolfia alkaloid, *reserpine*.
  - It may result in penile paralysis from prolonged protrusion resulting from stretching of the *pudendal* nerves.
  - It may result in priapism by blocking α-adrenergic impulses that mediate detumescence of an erect penis.
  - The likelihood of penile dysfunction after administration of *acepromazine* is ~1 in 10 000.
- General anesthesia may result in priapism.
  - The drugs administered for induction and maintenance of general anesthesia that are responsible for priapism have not been elucidated.

## III   Signs of paraphimosis

- Edema, primarily of the internal lamina of the prepuce.
  - From compromised venous and lymphatic drainage.
- The preputial ring may swell from edema, and the swollen ring may act as a constricting cuff, exacerbating swelling distal to it by impairing venous and lymphatic drainage (see Figure 38.6).
- The pudendal nerves eventually become damaged, presumably from becoming stretched, resulting in loss of sensation to the penis.
- A stallion may develop erectile dysfunction from nerve damage, but ejaculatory capability is usually preserved.
- The penis may become slightly turgid after two to five hours, because of clotting of blood in the corpus cavernosum penis (CCP), making paraphimosis not caused by priapism difficult to differentiate from priapism.
- The edematous penis and internal lamina of the prepuce become excoriated from trauma, leading to bacterial infection and fibrosis (see Figure 38.7)
- The penis eventually curves caudally (see Figure 38.8).

Figure 38.6   Swelling of the distal portion of the penis secondary to constriction caused by swelling of the preputial ring which is part of the internal lamina of the prepuce.

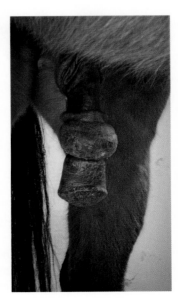

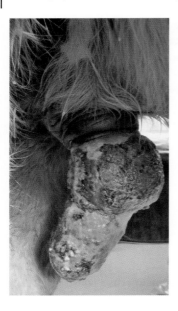

**Figure 38.7** Fibrosis of the penis subsequent to trauma and infection following paraphimosis.

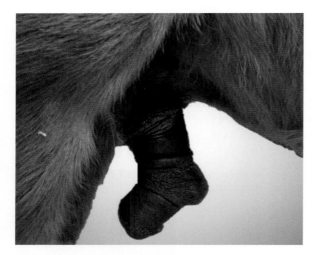

**Figure 38.8** Caudal curvature of the penis as a consequence of fibrosis.

## IV Signs of priapism

- Primarily affects stallions, but geldings can also be affected.
- Persistent erection.
  - Caused by a disturbance of venous outflow of blood from the CCP, usually from altered neural impulses that mediate detumescence.
- Penile paralysis and insensitivity.

- Unless rapidly corrected, priapism results in damage to the pudendal nerves, causing:
  - Dysuria (infrequently).
  - Impotence late in the disease.
  - Inability to achieve a firm erection because of damage to trabeculae within the CCP.

## V  Treatment for paraphimosis

Aims of treatment are to control edema of the penis and internal lamina of the prepuce and prevent trauma. This is done by:
- Applying hydrotherapy.
- Massage.
  - It is more effective than hydrotherapy.
- Bandaging the penis against the abdomen if it cannot be placed into the preputial cavity (see Figure 38.9).
- Applying *glycerin*, or another emollient, directly to the penis and internal lamina of the prepuce, beneath the bandage.
- Applying an antibiotic cream (e.g. *silver sulfadiazine*) to abrasions.
- Applying *lanolin* or *petroleum-based ointment* to keep the integument from desiccating.
- Applying 2% *testosterone cream* added to an equal amount of emollient and applied daily to help maintain the health of the penile and preputial epithelium.
- Firmly applying an *Esmarch bandage* to the penis, starting at the distal end of the penis and wrapping proximally to the preputial orifice.
- Applying a pneumatic infusion bag or a pneumatic bandage.
- Administering a NSAID.
- Walking exercise to facilitate lymphatic drainage.
- Securing the penis within the preputial cavity:
  - Towel clamps or purse-string suture at preputial ring or preputial orifice (short-term usage only) to maintain the penis within preputial cavity.

**Figure 38.9**  Bandaging of the penis to the abdomen to reduce edema formation.

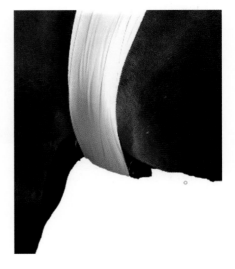

*Probang*

- ○ Using a *probang* to repel the penis into the internal and external preputial cavities (see Figures 38.10 and 38.11).
- ○ Composed of an endotracheal tube or other large-bore flexible tubing (~5-cm outside diameter) and a large wad of rolled cotton, covered with a latex glove attached to one end of the tube.
- ○ The penis is replaced into the preputial cavities and held there by pushing the latex-covered wad of cotton through the preputial orifice. The latex-covered wad of cotton is held in place by bandaging the attached tube to the abdomen. The latex glove covering the cotton wad is covered with an emollient before the end of the probang is inserted into the preputial orifice. The wad of cotton prevents the penis from exiting the preputial orifice.
- ○ The horse is able to urinate unimpeded around the wad of cotton.

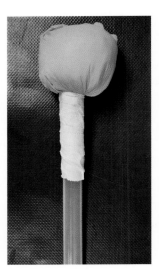

Figure 38.10   Probang ready for insertion into prepuce.

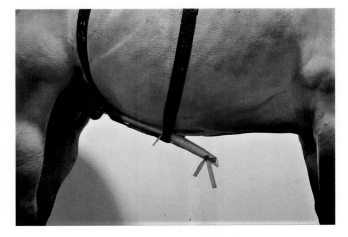

Figure 38.11   Probang in position to retain the penis in the preputial cavity.

Figure 38.12   Image of retainer bottle to be used as a probang.

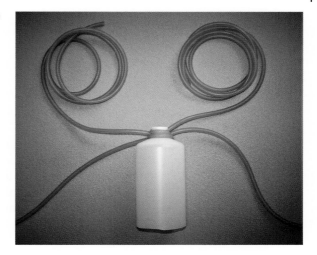

Figure 38.13   Image of retainer bottle in position in prepuce.

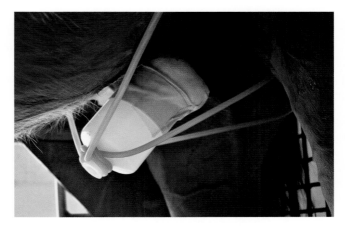

*Retainer bottle apparatus* (see Figures 38.12 and 38.13)

- ○ Composed of a 500-ml plastic bottle, the bottom of which has been removed, and 2 lengths of rubber tubing (each about 8 ft long [2.5 m]). Each length of tubing is tied at its center to the neck of the bottle. The cut edge of the bottom of the bottle is padded slightly with gauze swabs, which are held in place with duct tape.
- ○ The end of the penis is placed into the bottle, and the penis and bottle are inserted into the preputial cavity and held in place with tubing used as a *crupper* and *surcingle*.

## VI   Treatment for priapism

- • Control edema and prevent trauma, as for paraphimosis (as described above).
- • Cholinergic blockade (*acetylcholine antagonist*)
  - ○ *Benztropine mesylate* (8 mg, IV, administered slowly)
    - – It is composed of the active portions of *atropine* and *diphenhydramine*.
    - – Most effective if administered soon after the onset of priapism.

- $\alpha_1$ adrenergic receptor agonists – effective only in early stages of the disease.
  - *Phenylephrine* HCl: 5–10 mg diluted in 10 ml of physiological saline solution (PSS) injected into CCP.
    - Results are usually instantaneous, but the erection may return if collecting veins are occluded.
    - Can be repeated every 15 minutes for five to six treatments until resolution.
  - *Epinephrine* (if phenylephrine is not available) – 100 µg (0.1 ml of a 1 : 1000 solution) diluted in 10 ml of PSS injected into the CCP.
- *Irrigation of the CCP* to remove sludged blood if no response to above treatments.
  - Prepare the penis and perineum for aseptic centesis of the CCP.
  - Lavage the CCP with 1 L heparinized PSS (10 U heparin/ml).
  - Irrigate the CCP through a large-bore needle (e.g. 12- or 14-ga.) into CCP slightly distal to attachment of the internal lamina of the prepuce.
  - Drain through a large-bore needle (e.g. 12- or 14-ga) or a stab incision, ~10–15 cm distal to the ischium.
  - Instill 5–10 mg of *phenylephrine* solution in 10 ml of physiologic saline solution into the CCP after lavage.
  - Suture stab incision in tunica albuginea after irrigation.
- Surgical creation of a permanent shunt between the CCP and the corpus spongiosum penis (CSP)
  - Provides a portal through which blood in the CCP can exit, *because the CSP is not involved in the erection.*

## A  Sequelae to priapism

  - Fibrosis of the CCP may result in impotence. Erectile function may be improved sufficiently, after resolution of priapism, to allow copulation by administering a vasoactive drug into the CCP.
    - *Papaverine* (15–80 mg).
    - *Phenoxybenzamine* (5 mg).
    - *Phentolamine* (0.25–1.5 mg).

*Note*: Penile sensitivity can be increased, after resolution of priapism, by administering an anti-depressive drug, e.g. *imipramine* (2 mg/kg, PO).

## Suggested Reading

Driessen, B., Zarucco, L., Kalir, B., and Berntolotti, L. (2011). Contemporary use of acepromazine in the anesthetic management of male horses and ponies: a retrospective study and opinion poll. *Vet. Anaesth. Analg.* 43: 88–98.

Hayden, S.S. (2012). Treating equine paraphimosis. *Compend. Contin. Educ. Vet.* 34: E1–E5.

## Anaphylactic and Anaphylactoid Reactions
*Rachel A. Reed*

## I   Anaphylactic reactions

- Defined as an antigen-antibody mediated type I immediate hypersensitivity reaction.
- Exposure of the subject to the antigen results in production of IgE antibodies. This process of antibody production can take up to 10–14 days to occur.
- Antibodies subsequently attach to the cell wall of *basophils* and *mast cells*.
- With repeated exposure, the antigen binds to the IgE antibodies and causes release of inflammatory mediators including *histamine, tryptase, leukotrienes,* and *bradykinin*.

*Incidence*
- Appears to be rare in horses.
- In human beings, the estimated incidence in anesthetic patients is 1 in 10 000 to 1 in 20 000.

*Causes*
- Exposure to venomous animals, food allergens, drugs including ivermectin, antibiotics, and neuromuscular blocking agents (e.g. *rocuronium*).

## II   Anaphylactoid reactions

- Previous exposure of the subject to the antigen is *not* required.
- Considered a "*non-immune mediated*" phenomenon.
- The antigen directly activates *mast cells* resulting in release of the same inflammatory mediators.
- Observed with some opioids (e.g. *morphine, meperidine*).
  - More likely to occur if *meperidine* is administered IV.
- The incidence and severity of the reaction is related to the dose, route, and rate of administration. Rapid IV administration of these agents is more likely to cause an anaphylactoid reaction, whereas IM or subcutaneous administration is less likely to cause a reaction.

*Incidence*
- Appears to be uncommon.

*Causes*:
- Opioids (e.g. *morphine, meperidine*).
- Neuromuscular blocking agents (e.g. *atracurium*).
- Antibiotics.

## III   Clinical manifestations

- Similar presentations can be observed with *anaphylactic* and *anaphylactoid* reactions.
  - *Cardiovascular* compromise/collapse and *bronchospasm* are more common with *anaphylactic reactions*.

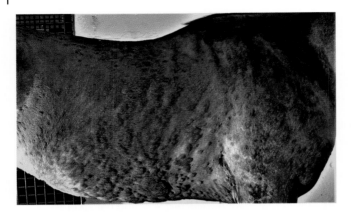

Figure 38.14 Urticarial lesion on a horse. The horse was sedated with xylazine, and anesthesia was induced with ketamine and midazolam. Thereafter, anesthesia was maintained for approximately 40 minutes with ketamine, xylazine, and guaifenesin. No respiratory or cardiovascular effects were noticed, and the urticaria resolved without treatment in approximately one hour. This was presumed to be an anaphylactoid reaction.

- *Cutaneous* reactions are more common with *anaphylactoid* reactions.
  - ○ Reactions can be mild or severe.
  - ○ *Mild* reactions may only present as urticarial (see Figure 38.14).
  - ○ *Severe* reactions may result in shock, coma, or cardiac arrest.
- Both anaphylactic and anaphylactoid reactions can be accompanied by acute systemic compromise including vasodilation, increased vascular permeability, hypotension, tachycardia, bronchospasm, and shock caused by mast-cell degranulation and histamine release.
  - ○ These reactions can be accompanied by the release of *catecholamines* which can counter the hypotensive effects of histamine.

## IV   Diagnosis

- Diagnosis of anaphylactic and anaphylactoid reactions is largely based on history and clinical signs including acute onset of respiratory distress, hypotension, urticaria, collapse, seizures, coma, and death.
- Blood samples can be obtained for determination of plasma *histamine* and *tryptase* concentrations and the presence of antigen specific *IgE*. These diagnostics are unlikely to be helpful in the immediate management of the case as these assays take time.
  - ○ *Histamine* and *tryptase* released from the activated mast cells reach peak concentrations in plasma within one hour of the inciting event.
  - ○ Therefore, sampling for these mediators should take place as quickly as possible after presentation. Unfortunately, a lack of increase in *tryptase* does not rule out the occurrence of mast cell degranulation.
  - ○ Intradermal skin or prick-tests can be performed six weeks after the reaction.

## V   Treatment

- The patient should be rapidly assessed to determine the degree of compromise to the cardiovascular and respiratory systems.

- The three primary goals of treatment are to:
  - Prevent/reverse continued damage.
  - Support the respiratory system.
  - Maintain cardiovascular stability.
- Prevent/reverse changes caused by inflammatory mediators.
  - Discontinue exposure to inciting cause, if known.
  - *Glucocorticoids* (see Table 38.1) will relieve bronchospasm, inhibit inflammatory cascade, and prevent late stage reactions.
  - *Antihistamines* (see Table 38.1) to prevent further activation of histamine receptors.
    - $H_1$ antagonists (e.g. *diphenhydramine, cetirizine, hydroxyzine*).
- Supporting the respiratory system
  - Monitor end-tidal carbon dioxide (if intubated), pulse oximetry, arterial blood gases.
  - Oxygen supplementation.
  - Intubation and/or emergency tracheotomy may be necessary.
  - *Epinephrine* (see Table 38.1) for bronchodilation. If the horse is anesthetized and intubated, administer positive pressure ventilation with 100% oxygen.
  - Bronchodilators (see Table 38.1) for management of bronchospasm.
- Secure and maintain cardiovascular stability
  - Monitor ECG, heart rate, blood pressure.

Table 38.1 Drugs used in management of anaphylactic and anaphylactoid reactions in horses.

| Drug | Class | Dose | Route[a] |
|---|---|---|---|
| *Anti-inflammatories* | | | |
| • Prednisolone sodium succinate | Glucocorticoids | 1–2 mg/kg | PO |
| • Dexamethasone | | 0.04–0.16 mg/kg | IV, IM |
| *Antihistamines* | | | |
| • Diphenhydramine | $H_1$ receptor antagonists | 0.5–1 mg/kg | IM or IV (slow) |
| • Cetirizine | | 1–2 mg/kg q12h | PO |
| • Hydroxyzine | | 0.2–0.4 mg/kg q12h | PO |
| | | 1–2 mg/kg q8-12h | PO |
| *Bronchodilators* | | | |
| • Albuterol | $\beta_2$ agonist | 2 µg/kg | Inhalation |
| *Vasopressors/Inotropes* | | | |
| • Epinephrine | α, β agonist | 0.01 mg/kg | IV, IM (2x dose), IT (5x dose) |
| • Norepinephrine | Primarily $\alpha_1$, some β agonism | 0.05–2 µg/kg/min | IV |
| • Dobutamine | $\beta_1$ agonist | 0.1–5 µg/kg/min | IV |
| • Ephedrine | α, β agonist | 0.05–0.1 mg/kg | IV |
| • Vasopressin | $V_1$ receptor agonist | 0.25 U/kg/min | IV |

[a] IV, intravenous; IM, intramuscular; PO, orally; IT, intratracheal.

- ○ Place/maintain a large-bore IV catheter in the jugular vein.
- ○ Isotonic crystalloid replacement solution for management of relative and absolute hypovolemia; consider *hypertonic saline* (4–6 ml/kg) for rapid volume resuscitation.
- ○ *Epinephrine* for cardiovascular support and bronchodilation.
- ○ Vasopressors and inotropes (e.g. norepinephrine, dobutamine, vasopressin) may be considered for management of hypotension. (see Table 38.1 and Intraoperative hypotension above)

## Intra-carotid and Perivascular Injections

*Rachel A. Reed*

- Intra-arterial injections involving the *carotid artery* are not uncommon, and occur during failed attempts to insert a hypodermic needle or catheter into a jugular vein.
- The jugular vein is generally palpable and visible following its occlusion (achieved by placing a thumb in the jugular furrow).
  - ○ However, it may not be visible in thick-necked horses with a dense hair coat.
    - – In these cases, the jugular vein may have to be located by digital palpation after occluding the blood flow.
    - – Clipping the hair will aid in locating the jugular vein.

## I   Factors contributing to intracarotid injection

- Improper control of the horse such that movement is occurring during injection or catheter placement.
- Poorly muscled horses and young foals in which the carotid is relatively superficial.
  - ○ Special care must be taken with jugular injections in these cases.
- Use of an unnecessarily long needle.
- Directing the needle too deeply and "*stabbing around*" to locate the jugular vein.
- Injections in the lower neck or high up on the neck may be more likely to strike the carotid.

## II   Verification of jugular puncture

- The color of the blood may *not* be helpful.
  - ○ Venous blood can resemble arterial blood once it contacts the air.
- Use of a long, narrow-bore needle or catheter may *not* give an indication of being in the carotid, as the blood may not be seen to pulse.
  - ○ Flow of blood through the needle or catheter depends on the *bore* and *length*.
- If a suitably sized needle or catheter is placed "*pointing downwards*" (toward the heart) in the jugular vein, blood will *not* flow from the tip unless the vein is being occluded (assuming that the horse's head is up); this is *not* the case with carotid placement.
  - ○ When the venous occlusion is removed, blood should flow back down the needle or catheter toward the heart; this is *not* the case with carotid placement.

– This is due to the pressure difference across the jugular vein.
*Caution*: It is important that *air* not be allowed to enter the circulation during this maneuver.

## III  Sequelae of failed jugular injection

### A  Hematoma formation

- Can develop rapidly after *carotid puncture* and distort the anatomy of the local tissues, making ipsilateral jugular venipuncture difficult or impossible.
  - Although unlikely, it is possible that a carotid hematoma may compress and deviate the trachea leading to a partial airway occlusion.
- If carotid puncture is suspected, the area should be compressed with the flat of one hand while the other hand applies pressure to the contralateral side of the neck.
  - Maintain pressure for at least 15 minutes.

### B  Recurrent laryngeal nerve damage

- Needle damage to the underlying recurrent laryngeal nerve can result in *airway closure* at the larynx on the affected side.
- Perivascular deposition of anesthetic drugs may cause a temporary paralysis of the nerve that may result in respiratory distress necessitating a *nasotracheal tube* or a temporary *tracheostomy*.
  - This would be expected in the event that a *local anesthetic* was deposited outside the jugular, but may also occur with an $\alpha_2$ *agonist*.

### C  Horner's syndrome

- Defined as ptosis, miosis, and enophthalmos.
- May result from damage to the underlying sympathetic nerve trunk.

### D  Esophageal injury

- Although possible, it is an unlikely consequence of failed jugular puncture.

### E  Tissue slough or abscess

- Either is possible following injection of an irritant substance.
- If inadvertent drug deposition of an irritant solution (e.g. *guaifenesin, thiopental*) occurs, it is important that every attempt be made to *lavage* the area immediately with copious volumes of warm isotonic saline solution.

## IV  Signs and sequelae of intracarotid injection

- Serious consequences result from intracarotid injections.
- Severity depends on the *substance* injected and the *volume* and *speed* of injection.

A **Responses to intracarotid injection**

- The CNS effects of arterial injection result from:
  - High concentrations of drug entering the brain.
  - Spasm of the carotid artery leading to cerebral hypoxia.
  - Cerebral injury may occur on the same side as the injection.
- *Immediate response* (e.g., excitement, staggering) indicates that the injection cannot have been into the jugular vein.
  - Stop any further drug administration.
  - This also emphasizes the importance of initially injecting slowly.
- Responses vary from mild *agitation* to excitement and *seizures*.
  - In most cases, the horse crashes to the ground with legs thrashing.
  - If the horse flips over backwards striking its poll on the ground this is likely to cause fracture of the occipital and basisphenoid bones, and the outcome is generally fatal.
  - There is a great risk of injury to handlers, especially in a confined space.
  - Once recumbent, the horse may continue to thrash around for a few minutes.
  - Trauma to the head and eyes may result.
- *Long-term response* – neurologic damage necessitating euthanasia in some cases.

B **Treatment**

- Treatment may not be necessary in some cases as the recumbent horse may be unconscious but continues to breathe adequately and have strong arterial pulses.
- Seizure activity, if occurring, should be controlled.
  - *α₂ agonists, diazepam/midazolam, propofol* or combinations of these drugs given to effect.
- Protect the airway and provide oxygen, if deemed necessary.

C **Prognosis**

- If the horse begins to calm down soon after the event and develops a normal breathing pattern, the prognosis is hopeful. The horse may spend 30 minutes or longer in recumbency, thus, attempts are needed to protect it from further injury by supplying padding to vulnerable areas, and, if possible, moving the horse to a more favorable position for recovery.
  - e.g., if the incidence occurs while the horse is in stocks, it should be moved out of the stocks to facilitate attempts at standing.
- Most horses seem to recover from an *α₂ agonist* intracarotid injection, but the prognosis is poor if *ketamine* is injected intracarotid.
- Accidental or intended (research) intracarotid injections of the following substances have resulted in fatalities: *promazine, chloral hydrate, calcium gluconate*.
- Accidental or intended (research) injections of the following substances have resulted in mild (e.g., head shakes) to severe (e.g., recumbency, violent behavior) reactions with no fatalities: *promazine, propiopromazine, acepromazine, thiopental, chloral hydrate, calcium gluconate*.
- Accidental or purposeful (research) injections of isotonic crystalloids and hypertonic saline does not cause an adverse reaction.

# Equine Cardiopulmonary Resuscitation
*Genevieve Bussieres*

## I Introduction

- The RECOVER (Reassessment Campaign On Veterinary Resuscitation) guidelines were published by the Veterinary Emergency and Critical Care Society in 2012 with the intent to standardize the approach to cardiopulmonary resuscitation (CPR) in small animals, and to identify the existing evidence and outline knowledge gaps persisting in that area.
- CPR in the equine species has not met with great success, and there is little evidence regarding the best approach to cardiopulmonary arrest (CPA) in horses. Studies looking at the survival rate to hospital discharge in horses experiencing CPA in a hospital setting are lacking. The guidelines published in the RECOVER initiative are largely applicable to foals and to some extent can be extrapolated to adult horses, taking into consideration the size of the adult horse and the energy required when performing CPR.
- Chest compressions are unable to generate sufficient CO to maintain life in adult horses but, by acting as a *thoracic pump*, compressions may help circulate the blood sufficiently to favor distribution of intravenously administered emergency drugs.
- It is recommended that small animals arresting while under general anesthesia and intubated should be intensively resuscitated as they have a much higher chance of survival in this scenario, and this recommendation should also apply to foals.

## II Causes of cardiopulmonary arrest in horses

- Cardiac arrest in horses is usually due to systemic conditions rather than by primary cardiac failure.
- There are various causes of cardiac arrest in horses, and recognizing the underlying condition helps determine the validity of initiating CPR and predicting the outcome. Causes of cardiac arrest include:
  - Anesthetic overdose in systemically compromised horses.
  - Body position changes, particularly during hoisting.
  - Endotoxemia.
  - Trauma leading to blood loss and hypovolemia.
  - Underlying respiratory conditions leading to hypoxemia and hypoxia.

*Foals*

  - Hypoxemia and hypoventilation due to primary lung disease, sepsis, hypovolemia, severe electrolyte imbalances (e.g. hyperkalemia), metabolic acidosis, hypoglycemia, hypothermia, vagally induced bradycardia, trauma to the thoracic cavity are more common causes of CPA in foals.
  - In CPA in newborn foals during the foaling process, poor or non-existent ventilation/oxygenation leading to respiratory arrest is most likely to precede cardiac arrest.

## III Components of CPR

- Following the RECOVER approach for small animals, CPR is divided into five domains:
  - ○ Preparedness and prevention.
  - ○ Basic life support (BLS).
  - ○ Advanced life support (ALS).
  - ○ Monitoring.
  - ○ Post-arrest care.

### A Preparedness and prevention

*Personnel training:*
  - ○ Training of personnel to identify signs of cardiac arrest improves their ability to recognize the need for CPA.
  - ○ In newborn foals, if resuscitation is started before a non-perfusing cardiac rhythm develops, the chances of survival are as high as 50%.
  - ○ Time is critical for successful resuscitation, and compressions should be instituted immediately while the rest of the personnel gathers drugs and equipment to intubate, if the patient is not already intubated.
  - ○ Delays of only three to four minutes to recognize a CPA are associated with a negative outcome.
  - ○ For compromised anesthetized horses, critical moments delaying recognition of CPA are most likely to occur during transitions from induction to the surgery table and when moving the horse from the surgery table to recovery. At these times monitoring equipment is unlikely to be in place.
    - − Therefore, it is recommended that the arterial pulse be palpated continually at these times.
    - − Alternatively, a Doppler probe can be placed over the coccygeal artery to give an audible signal of the pulse. A pulse oximeter placed on the tongue is another method to monitor the pulse, especially if it has a plethysmographic capabilities.

*Equipment:*
  - ○ Crash carts should be appropriately stocked with the necessary equipment and strategically located to be rapidly accessible in an emergency.
  - ○ A selection of endotracheal (ET) cuffed tubes, mouth gags, a demand valve, and an oxygen source should be at hand.
  - ○ The crash cart should contain emergency drugs (*epinephrine, vasopressin, atropine, lidocaine*), a dosage table, IV fluids bags, a long urinary catheter for intra-tracheal administration of drugs, and large-bore catheters for IV access, syringes and needles.
  - ○ Supplies to perform a tracheotomy should be available.

*Foals:*
  - ○ For foals, hospital, clinics and breeding/foaling facilities should be equipped with cuffed ET tubes of 7–12 mm ID and length of 55 cm for intranasal intubation.
  - ○ A self-inflating valve-bag (e.g. Ambu bag) device designed for adult human resuscitation (1600 ml) is ideal for ventilation.
  - ○ Equipment for aspiration of fluids and fetal membranes from the upper airway.
  - ○ Emergency drugs, IV access supplies, and fluids will be similar to what is needed for adult horses.

○ Monitoring equipment to assess the efficacy of CPR and to provide post-resuscitation care should also be available. An ECG is necessary to identify the cardiac rhythm, and monitoring the end tidal $CO_2$ ($ETCO_2$) with capnography can be used to monitor the adequacy of chest compressions and for the return of spontaneous circulation (ROSC).

## B   Basic life support

○ The first step is to recognize the need for CPR, and then decide if the patient is a good candidate for resuscitation based on the patient's status, comorbidities, welfare, owner wishes, and financial constraints.

○ In the *adult horse*, absence of a palpable pulse, dilated pupils and pupils unresponsive to a light stimulus, apnea, severe bradycardia (<18 beats/min), a sudden decrease in $ETCO_2$ or a value below 20 mmHg indicative of low CO, and any arrest rhythm noted on ECG (asystole, ventricular fibrillation, pulseless ventricular tachycardia), warrant intervention.

○ In *foals* during birth, neonatal foals, or hospitalized foals, the need for resuscitation includes foals gasping for longer than 30 seconds, no heartbeat or respiratory movement, apnea, heart rate of less than 40 bpm or less than 50 bpm and not increasing, dyspnea, absence of pulse at palpation, and decreased muscle tone for foals assessed while in the birth canal. If the patient being monitored is intubated, low $ETCO_2$ indicates the need for intervention.

*Chest compressions*:

○ CPR is initiated with the patient positioned in lateral recumbency on a firm, dry surface.

○ For anesthetized patients, discontinue anesthetic administration. Administer reversal agents for $\alpha_2$ agonists, benzodiazepines, and opioids.

○ In *adult horses*, chest compression is achieved by an individual delivering a blow with the knees immediately behind the horse's elbow.

  – To deliver the maximum force, the chest compressors must drop onto their knees from the standing position, and the compressors should be of large body mass.

  – Ideally, the compression rate should be 80 beats/min.

  – Despite maximum cardiac compressions and rate, CO is not higher than 50% of that reported for deeply anesthetized horses; therefore, it is insufficient to sustain life.

○ In *foals*, the thorax is compressed at its highest point at a rate of 100–120 beats/min in a fashion similar to that employed in a large dog.

  – For newborn foals with fractured ribs, place the side with the fractured ribs on the dependent aspect.

○ With more than one resuscitator is present, chest compressions are continuous and uninterrupted by the ventilation process.

○ The thorax should be compressed to one-third to one-half of its width and allowing full recoil of the chest between compressions. If possible, the person performing the compressions is replaced every two minutes to avoid fatigue and maintain efficiency. Chest compressions should not be stopped for more than 10 seconds every two minutes for needed interventions and to check the ECG.

*Ventilation*:

○ Establishment of a patent airway followed by ventilation is initiated at the same time as chest compressions if multiple persons are available.

○ In newborn foals, removal of fetal membranes or secretions obstructing the airway is an important first step. Intubation must be achieved rapidly, nasally (foals) or orally.

- If no tube is available, a mouth-to-nose ventilation can be attempted (neonates). Tracheostomy is another option if oro or naso-tracheal intubation is not possible. Once inserted, the proper position of the ET tube is confirmed (chest inflation, $ETCO_2$), the cuff is inflated and the ET tube is secured in place to prevent dislodgment during CPR.
- In foals, an inspiratory time of one second is preferred to a longer inspiratory time, thereby limiting the duration of increased intrathoracic pressure and its negative effect on venous return.
- A rate of 10 breaths/min in foals and 6–10 in adults, with a tidal volume of 10 mL/kg, while observing that the chest excursion is sufficient, is recommended.
- In foals, the aim should be to achieve normocapnia while avoiding hypoxemia.
- A self-inflating bag-valve device (e.g. Ambu bag) as used in human resuscitation is ideal for ventilating foals. In adult horses, a demand valve is useful for this purpose if the horse is not already connected to a mechanical ventilator.
- In the eventuality that there is only one resuscitator available for foal CPR, intubation, should be established as soon as possible and a compression-to-ventilation ratio of 30:2 has been recommended.

*Monitoring during CPR:*
- If the horse is intubated, monitoring during CPR is best accomplished with the observation of $ETCO_2$ as it helps identify ROSC, and can determine the efficacy of the chest compressions.
- ECG evaluation should be brief as it requires stopping the compressions, and this is detrimental to ROSC and maintenance of CPR efficiency.
- In the absence of $ETCO_2$ monitoring, the pupil size (neutral or responsive to light with adequate cerebral blood flow) can be used to assess the effectiveness of chest compressions.

## C Advanced life support (ALS)

- ALS includes:
  - Therapy with emergency drugs (vasopressors, positive inotropes, anticholinergics).
  - Reversal of anesthetic agents (e.g. $\alpha_2$ agonists, opioids, benzodiazepines).
  - Correction of electrolytes disturbances (e.g. hyperkalemia).
  - Intrathoracic cardiac compression.
  - Defibrillation, if indicated.
- Emergency drugs
  - Drugs should ideally be administered intravenously (IV).
  - Alternatively, intra-tracheal (IT) administration can be performed until venous access is achieved.

*Epinephrine*
- It should be administered at a dose of 0.01 mg/kg, IV (low dose) every three to five minutes.
- Intrathecal dose: 0.1 mg/kg. diluted in sterile water or saline and delivered via a catheter as far as possible down the tracheal tree.

*Vasopressin*
- The use of vasopressin alone or combined with epinephrine is still not clearly considered to be more beneficial than the use of epinephrine alone.
- Dose: a bolus dose of 0.2 IU/kg, IV. Doses of 0.3 and 1.0 IU/kg/min resulted in increases in arterial blood pressure in isoflurane-anesthetized hypotensive foals.

*Atropine*
  – There is no strong evidence supporting the use of atropine in CPR, but it has not been found to be harmful. It may be indicated in patients with a high vagal tone that may have contributed to the cardiac arrest. Consider its use in cases of asystole and PEA.
  – Dose: 0.02–0.04 mg/kg, IV.

*Lidocaine*
  – Lidocaine is a class 1-b antiarrhythmic agent. *Lidocaine* may be considered as a treatment for pulseless ventricular tachycardia and ventricular fibrillation unresponsive to CPR, defibrillation or vasopressor therapy. However, *lidocaine* is not considered to have short- or long-term efficacy in the treatment of cardiac arrest.
  – Dose: 1–2 mg/kg, IV.
○ Defibrillation
  – Defibrillation is currently used first for CPR in human beings. However, this is rarely indicated as a first intervention in the equine species.
  – It may be considered in equine patients weighing less than 200 kg.
  – In the presence of a shockable rhythm (ventricular fibrillation [VF] or pulseless ventricular tachycardia [VT]), immediate defibrillation is recommended if the arrhythmia is of less than four minutes in duration.
  – Preferably, a biphasic defibrillator (if available) should be used.
  – For CPA of more than four minutes duration, a first cycle of CPR prior attempting defibrillation can help improve the chance of success of defibrillation. A single defibrillation shock of 2–4 J/kg (100–200 J/50 kg foal) will immediately be followed by chest compressions and ventilation for a two-minute cycle, the ECG is then evaluated to determine if a second defibrillation attempt is necessary (energy increased by 50% for each attempt).
○ Intrathoracic cardiac compression
  – The RECOVER initiative states that intrathoracic cardiac compressions should not be delayed if it is an option for the patient and the client, in order to increase the chances of success.
  – However, in the equine species there is no evidence of positive outcomes following open chest CPR.
  – In CPA combined with significant intrathoracic disease (trauma, pneumothorax, pericardial effusion), intrathoracic compression may be more beneficial than standard CPR. In these cases, internal defibrillation paddles should also be readily available as internal defibrillation is more likely to be successful than external defibrillation in adult horses.
○ When to stop CPR
  – If, after 10–12 minutes of CPR, the spontaneous circulation and respiration are still absent, maneuvers should be stopped as survival is unlikely.
  – In foals, CPR maneuvers can be stopped specifically when a heart rate greater than 60 bpm is present and spontaneous breathing has resumed with over 16 bpm, regular breathing pattern and normal efforts.
  – It is noted in human medicine that premature withdrawal of ventilation is one of the most common mistakes in neonatal CPR.

### D Post-arrest care and monitoring

○ Key points of post-resuscitation care include maintenance of organ perfusion, normoxemia and potentially the use of mild hypothermia which would be applicable only in foals.

○ Avoidance of hypotension post-CPR with the use of fluid therapy, positive inotropes and vasopressors may increase the chance of survival. Efforts can be made at maintaining adequate perfusion throughout the monitoring of arterial blood pressure, central venous oxygen saturation, and lactate level.

○ A mild hypothermia may be beneficial in early post-resuscitation period (33 °C) for at least 12 hours. However, this is not feasible in equine patients.

○ If cerebral edema or elevated intracranial pressure is suspected post CPR, as it has been described to be the case in humans, mannitol and hypertonic saline administration can be used.

## IV Conclusion

- CPR in adult horses is going to have a poor chance of being successful.
- CPR should definitely be attempted in *foals*.
- Patients arresting under general anesthesia while tracheally intubated should be intensively resuscitated as they have the best of survival.
- In any case, CPR in equine species is extremely time sensitive. Early detection of bradycardia, hypotension or reduced respiratory rate and rapid efficient intervention by highly trained personnel are very critical points to the success of CPR in horses.

## Suggested Reading

Fletcher, D.J., Boller, M., Brainard, B.M. et al. (2012). RECOVER evidence and knowledge gap analysis on veterinary CPR. Part 7: clinical guidelines. *J. Vet. Emerg. Crit. Care 22 Supple.* 1: S02–S131.

Goldstein, M.A., Schwark, W.S., Short, C.E. et al. (1981). Cardiopulmonary resuscitation in the horse. *Cornell. Vet.* 71: 255–268.

Hallowell, G.D. (2016). Cardiopulmonary resuscitation: a waste of time? *Equine. Vet. Educ.* 28: 245–247.

Hopper, K., Epstein, S.E., Fletcher, D.J. et al. (2012). RECOVER evidence and knowledge gap analysis on veterinary CPR. Part 3: basic life support. *J. Vet. Emerg. Crit. Care 22 Supple* 1: S26–S43.

Hopster, K., Tuensmeyer, J., and Kastner, S.B. (2016). Resuscitation attempts in a foal with sudden cardiac arrest in the early recovery period. *Equine. Vet. Educ.* 28: 241–244.

Hubbell, J.A.E., Muir, W.W., and Gaynor, J.S. (1993). Cardiovascular effects of thoracic compression in horses subjected to euthanasia. *Equine. Vet. J.* 25: 282–284.

Jokisalo, J.M. and Corley, K.T. (2014). CPR in the neonatal foal. Has RECOVER changed our approach? *Vet. Clin. North Am. Equine. Pract.* 30: 301–316.

Rozanski, E.A., Rush, J.E., Buckley, G.J. et al. (2012). RECOVER evidence and knowledge gap analysis on veterinary CPR. Part 4: advanced life support. *J. Vet. Emerg. Crit. Care 22 Supple.* 1: S44–S64.

Ruiz, C.C. and Junot, S. (2018). Successful cardiopulmonary resuscitation in a sevoflurane anaesthetized horse that suffered cardiac arrest at recovery. *Front. Vet. Sci.* 5, article 138.

Steffey, E.P., Kelly, A.B., Hodgson, D.S. et al. (1990). Effect of body posture on cardiopulmonary function in horses during five hours of constant-dose halothane anesthesia. *Am. J. Vet. Res.* 51: 11–16.

Vieitez, V., Gomez de Segura, I.A., and Martin-Cuervo, M. (2017). Successful use of lipid emulsion to resuscitate a foal after intravenous lidocaine induced cardiovascular collapse. *Eq. Vet. J.* 49: 767–769.

39

# Recovery from Anesthesia

*Bernd Driessen*

## I Risk of morbidity and mortality during recovery

- The equine species has the highest risk of morbidity and mortality with general anesthesia, but perianesthetic mortality rates depend notably on whether professional oversight by anesthesiologists familiar with equine anesthesia is given or not.
  - < 0.1–1% mortality (up to 1 in 100 cases) for elective (mostly ASA I or II) cases.
  - 0.4–10% mortality (4 in 1000 to 5 in 50 cases) for emergency and after-hour (frequently ASA ≥ II) cases.
- The majority of complications occur in the recovery period and mortality is predominantly associated with the musculoskeletal system, the central nervous system, and the respiratory system.
  - Fractures in 71% of cases.
  - Respiratory obstruction in 14% of cases.
  - Myopathy in 7% of cases.
  - Neuropathy and myelomalacia in 7% of cases.
- Morbidity (non-fatal complication) is also frequent in the recovery period and associated with the same systems.
  - Postanesthetic myopathy/neuropathy.
  - Respiratory obstruction.

## II Predisposing risk factors

- Breed: heavy warmblood and draft horses are at a higher risk of developing hypoxemia in the recovery period, and myopathies due to poor muscle perfusion during anesthesia.
- The horse's behavior and instinct to assume a standing position as part of a *flight response*.
- Prolonged anesthesia time (> 90 minutes).
- Moderate-to-severe pain and associated premature attempts to stand.
- Fracture repair of a long bone.
- Metabolic disorders (e.g. hyperkalemic periodic paralysis, equine polysaccharide storage myopathy).

*Manual of Equine Anesthesia and Analgesia*, Second Edition. Edited by Tom Doherty, Alex Valverde, and Rachel A. Reed.

- Intraoperative hypotension.
  - Mean arterial pressures <70 mmHg over an extended period of time (> 30 minutes) are associated with a greater incidence of myopathy.
- Older horses (> 14 years of age) with musculoskeletal problems (e.g. osteoarthritis).
- Younger horses with excitable temperament.
- Lateral versus dorsal recumbency for the occurrence of myopathy.
- Dorsal versus lateral recumbency for *myelomalacia* and for airway obstruction.
- Inadequate positioning/padding of the horse on the surgery table.
- No prior recovery experience of the horse.

## III   Unassisted vs. assisted recovery

- There is no consensus as to whether an assisted recovery improves the quality of recovery over an unassisted recovery.
  - One study showed better recovery quality when head and tail ropes were used in ASA I or II horses undergoing soft-tissue or orthopedic surgeries under a balanced technique of *Triple Drip* infusion and isoflurane and no postanesthetic sedation.
  - In contrast, another study showed no difference between head and tail rope assistance vs. no assistance in horses of ASA status III or higher undergoing abdominal surgery with a balanced technique of *medetomidine* infusion and *isoflurane*, followed by *medetomidine* postanesthetic sedation.
- An appropriate environment (i.e. an adequately designed recovery stall) is a prerequisite to avoid injuries in the post-operative period.
- No method of assisted recovery will completely eliminate the risk of severe or fatal postanesthetic complications.

## IV   Recovery stalls

### A   Structural features designed to optimize conditions for recovery

- Close proximity to, but separate from, surgery room.
- Area: $4-5\,m^2$ ($\sim 43-54\,ft^2$) for average sized adult horses.
  - Avoid oversized stalls.
- Well-padded walls and doors at least 2.5–3.0 m ($\sim$ 8–10 ft.) high.
- Soft floor with non-slip surface (even when wet).
- Front and back doors locked by transverse bars and floor/ceiling bolts.
- Holes placed high in doors allowing head and tail ropes to be passed to the outside.
- Heating/AC system allowing for separate climate control within recovery stall.
- Light source equipped with dimmer function.

### B   Useful design features for various methods of assisted recovery

- Door windows, cameras, or observation platform to allow monitoring of the horse.
- Recessed wall outlets for oxygen supply, suction lines, and electrical power.
- Stout metal rings recessed into the wall of each corner, well above a horse's head height ($\sim$ 2.5 m or 8 ft. above floor).
- Ceiling hook centered over the stall to hold a hoist.
  - Alternatively, overhead monorail with hoist.

○ Escape route for personnel attending the horse within the stall during recovery.
○ Movable 30–40 cm (12–16 in.) thick, vinyl-covered foam mattress.

## V Pre-recovery preparation

- Efforts should be directed at minimizing predisposing risk factors (See Section II above), including:
  ○ Decreasing anesthesia time.
  ○ Maintaining stable cardiorespiratory function during anesthesia.
  ○ Assuring that the horse is well positioned and padded on the surgery table.
  ○ Administering appropriate intraoperative analgesia including loco-regional techniques of anesthesia and analgesia, and if necessary, for the recovery period.
  ○ Administering postoperative sedation including $\alpha_2$ *agonists* and *acepromazine* to allow time for residual inhalant anesthetic to be eliminated from the body and for the horse to regain more awareness and muscle strength before attempting to stand. (see Table 39.1)
  ○ Emptying the urinary bladder, especially when horses are receiving an infusion of an $\alpha_2$ agonist, before placement in the recovery room.
    – A urinary catheter should ideally be in place throughout the anesthesia time to collect the urine continuously and it can be removed when the horse is placed in the recovery room.

Table 39.1   Drugs commonly used for sedation and analgesia pre-recovery and during the recovery phase.

| Drug | Dose for intravenous (IV) administration | Indication |
|---|---|---|
| $\alpha_2$ agonists | | |
| • Xylazine | 0.1–0.3 mg/kg | To produce calming and analgesia |
| • Dexmedetomidine | 1–2 µg/kg alone or followed by CRI (0.01–0.03 µg/kg/min) | Prolong sleeping phase |
| | | Delay initial attempts to rise |
| • Detomidine | 2–4 µg/kg alone or followed by CRI (0.1–0.6 µg/kg/min) | |
| • Romifidine | 8–20 µg/kg | |
| Acepromazine | 5–20 µg/kg | Reduce excitement |
| | | Reduce risk of hypertension following $\alpha_2$-agonist administration |
| | | Inhibit opioid-induced central excitement |
| Propofol | 2 mg/kg alone or 0.75 mg/kg followed by CRI (0.125 mg/kg/min) | Prolong sleeping phase |
| Opioids | | |
| • Butorphanol | 0.01–0.02 mg/kg alone or followed by CRI (24 µg/kg/h) | Provide short-term pain relief |
| | | Prolong sedative action of $\alpha_2$-agonists |
| • Morphine | 0.05–0.15 mg/kg | |
| NSAIDs | | |
| • Flunixin meglumine | 1 mg/kg | Provide relief of muscle-skeletal pain |
| • Phenylbutazone | 4 mg/kg | Reduce inflammation |
| • Meloxicam | 0.6 mg/kg | |
| • Firocoxib | 0.09 mg/kg | |

# VI   Recovery phase

## A   Positioning and padding

- ○ Position the horse in the recovery stall on a pad of appropriate thickness (see Figure 39.1) or an air mattress (see Figure 39.2), where access to the horse and exit from the room is safe for personnel, and provides enough space for the horse to achieve the standing phase.
    - – Placing the horse on a thick pad or an air mattress generally delays first movement and attempt to stand.
    - – In addition, proper positioning (see Chapter 18) decreases the incidence of myopathy and neuropathy.
- ○ Protect limb extremities and the head from injury.
    - – Place padded bandages on the distal aspects of the limbs. (see Figure 39.3)

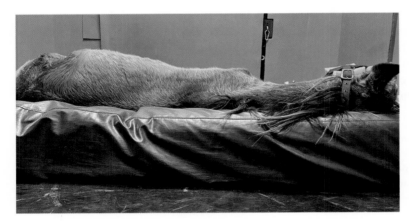

Figure 39.1   Horse lying in lateral recumbency in recovery from anesthesia on a thick pad.

(a)                                                              (b)

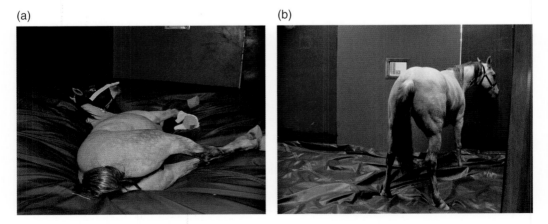

Figure 39.2   Air mattress. (a) Waking up a horse on a rapidly inflatable and deflatable air-cushion mattress installed in the recovery box. A nasotracheal tube ensures an open airway and, if necessary, allows oxygen insufflation. (b) Horse standing on deflated mat *Source:* Photos courtesy of Dr. David Hodgson, Kansas State University, Manhattan, KS.

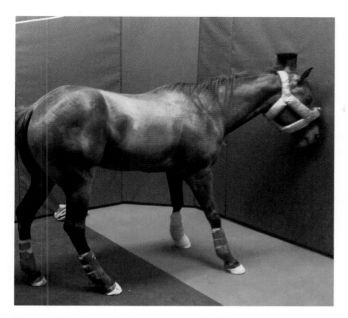

Figure 39.3   Horse in the recovery stall with padded bandages on limbs.

– Wrap the feet with tape (e.g. Elastikon) if the horse has shoes.
– Place a helmet when appropriate to protect surgical sites on the head or place a hood with an *eye cup* in the case of eye surgery.

## B   Sedation and analgesia

○ Administer a sedative ($\alpha_2$ agonist ± acepromazine ± opioid) to prolong the recumbency time to avoid premature attempts to rise, particularly when rapid nystagmus is present and return of proper proprioceptive function has not yet occurred. Recovery of the jaw-tongue reflex and alternating stretching and flexing of the hind limbs signify sufficient restore of proprioceptive function.

○ Dose and timing depends on whether the inhalant anesthetic was discontinued before the end of the surgery or continued until the end, and on whether an infusion of an $\alpha_2$ agonist was used intraoperatively.

○ Systemic analgesics, including NSAIDs and opioids, and locoregional anesthesia/analgesia (e.g. peripheral nerve blocks, epidural analgesia) may be administered as deemed necessary.

## C   Ensure a patent airway and administer oxygen (see "Airway Management" Chapter 3)

○ It is vital to maintain a patent airway.

○ This may involve keeping the endotracheal tube in place or replacing it with a nasotracheal tube or a nasal tube.

○ In cases of partial upper airway obstruction due to nasal edema, nasal instillation of *phenylephrine* or *norepinephrine* may suffice to maintain airway patency.

○ Administering supplemental oxygen at 15 l/minutes in an adult horse may increase the PaO$_2$; however, for this to be effective the oxygen line needs to be placed in the mid-tracheal area.

### D   Other

○ Dim the lights of the recovery room or cover the upper eye with a light towel and provide a quiet and calm environment to decrease the horse's awareness of the surroundings.

○ Place a towel under the penis or vulva to collect any leaked urine to avoid a slippery recovery stall floor.

○ Reversal of benzodiazepines (*midazolam, diazepam*) early in the recovery phase with *flumazenil* (0.02–0.04 mg/kg slowly IV or IM) maybe indicated, particularly if the benzodiazepine was administered in a dose >0.05 mg/kg and/or the anesthetic lasted <120 minutes.

○ If the recovery becomes prolonged due to repetitive or continuous administration of an α$_2$ agonist during the anesthesia and/or during the awakening phase, an α$_2$ antagonist (preferentially *tolazoline* 2–4 mg/kg slowly IV or IM; *yohimbine* 0.05–0.10 mg/kg, IM; or *atipamezole* 0.05–0.10 mg/kg, IM) may be given to facilitate recovery.

## VII   Methods of recovery

● A broad variety of options are available for recovery ranging from unassisted to assisted recovery. The latter includes simple methods to very sophisticated systems. (see Table 39.2)

● Many factors have to be considered when selecting the appropriate recovery system for an individual patient. (see Table 39.3)

### A   Unassisted recovery

○ Ideally the horse should remain in lateral recumbency long enough to allow for elimination of the inhalant anesthetic and for the horse to regain sufficient mental function, recover proper proprioception, and muscle strength.

○ The use of sedatives helps prolong the recumbency time.

○ Recoveries are best when the horse proceeds through the different phases of recovery, initially moving from lateral to sternal recumbency, and then from sternal recumbency to standing.

○ The horse may require some assistance during the different phases of recovery, such as helping it to become sternal, but for the most part the horse recovers unassisted.

### B   Personnel within recovery stall assisting horse manually

○ The concept is to keep the horse in lateral recumbency as long as possible (i.e. until signs indicate the horse has regained sufficient mental and proprioceptive function and muscle strength).

○ The method does not require special equipment but is not without risk to personnel.

○ *Only personnel familiar with recoveries should be allowed to "hand-recover" horses.*

Table 39.2 Common techniques of recovery in the horse.

| Method of recovery | Group of horses for which technique is suitable | Advantages | Disadvantages/Complications |
|---|---|---|---|
| Unassisted | General patient population<br>Well-tempered horses<br>Small equines (foals, ponies) | No extra equipment needed; patients are closely monitored from outside the room | Unpredictable mishaps |
| Personnel within recovery stall assisting patient manually | General patient population<br>Well tempered horses<br>Small equines (foals, ponies) | No extra equipment needed; patients are closely monitored | Potentially dangerous for attendants<br>Requires trained personnel |
| Head and tail rope recovery | General patient population Nervous or excited horses<br>Not well trained horses<br>Horses undergoing prolonged anesthesia<br>Horses with anticipated muscle weakness<br>Horses with mild to moderate neurological deficits | Better protection of attendants than "hand-recovery"<br>Allows for more than two attendants to help | Requires wall rings and/or holes in recovery stall doors<br>Loss of head or tail rope when head or tail rope attachment/knot fail<br>Horse fighting head restraint<br>Requires trained personnel |
| Deflating air pillow | General patient population<br>Nervous or excited horses<br>Not well trained horses<br>Horses undergoing prolonged anesthesia and anticipated muscle weakness | Prevents premature attempts to rise improving quality of recovery<br>Does not require special training of personnel | Additional expenses for air mattress and fan<br>Requires removal of horse shoes to prevent puncture of air pillow |
| Large animal vertical lift<br>● Large Animal Lift/Becker Sling[a]<br>● UC Davis Large Animal Lift[b] | Old and fatigued horses<br>Heavy (draft and large Warmblood horses)<br>Horses with mild to moderate neuropathies and/or myopathies | Lightweight equipment<br>Easy to put on down horse<br>Simple to use | Requires overhead hoist in recovery stall<br>Requires cooperative animal<br>Risk of tissue strangulation if narrow girths are used<br>Requires trained personnel |

(Continued)

Table 39.2 (Continued)

| Method of recovery | Group of horses for which technique is suitable | Advantages | Disadvantages/Complications |
|---|---|---|---|
| Sling recovery<br>• Sling-Shell System[c]<br>• Liftex Sling[c]<br>• Animal Rescue and Transportation Net (ARTN)[d]<br>• Anderson Sling[e] | Horses undergoing major orthopedic surgery (esp. long bone fracture repair)<br>Horses with major soft tissue trauma<br>Horses with neuropathies<br>Muscle fatigued horses<br>Horses in poor body condition | Prevents excessive weight loading in affected limb<br>Prevents injuries related to muscle fatigue or neuronal/ motor dysfunction<br>Dependent on sling design useful for long-term support of patient in recovery period (e.g. ARTN or Anderson Sling)<br>Significantly lower cost and less manpower required compared to pool recoveries | Requires overhead hoist(s)<br>Requires cooperative animal<br>Usually difficult to put on down horse<br>Rolling out of sling if sling doesn't match body size<br>Uneven body support (except Anderson Sling)<br>May limit chest excursions and thus breathing similar to a corset (esp. Liftex Sling)<br>Requires trained personnel |
| Pool recovery system<br>• Hydro-Pool<br>• Pool-raft System | Horses at high risk of unstable recovery:<br>• Primarily horses with long-bone, pelvic or scapular fracture<br>• Horses with major soft tissue trauma<br>• Horses with central or peripheral neuronal disease<br>• Horses with bad demeanor<br>• Horses with poor body condition | Significantly reduced incidence of recovery injuries to musculoskeletal apparatus in patients of the highest risk categories<br>Pool systems can also be used for physical therapy | Risk of pulmonary edema development (Hydro-Pool) Risk of incisional infections (esp. in Hydro-Pool)<br>Wet casts or bandages<br>Expensive systems to use and maintain<br>Labor intensive<br>Horse size limitations based on pool and/or raft size<br>Longer recovery time<br>Requires trained personnel |
| Tilt table | Horses undergoing major orthopedic surgery (esp. long bone fracture repair)<br>Horses with major soft tissue trauma<br>Horses with neuropathies<br>Muscle fatigued horses | Prevents excessive weight loading in affected limb<br>Prevents injuries related to muscle fatigue or neuronal/ motor dysfunction | Requires special set up room<br>Requires trained personnel<br>Some horses are reluctant to stand due to the pressure exerted by the chest and abdominal band |

[a] Large Animal Lift/Becker Sling: Häst, PSC, 10300 Wingfield Lane, Louisville, KY 40291-3655; phone: +1-502-267-7685 or +1-888-924-7685; Fax: +1-502-267-1395; http://www.hast.net.

[b] UC Davis Large Animal Lift (LAL): manufactured by Charles Anderson; distributed by Large Animal Lift Enterprises, 1026 Marchetti Court, Chico, CA 95926; phone: +1-530-320-2627; http://www.largeanimallift.com.

[c] Liftex Sling: Liftex, Inc., 443 Iviland Rd., Warminster, PA 18974; phone: +1-478-4651 or +1-215-957-0810; Fax: +1-215-957-9180; http://www.liftex.com.

[d] Animal Rescue and Transportation Net (ARTN), Ruedi Keller, Pferdeambulanzbau, Schützenhausstrasse 56, 8424 Embrach, Switzerland; phone: +41-44-865-2250, Fax: +41-44-865-2252; e-mail: ruedikeller@gmx.ch.

[e] Anderson Sling: manufactured by Charles Anderson; distributed by Care for Disabled Animals/CDA Products, 18385 Van Arsdale Road, Potter Valley, CA 95469; phone: +1-707-743-1300; Fax: +1-707-743-2530.

Table 39.3   Criteria for selecting method of assisted recovery.

---

*Patient-related factors*
    Size, weight, age, body condition, physical fitness
    Temperament and training status

*Injury- and/or disease related factors*
    Type and extent of soft tissue trauma
    Type of fracture and extent
    Presence of neuronal deficits affecting proprioception and/or motor function
    Presence of central neurological disease (e.g. history of seizure activity)

*Surgery-related factors*
    Surgical technique used
    Site and invasiveness of surgical procedure
    Location and size of cast or bandage
    Degree of surgery-related tissue trauma

*Anesthesia-related factors*
    Anesthetic protocol and drugs used (inhalant anesthesia, TIVA, balanced anesthesia)
    Duration of anesthesia
    Analgesia protocol used and adequacy of intraoperative pain control
    Options for post-operative/pre-recovery analgesia
    Occurrence of intraoperative complications (e.g. severe cardiopulmonary dysfunctions)

*Facility-related factors*
    Layout/design of available recovery stall
    Availability of equipment for assisted recovery techniques
    • Ropes
    • Mattress (size and thickness)
    • Slings/Animal Lifts (type and size)
    Availability and type of specially designed recovery systems

*Personnel-related factors*
    Manpower
    Familiarity with techniques of assisted recovery

---

*Technique*

- An experienced attendant kneels behind the horse's head with one knee pushing on its neck and both hands holding its head, raising the horse's nose and stretching it backwards.
- Restraining the head prevents the horse from swinging its head ventrally, thus preventing the horse from moving into sternal recumbency.
- A second person, if available, may stand behind the croup of the horse and grasp the tail at the moment the animal is allowed to get up.
- *Pre-recovery sedation* and *analgesia* is often helpful to minimize struggling in the early post-anesthetic period and the effects usually last 15–40 minutes.
- Once the horse is judged to be awake (i.e. by cessation of nystagmus, return of normal tongue tone and jaw-tongue reflex, chewing, normal responses to environmental stimuli) it should be allowed to roll sternal.
    - In this position, the two attendants may or may not be able to control the movement of the horse.

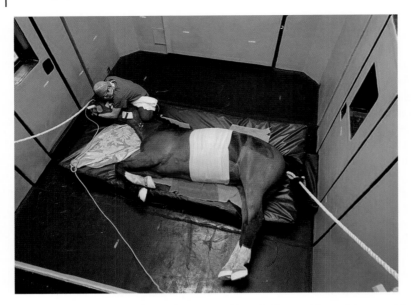

Figure 39.4   Head and tail rope in recovery. Use of a foam rubber mattress and head and tail ropes to assist a horse during recovery from anesthesia. The bottom front leg is pulled forward to lessen pressure on the dependent limb and all lower limbs are protected with gaiters against injury. Tubing entering one nostril provides oxygen supplementation. The horse is positioned so that it will roll off the mattress as it moves into sternal recumbency.

    ○ Once standing, the attendants should take hold of the halter and tail to keep the horse from moving until it has regained sufficient coordination to walk safely.

    ○ Most horses stand within one hour of discontinuing anesthetic drug administration.

C   Head and tail rope recovery (see Figure 39.4)

    ○ The method is very similar to manual assistance described above and is based on the same concept.

*Requirements*

    ○ The corners (or opposite walls) of the recovery stall must be equipped with recessed rings and/or the front and rear doors of recovery stall have holes through which head and tail rope can be passed.

    ○ Ropes should be strong but flexible enough to allow tying of knots for secure attachment to head (or halter) and tail and to ensure smooth gliding through rings and/or door holes.

    ○ A padded halter is recommended to prevent facial nerve damage. (see Figure 39.5)

*Technique*

    ○ Once the horse is considered to be awake, the attendant leaves the position behind the head and allows the horse to stand up when it next tries.

    ○ Two or more helpers can assist the horse in rising from lateral to sternal to standing by pulling on the ropes while keeping a safe distance from the recovering horse.

**Figure 39.5** Padded halter used to protect the face from the pressure of the halter straps and buckles.

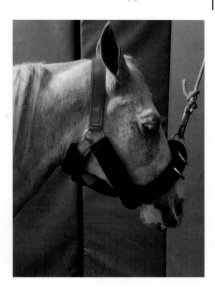

- Strain on head and tail rope provides some balance and support for the horse.
  - Tension on the *head rope* decreases the incidence of head strikes against walls or floor should the horse struggle.
  - Tension on the *tail rope* reduces forward momentum of the horse as it tries to stand.
- Once the horse is standing, head and tail ropes help keep it steady.
- This technique restricts the horse from using more than one-third of the recovery stall.

**D    Deflating air pillow** (see Figure 39.2)

- Recovery of horses on an air cushion significantly improves recovery quality.
- The concept behind the technique is to keep the horse recumbent until adequate mentation, proprioceptive function, and muscle strength have returned.
- With this method the recovery may be unassisted or assisted with head and tail ropes from outside the stall.
- The method is safe and without risk to personnel.

*Technique*

- A rapid inflation-deflation air pillow that is 46 cm (18 in.) thick is placed on top of a thick foam mat covering the entire recovery stall floor.
- Following surgery, the anesthetized horse is placed in the center of the recovery stall on the deflated air mattress.
- The pillow is rapidly filled with air from a fan located outside the recovery stall pumping air continuously through a hose-like duct into the mattress. (see Figure 39.6)
  - The soft pillow hinders the horse from rolling sternal and protects it from harming itself or causing pressure injury to dependent nerves and muscles.
- Once the horse is adequately awake, the fan is switched off and two 92-cm (36-in.) zippers along the sides of the air mattress are opened to allow for rapid deflation. Alternatively, some systems simply deflate through the inflation tube.
- When the air pillow is flat, the horse can attain sternal recumbency and safely stand with or without help from head or tail ropes.

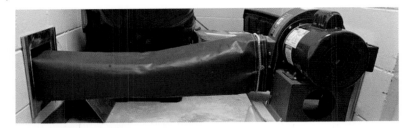

Figure 39.6    Fan used to keep air mattress inflated.

(a)                                                                          (b)

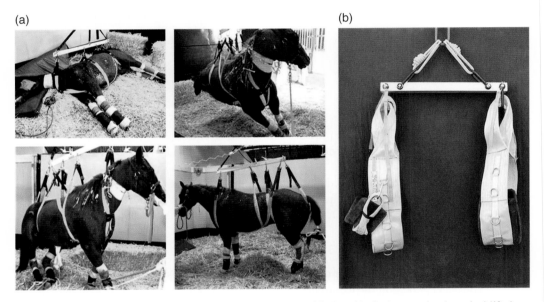

Figure 39.7    Large animal vertical lift. (a) Assisted recovery with the aid of a large animal vertical lift. As the horse attempts to move from lateral to sternal recumbency it is lifted off the ground into a standing position, with the head and tail rope helping to stabilize the patient during this process. (b) Alternative model of a "Large Animal Lift" with the so-called Becker sling *Source:* Photo courtesy Häst, PSC, 10300 Wingfield Lane, Louisville, KY 40291–3655, USA.

E    **Large animal vertical lift (LAL) or alternatively the Becker Sling** (see Figure 39.7)

- ○ The large animal vertical lift (LAL) and Becker Sling were developed as robust but simple and lightweight devices for assisting horses to stand.
- ○ They can easily be placed on a recumbent horse.
- ○ Principle components are an aluminum spread bar (keeps the front and rear parts of the lift separated), to which chest and body/pelvic slings are attached and which can handle body weights up to 1000 kg (2200 lbs).
- ○ The LAL and Becker Sling are particularly helpful in assisting very heavy and/or muscle fatigued horses.

F    **Sling recovery**

- ○ The high incidence of musculoskeletal system injury during recovery has stimulated the design of various sling systems in which the anesthetized horse may be placed.

- ○ Slings are used commonly for recovery of the following types of cases:
    - – Horses undergoing major orthopedic surgery in which any misstep or excessive weight loading of the affected limb may lead to implant failure.
    - – Horses that have an external skeletal fixation device or transfixation cast.
    - – Horses with neurologic or motor dysfunctions.
    - – Horses in poor body condition.

*Technique*

- ○ The sling is placed on the horse when it is still anesthetized or very sedate.
    - – Should the decision to use a sling be made after the horse has tried to stand, it should be re-anesthetized or heavily sedated unless the horse is very calm and cooperative.
- ○ Allow the horse to slowly wake up from sedation 60 minutes after the end of anesthesia.
    - – Treatment with an $\alpha_2$-agonist should be considered to keep the horse deeply sedated and pain-free while allowing time for elimination of residual anesthetic.
    - – If the recovery becomes prolonged, an $\alpha_2$-antagonist (*tolazoline* 2–4 mg/kg slowly IV or IM; *yohimbine* 0.05–0.10 mg/kg, IM; or *atipamezole* 0.05–0.10 mg/kg, IM) and/or the benzodiazepine antagonist *flumazenil* (0.02–0.04 mg/kg slowly IV or IM) may be given.
- ○ Once the horse looks bright and is trying to get up, it should be lifted in the sling with four legs being raised just off the ground and then lowered again.
    - – An awake horse will stand as soon as its feet contact the ground.

*Available sling systems*

1) **Sling-Shell Recovery System** (See Figure 39.8)
    - ○ This system was developed at the University of Berne.
    - ○ The sling system is suspended on four hoists affixed to overhead rails.
    - ○ Two customized glass-fiber enhanced plastic shells that match the contour of the front breast and the ventral part of the thorax support most of the horse's weight in

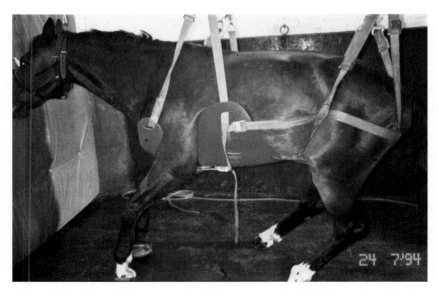

**Figure 39.8** Sling-shell system and with horse recovering in it. *Source:* Reproduced courtesy of Prof. Urs Schatzmann, University of Berne, Switzerland.

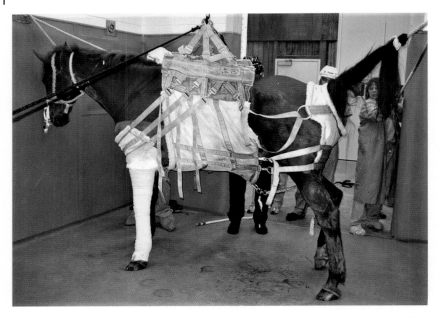

Figure 39.9    Liftex large animal sling. *Source:* Reproduced courtesy of Liftex, Inc. Warminster, PA.

the front without causing pressure damage to blood vessels or nerves or impairing expansion of the rib cage during breathing.
- Transverse girths passing in front and behind the thighs support the rear of the body.
- Transverse girths and straps attached to the edges of the shells and hooked up onto the hoists stabilize the body on the side.
- The sling system is easily mounted on the anesthetized horse after rolling the horse into dorsal recumbency for placement of breast and ventral thorax shells, and back into lateral recumbency for attachment of girths and straps to the four hoists.

2) **Liftex Large Animal Sling** (see Figure 39.9)
- Most widely used sling in North America.
- Commonly used in horses with major musculoskeletal trauma prior to surgery for safe induction of anesthesia and transport to the surgery table.
- Important features of its design:
  - It is difficult for the horse to back out of the sling or dog-sit in it.
  - Made of breathable nylon fabric that reduces sweating.
  - Can be adjusted to fit horses of different sizes.
  - Fulcrum of suspension from the lifting rings can be adjusted to promote sternal vs. abdominal support (point of lifting of the sling should be over the withers).
  - Offers flexibility in handling horses with injured shoulders or humeral fractures.

*Note*: It may impair breathing by acting like a narrow corset when horse is lifted to a standing position.

3) **Animal Rescue and Transportation Net** (ARTN) (see Figure 39.10a and b)
- Most widely used rescue, transportation, and recovery net (sling) in Europe.
- Commonly used in horses with major musculoskeletal trauma prior to surgery for safe induction of anesthesia, for transport to and from the surgery table, and for assisted recovery, for recovery in a hydropool, and for recovery of exhausted horses after abdominal surgery.

(a)

(b)

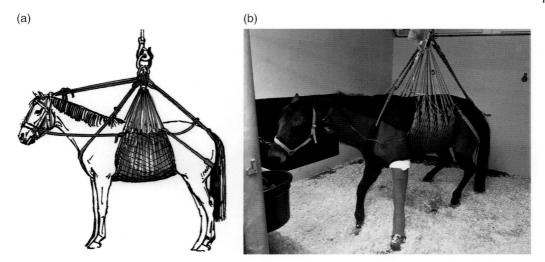

**Figure 39.10** (a) Animal Rescue and Transportation Net (ARTN). *Source:* Drawing courtesy of Matthias Haab, Pferdeambulanzbau, Embrach, Switzerland. (b) ARTN in place on a horse. *Source:* Photo courtesy of Ruedi Keller, Pferdeambulanzbau, Embrach, Switzerland.

- ○ Important features of its design:
  - – It is a lightweight knotless network (6 kg [13.2 lb]) made of extremely stable materials suitable for a maximum permissible load of 1100 kg (2425 lb.).
  - – It is washable in a regular laundry machine at 40 °C (104 °F).
  - – The animal rescue and transportation net (ARTN) exists in different sizes for draft or adult horses, ponies, and foals.
  - – To simplify the net placement on the animal, strings and ropes that shall meet at the attachment point of the overhead hoist are color-coded.
  - – Putting the ARTN on a horse is relatively easy, even on a down horse.
  - – Horses can remain in the ARTN for hours to days after recovery from anesthesia with little risk of developing decubitus wounds.
- *Note*: It impairs breathing when the horse is being lifted but less so than the Liftex sling.
- 4) **Anderson Sling** (see Figure 39.11)
  - ○ A specially designed sling system attached to a metal frame that can be affixed to either an overhead hoist or a hydraulic apparatus with a power supply.
  - ○ Useful for lifting and stabilizing a horse waking up from general anesthesia.
  - ○ Has *distinct advantages* over other slings:
    - – Supports the animal from the skeletal system (not by its chest and abdomen).
    - – Distributes the horse's weight much more evenly.
      - ■ More comfortable for the horse.
      - ■ Does not interfere with muscle, nerve, or respiratory function.
    - – Hydraulically controlled overhead frame provides an option for finely adjusting the weight distribution between front and rear as well as left and right limbs.
      - ■ Allows a horse to bear weight on only the front or rear limbs, or to adjust it to have only three limbs bear weight while one limb is kept suspended and restrained.
    - – Horses can be kept in the sling for extended periods of time (weeks to months).

(a)

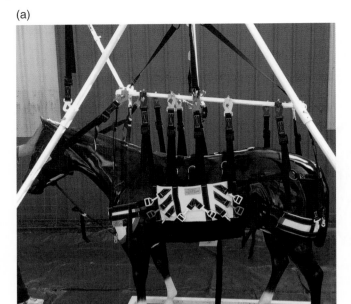

(b)

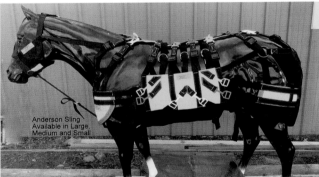

Figure 39.11 (a) Sling with hardware and (b) sling with no hardware on breast and rump. *Source:* Photo courtesy of Dr. Cora Anderson.

### G Pool Recovery

- Recovery in a pool system may offer advantages over recovery in a sling system.
- It can be lifesaving in horses that are at extremely high risk of unstable recovery due to the nature of the original trauma, prolonged and complicated surgical procedure, central or peripheral neuronal disease, and/or temperament.
- Two pool recovery systems are currently in use.

*Available pool systems*
1) Hydro-Pool (see Figure 39.12)
   - Uses a rectangular water pool approximately 3.7 m long, 1.2 m wide, and 2.6 m deep (12×4×8.5 ft.) and equipped with a hydraulic, stainless-steel grate floor that can be rapidly raised or lowered.

Figure 39.12  Hydro pool horse submerged in hydro-pool. *Source:* Reproduced courtesy of Dr. Martin Suarez, Biomedical Communications Unit, College of Veterinary Medicine, Washington State University.

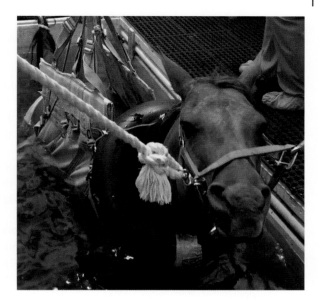

- Water is heated to 32–37 °C (90–100 °F) to avoid hypothermia.
- After surgery, the still anesthetized and intubated horse is lifted into the pool using a large animal sling or net and an overhead rail and hoist system.
- Two ropes are attached to the halter for subsequent cross-ties to support and restrain the head.
- The horse is then lowered into the pool with the body completely submerged.
- An air-filled tire inner tube is placed around the upper neck or, preferably, an air-filled flotation device placed *in front of* the neck, allowing the horse to rest its head without risk of aspirating water or drowning.
- The sling or net remains in place but is not bearing weight.
- An $\alpha_2$ agonist (e.g. *xylazine*) may be administered for sedation.
- Once the horse is judged to be awake, the floor of the pool is raised until it touches the horse's hoofs, allowing the horse to bear some weight.
- If the horse demonstrates sufficient weight bearing capability, the pool floor is raised further until the water level reaches the mid-thorax.
- At this point the inner tube or air-filled flotation device, cross-tie head ropes, and sling or net are removed.
- Finally, the floor is lifted to ground level and the horse walked from the recovery pool to a warm stall.

*Precautions and concerns:*
- Wound closure requires extra effort to provide a multilayered, water-tight closure.
- Use of *cyanoacrylate glue spray* enhances effectiveness of water-proof closure.
- Water-repellant bandage and cast material must be used.
  - Pulmonary edema (up to 17% incidence based on historic data) is the most common complication reported.
  - Horse may suffer skin abrasions when moving vigorously.
  - Horse may attempt to exit the pool if anxious, intolerant to the pool, or awake.
  - Horse must be dried after removal from pool.

2) Pool-Raft System (see Figure 39.13)
   ○ Uses a circular pool 6.7 m (22 ft.) in diameter, 3.4 m (11 ft.) deep, and surrounded by a cantilevered deck.
   ○ Water is heated to 36 °C (96 °F).
   ○ After surgery, the anesthetized horse is lifted using a large animal sling and overhead monorail/hoist system.
   ○ The horse is lowered into a large raft modified to accommodate the limbs and equipped with an additional air-cushion attachment at the front to protect the head from striking the pool deck or sinking into the water.
   ○ Once correctly positioned in the raft, horse and raft are lowered into the pool using two separate hoists (one carrying the horse in the sling, one carrying the raft).
   ○ The raft is secured to rings on the pool deck, while the horse's head is secured using cross-tied head ropes.
   ○ Sedation or tranquilization with *xylazine* or *acepromazine* may become necessary if the horse shows signs of severe anxiety or excitement early during the pool recovery phase or immediately before transfer from the pool to the recovery stall.
   ○ Once fully awake, the horse is blindfolded and lifted out of the raft and transferred to a nearby recovery box.
   ○ *Advantages* of this specific recovery system over the Hydro-Pool system include:
     – Use of a flotation device avoids complications associated with complete or partial water submersion of the animal's body.
     – Wounds and wound bandages/casts are less likely to get wet, reducing the risk of incisional infection.
     – Significantly lower, if any, risk for pulmonary edema.
     – Faster average recovery time.
     – Little risk of acquiring leg injuries while in pool raft.

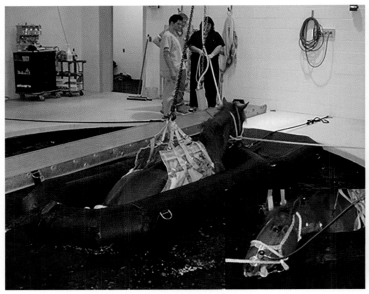
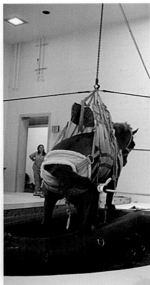

Figure 39.13  Pool raft. Horse being lifted into the pool raft, and horse floating in Pool-raft with head resting on raft with nasotracheal tube in place.

(a)

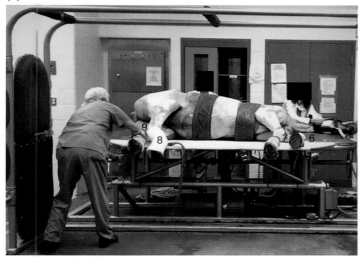

(b)

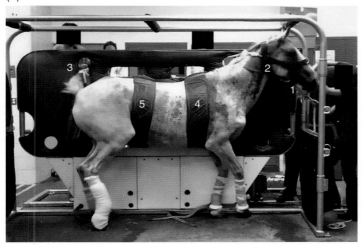

**Figure 39.14** Tilt table (a) Horse placed on a tilt recovery table (200Econ Stationary Model, Westwood Co., Ovando, MT) and (b) once standing. Notice in (a) anchor points 6–9 around the pastern, with anchor point 8 still not placed. Notice in (b) anchor points 1–4 still in place while the horse stabilizes and anchor points 6–9 removed from the legs prior to tilting the table to the vertical position.

H **Tilt table** (see Figure 39.14a and b)

- Uses an equine-padded tilt table with a hydraulic tilt. The table is bolted to the floor of a special recovery room.
- In a vertical position, the table is part of a chute with Dutch doors located on both ends of the chute and a squeeze gate that can be opened in either direction, which makes recovery in both right and left lateral recumbency possible.
- The table can also be used for induction.

*Technique*

- ○ The horse is transferred from the surgery table to the horizontally placed tilt table, by sliding it.
- ○ Nine anchoring points are used to restraint the horse on the table.
- ○ A halter and a recovery hood are placed on the head, and the head is secured to locks on the table from the halter with two lead shanks (anchor points 1 and 2), one from a ring located at the bridge of the halter and the other from the side of the halter.
- ○ The tail is secured to the table by means of a rope (anchor point 3).
- ○ The horse's body is secured to the table by two heavy girths, each with a width of 20 cm and length of 135 cm (1 chest band just behind the elbow and 1 abdominal band just in front of the tuber coxae) (anchor points 4 and 5).
- ○ Protective leg wraps are placed on all limbs and each limb is independently secured to the table by use of leather straps around the pastern (anchor points 6–9).
- ○ The horse is kept calm, and the use of sedatives is recommended to prolong the recumbency time, until the horse is considered to be awake.
- ○ Once the horse displays forceful, strong attempts to free itself from the anchoring points and is deemed ready for standing, the leg straps are then removed.
  - – One person controls the head, 1 person holds the tail rope, and another person controls the hydraulic lift.
  - – The table is slowly tilted into the vertical position, ensuring that the head and tail support remain secure.
  - – The horse is encouraged to stand once the table is fully vertical, and the chest and abdominal bands slowly loosen when the horse begins to support its own weight.

## Suggested Reading

Arndt, S., Hopster, K., Sill, V. et al. (2020). Comparison between head-tail-rope assisted and unassisted recoveries in healthy horses undergoing general anesthesia for elective surgeries. *Vet. Surg.* 49: 329–338.

Bidwell, L.A., Bramlage, L.R., and Rood, W.A. (2007). Equine perioperative fatalities associated with general anaesthesia at a private practice – a retrospective case series. *Vet. Anaesth. Analg.* 34: 23–30.

Brodbelt, D.V., Blissitt, K.J., Hammond, R.A. et al. (2008). The risk of death: the confidential enquiry into perioperative small animal fatalities. *Vet. Anaesth. Analg.* 35: 365–373.

Elmas, C.R., Cruz, A.M., and Kerr, C.L. (2007). Tilt table recovery of horses after orthopedic surgery: fifty-four cases (1994-2005). *Vet. Surg.* 36: 252–258.

Fürst, A., Keller, R., and von Salis, B. (2006). Entwicklung eines verbesserten Hängegeschirrs für Pferde: Das Tier - Bergungs- und Transportnetz (TBTN). *Pferdeheilkunde* 22: 767–772.

Kästner, S.B.R. (2010). How to manage recovery from anaesthesia in the horse - to assist or not to assist? *Pferdeheilkunde* 26: 604–608.

Niimura Del Barrio, M.C., David, F., Hughes, J.M.L. et al. (2018). A retrospective report (2003-2013) of the complications associated with the use of a one-man (head and tail) rope recovery system in horses following general anaesthesia. *Ir. Vet. J.* 71: 76. https://doi.org/10.1186/s13620-018-0117-1. eCollection 2018.

Ragno, V., Driessen, B., Bertolotti, L., and Zarucco, L. (2013). Perianesthetic morbidity and mortality in the equine: a retrospective study. *Vet. Surg.* 42: E68.

Rüegg, M., Bettschart-Wolfensberger, R., and Hartnack, S. (2016). Comparison of non-assisted versus head and tail rope-assisted recovery after emergency abdominal surgery in horses. *Pferdeheilkunde* 32: 469–478.

# 40

## Euthanasia
*Ron Jones and Tom Doherty*

- Euthanasia is often defined as "a quiet and gentle death" but it is probably better to refer to it as a "*quick and painless*" death.
- Euthanasia of horses is carried out by veterinarians under three different circumstances:
  - At *sporting events* when it is not feasible to treat a particular injury such as a compound fracture or a fracture of a proximal long bone of the limbs.
  - When horses have reached the end of their useful and productive life and are suffering from *crippling, debilitating, or untreatable conditions.*
  - When *incurable conditions are discovered during surgery* and the horse is not allowed to recover from anesthesia.
- Each of the three situations demands a different approach, and requires different interpersonal skills in dealing with the owners and attendants.
- In conscious horses, it is advisable to decrease distress and anxiety by administering a sedative prior to euthanasia.
- In most countries, euthanasia of an animal is not considered to be an act of veterinary surgery and hence can be performed by non-veterinarians.

## I  Important considerations

### A  Location

- Whenever possible, euthanasia should be performed in a quiet, uncluttered area with good footing, and which is readily accessible for removal of the body. The procedure should be performed quickly and quietly to decrease stress to the horse and personnel.
- In emergencies, it is generally preferable to perform euthanasia out of sight of the public. This can be achieved by moving the animal, preferably after the administration of sedative and analgesic drugs.
- However, in some emergency circumstances it is necessary to euthanize the horse promptly for humane reasons regardless of location. In such instances, screens may be used to conceal the horse from the public.
- If the euthanasia is a non-emergency, it is best to perform the procedure in surroundings familiar to the horse.

*Manual of Equine Anesthesia and Analgesia*, Second Edition. Edited by Tom Doherty, Alex Valverde, and Rachel A. Reed.

○ If the horse to be euthanized has a close bond with another horse or in the case where an unweaned foal has to be euthanized, it may be best to administer the euthanasia solution in the presence of the companion animal or its dam. In such cases, the body should remain at that location in the presence of the companion for a period so that they can accept the circumstances.

○ Safety is important; thus, it is best to minimize access to all but necessary personnel.

○ Proper *restraint* of the head is essential, and a suitable head collar or bridle should be used.

**B    Insurance**

○ It is important to ascertain whether the animal is insured and, wherever possible, to seek permission from the insurance underwriters.

**C    Permission**

○ If the owner of the horse or a responsible agent is available, permission for euthanasia should be obtained.

**D    Secondary veterinary opinion**

○ In an emergency and in the absence of the owner or agent, it is strongly recommended that the indications for euthanasia be documented by a second veterinarian.

**E    Welfare issues**

○ In all situations, it is important to stress that the welfare of the horse is the primary consideration.

**F    Written consent**

○ Under most circumstances, it is preferable to obtain written consent.

**G    Verbal consent**

○ Under certain circumstances, a verbal agreement in the presence of a *reliable witness* is adequate.

**H    Written records**

○ It is important to keep written records of the procedure.

**I    Postmortem examination**

○ A postmortem examination is warranted in some circumstances.

**J    Disposal of the body**

○ Disposal of the body may be subject to legal restrictions. It is also important to consider that the carcasses of horses euthanized by lethal injection are likely to be toxic to scavengers (see pentobarbital sodium).

### K Grief and owner considerations

- For some owners and handlers, the loss of a beloved horse may be equated to loss of a family member; thus, it is important to be empathetic.
- In the presence of a concerned owner or if circumstances dictate, it may be desirable to induce general anesthesia (e.g. $\alpha_2$ agonist followed by *midazolam/ketamine*) prior to administration of the euthanasia agent (e.g. pentobarbital sodium).
  – This will ensure that unconsciousness is attained in a tranquil, relaxed, and reliable manner.
  – It is prudent to advise a concerned owner that the horse may make agonal gasps or have involuntary limb movement for a brief period after euthanasia.

## II The ideal euthanasia solution

- Should produce relaxation allowing the horse to become recumbent in a natural manner and avoid crashing to and thrashing around on the ground.
- Is easy to administer in a relatively *small volume* through a relatively *small-bore* needle or catheter.
- Is capable of being administered as a *single dose*.
  - Placement of a jugular catheter is recommended to avoid repeated venipuncture and/or perivascular deposition of the drug.
- Must be "*reasonably safe*" for the personnel.
- *Work with certainty* on every occasion.
- Must not produce unpleasant and undesirable signs such as twitching, vocalizing, or gasping.
- Inexpensive.

## III Techniques

- Horses can be humanely killed by using either:
  - Drugs which produce hypoxia or depress the central nervous system.
  - *Physical methods* that damage the brain.
- Irrespective of the technique, the aim is to stop the flow of oxygenated blood to the vital tissues and, thereby, produce death.

### A Hypoxia-inducing agents

- Includes muscle relaxants such as *succinylcholine*.
- These should *never be used as sole agents* as it is inhumane.
- They produce muscle paralysis *without anesthesia*.
- Should only be used in combination with an anesthetic drug (e.g. a barbiturate).

### B Central nervous system (CNS) depressant drugs

- *Drugs of choice* (e.g. barbiturates) for euthanasia of horses.
  - *Pentobarbital sodium* is the barbiturate most commonly used.
  - Note: *Sodium thiopental* is no longer available in the USA and many other countries.
- Barbiturates produce cardiac and respiratory arrest.
- Inhalational drugs are rarely used, and are impractical due to the horse's physical size.
  - An exception is their occasional use to euthanize an anesthetized animal.

*Pentobarbital sodium*
- o This is the most common method of euthanasia of horses in North America and many countries.
- o It is a fast and humane method of euthanasia.
- o However, in some countries, barbiturates may not be readily available or may be illegal or cost prohibitive.
- o An intravenous (IV) dose of 50–75 mg/kg is generally sufficient to cause death.
- o *Phenytoin sodium* (50 mg/ml) is added to most commercial euthanasia preparations of pentobarbital sodium. It contributes to cardiovascular collapse and CNS depression.
- o Ideally, a large bore catheter should be placed in a jugular vein to facilitate rapid administration of the drug because concentrated solutions of pentobarbital sodium are viscous.
  - – Warming the drug solution will decrease viscosity and allow for more rapid administration.
  - – Pentobarbital *sodium* for euthanasia is available in concentrations in the range of 240–540 mg/ml.
- o Horses are generally sedated prior to pentobarbital administration.
- o *Note*: Sedation or general anesthesia does not cause a clinically important delay in the onset of loss of cerebral electrical activity (EEG) following *pentobarbital* administration, and irreversible loss of EEG activity usually occurs within 60 seconds of completion of the infusion.
- o In contrast to EEG activity, ECG activity may be present for many minutes after pentobarbital administration, although an arterial pulse and heart sounds are no longer detectable.
- o An important consideration when using pentobarbital sodium for euthanasia is the *disposal of the carcass*, as it is likely to be toxic to scavengers. For this reason, *adjunctive* methods are often used in place of pentobarbital sodium.

C   Adjunctive injectable methods of euthanasia

- o Adjunctive methods of euthanasia may be necessary when *pentobarbital sodium* is not available, is not cost effective, or is contraindicated for use, such as in situations when disposal of the carcass may risk endangering scavengers.
- o The horse should be anesthetized with a short-acting anesthetic regimen such as *xylazine* (1.0–1.5 mg/kg, IV) followed by *ketamine* (2.0–2.5 mg/kg, IV) and *midazolam* (0.05–0.1 mg/kg, IV). The adjunctive drugs should be administered as soon as possible after the horse assumes lateral recumbency.
- o The main adjunctive techniques for euthanasia are:
  - – *Potassium chloride* (KCl).
  - – *Magnesium sulfate* (MgSO$_4$).
  - – Intrathecally administered *lidocaine*.

*Potassium chloride* (KCl)
- o KCl is an acceptable "*adjunctive method of euthanasia*".
- o It can be used to produce cardiac arrest in the anesthetized horse. (see Figure 40.1)
- o It must *not be used as a sole euthanasia agent* as it does not cause anesthesia.
- o It is not a controlled substance, and is easily procured and prepared.
- o A KCl solution is inexpensive when prepared from the salts which are readily available commercially. It is important to use chemical or food grade KCl if making a solution. (see Box 40.1)

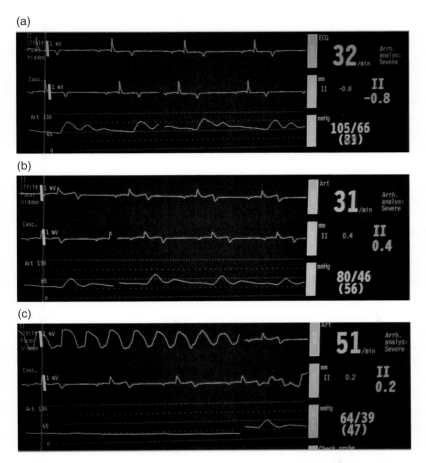

Figure 40.1   (a) ECG and blood pressure waveform of an anesthetized horse prior to administration of a KCl solution IV for euthanasia. The ECG shows a sinus rhythm and the horse is normotensive. (b) The QRS complex has widened and the T wave is enlarged. Hypotension is present. (c) Ventricular fibrillation is occurring.

| Box 40.1   Potassium Chloride (Preparation for Euthanasia) |
| --- |
| – Add 300 g KCl to container and bring to 1000 ml with sterile water.<br>– Let it sit overnight, or heat and stir (*do not autoclave*).<br>– Although not a super saturated solution, the KCl will enter solution much easier with heating and stirring.<br>  ○ Dose: 75–100 mg/kg<br>  ○ 125–150 ml per 500 kg horse. |

○ The carcass of a horse euthanized with KCl in association with a short-acting general anesthetic regimen is likely to be less toxic to scavengers than that of a horse euthanized with *pentobarbital sodium*. Thus, a KCl containing regimen may be an acceptable *adjunctive* method of euthanasia when facilities for disposal are not available.

- ○ A saturated solution of KCl is administered IV or intracardially.
  - − Intracardiac administration is technically more difficult and requires a long needle which may not be readily available; thus, this method is not commonly used.
  - ○ A KCl dose of 75–100 mg/kg IV is usually administered to induce cardiac arrest.
  - ○ Limb movements, mainly stretching movements, are common after KCl administration.

*Magnesium sulfate* ($MgSO_4$)
- ○ $MgSO_4$ is an acceptable *"adjunctive method of euthanasia"*
- ○ It should *not be used as a sole agent* for euthanasia.
- ○ Saturated solutions of $MgSO_4$ can be prepared by adding Epsom salts to water. (see Box 40.2)

---

**Box 40.2    Magnesium Sulfate (Preparation for Euthanasia)**

- Add 350 g $MgSO_4$ (e.g. Epsom salts) to container and bring to 1000 ml with sterile water.
- Heating the water increases solubility.
- Dose: 1–2 mg/kg IV.
  - ○ 500–1000 ml per 500 kg horse.

---

- − The solubility of $MgSO_4$ in water (20 °C) is approximately 400 g/l.
- − The solubility increases to about 500 g/l at 40 °C.
- ○ A dose of 1–2 ml/kg is sufficient to cause death in an anesthetized horse.
- ○ Involuntary limb movements are less likely to occur with $MgSO_4$ administration than with KCl administration.

*Intrathecal lidocaine hydrochloride*
- ○ This is considered to be an acceptable method of euthanasia of anesthetized horses.
- ○ Lidocaine HCl (4 mg/kg) injected intrathecally at the atlanto-occipital space is an effective method of causing brain death.
- ○ *Dose*: 100 ml of a 2% solution per 500 kg.
- ○ Brain death, as determined by loss of cerebro-cortical activity, occurs between 1 and four minutes after the infusion. The EEG activity is usually absent by four minutes.
  - − This is slower than the time of 60 seconds reported for *pentobarbital sodium*.
- ○ Respiratory arrest occurs within one to two minutes, but heart sounds may be audible up to 10 minutes. ECG activity may persist up to 20 minutes post-infusion.
- ○ Agonal gasps may occur.

  *Concerns with intrathecal injection*:
- ○ The procedure is technically more difficult than an IV injection, thus operator training may be necessary.
- ○ There are potential health risks associated with the procedure from exposure to infected spinal fluid (e.g. rabies).

**D    Physical method of euthanasia that result in brain damage**

*Free Bullet*
- ○ In some countries *shooting with a free bullet* is widely used.
- ○ If performed properly, this method is instantaneous, humane, and painless.

- ○ Nevertheless, this method may not be acceptable to all horse owners and is not widely accepted by the public in North America.
- ○ Use of a firearm has the disadvantages that the operator needs a license, and must be skilled in the use of the firearm. Additionally, there is a risk of accidental injury to personnel, especially if the gun is discharged in close quarters.
- ○ It has the advantage that there are no residues in the carcass.
- ○ When using a free bullet, it is important that the bullet should enter the skull just above the intersection of two imaginary lines each drawn from the base of the ear to the orbit on the opposite side of the head. (see Figure 40.2) Horses may be sedated beforehand, depending on the circumstances.

*Captive bolt* (see Figure 40.3)

- ○ In some countries, the captive bolt is never used to euthanize horses.
- ○ However, this is the method of euthanasia when horses are slaughtered for their meat.
  - – Under these circumstances, the animal is *exsanguinated* once it is rendered unconscious, as there is a small chance that the animal may regain consciousness.
- ○ Use of a captive bolt gun has the advantage that the operator does not need a license; however, the operator should be trained in its use.
- ○ It is important that the horse be restrained properly as the muzzle of the gun has to be placed firmly in contact with the head.
- ○ In most cases, it is prudent to sedate the horse.
- ○ Adjunctive methods, *apart from exsanguination*, to ensure death once the horse becomes unconscious includes the administration of KCl or $MgSO_4$.

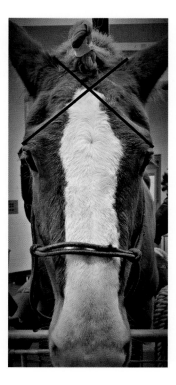

**Figure 40.2** Landmarks for entry of a bullet into the brain for euthanasia. The bullet should enter the skull just above the intersection of two imaginary lines each drawn from the base of the ear to the orbit on the opposite side of the head.

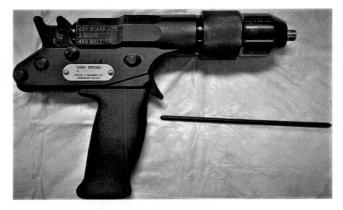

**Figure 40.3** Image of a captive bolt gun. The muzzle of the gun must be placed in direct contact with the head, using the landmarks depicted in Figure 40.2.

## IV   Confirmation of death

- Death should be confirmed before leaving the scene.
- This is done by noting:
  - The absence of *corneal reflexes.*
  - The absence of *cardiac* and *respiratory* activity.
    - No palpable arterial pulse or detectable heartbeat.
  - The presence of *muscle relaxation.*
- If the euthanasia was performed with KCl or pentobarbital while the horse was anesthetized and being monitored the following help to confirm death: (see Figure 40.1c).
  - Asystole or ventricular fibrillation.
  - Lack of $ETCO_2$ waveform on the capnogram.
  - Lack of an arterial pressure waveform.

## Suggested Reading

Aleman, M., Williams, D.C., Guedes, A., and Madigan, J.E. (2015). Cerebral and brainstem electrophysiologic activity during euthanasia with pentobarbital sodium in horses. *J. Vet. Intern. Med.* 29: 663–672.

Aleman, M., Davis, E., Williams, D.C. et al. (2015). Electrophysiologic study of a method of euthanasia using intrathecal lidocaine hydrochloride administered during intravenous anesthesia in horses. *J. Vet. Intern. Med.* 29: 1676–1682.

# Index